OBSTETRICS PROTOCOLS

OBSTETRICS PROTOCOLS

2nd Edition

L Krishna MD
Professor and Medical Superintendent
PES Institute of Medical Sciences and Research
Kuppam, Chittoor
Andhra Pradesh
India

Foreword
Kamini A Rao

JAYPEE BROTHERS MEDICAL PUBLISHERS
The Health Sciences Publisher
New Delhi | London

Jaypee Brothers Medical Publishers (P) Ltd

Headquarters
EMCA House
23/23-B, Ansari Road, Daryaganj
New Delhi 110 002, India
Landline: +91-11-23272143,
+91-11-23272703
+91-11-23282021, +91-11-23245672
E-mail: jaypee@jaypeebrothers.com

Corporate Office
Jaypee Brothers Medical Publishers (P) Ltd.
4838/24, Ansari Road, Daryaganj
New Delhi 110 002, India
Phone: +91-11-43574357
Fax: +91-11-43574314
E-mail: jaypee@jaypeebrothers.com

Overseas Office
JP Medical Ltd.
83, Victoria Street, London
SW1H 0HW (UK)
Phone: +44-20 3170 8910
E-mail: info@jpmedpub.com

EU GPSR Authorised Representative
Logos Europe, 9 rue Nicolas Poussin
17000, La Rochelle, France
Phone: +33 (0) 6 67 93 73 78
E-mail: Contact@logoseurope.eu

Website: www.jaypeebrothers.com
Website: www.jaypeedigital.com

Inquiries for bulk sales may be solicited at: jaypee@jaypeebrothers.com

Obstetrics Protocols

First Edition: 2013

Second Edition: 2016, Reprint: **2026**

ISBN: 978-93-5152-981-1

Printed in India

Dedicated to

My beloved father Late BJ Linge Gowda
My dear sister Late Mrs Leelavathi Dasappa
Our beloved Founder Chairman of PES Group of Institutions
Dr (Prof) MR Doreswamy, who has made me what I am today.
Also, to all my students, both from PES Institute of Medical Sciences, Kuppam; and Kempegowda Institute of Medical Sciences, Bengaluru, especially, Dr N Shailaja, who was just not another student but one who inspired and motivated me and worked hard to make my dream come true, and to all mothers, who deserve to get the best care during their pregnancy and childbirth.

Foreword

All pregnant women are at risk of obstetric complications. Many life-threatening complications occur during labor and delivery, and all of them cannot be predicted. They may occur at any time at any setting and are occurrences that every practicing obstetrician should be prepared for. Having a set of obstetrics protocols in place should be a fundamental necessity of any inpatient setting. To respond to these emergencies, it is important that obstetricians and gynecologists prepare themselves by assessing potential emergencies that might occur, creating plans that include establishing early warning systems, designating and training personnel to handle emergencies, and conducting emergency drills. Having such systems in place may prevent the severity of medical emergencies, thus, bringing down morbidity and mortality.

A practicing obstetrician and gynecologist may be faced with a sudden obstetric emergency at any time. Equipping the obstetrician with knowledge about normal labor and delivery is a must, but the doctor should also have adequate knowledge about the complications, which may arise the importance of early detection, analytical thinking, and on-the-spot decision-making. Whether it is shoulder dystocia, catastrophic postpartum hemorrhage, or an anaphylactic reaction to an injection in the office, it will require prompt response. Preparation for potential emergencies requires planning. This is where the importance of having standard operating procedures (SOPs) come into place. It is, therefore, a source of immense satisfaction for me to write the Foreword for this book. The book is a comprehensive account of the entire obstetric process—with sections covering Antepartum, Labor, Postpartum, Medical Disorders in Pregnancy, Infections in Pregnancy and Gynecological Disorders in Pregnancy.

Every effort has been made to consolidate the latest information on venous, physiological and pathological aspects of pregnancy, childbirth and women's health in a concise and easy-to-understand manner. The contents have been presented in a simple language, which will cover the basics as well as the practical clinical tips. I must commend Dr L Krishna and his assistants Dr N Shailaja and Dr Namrata Kulkarni, who have made a superlative effort in putting this book together. They have not only explained the principles but also succeeded in bringing out a book, which will serve as a practical guide to every practicing obstetrician. I hope that the book would make a difference to every obstetrician's clinical practice.

Kamini A Rao
DGO DORCP FRCOG FICOG FNAMS
Medical Director
Bangalore Assisted Conception Centre Pvt Ltd
Bengaluru, Karnataka, India

Preface to the Second Edition

It is gratifying to note the encouraging response to the first edition of this book. Encouraged by the enthusiasm of students and teachers, we embarked on revising all chapters thoroughly giving the latest information from updated standard guidelines. In this effort, I was ably assisted by my colleagues Dr N Shailaja, Associate Professor and Dr Kirtan Krishna, Assistant Professor. Although we have revised all the chapters, I cannot claim that we have been able to cover all the areas of this ever-growing field of obstetrics, but we have tried to give a comprehensive account of the entire obstetric process. I am sure this edition will receive even better response than the first edition.

L Krishna

Preface to the First Edition

As a teacher, I always felt that there is no uniformity in the management of obstetric cases; and individual consultants use to manage the case according to their experience and belief. I always felt that there should be no controversy in the management of obstetric cases, more so, with advancement in the field of medicine, as there is no room for "as per my experience, this is the best line of management". Such attitude might even be counterproductive, and a postgraduate student, who is in the pipeline to become a future specialist, gets confused as to what is the right approach in a given situation. I experienced this even while I was a postgraduate student at Vanivilas Women and Children Hospital, Bengaluru, India. Now, current practice is totally revolutionized, and we are in the era of evidence-based medicine. With this in mind, I got the idea of bringing out a protocol book in obstetrics for our departmental use, but the amount of effort that went into preparation of this was so much that we thought that this should benefit every student of obstetrics in following uniform and ethical practice. Our management, especially, Dr Suresh Krishnamoorthy, Medical Director, and Dr Roopa Suresh, Associate Medical Director, encouraged me to publish this, and M/s Jaypee Brothers Medical Publishers (P) Ltd, New Delhi, India, came forward to convert the idea into reality.

I could not have achieved this milestone in my career as a teacher, unless my favorite students Dr N Shailaja, Associate Professor; and Dr Namrata Kulkarni, Assistant Professor, who later on became my closed colleagues, made their hard effort in collecting material from various sources such that it would discuss comprehensively on every topic. I also remember the effort of my postgraduate students in compiling the data. I fondly hope that this effort will go a long way in fulfilling the need for standardization of management of obstetric cases.

Although the effort has been made to cover all important topics in obstetrics, some areas may not have been covered, and an effort would be made to fill the gap in the subsequent editions.

L Krishna

Acknowledgments

I sincerely thank the contributions of the following:

- All my colleagues—both the present and past
- All my postgraduate students

I thank my office Secretary, Mrs S Bhagyalakshmi, who was instrumental in typing the manuscript.

Last but not least, I thank M/s Jaypee Brothers Medical Publishers (P) Ltd, New Delhi, India, for publishing this book.

Contents

Section 1: Antepartum

Section 2: Labor

Abbreviations

A/REDV	–	Absent/Reverse end-diastolic volume
AED	–	Anti-epileptic drug
AFI	–	Amniotic fluid index
AFP	–	Alpha fetoprotein
ALT	–	Alanine transaminase
AMTSL	–	Active management of third-stage labor
APLA	–	Antiphospholipid antibody syndrome
aPTT	–	Activated plasma thromboplastin time
ARDS	–	Acute respiratory distress syndrome
ARF	–	Acute renal failure
ARM	–	Artificial rupture of membrane
ASD	–	Atrial septal defect
AST	–	Aspartate transaminase
ATD	–	Anti-thyroid drugs
ATN	–	Acute tubular necrosis
BMI	–	Body mass index
BMV	–	Balloon mitral valvoplasty
BPP	–	Biophysical profile
CBC	–	Complete blood count
CCF	–	Congestive cardiac failure
CCT	–	Controlled cord traction
CRD	–	Chronic renal disease
CSEA	–	Combined spinal epidural anesthesia
CS	–	Cesarean section
CVA	–	Cerebrovascular accident
DCT	–	Direct Coombs test
DFMC	–	Daily fetal movement count
DIC	–	Disseminated intravascular coagulation
DV	–	Ductus venosus
ECV	–	External cephalic version
EFW	–	Estimated fetal weight
ERCD	–	Elective repeat cesarean delivery
EROM	–	Early rupture of membrane

FFP	–	Fresh frozen plasma
GA	–	General anesthesia
HUS	–	Hemolytic uremic syndrome
ICT	–	Indirect Coombs test
IDDM	–	Insulin dependent diabetes mellitus
IUGR	–	Intrauterine growth restriction
LAM	–	Lactational amenorrhea
LDH	–	Lactate dehydrogenase
LFT	–	Liver function test
LUS	–	Lower uterine segment
MAP	–	Mean arterial pressure
MCA	–	Middle cerebral artery
MCA	–	Middle cerebral artery
MCH	–	Mean corpuscular hemoglobin
MOM	–	Multiples of median
MROP	–	Manual removal of placenta
MSAFP	–	Maternal serum alpha-fetoprotein
MTCT	–	Maternal to child transmission
NACO	–	National Aids Control Organisation
NST	–	Nonstress test
NYHA	–	New York Heart Association
OGCT	–	Oral glucose challenge test
OIs	–	Opportunistic infections
PCOS	–	Polycystic ovarian syndrome
PCT	–	Proximal convoluted tubule
PCV	–	Packed cell volume
PSV	–	Peak systolic velocity
PT	–	Prothrombin time
RDP	–	Random donor platelets
RFT	–	Renal function test
RUQ	–	Right upper quadrant
SDP	–	Single donor platelets
SGOT	–	Serum glutamate oxaloacetate transaminase
SGPT	–	Serum glutamate pyruvate transaminase
SLE	–	Systemic lupus erythematosis
STI	–	Sexually transmitted infection
TfR	–	Transferrin receptor
TOLAC	–	Trial of labor after cesarean delivery
TTP	–	Thrombotic thrombocytopenia
UA	–	Umbilical artery
UTI	–	Urinary tract infection
VE	–	Vaginal examination
VSD	–	Ventricular septal defect
VVF	–	Vesicovaginal fistula

SECTION 1

ANTEPARTUM

- Miscarriage
- Ectopic Pregnancy
- Gestational Trophoblastic Disease
- Hyperemesis Gravidarum
- Recurrent Pregnancy Loss
- Multiple Pregnancy
- Intrauterine Growth Restriction
- Rh-negative Pregnancy
- Oligoamnios
- Polyhydramnios
- Antepartum Hemorrhage
- Intrauterine Fetal Death
- Preterm Labor
- Premature Rupture of Membranes
- Preterm Premature Rupture of Membranes
- Prolonged Pregnancy
- Previous LSCS (Vaginal Birth after Cesarean Delivery)
- Resuscitation in Pregnancy and Puerperium

CHAPTER

1

Miscarriage

DEFINITION

It is expulsion or extraction of products of conception before fetal viability, i.e. before 20 weeks (28 weeks in India) of gestation or weight <500 grams (<1 kg in India).

Appropriate Terminology

- New terms–'Pregnancy of unknown location' and 'intrauterine pregnancy of uncertain viability'.

Previous term	Recommended term
Spontaneous abortion	Miscarriage
Threatened abortion	Threatened miscarriage
Inevitable abortion	Inevitable miscarriage
Incomplete abortion	Incomplete miscarriage
Complete abortion	Complete miscarriage
Missed abortion	Missed miscarriage
Anembryonic pregnancy	Early fetal demise
Blighted ovum	Delayed miscarriage/Silent miscarriage
Septic abortion	Miscarriage with infection (sepsis)
Recurrent abortion	Recurrent miscarriage

Term Definitions

- Biochemical pregnancy loss — Pregnancy not located on scan
- Empty sac — Sac with absent or minimal structures
- Fetal loss — Previous CRL measurement with loss of fetal cardiac activity
- Early pregnancy loss — Confirmed empty sac or sac with fetus but no FHA <12 weeks as 'early pregnancy loss'
- Delayed miscarriage/Late pregnancy loss — Loss of FHA >12 weeks
- Pregnancy of unknown location — No identifiable pregnancy on scan with positive hCG

Types

- Spontaneous miscarriage–Miscarriage occurring without medical or mechanical means to empty the uterus is referred to as *spontaneous.*
- Threatened miscarriage–Any bloody vaginal discharge or bleeding during 1st half of pregnancy. Pregnancy is so far intact but there is an obvious risk to its continuation.
- Inevitable miscarriage–Miscarriage where the changes have progressed to a state from where continuation of pregnancy is impossible.
- Incomplete miscarriage–Miscarriage where products of conception are partially expelled.
- Complete miscarriage–Miscarriage where products of conception are completely expelled.
- Missed miscarriage–When the fetus is dead and retained inside the uterus for a variable period of time.
- Septic miscarriage–Miscarriage associated with clinical evidences of infection of the uterus and its contents.

MOLAR PREGNANCY

Vaginal Bleeding in the First Trimester

Differential Diagnosis

Presenting symptoms	Clinical examination	Probable diagnosis
Spotting/minimal bleeding Bright red blood No pain in abdomen	Minimal bleeding through os Closed cervix Uterus corresponds to dates	**Threatened miscarriage**
Pain in abdomen Minimal bleeding per vagina With or without amenorrhea Syncopal attack Symptoms suggestive of hemorrhagic shock and/or hemoperitoneum	Vital parameters stable or unstable Minimal bleeding through os with closed cervix Tender adnexal mass/Cervical motion tenderness Uterus softer and slightly larger than normal size	**Ectopic pregnancy**
Amenorrhea followed by bleeding per vagina and pains in abdomen gradually subsiding on their own after the expulsion of products of conception	Minimal bleeding through os Closed cervix Uterine size normal	**Complete miscarriage**
Amenorrhea followed by bleeding per vagina and pain in abdomen Heavy bleeding per vagina and severe lower abdominal pain even after expulsion of products of conception	Bleeding through os present Cervix remains dilated Products of conception seen sometimes at the external os Uterus smaller than dates	**Incomplete miscarriage**
Amenorrhea followed by bleeding per vagina and pain in abdomen	Bleeding through os present Cervix remains dilated Products of conception seen	**Inevitable miscarriage**

Contd...

Contd...

No history of passing products of conception Amenorrhea followed by regression of pregnancy symptoms Brownish discharge per vagina	sometimes at the external os Uterus corresponds to dates	
No pain in abdomen usually Closed cervix usually	Brownish discharge per vagina Uterine size not corresponding to dates	**Missed miscarriage**
Amenorrhea followed by bleeding per vagina and pain in abdomen Partial expulsion of products of conception which resemble grapes	Uterus usually larger than dates No fetal parts felt No fetal cardiac activity Doughy feel of uterus White currant in red currant jelly	**Molar pregnancy**

Implantation Bleeding

Cyclical bleeding may occur up to 12 weeks of pregnancy until the decidual space is obliterated by the fusion of decidua capsularis with decidua vera.

Bleeding is usually scanty, lasts for shorter duration than the usual and roughly corresponds with the date of the expected period.

Pre-miscarriage Procedures

History

- Recent menstrual history (period of gestation)
- Prior obstetric and gynecological history
- Contraceptive history and future contraceptive desires
- Drugs (over-the-counter or prescription or recreational) currently being used including anticoagulants
- Complete medical history
- Acute or chronic illness

Clinical Examination

- A brief physical examination
- A thorough pelvic examination to determine size of pregnant uterus (whether it is corresponding to period of gestation, anteverted or retroverted), presence of any other pelvic pathology (leiomyoma or adnexal mass or ectopic pregnancy).

Laboratory Tests

1. Hemoglobin
2. Urine-routine for albumin and sugar
3. Blood grouping and Rh typing
4. HIV, HBSAg, VDRL
5. If there is reproductive tract infection–Optimally swabs should be taken for microbiological examination and antibiotic therapy started before miscarriage is performed.

6. A pelvic ultrasonography is unnecessary unless there is real doubt about the gestation, e.g irregular menstrual history or obesity making pelvic examination unreliable, disparity between period of gestation and uterine size, suspected pelvic pathology including ectopic pregnancy.
7. For medical method of MTP, pelvic ultrasonography is necessary.

COMPLETE MISCARRIAGE

Clinical Picture

- Symptoms and signs of pregnancy coincide with its duration.
- No vaginal bleeding.
- Pain is absent or slight.
- Cervix is closed.
- Pregnancy test is negative.

Management

- USG of pelvis should be done to check for presence of fetus.
- No antibiotics are needed.
- If pain is present, analgesic can be given.
- Post-miscarriage counseling.
- Contraceptive advice–cafeteria approach.

THREATENED MISCARRIAGE

Clinical Picture

- Symptoms and signs of pregnancy coincide with its duration.
- Vaginal bleeding slight or mild, bright red in color. Bleeding begins first followed by pain.
- Pain is absent or slight.
- Cervix is closed.
- Pregnancy test is positive.
- Ultrasonography shows a live fetus.

Prognostic Factors in Cases of Threatened Miscarriage

Favorable prognostic factors	Adverse prognostic factors
History Advancing gestational age	Maternal age >34 years Increasing number of previous miscarriages
Sonography Fetal heart activity at presentation	Fetal bradycardia Discrepancy between gestational age and crown to rump length Empty gestational sac >15–17 mm
Maternal serum biochemistry Normal levels of these markers	Low β hCG values Free β hCG value of 20 ng/ml β hCG increase <66% in 48 hrs Bioactive/immunoreactive ratio hCG<0.5 Progesterone <45 nmol/l in 1st trimester Inhibin A <0.553 multiples of median CA125 level ≥43.1 U/mL in 1st trimester

Treatment

- Rest in bed until one week after stoppage of bleeding.
- No intercourse.
- Sedatives: If the patient is anxious.
- Treatment of controversy: Progestogens, e.g. hydroxyprogesterone caproate
- Proluton depot 250 mg IM 1 dose (only if excessive bleeding). Micronized progesterone 200 mg vaginal OD up to 16 weeks (mandatory in case of women conceived after ART).

INEVITABLE MISCARRIAGE

Clinical Picture

- Symptoms and signs of pregnancy coincide with its duration.
- Vaginal bleeding is excessive and may be accompanied with clots.
- Pain is colicky, felt in the suprapubic region radiating to the back.
- The internal os of the cervix is dilated and products of conception may be felt through it.
- Rupture of membranes between 12–28 weeks is a sign of the inevitability of miscarriage.
- USG of pelvis may or may not show fetal cardiac activity.

Treatment

- Any attempt to maintain pregnancy is useless.
- On speculum examination if products are seen at the os—products are removed using sponge-holding forceps or ovum forceps.
- Pelvic USG should be done to check if the products are expelled completely. If incomplete, follow same protocol as in complete miscarriage.
- Prophylactic antibiotics should be given.
- Post-miscarriage counseling
- Contraceptive advice-cafeteria approach.

INCOMPLETE MISCARRIAGE

Retention of a part of the products of conception inside the uterus. It may be the whole or part of the placenta which is retained.

Clinical Picture

- The patient usually notices the passage of a part of the conception products.
- Bleeding is continuous.
- On examination, the uterus is less than the period of amenorrhea. The cervix is opened and products of conception are seen through the os.
- Ultrasonography shows the retained contents.

Treatment

- On speculum examination if products are seen at the os–products are removed using sponge-holding forceps or ovum forceps.

- Misoprostol 600 μg orally or 400 μg sublingually single dose.
- Wait for 1–2 weeks for the products to be expelled completely.
- Prophylactic antibiotics for 5 days should be given.
- Analgesics, antipyretics should be given, if required.
- Post-miscarriage counseling.
- Repeat scan after 2 weeks to check if products are expelled.
- Contraceptive advice–cafeteria approach.

MISSED MISCARRIAGE

Symptoms

- Regression of pregnancy symptoms as nausea, vomiting and breast symptoms.
- The fetal movements are not felt or cease if previously present.
- Milk secretion may start particularly in second trimester miscarriage (>16 weeks) because of the decline in estrogens secretion that were normally blocking the action of prolactin on the breasts.

Signs

- The uterus does not increase correspond to the period of amenorrhea.
- The cervix is closed.
- The fetal heart sounds cannot be heard by the Doppler.
- A dark brown vaginal discharge may occur (prune juice discharge).

Investigations

- Pregnancy test becomes negative within two weeks from the ovum death, but it may remain positive for a longer period due to presence of β HCG upto 6 weeks.
- Ultrasound shows either a collapsed gestational sac, absent fetal heart movement or fetal movement. Diagnosed if two ultrasound (T/V or T/A) at least 7 days apart showed an embryo of >7 weeks gestation (CRL >6 mm in diameter and gestational sac >20 mm in diameter) with no evidence of heart activity.
- Complete blood count (Platelets to rule out DIC).

Complications

- Disseminated intravascular coagulation (DIC) may occur if the dead conceptus is retained for more than 5 weeks.
- Superadded infection.

Treatment

The dead conceptus is expelled spontaneously in the majority of cases. Evacuation of the uterus is indicated in the following conditions:

- Spontaneous expulsion does not occur within five weeks
- Excessive bleeding
- Infection or DIC developed or patient is anxious.

Evacuation is carried out as follows:

- Surgical evacuation by D and C is the treatment of choice in 1st trimester missed miscarriage.
- Medical management–misoprostol 800 μg vaginally 3 hrly max. of 2 doses.

  Or

  Misoprostol 600 μg sublingually 3 hrly max. of 2 doses.
- Wait for 1–2 weeks for the products to be expelled completely.
- Prophylactic antibiotics for 5 days should be given.
- Analgesics and antipyretics should be given if required.
- Post-miscarriage counseling.
- Repeat scan after 2 weeks to check if products are expelled.
- Contraceptive advice–cafeteria approach.

SEPTIC MISCARRIAGE

It is an incomplete miscarriage which is complicated by infection of the uterine contents. This may be due to criminal interference.

Microbiology

Mixed Infection

The commonest organisms are:

- Gram -ve: *E.coli*, Strepto and Staphylococci
- Anaerobics: Bacteroides

Rarely *Cl. tetani*, which is potentially lethal if not treated adequately.

Types

- Grade 1–The infection is confined to decidua (80%).
- Grade 2–The infection extended to myometrium (15%).
- Grade 3–The infection extended to pelvis, generalized peritonitis, endotoxic shock are present.

Clinical Picture

General Examination

- Pyrexia and tachycardia
- General malaise
- Rigors suggest bacteremia
- A subnormal temperature with tachycardia is ominous and mostly seen with gas-forming organisms–endotoxic shock.
- Sweating, headache, and joint pain
- Jaundice and/or hematuria is an ominous sign, indicating hemolysis due to chemicals used in criminal miscarriage or hemolytic infection as *Clostridium welchii.*
- Dry tongue
- Decreased urine output

Abdominal Examination

- Suprapubic pain and tenderness

- Abdominal rigidity and distension indicates peritonitis due to perforation of the bowel.
- Absent bowel sound in paralytic ileus

Local Examination

- Vaginal bleeding
- Offensive vaginal discharge
- Uterus is tender.
- Products of conception may be seen at the os.
- Local trauma may be detected.
- Fullness and tenderness of pouch of Douglas indicates pelvic abscess which will be associated with diarrhea.

Complications

Endotoxic (septic) shock may develop with its serious sequelae as acute renal failure and DIC.

Investigations

- CBC, blood grouping, reserve 2 units of blood.
- Cervical swabs (not vaginal) for culture and sensitivity
- Coagulation profile, serum electrolytes and blood culture if pyrexia >38.5° C.

Treatment

- Isolate the patient. Bed rest in semi-prone position.
- An intravenous line is established for therapy. In case of shock, a central venous pressure (CVP) line to aid in the control of fluid and blood transfusion started, if required.
- Monitor vital signs: Pulse, temperature and blood pressure as well as fluid intake and urinary output.
- Antibiotic therapy: Give ampicillin 2 g IV every six hours + gentamicin 5 mg/kg body weight IV every 24 hours + metronidazole 500 mg IV every eight hours until the woman is fever-free for 48 hours.
- Fluid therapy, e.g. glucose 5% normal saline and/or lactated ringer solutions can be given as long as there is no manifestations of acute renal failure, particularly, the urinary output is more than 30 ml/hour.
- Blood transfusion – It is given if CVP is low (normal: 8–12 cm of water). It is of importance also to correct anemia, coagulation defects and infection. Packed cells, if severe anemia, platelets if <30,000, FFP if DIC.
- Oxytocin infusion: To control bleeding and enhance expulsion of the retained products 10–20 U in 500 ml RL. Misoprostol 600 μg oral.
- Surgical evacuation of the uterus can be done after 48 hours of commencing IV antibiotic therapy but may be earlier in case of severe bleeding or deteriorating condition in spite of the previous therapy. If done before 48 hrs, only major amount of products is to be removed.
- Hysterectomy may be needed in endotoxic shock not responding to treatment, particularly, due to gas gangrene (*Cl. welchii*).

The uterus is very soft, so evacuation should be gentle as chances of perforation are increased. It should be done by an experienced person and care should be taken to complete the procedure.

Other indications of surgical intervention (laparotomy) are:
- Injury to the uterus
- Suspected injury to the gut
- Pelvic abscess–posterior colpotomy, when the infection is localized in the POD
- Pyoperitoneum–In very sick patients, who are at a very high risk for anesthesia, percutaneous drainage can be done, but the risk of gut injury should be kept in mind.
- Septic shock or oliguria.

Even when nothing is found on laparotomy, simple drainage of the pus is effective.

Postoperative Care

- Pulse, BP, temperature, abdominal girth charting two hourly till general condition improves.
- Input output charting
- Daily electrolyte estimation
- Coagulation studies if evidence of coagulopathy

IV antibiotics continued till patient becomes afebrile for 48 hours and then orally for 14 days.

Post-Miscarriage Counseling

- Before discharge, tell a woman who has had a spontaneous miscarriage that spontaneous miscarriage is common and occurs in at least 15% (one in every seven) of clinically recognized pregnancies.
- Reassure the woman that the chances for a subsequent successful pregnancy are good unless there has been sepsis or a cause of the miscarriage is identified that may have an adverse effect on future pregnancies (this is rare).
- The woman should be encouraged to delay the next pregnancy until she is completely recovered, at least for 3 months.
- It is important to counsel the women who have had an unsafe miscarriage. If pregnancy is not desired, certain methods of family planning can be started immediately (within seven days) as ovulation can occur within 14 days of miscarriage.
- Give Anti-D injection to all women who are Rh negative. 50 μg before 12 weeks, and full dose of 300 μg after 12 weeks.

INDUCED MISCARRIAGE

Indications

- Continuation of pregnancy may threaten the life of a woman or seriously impair her health.
  - Persistent heart disease after cardiac decompensation (fixed pul. HTN).

- Advanced hypertensive vascular disease
- Invasive carcinoma of the cervix

- Pregnancy resulted from rape or incest.
- Continuation of pregnancy is likely to result in the birth of child with severe physical deformities or mental retardation.

MEDICAL METHODS

Antiprogesterone (RU 486)

Contraindications

- IUCD in situ
- Suspected ectopic pregnancy
- Hypertension, anemia, glaucoma, cardiovascular disease, smoker, asthmatic
- Woman on anticoagulant and glucocorticoid therapy
- Previous uterine scar
- Lactating woman
- Gestational age not greater than 49 days

Complications

- Nausea, vomiting, and gastrointestinal cramping
- Headache, malaise, skin rash, fever
- Failure to abort: 1%
- Adrenal failure
- Moebius syndrome: In fetus (congenital facial palsy, limb defects, bladder exstrophy, hydrocephalus). Termination of pregnancy is strongly recommended if medical termination fails.
- Surgery is required in case of failure or is incomplete. In case the woman starts bleeding profusely, emergency evacuation is a must.
- Subsequent menstruation may be delayed by 10–14 days.

Prostaglandins

- Used extensively to terminate pregnancies, especially in the 2nd trimester-PG E1, E2, F2α.
- Technique: Can act effectively on the cervix and uterus (86–95% effectiveness).

Protocol for Medical Method of Termination

- Written consent for MTP is required.
- Ultrasound is done to confirm uterine pregnancy and duration, and to exclude ectopic pregnancy.

Recommended Methods for Medical Termination of Pregnancy

For Pregnancies of Gestational Age up to 9 Weeks (63 Days)

The recommended method for medical miscarriage is mifepristone followed 1 to 2 days later by misoprostol.

Dosages and Routes of Administration for Mifepristone Followed by Misoprostol

- Mifepristone should always be administered orally. The recommended dose is 200 mg.

- Administration of misoprostol is recommended 1 to 2 days (24 to 48 hours) following ingestion of mifepristone.
- For vaginal, buccal or sublingual routes, the recommended dose of misoprostol is 800 μg.
- For oral administration, the recommended dose of misoprostol is 400 μg.
- With gestation up to 7 weeks (49 days), misoprostol may be administered by vaginal, buccal, sublingual or oral routes. After 7 weeks of gestation, oral administration of misoprostol should *not* be used.
- With gestation up to 9 weeks (63 days), misoprostol can be administered by vaginal, buccal or sublingual routes.

For Pregnancies of Gestational Age Between 9 and 12 Weeks (63–84 Days)

- The recommended method for medical termination of pregnancy is 200 mg mifepristone administered orally followed 36 to 48 hours later by 800 μg misoprostol administered vaginally.
- Subsequent misoprostol doses should be 400 μg, administered either vaginally or sublingually, every 3 hours up to four further doses, until expulsion of the products of conception.

For Pregnancies of Gestational Age Over 12 Weeks (84 Days)

- The recommended method for medical termination of pregnancy is 200 mg mifepristone administered orally followed 36 to 48 hours later by repeated doses of misoprostol.
- With gestations between 12 and 24 weeks, the initial misoprostol dose following oral mifepristone administration may be either 800 μg administered vaginally or 400 μg administered orally.
- Subsequent misoprostol doses should be 400 μg, administered either vaginally or sublingually, every 3 hours up to four further doses.
- For pregnancies beyond 24 weeks, the dose of misoprostol should be reduced, due to the greater sensitivity of the uterus to prostaglandins, but the lack of clinical studies precludes specific dosing recommendations.

Where Mifepristone is Not Available

For Pregnancies of Gestational Age up to 12 Weeks (84 Days)

- The recommended method of medical termination of pregnancy is 800 μg of misoprostol administered by vaginal or sublingual routes. Up to three repeat doses of 800 μg can be administered at intervals of at least 3 hours, but for no longer than 12 hours.

For Pregnancies of Gestational Age over 12 Weeks (84 Days)

- The recommended method of medical termination of pregnancy is 400 μg of misoprostol administered vaginally or sublingually, repeated every 3 hours for up to five doses.
- For pregnancies beyond 24 weeks, the dose of misoprostol should be reduced, due to the greater sensitivity of the uterus to prostaglandins, but the lack of clinical studies precludes specific dosing recommendations.

Recommended Methods of Termination of Pregnancy for Gestational Age Over 12 to 14 Weeks

- Dilatation and evacuation (D and E) and medical methods (mifepristone and misoprostol; misoprostol alone) are both recommended methods for miscarriage for gestation over 12 to 14 weeks.
- Facilities should offer at least one, and preferably both methods, if possible, depending on provider experience and the availability of training.

Recommended Methods for Surgical Termination

Vacuum aspiration is the recommended technique of surgical method of termination for pregnancies of up to 12 to 14 weeks of gestation. The procedure should not be routinely completed by sharp curettage.

Procedure

Vacum Evacuation

- Efficient till 12 weeks of gestation
- Better than suction and evacuation
- Under IV sedation, local infiltration
- Perform a pervaginal examination and assess the gestational age and uterine position
- Uterine sound is passed to assess the depth of uterine cavity, cervix is serially dilated using a series of metallic or plastic dilators. Dilatation is initially started using small dilators, later large dilators are used one after the other. The size of the suction cannula to be used for the procedure must be corresponding to the gestational age in weeks.
- A plastic Karman's cannula is inserted inside the uterine cavity, cannula is connected to suction machine, which generates pressure equivalent to 60–70 mm of Hg. Cannula is rotated at an angle of 360 and moved back by 1–2 cm, back and forth, till no further tissue is aspirated, grating sensation is felt all around the cavity, internal os begins to grip the cannula which reveals a blood stained froth.
- No need for sharp curettage.

Complications

Uterine perforation, cervical incompetence, uterine synechiae–Asherman's syndrome.

Management of Uterine Perforation

- Observation and antibiotic treatment
- Laparoscopy
- Laparotomy, if there is any suspicion of damage to the bowel, blood vessels or other structures.

RECOMMENDATIONS FOR CARE PRECEDING INDUCED MISCARRIAGE

1. ***Cervical preparation***
   Between 12 to 14 weeks of gestation
   Any one of these methods of cervical preparation before surgical miscarriage in the first trimester is recommended:

- Oral mifepristone 200 mg (24 to 48 hours in advance); or
- Misoprostol 400 μg administered sublingually, 2 to 3 hours prior to the procedure; or
- Misoprostol 400 μg administered vaginally 3 hours prior to the procedure; or laminaria placed intracervically 6 to 24 hours prior to the procedure.

After 14 weeks of gestation

Osmotic dilators or misoprostol are recommended.

2. ***Ultrasound scanning***

   Use of routine pre-miscarriage ultrasound scanning is not necessary.

3. ***Prophylactic antibiotics***
   - All women having surgical miscarriage, regardless of their risk of pelvic inflammatory infection, should receive appropriate prophylactic antibiotics pre- or peri-operatively.

     Pre-miscarriage prophylaxis (RCOG criteria):

     Metronidazole 1 g rectally at the time of miscarriage

     plus

     Doxycycline 100 mg orally twice daily for 7 days, commencing on the day of miscarriage

     or

     Metronidazole 1 g rectally at the time of miscarriage

     plus

     Azithromycin 1 g orally on the day of miscarriage
   - For women having medical miscarriage, routine use of prophylactic antibiotics is not recommended.

4. ***Pain management***
   - All women should be routinely offered pain medication (e.g. non-steroidal anti-inflammatory drugs) during both medical and surgical method of termination of pregnancy.
   - General anesthesia is not recommended routinely for vacum aspiration miscarriage or dilatation.

RECOMMENDATIONS FOR POST-MISCARRIAGE CARE

Contraception

- Women may start hormonal contraception at the time of surgical miscarriage, or as early as the time or administration of the first pill of a medical method of termination regimen. Following medical method of termination, an intrauterine device (IUD) may be inserted when it is reasonably certain that the woman is no longer pregnant.

Follow-up

- There is no medical need for a routine follow-up visit following uncomplicated surgical miscarriage or medical miscarriage using mifepristone followed by misoprostol. However, women should be advised that additional services are available to them if needed or desired.

Incomplete Miscarriage

- If uterine size at the time of treatment is equivalent to a pregnancy of gestational age 13 weeks or less, either vacuum aspiration or treatment with misoprostol is recommended for women with incomplete miscarriage. The recommended regimen of misoprostol is a single dose given either sublingually (400 μg) or orally (600 μg).

After-care and Follow-up

- For surgical method of termination, women can leave the health-care facility as soon as they feel able and their vital signs are normal.
- Following uncomplicated surgical and medical miscarriage using mifepristone with misoprostol, routine follow-up visits are not necessary. For women who wish to return to the clinic, a follow-up visit may be scheduled at 7–14 days after the procedure.
- Before leaving the health-care facility following the surgical termination of pregnancy or administration of medical termination of pregnancy pills, all the women should receive contraceptive information and, if desired, the contraceptive method of their choice or referral for such services.

Tissue Examination Following Surgical Miscarriage

- Routine analysis not essential
- Should be tested when ectopic/molar is suspected
- Should be tested in missed miscarriage.

Evaluation of Patients during Follow-up Visits

History

Since the elective miscarriage—
- Antibiotic use
- Use of other medications
- Fever, bleeding and cramping pain
- Pregnancy symptoms
- Activity level
- Sexual intercourse
- Contraceptive use and plans
- Emotional status and support system
- Any other questions or problems

Physical Examination

- Temperature, blood pressure, pulse
- Uterine size, shape, consistency, tenderness, position
- Adnexa.

Warning signs of post-miscarriage complications
- Fever >100° F or 38° C and/or chills
- Increasing severe abdominal pain
- Foul odor with discharge
- Prolonged (over two weeks) or heavy bleeding
- Passage of tissue

- Delay of menses >8 weeks
- Continued pregnancy symptoms—should be offered uterine evacuation
- Abdominal tenderness

THE MEDICAL TERMINATION OF PREGNANCY ACT, 1971

When pregnancies may be terminated by registered medical practitioners— Medical grounds when the continuation of pregnancy is likely to: (i) Endanger the life of the pregnant women or (ii) cause grevious injury to her physical and/or mental health, as in cases of severe hypertension, cardiac disease, diabetes, psychiatric illnesses, genital and breast cancer.

Eugenic grounds when there is a substantial risk of the child being born with serious physical or mental abnormalities.

Humanitarian grounds when the pregnancy is caused by rape or incest.

Social grounds when in the actual or reasonably forseeable future, her environment (social or economic) might lead to risk of injury to her health or (ii) pregnancy resulting from failure of contraceptive device or method.

Place Where Pregnancy may be Terminated—

No termination of pregnancy shall be made in accordance with this Act at any place other than—

a. A hospital established or maintained by Government, or
b. A place for the time being approved for the purpose of this Act by Government.

MEDICAL TERMINATION OF PREGNANCY REGULATIONS, 2003

Form of Certifying Opinion or Opinions

1. One or two registered medical practitioners, who form the opinion should certify the opinion in Form I.
2. Every registered medical practitioner, who terminates the pregnancy should certify such termination in Form I within three hours from the termination of the pregnancy.

Custody of Forms

1. The consent given by a pregnant woman for the termination of her pregnancy, together with the certified opinion recorded, and the intimation of termination of pregnancy, has to be placed in an envelope which has to be sealed by the registered medical practitioner or practitioners by whom such termination of pregnancy was performed and until that envelope is sent to the head of the hospital or owner of the approved place or the Chief Medical Officer of the State, it has to be kept in the safe custody of the concerned registered medical practitioner or practitioners.
2. On every envelope the serial number assigned to the pregnant woman in the Admission Register and the name of the registered medical practitioner or practitioners by whom the pregnancy was terminated, has to be noted and such envelope has to be marked "SECRET".

3. Every envelope has to be sent immediately after the termination of the pregnancy to the head of the hospital or owner of the approved place where the pregnancy was terminated.
4. The head of the hospital or owner of the approved place has to keep the receipt of the envelope in safe custody.
5. Every head of the hospital or owner of the approved place has to send monthly statement of cases where medical termination of pregnancy has been done to the Chief Medical Officer of the Sate, in form II.
6. On every envelope, the name and address of the registered medical practitioner by whom the pregnancy was terminated and the date on which the pregnancy was terminated have to be noted and such envelope shall be marked as "SECRET".
7. When the pregnancy is not terminated in an approved place or hospital, has to be sent by registered post to the Chief Medical Officer of the State on the same day on which the pregnancy was terminated or on the working day next following the day on which the pregnancy was terminated.

Maintenance of Admission Register

1. Every head of the hospital or owner of the approved place has to maintain a register in form III for recording the the details of the admissions of the women for the termination of their pregnancies and keep such register for a period of five years from the end of the calendar year it relates to.
2. The entries in the Admission Register have to be made serially and a fresh serial has to be started at the commencement of each calendar year and the serial number of the particular year has to be distinguished from the serial number of other years by mentioning the year against the serial number, for example, serial number 5 of 1972 and serial number 5 of 1973 shall be mentioned as 5/1972 and 5/1973.
3. Admission Register has to be maintained as secret document and the information should not be disclosed to any person.

Admission Register not to be Open to Inspection

The Admission Register should not be opened by any person for inspection except under the authority of the law:

Provided that the registered medical practitioner grants a certificate for the purpose of enabling the woman to obtain leave from her employer.

Provided further that any such employer should not disclose this information to any other person.

Entries in Registers Maintained in Hospital or Approved Place

No entry has to be made in any case-sheet, operation theater register, follow-up card or any other document or register other than the Admission Register.

FORM A

(To be filled by the head of the hospital or owner of the approved place)

Form of application for the approval of a place under the clause

1. Name of the place (in capital letters)
2. Address in full
3. Non-Governmental/Private/Nursing Home/Other Institutions*
4. State, if the following facilities are available at the place—
   i. An operation table and instruments for performing abdominal or gynecological surgery.
   ii. Drugs and parenteral fluid in sufficient supply emergency cases.
   iii. Anesthetic, resuscitation and sterilization equipment.

Place:
Date:
Signature of the owner
of the place
*Strike out whichever is not applicable.

FORM B

(To be filled by the Government)

Certificate of approval.
The place described below is hereby approved for the purpose of the Medical Termination of Pregnancy Act, 1971 (34 of 1971).
Name of the Place
Address and other descriptions
Name of the owner
Place:
Date:
To the Government of the ....

FORM C

(To be filled by the woman who is willing to terminate her pregnancy)

I .... daughter/wife of ....aged about .... years of .... (here state the permanent address) at present residing at .... do hereby give my consent to the termination of my pregnancy at ....
(State the name of place where the pregnancy is to be terminated).
Place:
Date:
Signature
(To be filled in by guardian when the woman is a lunatic or minor).
I .... son/daughter/wife of .... aged about .... years of .... at present residing at .... (permanent address) .... do hereby give my consent to

the termination of my pregnancy of my ward .... who is a minor/lunatic at ....

(Place of termination of pregnancy)

Place:

Date:

Signature

FORM I

(To be filled by the registered medical practitioner who terminated the pregnancy)

I____

(Name and qualifications of the Registered Medical Practitioner in block letters)

____

(Full address of the Registered Medical Practitioner)

I____

_______ (Name and qualifications of the Registered Medical Practitioner in block letters) __________________________________

______________ (Full address of the Registered Medical practitioner) hereby certify that *I/We am/are of opinion, formed in good faith, that it is necessary to terminate the pregnancy of ______________________________

___________________________ (Full name of the pregnant woman in block letters) resident of __________________________________

________________________ (Full address of pregnant woman in block letters) for the reasons given below**.

* I/We hereby give intimation that *I/We terminated the pregnancy of the woman referred to above who bears the serial no. ______________ in the Admission Register of the hospital/approved place.

Signature of the Registered Medical Practitioner(s)

Date:

*Strike out whichever is not applicable,

**Of the reasons specified as items (i) to (v) below write the one which is appropriate.

i. In order to save the life of the pregnant woman,
ii. In order to prevent grave injury to the physical and mental health of the pregnant woman,
iii. In view of the substantial risk that if the child was born it would suffer from such physical or mental abnormalities as to be seriously handicapped,
iv. As the pregnancy is alleged by the pregnant woman to have been caused by rape,
v. As the pregnancy has occurred as the result of failure of any contraceptive device or methods used by married woman or her husband for the purpose of limiting the number of children.

Note: Account may be taken of the pregnant woman's actual or reasonably foreseeable environment in determining whether the continuance of her pregnancy would involve a grave injury to her physical or mental health.

Place:

Date:

Signature of the Registered Medical Practitioner

FORM II

(To be filled by the head of the hospital or owner of the approved place)

1. Name of the State
2. Name of the Hospital/approved place
3. Duration of pregnancy (give total No. only)
   a. Up to 12 weeks
   b. Between 12–20 weeks
4. Religion of woman
   a. Hindu
   b. Muslim
   c. Christian
   d. Others
   e. Total
5. Termination with acceptance of contraception
   a. Sterilization (b) IUD
6. Reasons for termination: (give total number under each sub-head)
   a. Danger to life of the pregnant woman
   b. Grave injury to the physical health of the pregnant woman
   c. Grave injury to the mental health of the pregnant woman
   d. Pregnancy caused by rape
   e. Substantial risk that if the child was born, it would suffer from such physical or mental abnormalities as to be seriously handicapped
   f. Failure of any contraceptive device or method

Signature of the Officer Incharge with Date

FORM III

(To be destroyed on the expiry of five years from the date of the last entry in the register)

(To be filled by the head of the hospital or owner of the approved place)

1	2	3	4	5	6	7
S. No.	Date of admission	Name of patient	Wife/ daughter of	Age	Religion	Address
8	**9**	**10**	**11**	**12**	**13**	**14**
Duration of pregnancy	Reasons on which pregnancy is terminated	Date of termination of pregnancy	Date of discharge of patient	Results and Remarks	Name of Registered Medical Practitioner (s) by whom the opinion is formed	Name of Registered Medical Practitioner (s) by whom pregnancy is terminated

CHAPTER

2

Ectopic Pregnancy

DEFINITION

Any pregnancy where the fertilized ovum gets implanted and develops in a site other than normal uterine cavity.

RISK FACTORS

Risk factors	Relative risk%
• Previous ectopic pregnancy	3–13
• Tubal corrective surgery	4
• Tubal sterilization	9
• Intrauterine device	1–4.2
• Documented tubal pathology	3.8–21
• Infertility	2.5–3
• Assisted reproductive technology	2–8
• Previous genital infection	2–4
– Chlamydia	2
– Salpingitis	1.5–6.2
• Smoking	1.7–4
• Prior miscarriage	0.6–3
• Multiple sexual partners	1.6–3.5
• Prior cesarean delivery	1–2.1

SITES OF ECTOPIC PREGNANCY

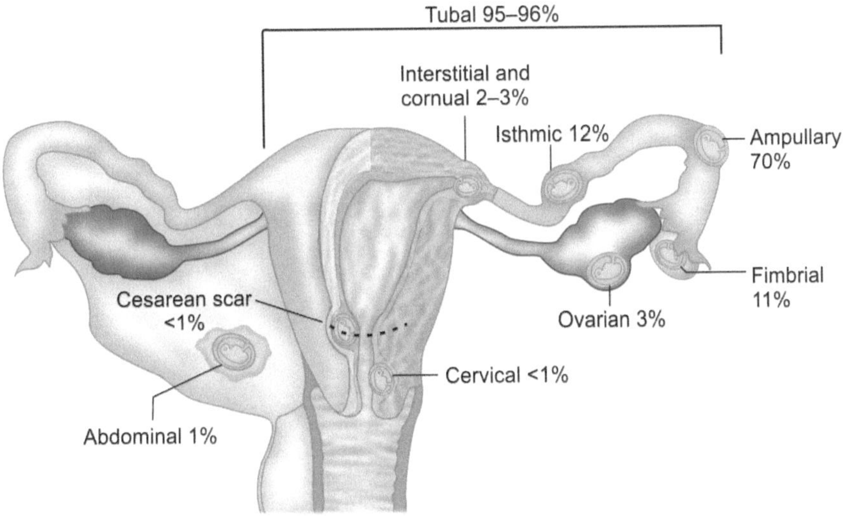

Figure 2.1: Sites of ectopic pregnancy

Tubal Ectopic Pregnancy

- Most common site of ectopic.
- The ampulla is the most frequent site, followed by the isthmus. Interstitial pregnancy accounts for only about 2 percent.

CLINICAL FEATURES

- Pelvic and abdominal pain (95%)
- Abnormal bleeding: Amenorrhea followed by vaginal bleeding/ spotting (60–80%)
- Abdominal and pelvic tenderness: Uncommon in unruptured ectopic, seen in 75% cases of ruptured ectopic pregnancy.

SYMPTOMS AND SIGNS

Acute ectopic	Unruptured ectopic	Chronic ectopic
Symptoms	**Symptoms**	**Symptoms**
Nausea, vomiting, syncopal attacks	• Spotting • Uneasiness on one side of the flanks	• Amenorrhea • Lower abdominal pain • Vaginal bleeding • Features of bladder irritation
Signs	**Bimanual examination**	**Signs**
• Pallor, Feeble pulse, BP, Cold clammy extremities	• Uterus seems normal in size. • A pulsatile small well-circumscribed tender mass felt	Pt. looks ill, pallor, high pulse rate, ↑ temp

Contd...

Contd...

Abdominal examination		Abdominal examination
• Tense, tumid, tender		• Tenderness and guarding • Irregular and tender mass • Cullen's sign
Bimanual examination		**Bimanual examination**
• Uterus seems normal in size. • Extreme tenderness on fornix palpation. • No mass is felt in fornices. • Uterus floats as if in water. • Vaginal mucosa blanched white		• Pale vaginal mucosa • Extreme tenderness on movement of cervix • An ill-defined boggy, extremely tender mass felt through posterolateral fornix

INVESTIGATIONS

Laboratory Tests

- Blood routine
- Urine pregnancy test
- Serum beta hCG level (useful in conservative line of management)
- Serum progesterone—the clinical utility is limited because in most ectopic pregnancies, progesterone levels range between 10 and 25 ng/mL.

Imaging Studies

Transvaginal Sonography/Transabdominal Sonography

- Absence of intrauterine pregnancy with positive test
- Ectopic cardiac activity
- Ectopic gestational sac
- Ectopic mass
- Fluid in POD
- Blob sign

Doppler

- Beigel's sign—Ring of fire.

DIAGNOSIS

1. **Quantitative β-hCG + Sonography**
   - TVS + β hCG levels >1500 IU/L
   - Failure in doubling of β hCG in 48 hrs
2. **Surgical diagnosis**
   - Laparoscopy
   - Laparotomy
   - Culdocentesis
   - Curettage

MANAGEMENT

Flow chart 2.1: Management of suspected ectopic pregnancy

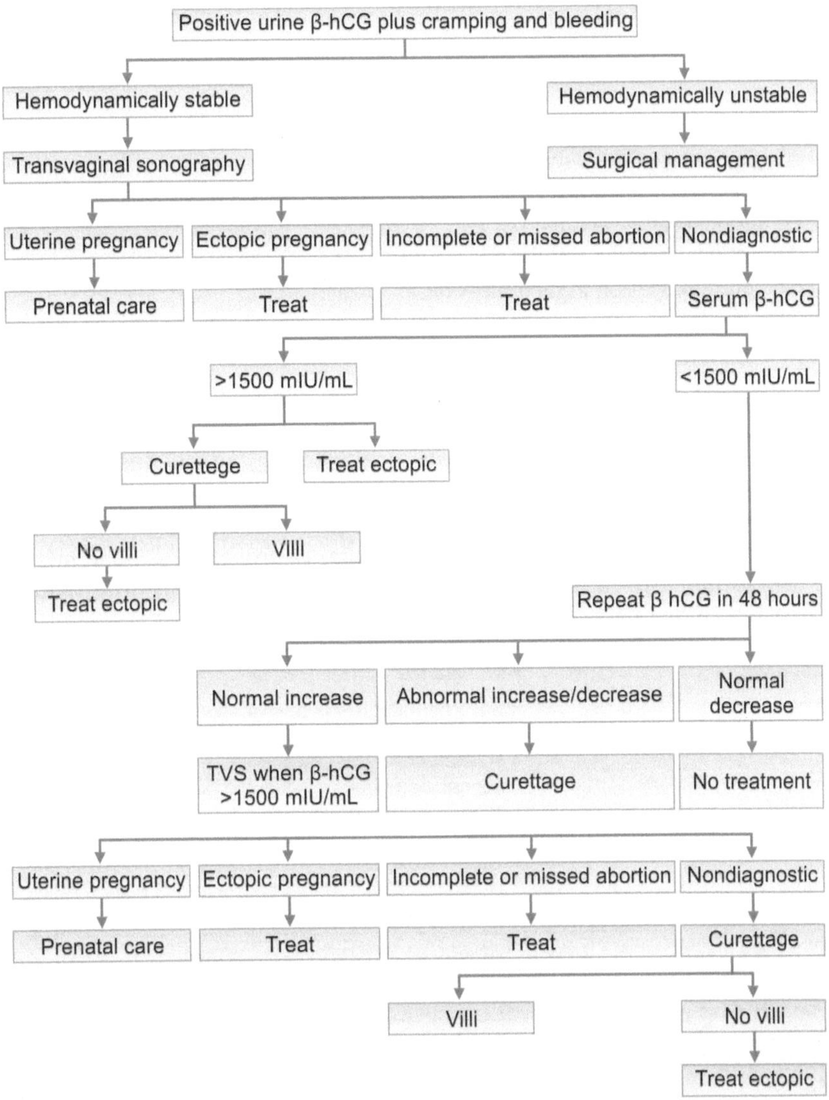

EXPECTANT MANAGEMENT OF TUBAL ECTOPIC PREGNANCY

Restrict expectant management to women with these criteria (Stovall and Ling)

- Tubal ectopic pregnancies only
- Decreasing serial β-hCG levels (<1000 IU/L)
- Diameter of the ectopic mass <3.5 cm
- No evidence of intra-abdominal bleeding or rupture by transvaginal sonography
- Patient with good compliance

Follow-up: Twice weekly hCG measurement and weekly TVS to ensure a rapidly decreasing hCG level (ideally <50% decrease in 7 days) and a reduction in the size of adnexal mass in 1 week, later weekly hCG and TVS until serum hCG becomes <20 IU/L

MEDICAL MANAGEMENT OF ECTOPIC PREGNANCY

Criteria

- Asymptomatic (Hemodynamically stable)
- β hCG levels <5000 mIU/ml
- Gestational sac <3.5 cms
- Absent fetal cardiac activity
- No contraindication to methotrexate

Methotrexate

- Folic acid antagonist, highly effective against rapidly proliferating trophoblastic tissue
- Contraindications: Active intra-abdominal bleeding, intrauterine pregnancy; breastfeeding, immunodeficiency, alcoholism; chronic hepatic, renal, or pulmonary disease, blood dyscrasias; and peptic ulcer disease.
- Side effects: Liver involvement, stomatitis, gastroenteritis, bone marrow depression, life-threatening neutropenia, fever, transient drug-induced pneumonitis and alopecia.

Regimen	Surveillance
Single dose Methotrexate,50 mg/sq m IM	Measure β-hCG levels days 4 and 7: • If difference ≥15%, repeat weekly until undetectable • If difference ≤15% between day 4 and day 7 levels, repeat methotrexate dose and begin new day 1 • If fetal cardiac activity present day 7, repeat methotrexate dose, begin new day 1 • Surgical treatment if β-hCG levels not decreasing or fetal cardiac activity persists after 3 doses methotrexate
Two dose Methotrexate, 50 mg/ m_2 IM on days 0.4	Follow-up as for single dose regimen
Variable dose (up to 4 doses) Methotrexate 1 mg/kg IM days 1,3,5,7 Leucovorin 0.1 mg/kg IM days 2,4,6,8	Measure β-hCG levels day 1, 3, 5 and 7. Continue alternate day injections until β-hCG level decreases ≥15% in 48 hrs or four doses of methotrexate given. Then weekly β-hCG level until undetectable.

SURGICAL MANAGEMENT

- Conservative surgeries.

Salpingostomy

- This procedure is used to remove a small pregnancy, usually less than 2 cm in length and located in the distal third of the fallopian tube.

- A 10 to 15 mm linear incision is made with unipolar needle cautery on the antimesenteric border over the pregnancy, products usually will extrude from the incision which are removed or flushed out using high-pressure irrigation that more thoroughly removes the trophoblastic tissue.
- Control the small bleeding sites by needle point electrocoagulation or laser, the incision is left unsutured to heal.
- 75% will experience abdominal pain (separation pain due to tubal miscarriage), needs admission.
- Side effects: conjunctivitis, stomatitis, gastrointestinal upset.
- Advice on discharge:
    - Abstinence
    - Hydration
    - Contraception for 3 months because of teratogenic risk.

Salpingotomy

Seldom performed now-a-days.

Radical Surgery

Salpingectomy

- Tubal resection: Used for both ruptured and unruptured ectopic pregnancies.
- Cornual resection (excision of wedge of the outer third (or less) of the interstitial portion of the tube) is done in an effort to minimize the rare recurrence of pregnancy in the tubal stump.

Indications for oophorectomy: It is when bleeding from tubo-ovarian anastomosis is not controlled/diseased ovary.

CERVICAL PREGNANCY

- The endocervix is eroded by trophoblast, and the pregnancy proceeds to develop in the fibrous cervical wall. The higher the trophoblast is implanted in the cervical canal, the greater is its capacity to grow and hemorrhage.

Diagnosis

Clinical Diagnostic Criteria (Rubins Criteria)

a. Soft, enlarged cervix equal to or larger than fundus
b. Uterine bleeding following amenorrhea, without cramping pain
c. Poducts of conception entirely confined within and firmly attached to endocervix
d. Closed internal cervical os and partially opened external os.

Symptoms

- Painless vaginal bleeding
- Massive hemorrhage
- Abdominal pain with bleeding

Signs

- As pregnancy progresses, a distended, thin-walled cervix with a partially dilated external os. Above the cervical mass, a slightly enlarged uterine fundus may be palpated.
- Closed internal os, partially dilated external os.

Investigations

Serum β-hCG levels – 2800 to 10,000 mIU/mL.
Sonography – Gestational sac in the cervix with empty uterine cavity.

Management

Medical Management

- Methotrexate first line of management. Same dosage used for medical management of tubal pregnancy. Potassium chloride can be injected directly into the gestational sac.

Cerclage

- Hemorrhage associated with cervical pregnancy can be managed successfully by placing a heavy silk ligature around the cervix.

Curettage and Tamponade

- Placement of hemostatic cervical sutures at 3 and 9 o'clock to ligate descending cervical branches of the uterine artery. Suction curettage is then performed, followed immediately by insertion of a Foley catheter into the cervical canal. A 30 ml catheter bulb is inflated, and the vagina is packed tightly with gauze to further tamponade bleeding. A suction catheter tip may be left above the vaginal packing to ensure adequate drainage and to monitor blood loss.

Arterial Embolization

- Combination of laparoscopically assisted uterine artery ligation followed by hysteroscopic endocervical resection.
- Hysterectomy if bleeding is uncontrolled.

OVARIAN PREGNANCY

Spiegelberg's Criteria

1. Tube on the affected side must be intact.
2. The gestation sac must be in the position of ovary.
3. Gestation sac is connected to the uterus by ovarian ligament.
4. Ovarian tissue must be found on its wall on histological examination.

Management

- Findings are likely to mimic those of a tubal pregnancy or a bleeding corpus luteum.
- Early bleeding for small lesions-managed by ovarian wedge resection or cystectomy.
- Larger lesions – oophorectomy is most often performed, and laparoscopy has been used to resect or to perform laser ablation.
- Unruptured ovarian pregnancies – methotrexate (similar to tubal ectopic)

INTERSTITIAL PREGNANCY AND CORNUAL PREGNANCY

- Cornual implantation describes those in the upper and lateral uterine cavity, whereas interstitial denotes those implanted within the proximal intramural portion of the tube.

Management

- Ruptured cornual pregnancy – Cornual resection via laparotomy.
- Conservative – Uterus sparing hysterolaparoscopic surgery or methotrexate.

ABDOMINAL PREGNANCY

- Abdominal pregnancy is an implantation in the peritoneal cavity exclusive of tubal, ovarian, or intraligamentary implantations.

Diagnosis

Studdiford Criteria

1. Both the tubes and ovaries are normal without evidence of recent injury
2. Absence of utero-peritoneal fistula
3. Presence of a pregnancy related exclusively to the peritoneal surface and young enough to eliminate the possibility of secondary implantation following primary nidation in the tube.

Symptoms

- Abdominal pain and vaginal bleeding
- Nausea, vomiting, constipation, bleeding, decreasing to absent fetal movements.

Signs

- Uterine contour not well defined.
- Braxton Hicks contraction is absent.
- Fetal parts are felt easily and persistent abnormal attitude and position.
- Per-vaginal examination–Cervix displaced, depending on the the fetal position.

Investigations

- Sonography–Oligoamnios is common but nonspecific. Absence of uterine wall around the fetus. Abnormally high position of the fetus with abnormal attitude. The fetal head may be seen to lie immediately adjacent to the maternal bladder with no interposed uterine tissue.

Management

- Clinical management depends on the gestational age at diagnosis.
- Waiting until fetal viability within hospital observation if pregnancy is diagnosed after 24 weeks.
- Patient attenders counseled about catastrophic hemorrhage, fetal death, increased fetal malformations, increased neonatal loss.
- Once fetus is viable, emergency laparotomy. Delivery of the fetus and careful assessment of placental implantation without provoking hemorrhage.
- If the placenta can be safely removed or if there is already hemorrhage from its implantation site, then removal begins immediately. When possible, blood vessels supplying the placenta should be ligated first.
- If the placenta is left, its involution may be monitored using sonography and serum β -hCG levels. Methotrexate use is controversial.

CHAPTER

3

Gestational Trophoblastic Disease

DEFINITIONS

Refers to benign and malignant trophoblastic diseases–Hydatidiform mole, Invasive mole, Choriocarcinoma (CCA) and Placental site trophoblastic tumor (PSTT).

Gestational Trophoblastic Tumor/Neoplasia: Refers to the subset of gestational trophoblastic disease that develops malignant sequela. They require staging and respond to chemotherapy (and/or excisional surgery).

Flow chart 3.1: Progression of GTD to GTN

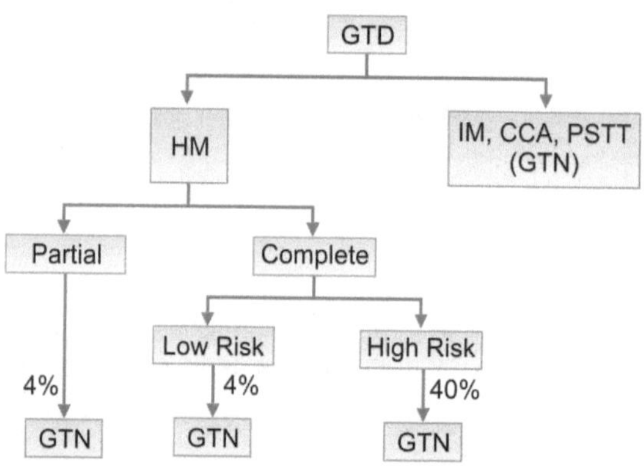

HYDATIDIFORM MOLE

Incidence

Complete mole: 1 per 1,945.
Partial mole: 1 per 695 pregnancies.

Features	Complete mole	Partial mole
Fetal tissue	Absent	Present
Hydatidiform swelling of chorionic villi	Diffuse	Focal
Trophoblastic hyperplasia	Diffuse	Focal
Scalloping of chorionic villi	Absent	Present
Trophoblastic stromal inclusions	Absent	Present
Karyotype	46 XX or XY	69 XXX or XXY

Symptoms

- Vaginal bleeding (84%)
- Symptoms of anemia (5%)
- Lower abdominal pain
- Constitutional symptoms
- Excessive vomiting (8%)
- Breathlessness (2%) {Trophoblastic emboli}
- Thyrotoxicosis (7%)
- Expulsion of grape-like vesicles per vagina
- H/o quickening absent

Diagnosis

Abdomen examination:

1. Uterine size
   - Uterus enlarged more than corresponding weeks of gestation (>70%)
   - Uterine size corresponding to period of amenorrhea (20%)
   - Uterine size lesser than period of amenorrhea (<10%)
2. Doughy feel of abdomen
3. Fetal parts not felt, absence of FHS in complete mole. In partial mole, fetus present, may show features of IUGR.
4. P/S: Presence of grape-like vesicles in discharge.
5. U/L or B/L theca lutein cysts

Investigation

- Complete blood count
- Chest X-ray
- Hepatic, renal, thyroid function tests (when indicated)
- Ultrasonography
  - Complete mole—Vesicular pattern {diffuse hydropic swelling of chorionic villi}, Snowstorm or granular appearance of multiple echogenic foci.
  - Partial mole—Focal cystic spaces in placental tissue
    - Increase in transverse diameter of gestational sac
    - T: AP dimension–1.5:1 (PPV–90 %)
    - Rapidly increasing serum hCG levels (>1 lac m IU/ml)
- Chest X-ray—Pulmonary metastasis

Treatment

- Arrange adequate amount of blood and consent to be taken.
- Suction evacuation irrespective of gestational age with 12 mm Karman's cannula after dilatation of cervix irrespective of gestational age.
- Cervical preparation with misoprostol, immediately prior to evacuation is safe.
- If the woman is experiencing significant hemorrhage prior to evacuation, surgical evacuation should be expedited and the need for oxytocin infusion weighed up against the risk of tumor embolization.
- Anti-D prophylaxis is required following evacuation of a molar pregnancy.

- Sharp curettage, or medical evacuation of complete molar pregnancy is not recommended.
- In partial mole or twin pregnancy (there is 1 normal pregnancy with 1 molar pregnancy) and the size of the fetal parts deters the use of suction curettage, then medical evacuation can be used.

Management after Evacuation of the Mole

- Meticulous follow up with serial hCG estimation.

Follow-up after GTD is increasingly individualized.

- If hCG has reverted to normal within 56 days of the pregnancy event, then follow up will be for 6 months from the date of uterine evacuation.
- If hCG has not reverted to normal within 56 days of the pregnancy event, then follow-up will be for 6 months from normalization of the hCG level.
- All women should notify the screening center at the end of any future pregnancy, whatever the outcome of the pregnancy. hCG levels are measured 6–8 weeks after the end of the pregnancy to exclude disease recurrence.

The histological assessment of material obtained from the medical or surgical management of all failed pregnancies is recommended to exclude trophoblastic neoplasia.

Flow chart 3.2: Management and follow up after evacuation of molar pregnancy

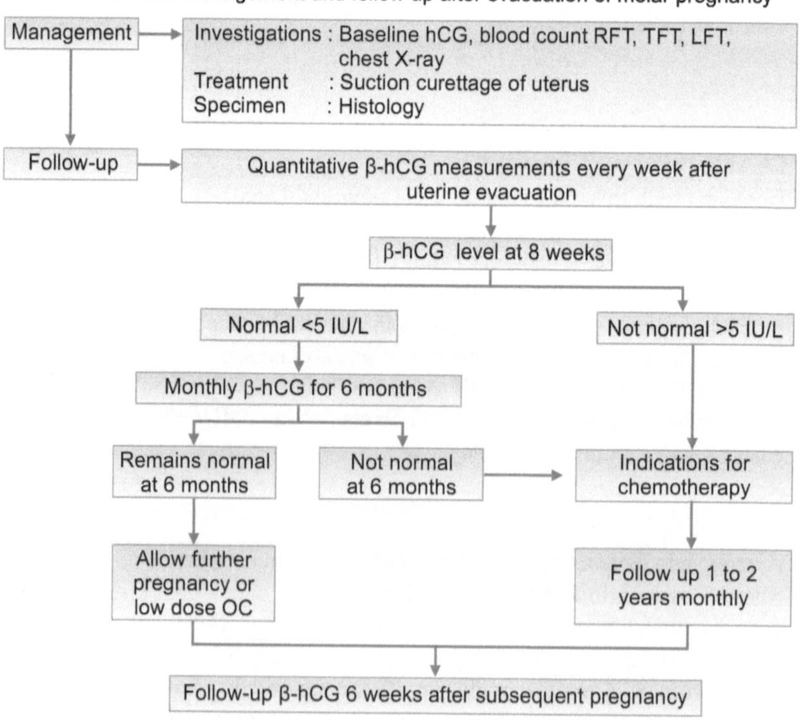

There is no need to routinely send products of conception for histological examination following therapeutic termination of pregnancy, provided that fetal parts have been identified on prior ultrasound examination.

Complications

Immediate

- Hemorrhage and shock
- Sepsis
- Perforation of uterus
- Early onset preeclampsia
- Acute pulmonary insufficiency
- Thyroid storm

Late

- Choriocarcinoma–5%
- Dyspnea and abnormal neurology–rarely

Any woman who develops persistent vaginal bleeding after a pregnancy event is at risk of having GTN. A urine pregnancy test should be performed in all cases of persistent or irregular vaginal bleeding after a pregnancy event.

Risk Factors for Malignant Change

The points listed below are for high change:

- Risk varies from 3–25% (Partial mole 2–4%, Complete mole 20%)

Clinical factors associated with risk for post-molar GTD:

- High hCG levels (>1,00,000 m IU/ml)
- Uterine size >20 weeks
- Bilateral theca lutein cyst >6 cm
- RDS after molar evacuation
- Associated medical factors (PE, hyperthyroidism, trophoblastic embolism)
- Maternal age >40 years
- Previous history of molar pregnancy

Hydatidiform mole - high risk

- Uterine size > period of gestation
- Serum β hCG >100,00 m IU/ml
- Large theca-lutein cysts (>6 cm)
- PIH, thyrotoxicosis, pulmonary embolism, previous mole.

Prophylactic chemotherapy: For unreliable patient with high-risk molar pregnancy.

- hCG level fails to become normal by stipulated time (8 weeks) or re-elevation (>20,000 m IU/ml) at 8 weeks
- Evidence of metastasis irrespective of hCG level
- Presence of risk factors for malignant change
- Proper follow-up facilities are not available.

Regimen–MTX 1 mg/kg IM on days 1, 3, 5 and 7 with folinic acid or leucovorin-0.1 mg/kg on days 2, 4, 6 and 8.

- Women should be advised not to conceive until their follow-up is complete.
- Women who undergo chemotherapy are advised not to conceive for 1 year after completion of treatment.
- Women who receive chemotherapy for GTN are likely to have an earlier menopause.
- Women with high-risk GTN who require multi-agent chemotherapy, which includes etoposide, should be advised that they may be at increased risk of developing secondary cancer.

Prophylactic Hysterectomy

- Unreliable multiparous patient aged >39 years.
- Uncontrolled excessive bleeding
- Sepsis
- Invasive mole
- Evidence of uterine perforation
- Hysterectomy does not eliminate but reduces risk of metastatic disease from 20 to 3.5%.
- Large theca lutein cyst encountered at hysterectomy—decompressed by aspiration.

Twin Pregnancy–One Viable Fetus and Molar Pregnancy

- In the situation of a twin pregnancy where there is one viable fetus and the other pregnancy is molar, the woman should be counseled about the increased risk of perinatal morbidity and outcome for GTN.
- Prenatal invasive testing for fetal karyotype should be considered in cases where it is unclear if the pregnancy is a complete mole with a coexisting normal twin or a partial mole. Prenatal invasive testing for fetal karyotype should also be considered in cases of abnormal placenta, such as suspected mesenchymal hyperplasia of the placenta.

Contraception

- Women with GTD should be advised to use barrier methods of contraception until hCG levels revert to normal.
- Once hCG levels have normalized, the combined oral contraceptive pill may be used. There is no evidence as to whether single-agent progestogens have any effect on GTN.
- If oral contraception has been started before the diagnosis of GTD was made, the woman can be advised to remain on oral contraception but she should be advised that there is a potential but low increased risk of developing GTN.
- Intrauterine contraceptive devices should not be used until hCG levels are normal to reduce the risk of uterine perforation.

Future Conception

- Repeat molar pregnancy–3%, which increases to 30% after two consecutive molar pregnancies.

- Early USG during the subsequent conceptions
- Placenta should be sent for HPE
- β hCG level after 6 weeks.

Follow-up

Symptoms

- Amenorrhea
- Irregular bleeding
- Hematuria
- Abdominal pain—uterine perforation
- Difficulty in breathing
- Persistent cough
- Hemoptysis
- Headache, seizures

Signs

- Uterine enlargement
- Ovarian masses
- Nodules in vagina
- Pulmonary HTN
- Shadows on chest X-ray
- Localizing neurological signs

Investigations

- hCG in serum
- Chest X-ray—Before treatment and 4 weeks after evacuation, then at 3, 6, and 12 months only if 4 weeks report shows embolization/symptomatic.
- Complete blood count, liver, renal and thyroid function, if indicated.

Prognosis

- Persistent GTN: 15–20%
- Metastatic disease: 4–5%
- Recurrence in future pregnancy: 1–4%

Is hormone replacement therapy safe for women to use after GTD?
Hormone replacement therapy may be used safely once hCG levels have returned to normal.

GESTATIONAL TROPHOBLASTIC NEOPLASIA (GTN)

Invasive Mole

Hydatidiform mole that has invaded the myometrium or metastasized.

- It is seen in early months following evacuation of H. mole
- Common in women >40 years.

Symptoms

- Vaginal bleeding
- Amenorrhea
- Infertility

- Abdominal pain
- Symptoms resulting from uterine perforation.

Choriocarcinoma

- Differs from invasive mole in that the villous pattern is lost 1/20,000–1/40,000
- Develop from term pregnancies (50%)
- Develop after molar pregnancies (25%)
- Develop after other gestations (25%).

Placental Site Trophoblastic Tumor

- Composed mainly of cytotrophoblast
- hPL is raised >hCG
- Less responsive to chemotherapy, hence hysterectomy to be considered
- Arises commonly after term pregnancy.

Diagnosis of GTN

- Serum hCG >20,000 mIU/ml at 4 weeks after evacuation of mole
- Rising hCG titers
- Plateauing of hCG
- Histopathological evidence of invasive mole, choriocarcinoma and placental site trophoblastic tumor
- Evidence of metastases

Staging of GTN

Stage I: Disease confined to uterus
Ia: Disease confined to uterus with no risk factors
Ib: Disease confined to uterus with one risk factor
Ic: Disease confined to uterus with two risk factors

Stage II: Outside uterus but limited to genital structures (adnexa, vagina, broad ligament)
IIa: Genital structures without risk factors
IIb: Outside uterus but limited to genital structures with one risk factor
IIc: Outside uterus but limited to genital structures with two risk factors

Stage III: Extending to lungs with or without known genital tract involvement
IIIa: Lungs with or without genital tract involvement and with no risk factors
IIIb: Lungs with or without genital tract involvement and with one risk factor
IIIc: Lungs with or without genital tract involvement and with two risk factors

Stage IV: All other metastatic sites
IVa: All other metastatic sites without risk factors
IVb: All other metastatic sites with one risk factor
IVc: All other metastatic sites with two risk factors

WHO Scoring System

Score	0	1	2	4
Age (yrs)	<39	>39		
Antecedent pregnancy	H. mole	Abortion	Term	
Interval (months)	<4	4–6	7–12	>12
Pre-treatment β hCG mIU/ml	$<10^3$	10^3–10^4	10^4–10^5	$>10^5$
Tumor size (cms)	<3	3–4	≥5	—
Site of metastasis	Vagina, lungs	Spleen, kidney	GIT	Brain, liver
No. of metastasis	0	1–4	5–8	>8
Previous failed chemotherapy			Single drug	2 or more drugs

Two risk groups: ≤6 (low risk) and ≥ (7 high risk).

Scoring and Diagnosis of Metastasis

- Clinical history and serum hCG estimation
- Chest X-ray/CT scan for diagnosis of lung metastases
- USG/CT scan for diagnosis of intra-abdominal metastases
- MRI/CT scan for brain metastases

Management

Stage 1

Initial—Single-agent chemotherapy or hysterectomy with adjunctive chemotherapy
Resistant—Combination chemotherapy
Hysterectomy with adjunctive chemotherapy

Stages II and III

Low-risk

- *Initial*—Single-agent chemotherapy
- *Resistant*—Combination chemotherapy

High-risk

- *Initial*—Combination chemotherapy
- *Resistant*—Second-line combination chemotherapy

Stage IV

Initial—Combination chemotherapy
Brain—Whole-heat irradiation (3,000 Gy)
Craniotomy to manage complications
Liver—Resection to manage complications
Resistant—Second-line combination chemotherapy

Hepatic arterial infusion

- Low-risk GTN is mostly cured with single-agent chemotherapy
- High-risk GTN should be always treated with combination chemotherapy

Low-risk

- Inj. Methotrexate 1 mg/kg on day 1, 3, 5 and 7
- Inj. Leucovorin 0.1 mg/kg on day 2, 4, 6 and 8
    - Repeat cycle on day 15 (if no toxicity).
    - Estimate serum hCG serially weekly.
    - Continue CT for 1–2 cycles after three consecutive levels of hCG are normal.
    - Change CT if hCG values plateau or rise.
    - In case of abnormal LFT/RFT, consider actinomycin D in place of methotrexate
    - Actinomycin D: 1.25 mg/m^2 IV or 12 ugm/kg/day x 5 days
    - Act-D every other week as a 5-day regimen or pulsatile fashion.

High-risk

EMA-Co-Regimen

- EMA on day 1 and 2, CO on day 8.

Day 1

- Etoposide 100 mg/m^2 IV infusion in 200 ml NS over 30 min
- Actinomycin D 0.5 mg IV bolus
- Methotrexate 100 mg/m^2 IV infusion over 12 hr.

Day 2

- Etoposide 100 mg/m^2 IV infusion in 200 ml NS over 30 min
- Actinomycin D 0.5 mg IV bolus
- Folinic acid 15 mg IM every 12 hrs for 4 doses beginning 24 hr after starting methotrexate.

MAC

- Day 1, 3, 5, 7–Methotrexate 1 mg/kg IM
- Day 2, 4, 6, 8–Folinic acid 0.1 mg/kg IM
    - Day 1–5
      –Actinomycin 12 ugm/kg IV
      –Cyclophosphamide 3 mg/kg IV
- Repeat cycle on day day 15 (if no toxicity).
    - Estimate serum hCG serially weekly.
    - Continue chemotherapy for 3–4 cycles after normalization of hCG.
    - Change chemotherapy if hCG values plateau or rise.
    - Consider excisional surgery for localized tumor.

Supportive therapy—It is important in patients with extensive brain/lung metastases-steroids to decrease brain/lung edema.

- Positive pressure ventilation
- Hemostatic radiotherapy to brain.

Follow-up

- Stages I, II, III
    - Weekly measurement of hCG levels until they are normal for 3 consecutive weeks.

- Monthly measurement of hCG values until levels are normal for 12 consecutive months.
- Stage IV
  - Weekly determination of hCG levels until they are normal for 3 consecutive weeks.
  - Monthly determination of hCG levels until they are normal for 24 consecutive months.
- Monthly hCG-until normal for 1 year (low risk) and 2 years (high risk).
- If at any time serum levels are increased—Rule out relapse/recurrence.
- RFT, LFT, CBC after every cycle of chemotherapy.

CHAPTER

4

Hyperemesis Gravidarum

Hyperemesis is defined as persistent vomiting in the first trimester pregnancy not due to other causes with the inability to maintain adequate hydration, fluid and electrolyte balance and nutritional status (large ketonuria) and some discrete measure of severity which is 5% loss of pre-pregnancy weight or requirement for hospitalization and intravenous hydration.

Nausea and vomiting present in the first trimester in about 80% and 50% of pregnant women, respectively. They may persist beyond 20 weeks in 13% of cases. Hyperemesis gravidarum occurs in 0.1–1% of pregnancies.

RISK FACTORS/ASSOCIATED FACTORS

- Family history
- Female gender of the fetus
- H/o migraine
- Multiple gestations
- Down syndrome
- Molar gestation
- Hyperthyroidism
- UTI
- Viral hepatitis
- Other liver disorders
- Bowel obstruction
- Raised intracranial pressure
- Gastroenteritis

SYMPTOMS

- Onset is always in the first trimester (usually weeks 6–8)
- Nausea and vomiting
- Ptyalism (excessive salivation)
- Increased olfactory and gustatory aversion
- Changes in taste sensitivity
- Weight loss (up to 20%) +/- muscle wasting.

FEATURES OF DEHYDRATION AND KETOACIDOSIS

- Dry, coated tongue
- Sunken eyes
- Acetone smell in breath
- Tachycardia
- Hypotension
- Rise in temperature
- Decreased urine output

It is a diagnosis of exclusion. Vomiting refractory to treatment and new symptoms appearing after the 12th week should not be attributed to hyperemesis gravidarum. Urinary tract infection, peptic ulceration, pancreatitis, hyperthyroidism, hypercalcemia or Addison's disease (rare) should be excluded.

INVESTIGATIONS

- Hb, PCV—raised hematocrit.
- Urine—ketone bodies to be sent every 8 hrly and increased specific gravity of urine.
- LFT—If patient appears icteric. It is abnormal in ≤50% of cases. Moderate rise in transaminases (>50 mmol/l but <200 mmol/l) and in bilirubin (but not frank jaundice).
- Serum electrolytes–If patient appears dehydrated, signs of ketoacidosis are present.
- Serum amylase and lipase–If intractable vomiting with severe pain in abdomen
- Free T_3 T_4, TSH–If intractable vomiting. Shows a picture of biochemical hyperthyroidism in 75% of cases, with a raised free thyroxine and/or suppressed thyroid-stimulating hormone. These patients are clinically euthyroid without thyroid antibodies. Abnormal TFTs do not require treatment and resolve as hyperemesis improves.
- Calcium is tested to exclude hypercalcemia.
- USG–To confirm pregnancy and rule out hydatidiform mole, multiple pregnancy.
- Arterial blood gases are rarely carried out and test for metabolic hypochloremic alkalosis.

TREATMENT

Nausea or vomiting interfering with daily routine activity

- Ginger root (250 mg q.d.s) reduces the incidence of nausea and vomiting.
- The results of acupuncture or accupressure are equivocal.
- Doxylamine 12.5 mg start with 1 HS, if not controlled, then 2 HS + oral vitamin B6 10–30 mg tid/qid oral.

Outpatient Advice For Emesis Gravidarum

- Morning 30–45 min before waking up from bed, eat a toast or biscuits and free hand exercises
- Small frequent meals of whatever is appealing
- Avoid spicy meals
- Vitamin supplements

Hospitalization

Indications
- Vomiting not controlled with drugs
- Evidence of dehydration and ketonuria

MANAGEMENT

Investigations

- Urea and electrolytes, full blood count, liver function tests, thyroid function tests, calcium.
- Mid-stream urine.
- Ultrasound scan pelvis

Intravenous Fluids

1 L 0.9% normal saline with 20 mmol potassium chloride over 2 h
1 L 0.9% normal saline with 20 mmol potassium chloride over 4 h.

Followed by—
1 L 0.9% normal saline every 8 h with potassium replacement dependent on serum level.

Thiamine

Orally, if tolerated (thiamine hydrochloride 25–50 mg; t.d.s.); otherwise 100 mg in 100 ml 0.95 saline (IV) over 30–60 min weekly or pabrinex.

Much higher doses needed to treat Wernicke's encephalopathy.

Iron

Stop iron (PO) and provide psychiatric and emotional support.

Symptom Control

Anti-emetics are safe in the first trimester.
Possible regimens include:
- **Antihistamines** (cyclizine 50 mg PO/IM/IV; TDS) or promethazine (25 mg PO Nocte).
- **Phenothiazines** (prochlorperazine 5 mg PO TDS; 12.5 mg IM/IV TDS) or chlorpromazine (10–25 mg PO; 25 mg IM TDS)

- **Dopamine antagonists** (metoclopramide 10 mg PO/IM/IV TDS) or domperidone (10 mg PO QDS; 30–60 mg PR TDS)
- **5HT3-selective serotonin antagonist** (ondansetron 8 mg PO BD)

H_2-receptor blockers may be used for dyspeptic symptoms.

A Cochrane review of seven underpowered randomized controlled trials comparing antiemetics versus placebo could not demonstrate any significant effect of antiemetic agents.

Refractory Cases

Prednisolone (P.O.; 40–50 mg daily in divided doses) or **hydrocortisone** (IV; 100 mg b.d.) may provide rapid resolution of symptoms. Following response to treatment, tapering of the dose should be gradually instigated until the gestation of anticipated resolution.

Thromboprophylaxis

Anti-embolic stockings
Low molecular weight heparin, e.g: Enoxaparin 40 mg OD (<90 kg) or 60 mg OD (>90 kg). Life-threatening cases –

- Patient is kept nil per oral.
- Do not use Dextrose saline due to the risk of Wernicke's encephalopathy, also low in sodium (30 mmol/l Na).
- Do not use double strength saline even in cases of severe hyponatremia as this will result in too rapid a correction of serum sodium with risk of pontine myelinolysis.
- Ketone bodies to be repeated 8 hrly.
- Strict input/output charting
- If vomiting not controlled with Inj metaclopramide, switch over to Inj ondansetron, if still not controlled, Inj promethazine, not controlled Inj methylprednisolone.
- If 24 hrs of no vomiting, ketone bodies negative, start dry toast and biscuits, if tolerated soft diet to be started.
- If patient appears dehydrated, send serum electrolytes.
- If potassium 3–3.5 mEq/ml, RL to be started and syp Potchlor 15 ml tid.
- If 2.5 mEq/ml—3.0 mEq/ml-IV supplementation 40 mEq of KCl in 500 ml NS.
- If <2.5 mEq/ml—80 mEq of KCL in 500 ml NS.
- **Life-threatening cases** may require total parenteral nutrition, enteral feeding or, as last resort, termination of the pregnancy.

DISCHARGE CRITERIA

- If the woman has tolerated at least two meals without vomiting
- Follow-up as outpatient within two days.
- Consider eliminating precipitating factors and offer reassurance of self-limiting condition and no specific fetal risk factors.

COMPLICATIONS

1. **Wernicke's Encephalopathy**
   - Delay in or inappropriate treatment may result in serious morbidity and mortality. Deficiency of vitamin B1 (thiamine) and Wernicke's encephalopathy.
   - Characterized by diplopia, abnormal ocular movements, ataxia and confusion.
   - Wernicke's encephalopathy is potentially precipitated by intravenous fluids containing dextrose and is more common in women with hyperemesis gravidarum and abnormal liver function tests.
   - Wernicke's encephalopathy may be confirmed by low red cell transketolase (thiamine-dependent enzyme). MRI may reveal symmetrical lesions around the aqueduct and fourth ventricle, which resolve after treatment with thiamine.
   - If it progresses to retrograde amnesia, impaired ability to learn and confabulation (Korsakoff psychosis); the recovery rate is only about 50%.
2. **Other vitamin deficiencies**—Deficiency of vitamin B12 and B6 may cause anemia and peripheral neuropathy.
3. **Hyponatremia**
   - Plasma sodium <120 mmol/l causes lethargy, seizures and respiratory arrest.
   - Severe hyponatremia (and particularly its rapid reversal) may precipitate central pontine myelinolysis. This is associated with symmetrical destruction of myelin at the center of the basal pons and causes pyramidal tract signs, spastic quadraparesis, pseudobulbar palsy and impaired consciousness.
4. **Thrombosis**–Dehydration and bed rest are risk factors for thromboembolism.
5. **Other**–Prolonged vomiting can cause Mallory-Weiss esophageal tears and hematemesis. Infection and pneumothorax complicate total parenteral nutrition.

Fetal Complications

- No increased risk of congenital malformations.
- Severe HG (abnormal biochemistry and/or Wernicke's) can result in intrauterine growth restriction (IUGR) or even intrauterine death (IUD), but overall there are lower risks of miscarriage, stillbirth and pre-term delivery.
- Wernicke's encephalopathy is associated with a 40% incidence of fetal death.

Termination of pregnancy if complications develop as—

- Emaciation
- Apathetic, drowsy, confused and euphoric
- Squint, diplopia, nystagmus, retinal hemorrhages
- Peripheral neuritis
- Wernickes encephalopathy
- Coma

CHAPTER

5

Recurrent Pregnancy Loss

DEFINITION

A recurrent miscarriage is 3 or more consecutive, spontaneous pregnancy losses, before 20 weeks gestation.

Primary Recurrent Miscarriage Group

This group consists of women with three or more consecutive miscarriages with no pregnancy progressing beyond 20 weeks' gestation.

Secondary Recurrent Miscarriage Group

This group consists of women who have had three or more miscarriages after a pregnancy that, having gone beyond 20 weeks' gestation, may have ended in live birth, stillbirth, or neonatal death.

Tertiary Recurrent Miscarriage Group

This is a group that has not been well-characterized or studied, and consists of women who have had at least three miscarriages that are not consecutive but are interspersed with pregnancies that have progressed beyond 20 week's gestation (and may have ended in live birth, stillbirth, or neonatal death).

INCIDENCE

10–15% of all clinically recognized pregnancies end in a miscarriage
True early pregnancy loss = clinically recognized + occult early miscarriages

- Risk of clinically recognized spontaneous miscarriage increases with age

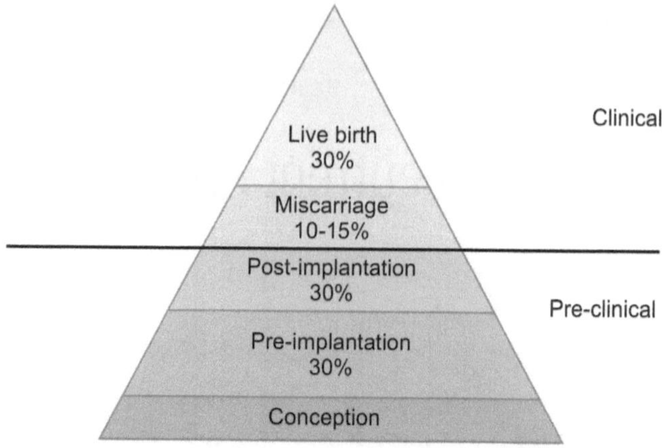

Age	Risk
<30 yrs	7–15%
30–34 yrs	8–21%
35–39 yrs	17–28%
>40 yrs	34–52%

H/o previous loss with age >40 yrs–52%
Age <30 yrs–25%
Total pregnancy wastage >40 yrs–75%

	Number of prior miscarriages	% risk of miscarriage in next pregnancy
Women who have had at least one live-born infant	0	12%
	1	24%
	2	26%
	3	32%
	4	46%
	6	53%
Women who have not had even one live-born infant	2 or more	40–45%

ETIOLOGY

I trimester
- Genetic
- Endocrine and metabolic
- Infection
- Inherited thrombophilia
- Immunological

II trimester
- Anatomical
- Chronic maternal diseases
- Infections
- Unexplained

ETIOLOGICAL FACTORS IN RECURRENT PREGNANCY LOSS

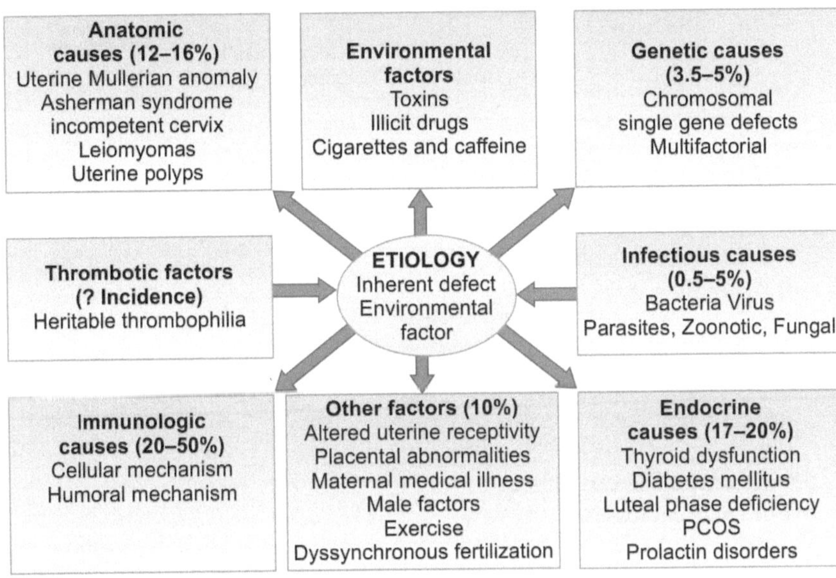

HISTORY

- Pattern, trimester, and characteristics of prior pregnancy losses
- History of subfertility or infertility
- Menstrual history
- Prior or current gynecologic or obstetric infections
- Signs or symptoms of thyroid, prolactin, glucose tolerance and hyperandrogenic disorders (including PCOS)
- Personal or familial thrombotic history
- Features associated with the antiphospholipid syndrome (thrombosis, false positive test for syphilis)
- Other autoimmune disorders (joint pains, skin rash, allergy)
- Medications
- Environmental exposures, illicit and common drug use (particularly caffeine, alcohol, cigarettes, and in utero DES exposure)
- Genetic relationship between reproductive partners
- Family history of recurrent spontaneous abortion, obstetric complications, or any syndrome associated with embryonic or fetal losses
- Previous diagnostic tests and treatment

Basic Diagnostic Algorithm for Early Pregnancy Loss

Flow chart 5.1: Diagnosis of early pregnancy

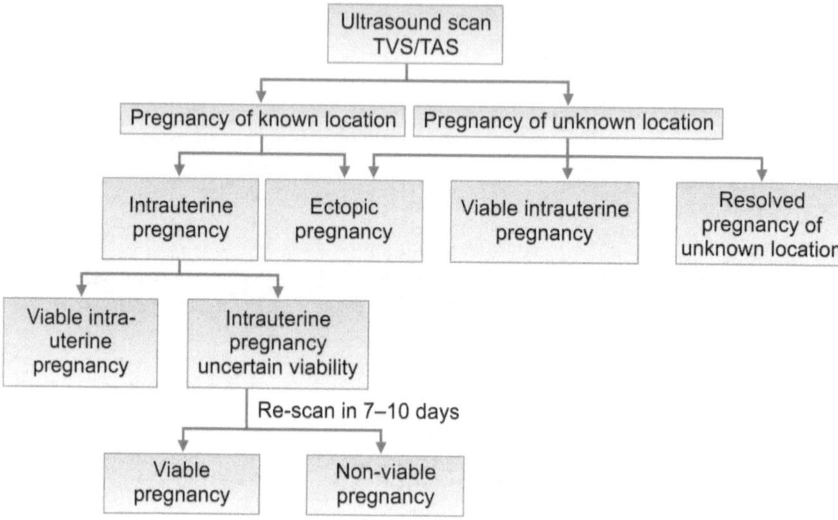

GENETIC ABNORMALITIES

- 55% of occult and early losses
- 5% of recurrent losses.

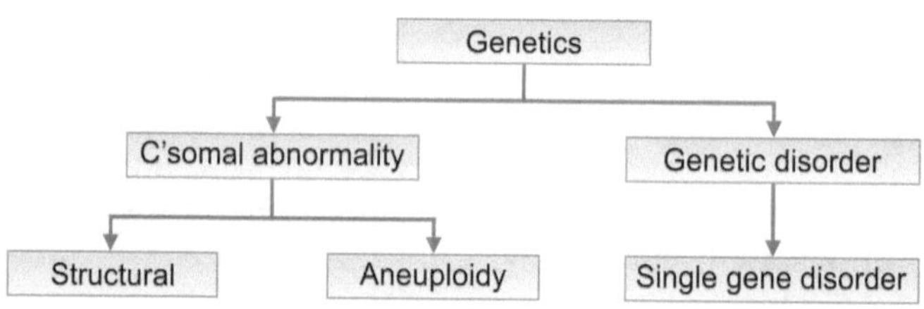

Structural Abnormalities

- Translocation (commonest) (1in 500)
  - Reciprocal (50%)
  - Robertsonian (24%)
- Mosaicism for a numeric aberration (12%)
- Inversion
- Deletions

Translocations

Reciprocal translocations occur when two different chromosomes exchange segments (46 chromosomes with two variants)	**Robertsonian translocations** occur when two chromosomes fuse together, creating one chromosome that contains most of the original two (45 chromosomes with one variant)

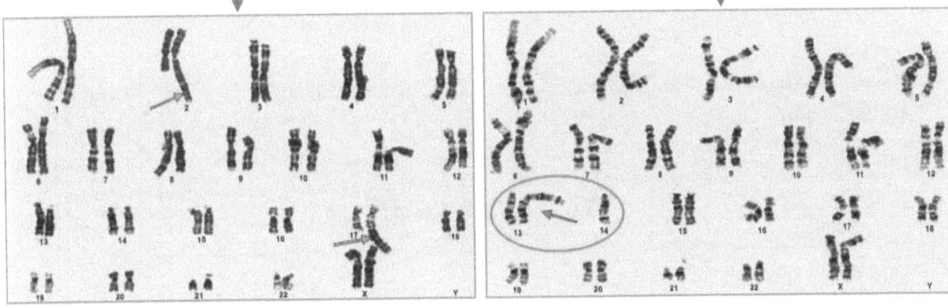

- All couples with a history of recurrent miscarriage should have peripheral blood karyotyping, cytogenetic analysis of products of conception if next pregnancy fails.
- If abnormal parental karyotype, refer to a clinical geneticist.
- No therapies are presently available to treat those parental chromosomal anomalies that potentially contribute to recurrent abortion.
- Preimplantation genetic diagnosis involves the removal of a single cell from an in vitro—matured embryo and rule out gross chromosomal abnormalities or the presence of specific genetic diseases.
- Use of either donor oocyte or donor sperm, depending on the affected partner, is recommended.

Preimplantation Genetic Diagnosis

- FISH (Fluorescent in situ hybridization)
  - Easy to perform
  - Yields results in 2 days
  - Detects 80% of all chromosome abnormalities
  - Provides information about presence or absence of very small segment of chromosome
- CGH (Comparative genomic hybridization)–
  - Yields results in 5 days
  - Allows analysis of all chromosomes
- Karyotype–
  - Yields results in 2 weeks.

Flow chart 5.2: Management of genetic causes of RPL

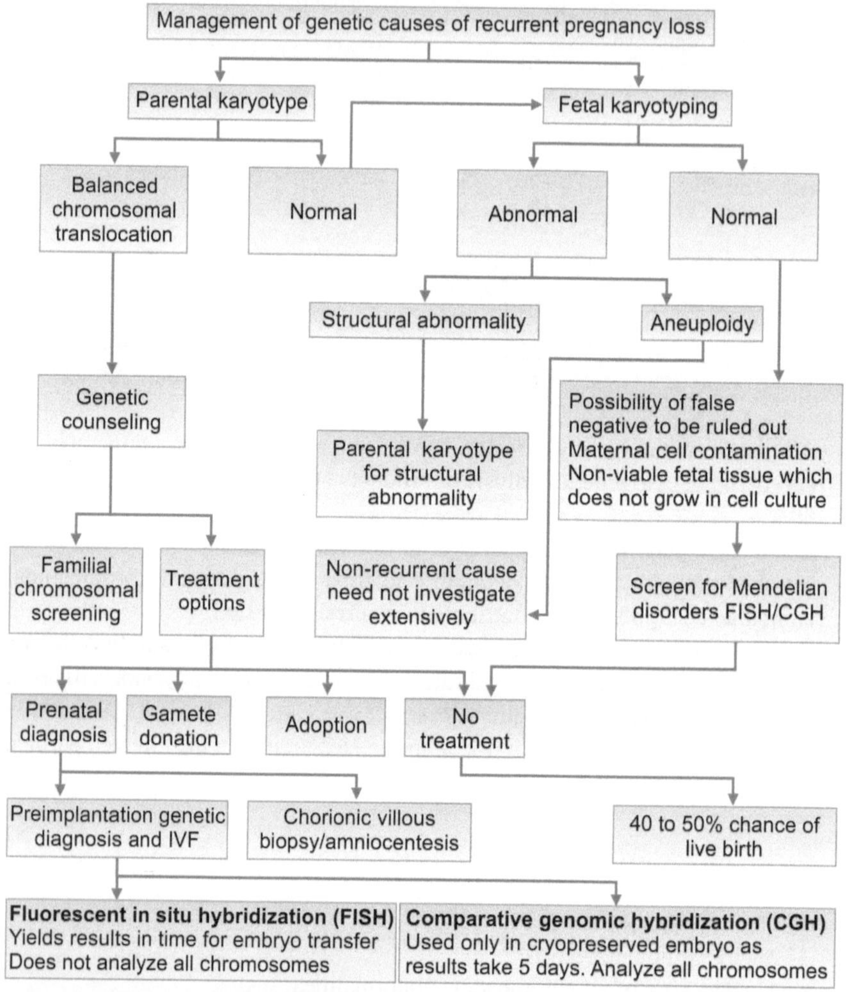

ANATOMIC ABNORMALITIES

- One in six to ten women with recurrent miscarriages has a structural defect like uterine septum or adhesions.
  - Mullerian anomalies
  - Cervical insufficiency
  - Fibroid uterus
  - Asherman syndrome
- The prevalence of uterine anomalies in recurrent miscarriage populations—1.8% and 37.6%.
- It is higher in women with late miscarriages.
- Investigations
  - Hysterosalpingogram (HSG)
  - Two-dimensional pelvic ultrasound with (or without) sonohysterography

  - 3D ultrasound
  - Laparoscopy
  - Hysteroscopy
- Submucous leiomyomas, intrauterine adhesions, and intrauterine septa–hysteroscopic resection
- Septate uterus.

Indication for Surgery (Septal Incision)

- Recurrent miscarriage
- Preterm delivery
- Infertility
- Other-dysmenorrhea, abnormal uterine bleeding

Three different approaches to hysteroscopic metroplasty:

1. Mechanical divison of septum with hysteroscopic microscissors
2. Resectoscopic divison with electrosurgery
3. Fibreoptic laser [neodymium yttrium aluminium garnet, KTP/532, argon, or krypton lasers] divison of the uterine septum

- Septal incision not septal resection

  Two basic techniques:

1. Shortening technique (thin septa)—septum is incised across its apex, causing gradual shortening
2. Thinning technique (wide septa)—incisions are made along each side of the septum alternatively, gradually thinning the septum until a short, broad notch remains that is then incised beginning at one cornual end and progressing to the other.

Best time for surgery—early follicular phase to avoid thick endometrium

Postoperative treatment

- Estrogen therapy—conjugated estrogen 2.5 mg 2–3 times per day for 4 weeks after surgery
- Combined with medroxy progesterone acetate 10 mg in 3rd and 4th week
- Estrogens will help re-epithelialization and proliferation and thereby preventing development of scar tissue

- Cervical insufficiency is suspected—TVS is to be done.

  Findings—Shortening of endocervical canal <25 mm–best predictor of spontaneous pre-term before 34 weeks
  - Funnelling of the internal os
  - Sacculation or prolapse of membranes into cervix either spontaneously or as a result of fundal pressure.
- Women are divided into 2 risk groups—medium risk and high risk.

High risk—2 or more 2nd trimester miscarriages without bleeding or clear signs of labor preceding the miscarriage.

- Benefit from prophylactic stitch at 13–16 weeks, with removal at 37–38 weeks.
- Short course of antibiotics and bed rest for 24 hrs.

Medium risk—One 2nd trimester loss.

- Serial ultrasound beginning at 12 weeks and performed every 2 weeks until 23 weeks to measure cervical length.
- Therapeutic cerclage to be offered when cervical length < 25 mm or progressive funnelling.
- No role of rescue cerclage.

McDonald suture: Simple purse string suture placed around cervix at the level of internal os.

- Mersilene tape, nylon, black silk.
- Knots tied anteriorly, as pregnancy progresses uterus anteverts making the access to posterior aspect difficult.
- Removed at 37 weeks of gestation or earlier if she goes into labor.

Shirodkar suture: Not routinely followed because stitch is placed at the base of the bladder. So bladder has to be dissected.

Transabdominal cervicoisthmic cerclage: Suture at the internal os via abdominal approach.

Indications: Previous failed vaginal suture.

- Traumatic or surgical damage making a vaginal approach difficult.
- Severe scarring or chronic cervitis, cervicovaginal fistula.
- At 12 weeks, with prior USG screening for fetal anomaly.

Under GA

- Pfannenstiel incision is appropriate.
- Mersilene tape and double stranded nylon is used.
- Scanning to confirm fetal life and intact membranes.
- Intraoperative antibiotics, NSAIDS for pain relief.
- Preoperative thromboprophylaxis is recommended, using LMWH.

ENDOCRINE ABNORMALITIES

- No direct evidence that thyroid disease is associated with RPL. The two proposed theories:
    - The presence of thyroid autoantibodies in women with normal thyroid function could be associated with a subtle deficiency in the availability of thyroid hormones or a lower capacity of the thyroid gland to adequately rise to the demand for augmented synthesis of thyroid hormones required in pregnancy.
    - Thyroid autoantibodies might be an indicator of an underlying enhanced global autoimmune state. This itself can have a direct adverse effect on placental or fetal development.
- Routine screening for occult diabetes and thyroid disease with oral glucose tolerance and thyroid function tests in asymptomatic women presenting with recurrent miscarriage is not needed.
- Thyroid hormone replacement with *L-Thyroxine* in cases of hypothyroidism.
- Metformin and insulin reduction, increases glycodelin, IGFBP in the luteal phase endometrium—enhances vascularity—improved endometrial milieu for the establishment and maintenance of pregnancy.

- There is insufficient evidence to evaluate the effect of progesterone supplementation and human chorionic gonadotropin (hCG) in pregnancy to prevent miscarriage.
- Prepregnancy suppression of high luteinizing hormone (LH) concentration among ovulatory women with recurrent miscarriage and polycystic ovaries who hypersecrete LH does not improve the live birth rate.
- Polycystic ovary morphology itself does not predict an increased risk of future pregnancy loss among ovulatory women with a history of recurrent miscarriage who conceive spontaneously.
- There is insufficient evidence to assess the effect of hyperprolactinemia as a risk factor for recurrent miscarriage.

INFECTIONS

- TOCH (toxoplasmosis, other [congenital syphilis and viruses], cytomegalovirus and herpes simplex virus) screening is not neededed in the investigation of recurrent miscarriage.
- Rubella screening should be done routinely in all women with recurrent miscarriage.
- Screening for and treatment of bacterial vaginosis in early pregnancy among high-risk women with a previous history of second-trimester miscarriage or spontaneous preterm labor may reduce the risk of recurrent late loss and preterm birth.
- Empirical antibiotics are not needed.

IMMUNE FACTORS

Guidelines for measurement of Thyroid Stimulating Hormone Receptor Antibodies in Pregnancy

1. A euthyroid pregnant woman without medication but who has previously received antithyroid drugs for Graves disease. The risk for fetal and neonatal hyperthyroidism is negligible. Measurement of TRAbs is not necessary.
2. A euthyroid pregnant women (with or without thyroid hormone substitution therapy) who has previously received radioiodine therapy or undergone thyroid surgery for Graves disease—measure TRAbs in the first trimester.
   - If absent or low—no further evaluation is recommended
   - If high—fetus should be followed carefully for the signs of hyperthyroidism, again measure TRAbs in the last trimester to evaluate the risk of neonatal hypothyroidism
3. A pregnant woman who takes antithyroid drugs for Graves diasese, TRAbs should be measured in the last trimester
   - If absent or low—neonatal hyperthyroidism is unlikely
   - If high—evaluation for neonatal hyperthyroidism is needed (clinical evaluation and thyroid function tests on cord blood and again after 4 to 7 days).

IMMUNOLOGY OF PREGNANCY

- HLA compatibility between partners should be absent
- Prevents the formation of blocking antibody—rejection by the mother—fetal loss
- Depressed response of maternal lymphocytes to stimulation by Paternal antigens
- HLA-G and HLA-E polymorphism—suppress cytotoxic T cells and NK cells activity—protects the fetus
- For a normal pregnancy Th2 >Th1

  Th1 cytokines-IFN-γ, TNF- α, β, IL 2,– macrophages and cell mediated reactions – delayed hypersensitivity–intracellular pathogens

  Th2 cytokines-IL4, IL5, IL6, IL10, IL13 – humoral vigorous antibody production and are found in association with strong Ab responses–extracellular organisms

  Th3–TGF–β secreting CD4 cells, mucosal T helper function
- Progesterone may be responsible for a switch from Th1 to Th2 at the maternal fetal interface by production of PIBF (Progesterone Induced Blocking Factor).

THROMBOPHILIAS

Acquired Thrombophilia

- Antiphospholipid antibody syndrome (APS)
- Hyperhomocystinemia
- Activated protein C resistance.

Inherited Thrombophilia

- Factor V Leiden mutation
- Prothrombin G20210A mutation
- Antithrombin III deficiency
- Protein S deficiency
- Protein C deficiency
- Methyl tetrahydrofolate reductase.

Thrombogenic changes of pregnancy exaggerate an inherent predisposition to thrombosis-reduced placental blood flow–pregnancy loss.

Coagulation Factors

Factors which favors clotting when increased
- Factor VII, VIII, X
- Fibrinogen

Factors which favor clotting when decreased
- Antithrombin III
- Protein C, S

Fibrinolysis Factors

Factor which favor clotting when increased
- Plasminogen activator inhibitor-1 (PAI 1)

Factor which favor clotting when decreased

- Antiplasmin

Flow chart 5.3: Pathophysiology of thrombophilia

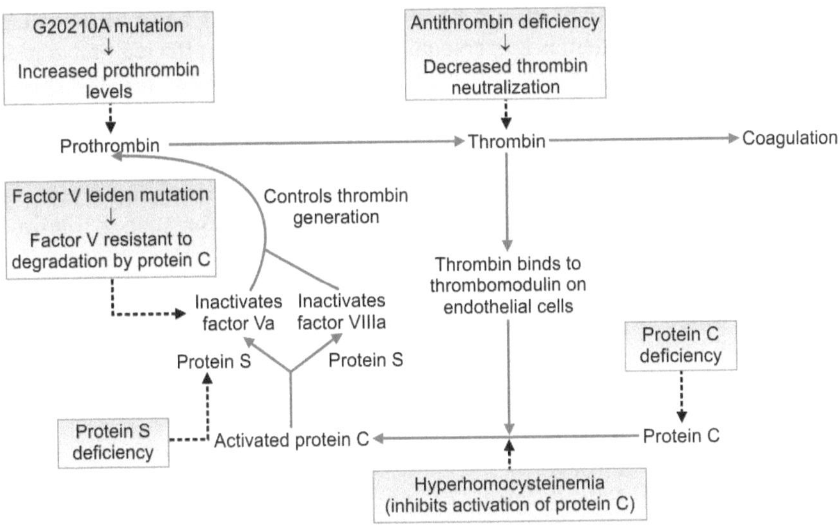

Management

Screening

- Screening should be considered in patients with personal history of VTE or a strong family of VTE
- Population screening should not be done
- Screening for inherited thrombophilias is not recommended in patients with history of adverse pregnancy outcome
- Laboratory testing should ideally be done in the nonpregnant patient who is not receiving hormonal or anticoagulation therapy and is remote (more than 6 months) from a history of VTE.

Thrombophilia Work-up
Activated protein C resistance screen (95% of positives due to Factor V Leiden) or Factor V Leiden (DNA)
Antithrombin activity
Prothrombin gene mutation G20210A (DNA)
4G/4G PAI–1 mutation (DNA)[a] (if not available, quantitative assay for plasma PAI–1 protein levels)
Protein C activity (if low, measure free and total antigen levels)
Protein S activity (if low, measure free and total antigen levels)
Lupus anticoagulant
Anticardiolipin antibodies
MTHFR mutation screen and/or fasting plasma homocysteine levels
[a]Testing should be remote from thrombotic event and while off anticoagulants, except DNA tests.

Prevention of Venous Thromboembolism

- High-risk women (more thrombogenic) thrombophilia (AT deficiency, FVL homozygosity, and PGM homozygosity and FVL/PGM compound

heterozygosity) should be treated with full therapeutic anticoagulation during pregnancy and for at least 6 weeks postpartum, regardless of the history.
- Low-risk women (less thrombogenic) thrombophilia (FVL heterozygosity, PGM heterozygosity, PC or PS deficiency) do not need antepartum anticoagulation if there is no personal history of VTE or affected first degree relative.

Prevention of Recurrent Venous Thromboembolism

- Women with history of VTE during current pregnancy should receive therapeutic anticoagulation for at least 4 months during the pregnancy, followed by prophylactic therapy for 6 weeks postpartum.
- Women with history of VTE associated with nonrecurrent risk factors but without acquired or inherited thrombophilia prophylaxis during antepartum period is unnecessary, prophylaxis should be used during the higher risk post-partum period.

VTE prophylaxis and inherited thrombophilia

Previous VTE	Inherited thrombophilia	Antenatal prophylaxis	Postnatal prophylaxis
Yes	Antithrombin III deficiency	Yes LMWH	Yes LMWH
No	Antithrombin III deficiency	Yes LMWH	Yes LMWH
No	Protein C deficiency	Yes LMWH	Yes LMWH
No	Homozygous factor V Leiden	Yes LMWH	Yes LMWH
No	Homozygous prothrombin gene	Yes LMWH	Yes LMWH
No	Protein S deficiency	No	? consider aspirin
No	Heterozygous factor V Leiden	No	? consider aspirin
No	Heterozygous prothrombin gene	No	? consider aspirin
Yes	Any other thrombophilic defect, example: APS	Yes LMWH	Yes LMWH

LMWH, Low molecular weight heparin; APS–Anti-phospholipid syndrome

Prenatal

- Unclear benefit of treatment for a history of adverse pregnancy outcome with anticoagulation
- Provide therapeutic heparin or low-molecular weight for a history of VTE during pregnancy
- Provide prophylactic or therapeutic heparin or low-molecular weight heparin for a history of VTE, depending on the level of risk and recurrent features
- Provide folate and vitamin B12 supplementation for homocysteinemia.

Intrapartum

Reduce or stop heparin for labor and delivery; restart after 6 hours.

Postnatal

Switching to warfarin postpartum is an option.

Various heparin dosing regimens
Therapeutic anticoagulation
1. Unfractionated heparin (UFH) A. Initial treatment i. IV heparin for at least 5 days a. Weight-adjusted: Bolus with 80 U/kg followed by 18 U/kg/hr (target aPTT of 1.5–2.5 x control) or b. Bolus with 5,000 U followed by infusion of at least 30,000 U for the first 24 hours B. Maintenance therapy i. Adjusted dose SC heparin injections a. ≥ 10,000 U every 8–12 hours titrating to 1.5–2.5 x control aPTT b. Treat for the remainder of pregnancy and at least 6 weeks postpartum ii. LMWH C. Weight adjusted 1. Enoxaparin 1 mg/kg SC every 12 hours 2. Dalteparin 100 U/kg SC every 12 hours Tinzaparin 175 U/kg SC every day Prophylactic anticoagulation i. Unfractionated heparin A. By trimesters 1. 1st trimester: UFH 5,000 U SC every 12 hours 2. 2nd trimester: UFH 7,500–10,000 U SC every 12 hours 3. 3rd trimester: UFH 10,000 U SC every 12 hours unless aPTT is elevated ii. LMWH A. Enoxaparin 30 mg SC every 12 hours (or 40 mg SC daily)[a] B. Dalteparin 5,000 U SC daily C. Tinzaparin 4,500 U SC daily

[a]Twice daily dosing is preferred in pregnancy. SC, subcutaneous.

HYPERHOMOCYSTEINEMIA

Homocysteine

- Naturally occuring sulphur containing nonessential amino acid
- Produced as an intermediate during metabolism of other amino acids (methionine)
- 50% is re-methylated back into methionine
- 50% is trans-sulfurated to cystathionine, a source of cysteine
- Methylcobalamin, folic acid and pyridoxine keep homocysteine normal.

Vitamin B_{12}

- Important cofactor methionine synthetase (MS) in methylation of homocysteine
- Plays a key role in the remethylation of homocysteine to methionine
- In Vitamin B_{12} deficiency, folate is trapped as unusable MTHF causing functional folate deficiency.

Vitamin B_6

- Important cofactor pyridoxal phosphate in methylation of homocysteine
- Reduces the level of homocysteine by the process of transulphuration to cysteine.

Folic Acid

- L methyl folate (Natural Folate) is the primary biologically active form of folate in circulation
- Folic acid, the synthetic form of folate, must undergo enzymatic reduction by methylene tetrahydrofolate reductase (MTHFR) to become biologically active
- Methyltetrahydrofolate is the active form of folic acid.

ANTIPHOSPHOLIPID SYNDROME

Antiphospholipid syndrome (APS)—Autoimmune disorder defined by presence of characteristic clinical features and specified levels of circulating antiphospholipid antibodies.

Primary APS: APS in the absence of lupus or other (53%) connective tissue disorder.

Secondary APS: APS with lupus or other connective (47%) tissue disorders.
- Systemic lupus erythematosus
- Rheumatoid arthritis
- Scleroderma
- Polymyositis
- Sjogren's syndrome.

Antiphospholipid Antibody Syndrome (APLA)

To diagnose APLA, it is mandatory that the patient should have two positive tests at least 12 weeks apart for either lupus anticoagulant or anticardiolipin (aCL) antibodies of IgG and/or IgM class present in medium or high titer.

Sapporo Criteria (Wilson's Diagnostic Criteria)

For a patient to be diagnosed with APLA, one or more clinical and one or more laboratory criteria must be present on 2 occasions 3 months apart.

Clinical Criteria

Thrombosis: One or more confirmed episodes of venous, arterial or small vessel disease.

Adverse Pregnancy Outcomes (APO)

a. Three or more consecutive miscarriages before ten weeks of gestation
b. One or more morphologically normal fetal deaths after the tenth week of gestation, and

c. One or more preterm births before the 34th week of gestation due to severe pre-eclampsia, eclampsia or placental insufficiency.

Laboratory Criteria

1. ACL–nonspecific, diagnosed by ELISA
   Negative <10 GPL units
   Low positive 10–20 GPL units
   Moderate positive 20–100 GPL units
   Strong positive >100 GPL units
2. Anti β2 GPI antibody IgG or IgM (>99 percentile), OR
3. LA–more specific

Step I—APTT, dRVVT-use both
Step II—Demonstration of inhibitor-mix patient and normal plasma, prolonged screening test
Step III—Demonstration of phospholipid dependence of inhibitor.

Antibody	Directed against	Test of detection	Sensitivity (%)	Specificity (%)
Lupus anticoagulant	Plasma prot. bound to phospholipids	dRVVT	83	95
Anti-cardiolipin (IgG, IgM)	Phospholipids	ELISA	95	75 (IgG is specific)
Anti-B2 Glycoprotein I (IgG, IgM)	Phospholipid binding prot.	ELISA	81	91

Obstetric Manifestations

- Infertility (?implantation failure)
- Increased risk of DVT and PE
- Increased risk of thrombocytopenia
- Increased risk of PE and E
- Abruptio placenta
- Early miscarriage, IUGR, prematurity, stillbirth
- ?Increased risk of neonatal neuropsychological disorder.

Other Clinical Features

- Thrombocytopenia, hemolytic anemia (DCT +ve)
- Livedo reticularis (25%) – high risk for arterial thrombosis
- Cardiac valve disease-MV > AV, MR > MS, asymptomatic
- Nephropathy–Thrombotic microangiopathy (HT, non-nephrotic proteinuria, renal impairment)
- Neurologic manifestations: Myelopathy, Chorea, Epilepsy, Migraine, Cognitive impairment (MR white-matter lesions).

Treatment

- As soon as pregnancy is diagnosed, start aspirin 1.2 mg/kg/day.
  - It acts by preventing thrombosis and damage to trophoblast.
  - Add heparin 5000 units SC daily in the following indications:

Flow chart 5.4: Management of APS

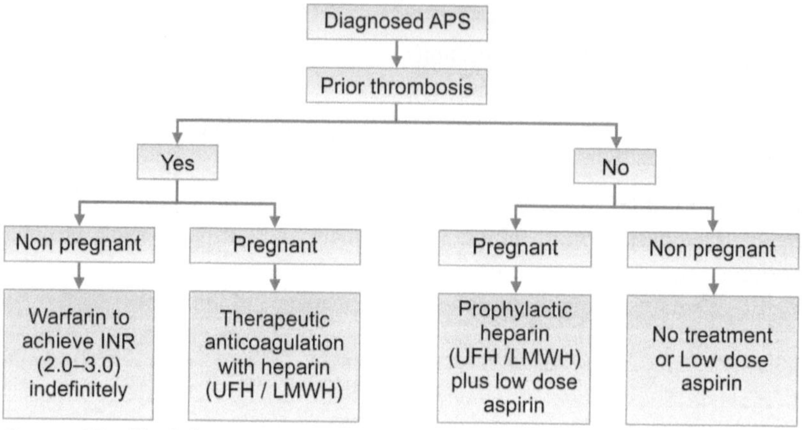

Source: Clin Obs & Gyne. JAMA 2006;49(4)295:1050

  1. In subjects who test high positive
  2. In subjects who test positive for both lupus anticoagulant and anti-cardiolipin antibody
  3. Low positive but refractory to only aspirin in previous pregnancy.
  - Besides, antithrombotic acts by blocking complement activation (immunomodulation), prevents binding of aPL, decreases inflammation and facilitates implantation.

  Continue both till 36 weeks.

  Induce at 37 completed weeks.
- Calcium supplementation and weight-bearing exercises to prevent osteoporosis.
- Immunosuppressive therapy–IV immunoglobulin and steroids are not recommended (Cochrane analysis–IV Ig is associated with increased risk of pregnancy loss or premature birth).

Dosage Regimens

- Therapeutic and prophylactic heparin dosage as previously mentioned.
- Low titers of anti-cardiolipin antibodies: no treatment is required.
- Regular heparin—PT and APTT to be tested every 3 weeks.
  If increased by more than double the controls, stop heparin for a week.
  Repeat PT and APTT, if <2 times the control, restore heparin.
- Patient should be councelled about risk of placental abruption, retroplacental hemorrhage, heparin-induced thrombocytopenia (HIT) and osteoporosis which is seen with heparin usage and bleeding, neutropenia, thrombocytopenia are seen with aspirin.

- Currently there is no reliable evidence to show that steroids improve the live birth rate of women with recurrent miscarriage associated with aPL when compared with other treatment modalities; increased risk of preeclamsia, PROM, GDM. Their use may provoke significant maternal and fetal morbidity.

Subcutaneous Heparin Regimens for Treatment of APLA in Pregnancy

1. APLA syndrome without prior thrombosis
   Recurrent early (preembryonic or embryonic) miscarriage
   - Unfractionated heparin 5000–7500 U, subcutaneously 12 hourly
   - Low molecular weight heparin
     Enoxaparin 40 mg or dalteparin 5000 U subcutaneously, once daily
     OR
     Enoxaparin 30 mg or dalteparin 5000 U subcutaneously, 12 hourly
     Fetal death (>10 weeks gestation) or prior early delivery (<34 weeks gestation) due to severe preeclampsia or placental insufficiency
   - Unfractionated heparin 7500–10000 U, SC,12 hourly in the first trimester; 10000 U SC, q12h in the 2nd and 3rd trimesters,
     OR
     q8–12h adjusted to maintain the midinterval aPTT 1.5 times the control mcan
   - Low molecular weight heparin
     Enoxaparin 30 mg or dalteparin 5000 U, SC q12h
2. APLA with thrombosis
   - Unfractionated heparin -q8–12h adjusted to maintain the midinterval aPTT or heparin level (anti-Xa activity in the therapeutic range)
   - Low molecular weight heparin—Weight adjusted, e.g. 1 mg or dalteparin 200 U/kg SC q-12h with monitoring of anti-Xa activity

Future Therapies

1. Combination anti-aggregant therapy (aspirin + clopidogrel or dipyridamole): especially when warfarin is contraindicated
2. Oral anti-factor Xa drugs (rivaroxaban, apixaban) - As effective as warfarin
3. Direct thrombin inhibitors (dabigatran) - RE-LY trial (AF), Recover trial (DVT)
4. Statins (fluvastatin, rosuvastatin)
   - Inhibition of tissue factor production by APLA
   - Prevent increased adhesiveness of endothelial cell by anti-β_2
   - Decreased risk of DVT in healthy people with normal cholesterol

Antenatal Management

- Monitor platelets every week first 2–3 weeks after starting heparin
- Prenatal visits 2–4 weeks till 24 weeks 1–2 weeks thereafter
- Fetal growth monitoring every 3-4 weeks by USG after 17–18 weeks,
- Uterine artery Doppler at 24 weeks: decreased diastolic flow, protodiastolic notching are predictors for fetal growth restriction and preeclampsia.
- Antepartum fetal surveillance after 28 weeks includes DFMC, weekly NST and AFI measurement.

Labor

- Induction before 38 weeks.
- Withhold anticoagulation 24 hrs prior induction. Regional anesthesia not to be within 12 hrs of LMWH and 6 hours of unfractionated heparin.
  - 12hrs after last prophylactic dose
  - 24 hrs after last therapeutic dose
- If postoperative LMWH is to be given to patient who had spinal or epidural anesthesia.
  - 24 hrs postoperatively, if on therapeutic infusion
  - 6–8 hrs postoperatively, if prophylactic dose is used
- Epidural cannula not removed within 10–12 hrs of most recent injection.

Postpartum

- No routine prophylaxis in APLA without thrombotic risk factors
- Resume anticoagulation 4–6 hrs after vaginal delivery and 8–12 hrs after cesarean section till 6 weeks.
- Only if family h/o thrombophilia or thrombotic risk factors Warfarin can be substituted, adjust the dose to achieve an INR of 2 to 3.
- Finally oral contraceptives containing estrogen are contraindicated.

Unexplained Recurrent Miscarriage

- Despite extensive testing approximately 50% couples with recurrent miscarriage no cause is identified.
- Aspirin doesn't improve live birth rate in unexplained miscarriage.
- 2–3 fold increased risk of gastroschisis in mothers taking aspirin during 1st trimester.
- Psychological support.
- All professionals should be aware of the psychological sequelae associated with miscarriage and should provide support and follow-up, as well as access to formal counseling when necessary.
- These women should be reassured that the prognosis for a successful future pregnancy with a supportive care alone is 75%, however the prognosis worsens with increase in maternal age and the number of previous miscarriages.
- Plans for follow-up should be clearly recorded in the discharge letter.
- Empirical treatment is unnecessary and should be avoided. Some empirical drugs are—
  - Low dose asprin
  - Subcutaneous heparin
  - Folic acid
  - Progesterone
  - Solcoseryl (increase oxygen supply)
  - Nitroglycerin (increase implantation by increase uterine blood flow)
  - Tocolytic

Treatment of Miscarriage

- Surgical uterine evacuation—Suction curettage.
- Surgical uterine evacuation—Screen for Chlamydia trachomatis.
- Medical and expectant methods are also effective in the management of confirmed miscarriage.
- Tissue obtained at the time of miscarriage should be examined histologically to confirm pregnancy and to exclude ectopic pregnancy or gestational trophoblastic disease.
- Non-sensitized rhesus (Rh) negative women should receive anti-D immunoglobulin in the following situations: ectopic pregnancy, all miscarriages over 12 weeks (including threatened), all miscarriages where the uterus is evacuated, and for threatened miscarriages under 12 weeks when bleeding is heavy or associated with pain.
- A woman who has suffered a single sporadic miscarriage has an 80% chance and a woman with three consecutive miscarriages a 60% chance of her next pregnancy being successful.

Chromosomal Analysis of Products of Conception

General—it is good practice–legal reguirement, to obtain patient consent prior to tissue collection.

Collection:
1st trimester–collect all fetal tissue and placental villi
2nd trimester–small piece of full thickness fetal skin with subepidermal layers.

- IUD and macerated fetus—send placental biopsy, wedge from cord insertion site include membranes.
- Container—sterile universal container, sterile saline or transport media. Do not add formalin.
- Labeling—Name, date of birth, hospital number.
- Transport and storage—Send sample immediately at room temperature, sample can be refrigerated at 4°C.
- Causes for rejection—Gross contamination, necrotic tissue, specimen in formalin fixative.
- Limitations—Sample may contain maternal tissue and trophoblastic tissue cantaining mosaicism or aneuploidy which is not present in fetus.
- Comparison of three protocols for the investigation and treatment of recurrent pregnancy loss.

Management During Subsequent Pregnancy

USG is valuable in management of early pregnancy to confirm viability and fetal heart activity. TVS–intrauterine gestational sac will be visible at 5 weeks, yolk sac at 5.5 weeks, cardiac activity at 6 weeks. Thereafter to check fetal heart activity scan to be done every week or every 2 weeks till the end of 1st trimester.

Investigation or treatment	RCOG protocol	ACOG protocol	ESHRE protocol
Parental karyotyping	Recommended	Recommended	Recommended
APS assessment (ACL and LA)	Recommended	Recommended	Recommended
Fetal karyotyping	Recommended	Insufficient evidence	Trial required
Uterine cavity assessment	Recommended by USG or hydrosonography	Insufficient evidence	Recommended by ultrasound or hysterosal-pingography
Resection of uterine septum	Insufficient evidence	Recommended despite lack of evidence	—
Treatment of APS with heparin and aspirin	Recommended	Recommended	Insufficient evidence
Luteal phase investi-gation required	—	Insufficient evidence	Insufficient evidence: trials
Progesterone or hCG supplementa-tion RCTs required	Insufficient evidence	Insufficient evidence	Insufficient evidence: more
Bacterial vaginosis	Insufficient evidence	Not recommended	—
Hereditary thrombophilias investigation	Insufficient evidence	Insufficient evidence	Recommended as advanced
Anticoagulants for hereditary thrombophilia	Insufficient evidence	Insufficient evidence	Insufficient evidence
Thyroid function	Not recommended	Not recommended	Recommended
Glucose challenge test	Not recommended	Not recommended	Recommended
TORCH testing	Not recommended	Not recommended	Not recommended
Alloimmune testing	Not recommended	Not recommended	Insufficient evidence
Immunotherapy for IVIG and third-party leukocytes	Not recommended	Not recommended	Insufficient evidence: RCT required
'Tender loving care'	Insufficient evidence	—	Recommended
Diet, smoking, alcohol reduction	—	—	Recommended
Folic acid for hyper-homocysteinemia	—	—	Insufficient evidence
Vitamin supplementation	—	—	Not recommended
Steroids	Not recommended	—	Not recommended

CHAPTER

6

Multiple Pregnancy

Twin fetuses usually result from fertilization of two separate ova—dizygotic or fraternal twins and less often, twins arise from a single fertilized ovum that subsequently divides—monozygotic or identical twins.

Incidence—Multiple pregnancy rates vary worldwide—6.7/1000 in Japan, 40/1000 in Nigeria.

Monozygous twins–3.5 per 1000 births

Hellin's rule–Twins – 1 in 80

Triplets–1 in 80[2]

Quadruplets–1 in 80[3]

DIAGNOSIS

Symptoms

- Hyperemesis
- Excessive fetal movements
- Cardiorespiratory embracement—palpitations, shortness of breath
- Tendency of swelling of legs, varicose veins, hemorrhoids
- Unusual enlargement of abdomen

Signs

- Uterine height more than period of gestation
- Abdominal girth >100 cm at term
- Multiple fetal parts
- Two fetal heads or three poles
- Polyhydramnios
- Two fetal heart sounds heard 10 cm apart, rate differs by 10 bpm by 2 examiners simultaneously

Ultrasound in Multiple Pregnancy

First trimester

- Diagnosis of multifetal pregnancy
- Determination of chorionicity and amnionicity
- Accurate pregnancy dating (crown-rump length)
- Screening for some anomalies (nuchal translucency)
- Guidance for chorionic villous sampling and multifetal pregnancy reduction

Second trimester

- Screening for fetal anomalies
- Guidance for amniocentesis
- Determination of chorionicity and amnionicity
- Determination of placental cord insertion
- Biometry to screen for early fetal growth restriction or discordance
- Assessment of cervical length

Third trimester

- Biometry to screen for fetal growth restriction and discordance
- Assessment of cervical length
- Fetal status assessment
  - Amniotic fluid volume
  - Biophysical profile
  - Doppler flow studies
- Fetal presentation

Intrapartum

- Fetal presentation
- Guidance for external cephalic version of second twin.

Ultrasound Prediction of Amnionicity and Chorionicity

- Chorionicity is most accurate in the first trimester
- 6 to 10 weeks: Counting the number of gestational sacs and evaluating the thickness of the dividing membrane determines chorionicity.
- 11 to 14 weeks gestation:
  - In dichorionic pregnancies, inter-twin membrane is thick and easy to identify at the attachment to the placenta as a triangular projection: lambda or twin peak sign.
  - Two separate gestational sacs, each containing fetus and a thick dividing membrane.

Dichorionic Diamniotic Pregnancy

- Dividing membrane appears "thick" measures diameter of ≥2 mm, and 3 or 4 layers can be identified -"Twin peak sign" or "Lambda sign".
- One gestational sac with a thin dividing membrane and two fetuses.

Monochorionic Diamniotic Pregnancy

Two layers of membranes identified, membrane appears as "T" sign (a point at which amnions meet placenta).

COMPLICATIONS

Maternal

- Anemia
- Pressure symptoms: Edema of legs/vulva/abdominal wall, shortness of breath.
- Hyperemesis

- Hypertensive disorders of pregnancy: Gestational hypertension, preeclampsia-increased 2–3 fold. Atypical forms like HELLP syndrome and placental abruption.
- Placenta previa
- Polyhydraminos
- PROM/PPROM
- Preterm labor

Fetal

- Vanishing twin
- Malformations: Structural defects, chromosomal anomalies
- Monochorionic twins:
  - Discordant growth/Twin to twin transfusion syndrome
  - Acardiac twin
  - Single fetal demise
  - Conjoined twins

Antenatal Management

- Diet–Increased calorie intake by 2800 kcal/day, proteins-175 gm/day
- Supplements–Iron to be increased to 100 mg/day. Additional vitamins, calcium and folic acid (5 mg) to be given over those prescribed for a singleton.
- Frequency of antenatal visits–Once a month till 20 weeks, once in 15 days from 20 weeks–28 weeks, Weekly–from 28 weeks till delivery.
- Fetal surveillance–Monthly ultrasound from 24 weeks to assess fetal growth, amniotic fluid volume, fetal well-being.

Key events in antenatal and postnatal care to be offered for dichorionic twins:
Multiple pregnancy clinic: lead clinician with multidisciplinary team

- Ultrasound at 10–13 weeks: (a) viability, (b) chorionicity, (c) nuchal translucency: aneuploidy
- Structural anomaly scan at 20–22 weeks
- Serial fetal growth scans, e.g. at 24, 28 and 32 weeks and then every 2–4 weeks
- Blood pressure and urinalysis at 20, 24 and 28 weeks and then every 2 weeks
- Discussion of woman's /family's needs relating to twins
- 34–38 weeks: discussion of mode of delivery and intrapartum care
- Elective delivery at 37–38 completed weeks
- Postnatal advice and support (hospital and community-based) to include breastfeeding and contraceptive advice

Key events in antenatal and postnatal care to be offered for monochorionic twins:

- Multiple pregnancy clinic: lead clinician with multidisciplinary team
- Ultrasound at 10–13 weeks: (a) viability, (b) chorionicity, (c) nuchal translucency: aneuploidy/TTTS
- Ultrasound surveillance for TTTS and discordant growth: at 16 weeks and then every 2 weeks
- Structural anomaly scan at 20–22 weeks (including fetal echocardiography)

- Serial fetal growth scans every 2 weeks until delivery
- Blood pressure and urinalysis at 20, 24 and 28 weeks and then every 2 weeks
- Discussion of woman's/family needs relating to twins
- 32–34 weeks: discussion of mode of delivery and intrapartum care
- Elective delivery at 36–37 completed weeks (if uncomplicated)
- Postnatal advice and support (hospital and community-based) to include breastfeeding and contraceptive advice
- Weekly NST from 36 weeks.
- Avoid strenuous work from 24 weeks upto 34 weeks to reduce risk of preterm birth.
- Use of tocolysis, encirclage, corticosteroids–no benefit. Twins develop lung maturity 3–4 weeks earlier than singletons.
- Aspirin 75 mg from 12 weeks till delivery to be added in the following criteria in order to prevent PIH:
  1. Age >40 years.
  2. BMI >35 kg/m^2
  3. First pregnancy
  4. Pregnancy interval >10 years
  5. Family history of preeclampsia
- Be vigilant for early symptoms of preterm labor.
- Therapeutic amniocentesis if extreme polyhydramnios or maternal distress.
- Preterm labor—A mean cervical length of 25 mm (compared with 15 mm for singletons) is a good predictor of preterm labor before 32 weeks of twin gestation. The use of fetal fibronectin is less predictive of preterm delivery of twins compared with singletons, with only 50% of deliveries before 35 weeks predicted at 28 weeks of gestation.
- Optimal timing of delivery:
  - Monochorionic diamniotic–36 weeks with steroids.
  - Monochorionic monoamniotic–32 weeks due to risk of cord entanglement.
  - Dichorionic–37 weeks
  - Triplets–35 weeks.

MANAGEMENT DURING LABOR

Confirm Diagnosis of Twins and Labor

In Case of Unbooked Patient

- Note: History suggestive of complications such as bleeding, headache, etc.
- Height of uterus > period of gestation, multiple fetal parts, 3 fetal poles felt.
- USG to confirm diagnosis and rule out higher order multiple pregnancy.

In Case of Booked Patient

- Go through previous records and date pregnancy.
- Note chorionicity of twins.

Examination

- Maternal condition—Pulse, BP, hydration, pallor, pedal edema, jaundice
- Height of the uterus

- Presentation of 1st twin
- Presentation of 2nd twin
- FHS of both babies
- Uterine activity
- Look for complications like:
    - Anemia
    - PIH
    - Prematurity
    - APH
    - Abnormal presentation
    - Gross congenital anomalies

Investigations–CBC, blood grouping and cross-matching and USG if not already done.

Mode of Delivery

- Twin 1 vertex (criteria as for singleton)—vaginal delivery unless contraindicated. Cesarean delivery only for obstetric indications.
- Twin 1 transverse or oblique or complicated breech–LSCS
- Monoamniotic twins: elective cesarean because of complications such as cord entanglement, TTTS, IUD.

Indications for Cesarean in Twin Pregnancy

- Twin 1 noncephalic presentation
- Twin 2 significantly larger than twin 1 and likely to cause CPD and difference more than 500 gm
- Monoamniotic twins
- Conjoint twins
- Monochorionic twins with TTTS

Obstetric indications–
- Placenta previa
- Severe preeclampsia with unfavorable cervix
- Previous cesarean section
- Cord prolapse of 1st twin
- Inco-ordinate uterine action
- Contracted pelvis

Labor Management

General measures
- Watch for APH, incoordinate uterine action, cord prolapse, PPH
- Establish IV access
- Emergency Hb, blood group and cross-match
- Arrange 1 or more units of compatible blood according to Hb level
- Appropriately trained obstetric attendant, preferably two obstetricians
- Inform staff nurse (double set of instruments including forceps and vacuum to be kept ready)

- Two pediatricians trained in neonatal resuscitation
- Anesthetic back up.

First Stage of Labor

- Maintain maternal hydration, appropriate analgesia
- Clear fluids only
- Partogram after she enters active phase of labor
- Monitoring of both FHS separately
- Augmentation, if required.

Second Stage of Labor

- Two obstetricians and two pediatricians
- Appropriate analgesia—local infiltration, pudendal block
- Liberal episiotomy
- Deliver 1st baby, no prophylactic oxytocics/methergin
  - Cut the cord in between 2 clamps
  - Handover twin 1 to pediatrician
  - Early cord clamping to prevent transfer of 2nd twins blood to 1st twin.
- Examine the patient—pulse, BP, determine lie and presentation of 2nd twin by PA and PV examination (take care not to rupture membranes), use USG, if necessary
- If second twin cephalic or breech
  - Augment with syntocin if uterine activity less after delivery of twin 1
  - Await spontaneous delivery unless fetal distress/bleeding PV/cord prolapse
  - ARM only after presenting part enters pelvis
- If second twin transverse or oblique, ECV to be attempted
  ECV:
  - If successful—once fetus enters pelvis, ROM and await spontaneous delivery
  - If unsuccessful—breech extraction (for breech presentation), IPV and breech extraction (for transverse lie) under GA unless LSCS indicated (See indications).

Interval between delivery of two twins—Usually up to 30 min
- Delay beyond this is acceptable if progress is being made, bleeding is minimal and FHS is normal.

Indications for urgent delivery of 2nd twin
- Severe vaginal bleeding
- Cord prolapse of 2nd twin
- Use of ergometrine after delivery of 1st twin
- Fetal distress

Management of fetal distress of second twin
- Cephalic presentation—Ventouse or forceps if prerequisites are fulfilled.
- Breech—Breech extraction
- Transverse lie—LSCS

Indications of CS for Second Twin

- Persistent transverse lie
  - Failed IPV
  - Obstetrician not experienced in IPV
- Second twin bigger than first causing CPD
- Excessive bleeding after delivery of twin 1

Third Stage of Labor

- Active management of 3rd stage of labor
- Prophylactic oxytocin after delivery of second twin and 20–40 units oxytocin in infusion for 4 hours and 10 units IM.
- Keep second line drugs—methyl ergometrine
- Placenta to be delivered by controlled cord traction.
- Tab misoprostol 800 μg oral, sublingual or per-rectally
- Massaging of the uterus

Triplets

- Develop from fertilization of a single ovum or 2 or 3 ova.
- Diagnosed accidentally by ultrasound.
- Clinical course and complications are intensified compared to twins.
- Pre-term delivery is common and usually occurs by 32–34 weeks.
- Discordance of fetal growth more common than twins.
- Perinatal loss is inversely related to birth weight.
- Management similar to twins

DISCORDANT TWINS

- Discordant growth causes a difference in weight of twins.
- Difference is expressed as a percentage of larger twin weight.
- Discrepancy of 20% or more: Significant.
- Earlier discordancy is usually symmetrical and indicates higher risk for fetal demise.
- Discrepancy in EFW >25%: Significant.
- Most accurate parameter for measurement is abdominal circumference.
- Earlier discordancy is usually symmetrical and indicates higher risk for fetal demise.

  Grading Grade 1: difference of 15–25%
  Grade 2: difference >25%
- Monochorionic twins—Both fetuses have the same growth potential. Hence discordance will be more severe and worse prognosis
- Dichorionic twins—different growth potential. The onset will be later and prognosis is better.

Management

- Prenatal diagnosis of both twins to rule out aneuploidy.
- Ultrasonographic monitoring of growth of twins.

- Depending on degree of discordancy and the gestational age: fetal surveillance is indicated: Doppler, weekly from 28 weeks or from the time of diagnosis. Admission of those with abnormal Doppler findings.
  - Twice daily CTG
  - Twice weekly BPP and Doppler
  - Inj. Betamethasone is given.
- Expectant management till 32 weeks. The smaller growth restricted twin must be sacrificed and pregnancy should be prolonged till maturity of other twin. Risk of IUD must be balanced against iatrogenic pre-term birth.
- However, risk of other fetal death (12%) and neurological impairment (18%) following death of 1 twin must be explained to the couple.
- Umbilical cord occlusion may be done at the time of imminent fetal death. This may protect the surviving twin. Survival rate 50%.
- Route of delivery is controversial: Cesarean or vaginal depends on the Doppler and NST findings at the time of delivery.

TWIN TO TWIN TRANSFUSION SYNDROME

In this syndrome, blood is transfused from a donor twin to its recipient sibling such that the donor becomes anemic and its growth may be restricted. In contrast, the recipient becomes polycythemic and may develop circulatory overload manifesting as hydrops.

Quintero's Staging System

Stage I–Discordant amnionic fluid volumes but urine still visible sonographically within the donor twin's bladder.

Stage II–Criteria of stage I, but urine is not visible within the donor's bladder.

Stage III–Criteria of stage II and abnormal Doppler studies of the umbilical artery, ductus venosus, or umbilical vein. At least one of the following:

Absent or reversed diastolic flow in umbilical artery of donor twin.
Reversed flow in ductus venosus of donor twin.
Pulsatile flow in umbilical vein of recipient twin.

Stage IV–Ascites or frank hydrops in either twin.

Stage V–Demise of either fetus.

3A: Presence of arterio-arterial anastomosis—fetal survival rate (83%)
3B: Absence of arterio-arterial anastamosis—fetal survival rate (52%)

Criteria for Diagnosis

- Only one placenta is seen by ultrasound (Concordant gender).
- Twins are of same sex.
- There is thin membrane between twins.
- 20% or larger discordancy in estimated fetal weight between twins.
- Difference in Hb is >5 g%.
- Severe discrepancy in amniotic fluid volume (one sac with maximum vertical pocket 2 cm vs 8 cm in the other sac).
- Fetal hydrops in one or both twins.
- Umbilical cords are of different length.
- Gestational age more than 28 weeks.

Management

- Bed rest and early delivery.
- Serial amnioreduction–Removal of fluid will reduce intra-amniotic pressure improving placental perfusion. Fluid drained should be 1000 ml in 30 minutes and not more than 5000 ml in each session and to reduce largest pocket of fluid to diameter of 5–8 cm.
  Complications: Rupture of membranes, preterm labor, chorioamnionitis.
- **Septostomy**—Intentional creation of a communication in the dividing amniotic membrane.
  22G amniocentesis needle is used for procedure.
  Size of perforation should be small to avoid formation of monoamniotic pregnancy.
- **Laser photocoagulation**—Laser photocoagulation of placental vascular anastomosis.
  Vascular anastomosis are photocoagulated with YAG laser which is inserted through operative channel of a fetoscope.
  Complications: PROM, sudden reverse transfusion, abruptio-placenta, pulmonary edema, fetal ischemic lesions.
- Selective fetal reduction–Done after 20 weeks. Indication is fetal hydrops in TTTS.
  Feticidal techniques—Saline cardiac tamponade followed by intracardiac potassium chloride injection of an occlusive substance into the umbilical vein and fetoscopic ligation, laser coagulation, monopolar coagulation, or bipolar cautery of the umbilical cord.

Timing of delivery: Vaginal delivery at 36–37 weeks if no complications.

Single Fetal Demise

- Effect of death of one twin upon survival varies depending on gestational age at the time of death.
  GA <14 weeks—No increased risk on survival
  GA >14 weeks—Severe morbidity on surviving twin
- Survivor twin at high risk of renal [renal corticonecrosis], cardiac and neurological morbidity.
- At delivery, dead fetus may be identifiable but may be compressed appreciably (fetus compresses) or may be flattened remarkably through loss of fluid and most of the soft tissues (fetus papyraceous).

Dichorionic Twins

- Check for signs of threatening miscarriage and severe pre-term delivery.
- Continue fetal surveillance in survivor.

Monochorionic Twins

- Check for signs of threatened miscarriage and pre-term delivery.
- Continue fetal surveillance in survivor.
- Doppler of the middle cerebral artery—peak systolic velocity to detect anemia
- Ultrasound or MRI to rule out multiple encephalomalacia 2–3 weeks after demise.

- Baseline maternal coagulation profile with periodic follow up.
- It is suggested that surveillance of uncomplicated MC twins should occur at intervals of every 2–3 weeks from 16 weeks, and should include: (minimum)
  1. Abdominal circumference (AC) measurements.
  2. Imaging of the fetal brains with or without head circumference measurement
  3. Measurement of maximum pool depth of both sacs and umbilical artery Doppler studies (after 24 weeks).
  4. Identify the dividing membrane and to ensure that each cord is studied separately.

There is no necessity to terminate the pregnancy. Longer the death to delivery interval, better is the prognosis.

MONOZYGOUS TWINS

Acardiac Twin/TRAP Sequence

Twin reversed-arterial-perfusion (TRAP) sequence is rare—1 in 35,000 births.

In the TRAP sequence, there is usually a normally formed donor twin who has features of heart failure as well as a recipient twin who lacks a heart (acardius) and other structures.

- Since the circulation of both infants is maintained by healthy twins, the circulatory load may be so large that normal twin develops high output heart failure.
- Mortality of normal twin is 50%.
- *Acardius acephalus:* Failure or disrupted growth of the head.
- *Acardius myelacephalus:* A partially developed head with identifiable limbs.
- *Acardius amorphous*: Failure of any recognizable structure.
- *Acardius acormus*: Only fetal head develops.

Management

Interruption of the vascular communication between the donor and recipient twins

- Coagulation of cord to acardiac twin—before 21 weeks—laser and bipolar
- Ligation of cord to acardiac twin
- Intra fetal coagulation of fetal vessels
- Expectant management with close fetal surveillance

CONJOINT TWINS

- It results from incomplete fusion of embryonic inner cell mass rather than partial fusion of two separate centers of growth.
- Occurs in early gestation probably before 2nd week of gestation.

Antepartum diagnosis: Ultrasound

1. Twins face each other.
2. Heads are at same level and plane.
3. Thoracic cages are in unusual proximity.
4. Both fetal heads are hyperextended.
5. No change in relative position of fetus with movement, manipulation or in repeat examination obtained hours or days later.

Management

- Careful evaluation of point of connection and the organs involved: Essential before counseling.
- Surgical separation of nearly completely joined twins may be successful when organs essential for life are not shared.
- Consultation with pediatric surgeon who assists antenatal parental decision making.
- Conjoint twins with discordant structural anomalies further complicate decisions about whether or not to continue the pregnancy
- Viable conjoined twins should be delivered by cesarean.
- Vaginal delivery of conjoined twins for the purpose of pregnancy termination is possible because union is most often pliable.

CHAPTER

7

Intrauterine Growth Restriction

DEFINITION

Any baby with birth weight below 10th percentile for gestational age who fails to achieve its genetic growth potential with signs of chronic hypoxia or failure to thrive.

All IUGR babies are not low-birth weight.

Small for Gestational Age: Infants whose weights were below 10th percentile for the gestational age.

It is used as a synonym for IUGR but it also includes constitutionally small babies.

Small size (Healthy) fetus	IUGR
Constitutionally small	Due to various etiological factors
Always symmetrical	Symmetrical or asymmetrical
Normal subcutaneous fat	Decreased fat
Weight <2500 gms always	Weight can be >2500 gms in full term IUGR cases
Perinatal mortality normal	Perinatal mortality increased
Growth is maintained	Growth is retarded when serially measured

Incidence: 3–15%.

CLASSIFICATION

Campbell S and Thomas A (1965): Introduced the concept of classifying IUGR into:

- Symmetrical: 20–30%
- Asymmetrical: 70–80%

Symmetrical/Type I	Asymmetrical/ Type II
Intrinsic (hypoplastic–decrease in cell number)	Extrinsic (hypotrophic–decrease in cell size)
All organs symmetrically small	Sparing of brain and long bones
Causes– 1. Congenital–Chromosomal and structural anomalies 2. Infections–TORCH, malaria, syphilis 3. Toxins–Alcohol, smoking, cocaine 4. Drugs–Warfarin, phenytoin, Antiphospholipid antibodies	Causes– 1. Nutritional 2. Placental insufficiency due to medical or obstetrical causes

Contd...

Contd...

Ratio of HC/AC and FL/AC normal	Ratio of HC/AC and FL/AC increased
Ponderal Index (PI) is usually normal	Ponderal Index (PI) is low
Growth restriction occurs in 1st trimester and early 2nd trimester	Growth restriction occurs in late 2nd trimester and 3rd trimester

ETIOLOGY

Fetal Factors

- Infection
- Heart disease
- Malformations
- Chromosomal abnormalities
- Osteogenesis imperfecta

Maternal Factors

Maternal characteristics

- Extremes of age
- Nulliparity or grand multiparity
- Low BMI

Diseases

- Hypertension
- Diabetes with vasculopathy
- Chronic renal disease
- Cyanotic heart disease
- Autoimmune disorders
- Hyperthyroidism
- Respiratory diseases—cystic fibrosis/bronchiectasis/asthma
- Thrombophilias
- Drugs (diethylstilbestrol, anticancer agents, narcotics)
- Smoking (infants weigh 100–300 g less than the non-smokers)
- Alcohol (crosses the placenta and reduces the cell growth potential)

Uterine Factors

- Decreased uteroplacental blood flow
- Atheromatosis, arteriosclerosis of decidual spiral arteries
- Connective tissue disorders
- Fibromyomas
- Morphologic abnormalities

Placental Factors

- Abruptio placentae, placenta previa
- Thrombosis, infarction

- Deciduitis
- Placentitis, vasculitis, edema
- Chorioamnionitis
- Placental cysts, chorioangioma

IDENTIFICATION OF PATIENTS AT RISK

- Risk factors:
  - Chronic hypertension
  - Preeclampsia
  - Multiple gestation
  - Hematological conditions
  - Chronic renal disease
  - IDDM with microvascular disease
  - Previous h/o IUGR baby—With 1 IUGR baby—25%
—With 2 IUGR babies—4-fold increase

Screening

Clinical

- Detects only 40% of IUGR cases:
- Fundal height—after 20 weeks of gestation approximates with weeks of gestation. Discrepancy of 3 cm suggests IUGR if abnormal lie and uterine anomalies are excluded (sensitivity 60–85%, PPV: 20–80%).

Biochemical

- Estriol, human placental lactogen (hPL), human chorionic gonadotropin, and AFP measured in the maternal serum early in the 2nd trimester are associated with subsequent IUGR.
- These markers are not used in clinical practice.

Ultrasonography

- If the GA is certain, the methods most commonly used to diagnose FGR are Biparietal diameter (BPD), Estimated Fetal Weight (EFW), Fetal abdominal circumference (AC) and head circumference/abdominal circumference ratio (HC/AC).
- AC–The best single measurement to diagnose FGR in women with accurate LMP
- If diagnosis of GA is uncertain, then following are taken into consideration:
  - Trans-cerebellar diameter/abdominal circumference (TCD/AC)
  - Femoral length/abdominal circumference (FL/AC)
  - Fetal ponderal index

1. HC/AC ratio → HC >AC upto 32 weeks
normally HC=AC from 32 to 36 weeks
AC >HC after 36 weeks

If HC > AC after 32 weeks it suggests asymmetrical IUGR

2. FL/AC ratio 0.22 ± 0.02 (normal)
>0.24 (asymmetrical IUGR)

Ultrasound Markers of Chromosomal Abnormalities

- Mild ventriculomegaly
- Choroid plexus cyst
- Short humerus
- Polydactyly
- Echogenic focus in left ventricle
- Echogenic bowel
- Renal pyelectasis
- Club foot
- Single umbilical artery

Uterine Artery Doppler

Not for diagnosis of IUGR, used in antepartum fetal surveillance of IUGR babies.

Flow chart 7.1: Doppler sequence in IUGR

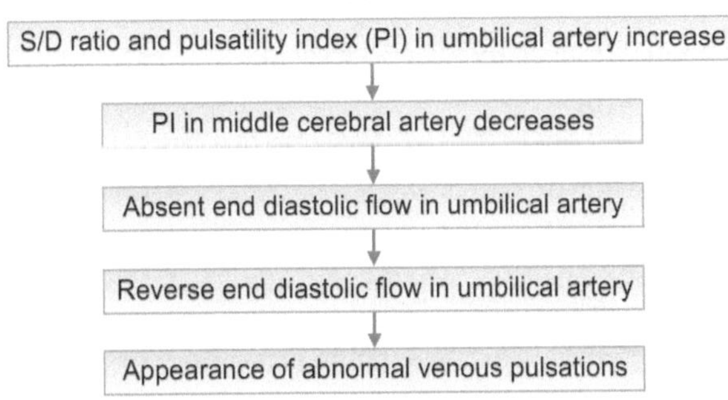

MANAGEMENT

First Trimester Screening

- Uterine artery Doppler is done in high-risk cases.
- Give low dose aspirin (75–100 mg/day) if bilatreral notching occurs.

Second Trimester Screening

- If bilateral uterine artery notching persists until 24 weeks, there is only a marginal benefit of low dose aspirin in selected patients, there is no evidence of harmful effect.

Prophylaxis

- Stop smoking
- Reduce stress
- Rest in left lateral position
- Low dose aspirin after diagnosis of placental based mild IUGR
- Maternal hyperoxygenation, intravascular volume expansion and hyperalimentation are experimental

- L-arginine 3 gms sachet TID from first trimester onwards or whenever IUGR is diagnosed as part of treatment. Not evidence-based but not harmful to the mother or the fetus.

On Clinical Suspicion of IUGR

- Two abdominal circumference measurements are obtained at least 14 days apart, with umbilical artery Doppler, to distinguish between normally grown small fetus and growth-restricted fetuses (growth trend is important—customized growth chart is useful taking into consideration parental height and weight and indigineously designed for that population).

Follow for IUGR, if:
- Abdominal circumference <5th percentile or growth rate <11 mm in 2 weeks
- Umbilical artery Doppler index is elevated.
- Cerebroplacental ratio is decreased.
- Middle cerebral Doppler index is decreased (centralization) even if uterine artery.
  Doppler is normal (especially after 34 weeks).

Flow chart 7.2: Diagnosis of IUGR

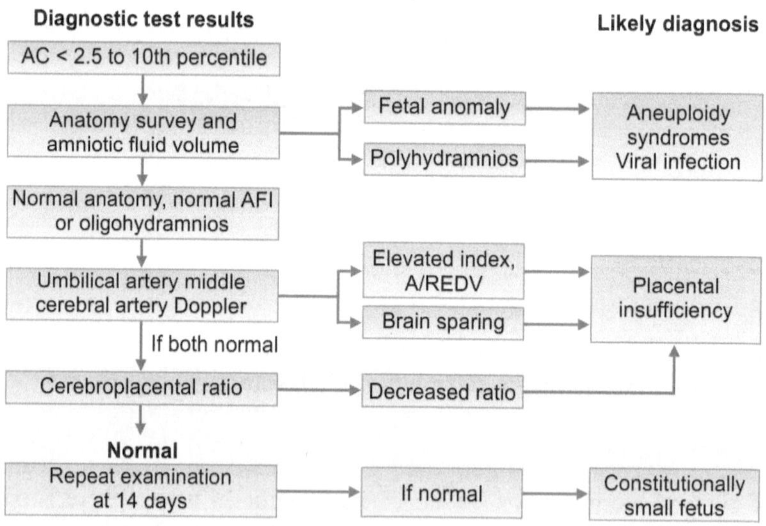

With a Diagnosis of IUGR

- The most accurate assessment of fetal status is obtained with combined Doppler and biophysical assessment (AFI + NST-modified biophysical profile)
- Administer betamethasone when delivery is anticipated before 34 weeks
  Antepartum Fetal Surveillance
  - Daily fetal movement count
  - USG for growth assessment every 2 to 3 weeks
  - Modified BPP
  - Fetal Doppler study

Flow chart 7.3: Management of IUGR

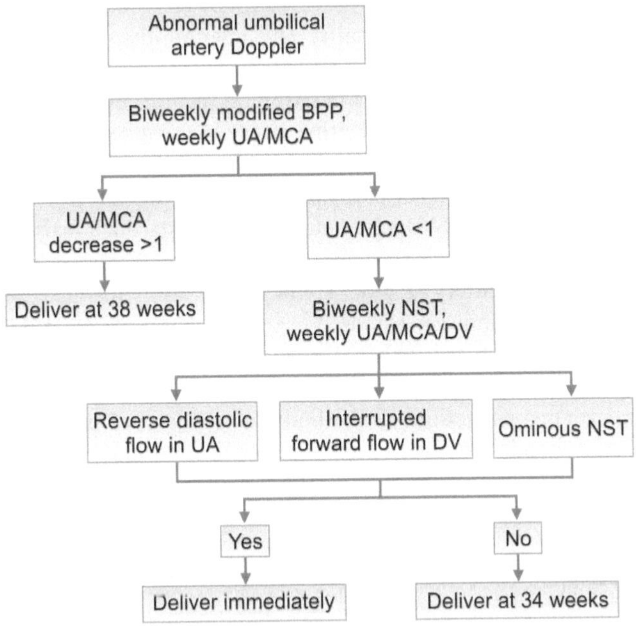

Labor and Delivery

- Route of delivery is determined by fetal status before the onset of labor as well as maternal and obstetric factors. Delivery route is tailored to the cervical Bishop's score.

  Cesarean delivery without a trial of labor is indicated when–
  - Presence of evidence of fetal distress by NST
  - Reversed diastolic flow in umbilical artery Doppler
  - Prelabor evidence of fetal acidemia
  - Spontaneous late decelerations
  - Abnormal DV waveforms
- Timing of delivery:
  - Pregnancy should be terminated at 38 weeks.
  - If abnormalities in AFI or other indicators of fetal status such as umbilical artery, Doppler delivery should be planned in <38 weeks.

Induction of labor:
- Preferable method is Foley's bulb
- Judicious use of prostaglandins
- Consider low dose oxytocin for augmentation.

PRACTICE POINTS

- Clinical examination remains the mainstay of screening for IUGR.

- Ultrasound biometry should be repeated no more frequently than every 2 weeks, and is required only every 4 weeks if growth velocity is normal.
- The possibility of fetal abnormality and aneuploidy must be considered, particularly in early-onset IUGR.
- Uterine artery Doppler at 24 weeks is a useful screening test for IUGR requiring preterm delivery, with bilateral uterine artery notches representing a relative risk of 33.7.
- Umbilical artery Doppler is of no value in low-risk pregnancies.
- Abnormal umbilical artery Doppler studies reflect placental resistance and are often long-standing.
- Abnormal umbilical artery Doppler studies alone rarely mandate delivery.
- Further fetal compromise is assessed by examination of the middle cerebral artery, ductus venosus and umbilical vein, and such assessments permit fine-tuning of the management of severe IUGR.
- Umbilical venous pulstations in the cord and reversal of the 'a' wave in the ductus venosus indicate severe fetal compromise but may occur before CTG abnormalities.

Neonatal Risks

- Hypoglycemia
- Hypothermia
- Hypocalcemia
- Hyperviscosity
- Hyperbilirubinemia
- Necrotizing enterocolitis

IUGR	**Preterm**
<10th percentile	Less than 37 weeks
Same complications	
Birth asphyxia	✓
Hypothermia	✓
Hypoglycemia	✓
Hyperbilirubinemia	✓
Opposite	
Meconium	Uncommon
Cord problems	More common
No long-term sequelae	More common
Apneic spells not common	More common
No feeding problems	
No such	Less resistance to infections
ICH less common	More common

CHAPTER

8

Rh-negative Pregnancy

Incidence of iso-immunization in India 5–10%: South India (5%), North India (10%).

ABO incompatibility reduces isoimmunization from 16 to 2%.

NON-IMMUNIZED MOTHER

Antenatal Period

First prenatal visit:

- Check partner's blood group if woman is Rh negative.
- If partner is Rh negative—no further evaluation required.
- If partner is Rh positive—ICT to be done.
- If ICT is positive, treat as isoimmunized pregnancy.
- If ICT is negative, repeat it at 28, 34 weeks in primigravida and monthly after 24 weeks in multigravida.

Antepartum Prophylaxis

- 1–2% mothers sensitized within 20–40 weeks due to silent bleeds.
- Reduces isoimmunization from 1.5–1.8% to 0%.
- Anti-D immunoglobulin:
  300 μg of Anti-D = 30 ml of fetomaternal bleed = 15 ml of RBC.

Dose determined by Kleihauer-Betke test

Estimated blood loss = Fetal cells /Number of maternal cells x Estimated maternal blood volume (ml).

Indications for Antepartum Anti-D Prophylaxis

1. Invasive prenatal diagnosis
   - Chorionic villous sampling
   - Amniocentesis
   - Fetal blood sampling
2. Miscarriage
   - All miscarriages >12 weeks including threatened abortion.
   - All miscarriages where uterus is evacuated medically/surgically.
   - <12 weeks in threatened abortion if pain or bleeding is heavy.

Prophylaxis not recommended for complete miscarriage <12 weeks where there is no intervention done.

3. Ectopic pregnancy
4. Intrauterine procedures
   - Embryo reduction
5. External cephalic version
6. Closed abdominal injury
7. Intrauterine death
8. Antepartum hemorrhage: Feto-maternal hemorrhage (FMH) occurs due to abruptio placentae, abdominal trauma, IUD, placenta previa—Anti-D dose should be determined after estimation of FMH.
9. Where bleeding continues intermittently after 12 weeks' gestation, anti-D Ig should be given at 6-weekly intervals. However, it may be prudent to administer anti-D Ig where bleeding is heavy or repeated or where there is associated abdominal pain, particularly, if these events occur as gestation approaches 12 weeks.

Indications	Recommended dose
First trimester—induced or spontaneous abortion	50 µg
Unruptured ectopic pregnancy	50 µg
CVS	50 µg
2nd trimester abortion	300 µg
Ruptured ectopic pregnancy	300 µg
Routine prophylaxis at 28 weeks	300 µg
Postpartum	300 µg (baby is Rh positive)
Antepartum hemorrhage	FMH to be calculated
Amniocentesis	300 µg

- 99.2–99.3% of women have an FMH less than 4 ml at delivery.
- Up to 50% of larger FMHs occur after normal deliveries.
- However, the following clinical circumstances are more likely to be associated with large FMH:
  - Traumatic deliveries including cesarean section
  - Manual removal of the placenta
  - Stillbirths and intrauterine deaths
  - Abdominal trauma during the third trimester
  - Twin pregnancies (at delivery)
  - Unexplained hydrops fetalis.

Antenatal Prophylaxis

- A woman's decision not to be given routine antenatal anti-D prophylaxis should always be respected. This should be clearly documented after full discussion
- Routine antenatal prophylaxis anti-D immunoglobulin 500 IU (100 µg) given intramuscularly (IM) at 28 and 34 weeks gestation (if 300 µg is given only one

dose at 28 weeks is sufficient, if delivered within 3 weeks of 300 μg anti-D, then we need not repeat anti-D if pregnancy is continued beyond 12 weeks of 300 μg of anti-D, repeat another dose of anti-D 300 μg).

- A blood sample should be taken for antibody screening (and full blood count) at 28 weeks gestation prior to anti-D injection. However, there is no need to take blood sample for antibody screening at 34–36 weeks.
- Women should still be given further anti-D after a sensitizing event even if they have received routine antenatal prophylaxis.
- Use of routine antenatal anti-D prophylaxis at 28 weeks should not be affected by whether she has already had antenatal anti-D prophylaxis for a potentially sensitizing event early in pregnancy.

Labor and Delivery

- Avoid pregnancy beyond EDD. Induce labor at 40 weeks, method of induction is determined by Bishop's score.
- PGE1/E2/oxytocin can be used depending on cervix favorability.
- Cesarean section is indicated only in obstetric situations.
- Continuous CTG monitoring—sinusoidal pattern (fetal anemia) late deceleration (placental insufficicncy).
- Prophylactic instrumental delivery to cut short second stage of labor.
- Early cord clamping, no milking of the umbilical cord.
- Avoid methergine.
- No manual removal of placenta.
- Cord kept long.
- Take cord blood for CBC, DCT, blood grouping and Rh typing, total bilirubin, manual reticulocyte count.
- If baby is Rh negative, no prophylaxis is required.
- If baby is Rh positive, ICT and DCT are negative, then anti-D immunoglobulin is given within 72 hrs of delivery to the mother.
- **The recommended policy is to obtain an anticoagulated blood sample as soon as possible (within two hours) after delivery and to undertake a Kleihauer screening test to identify women with a large FMH who need additional anti-D Ig.**
- Intramuscular anti-D Ig is best given into the deltoid muscle as injections into the gluteal region often only reach the subcutaneous tissues and absorption may be delayed.
- For successful immunoprophylaxis, anti-DIg should be given as soon as possible after the sensitizing event but always within 72 hours.
- If it is not given before 72 hours, every effort should still be made to administer the anti-D Ig, as a dose given within 9–10 days may provide some protection *(Grade B recommendation)*.
- A woman's use of postpartum anti-D prophylaxis should similarly not be affected by whether she has had routine antenatal anti-D prophylaxis or anti-D prophylaxis following a sensitizing event during the antenatal period.

- In women with bleeding disorders, anti-D should be given by SC/IV instead of giving IM after taking consent from the patient.
- Anti-D administration in a woman undergoing sterilization: should be guided by the patient's desire for protection against any chance of alloimmunization.

Blood Transfusion

- It should usually be possible to provide RhD negative platelets for women of child-bearing age who need a platelet transfusion. Occasionally, if an appropriate product is not available, it may be necessary to use RhD positive platelets. In these circumstances, prophylaxis against possible Rh alloimmunization by red cells contaminating the platelet product should be given *(Grade B recommendation)*.
- 250 IU (50 mcg) anti-D Ig should be given following every three units of platelets administered.
- Patients who have marked thrombocytopenia should be given the anti-D Ig subcutaneously to avoid the possibility of a hematoma following intramuscular injection.
- Inadvertent transfusion of RhD positive blood: Larger amounts of anti-D are required and occasionally exchange transfusion but this must be discussed with the consultant hematologist.

Other Methods to Prevent or Minimize FMH

- Precautions during cesarean section (Pack the abdominal cavity, early cord clamping, avoid manual removal of placenta).
- No prophylactic ergometrine.
- Amniocentesis under sonological guidance.
- To refrain from abdominal palpation, in abruption
- Avoid forcible attempt of ECV under anesthesia.
- Avoid Rh positive blood transfusion to Rh negative female from birth to menopause.

Failure of Prophylaxis

- Small percentage of failures—due to large FMH.
- Prevented by calculation of anti-D depending on FMH.
- Some women, who have received anti-D Ig during pregnancy may have detectable anti-D in their blood at delivery. The report may read presumed passive anti-D. It is important to document on the Kleihauer form when a woman received antenatal prophylaxis.
- Because it may be difficult or impossible to distinguish between such passive anti-D Ig and weak anti-D resulting from early immunization, anti-D Ig should be given to any eligible woman with weak anti-D antibody at delivery unless it has been clearly confirmed that she is already sensitized.

Adverse Reaction

- Local swelling, headache, chills, urticaria, itching, maculopapular rash.

Flow chart 8.1: Management of Rh negative pregnancy

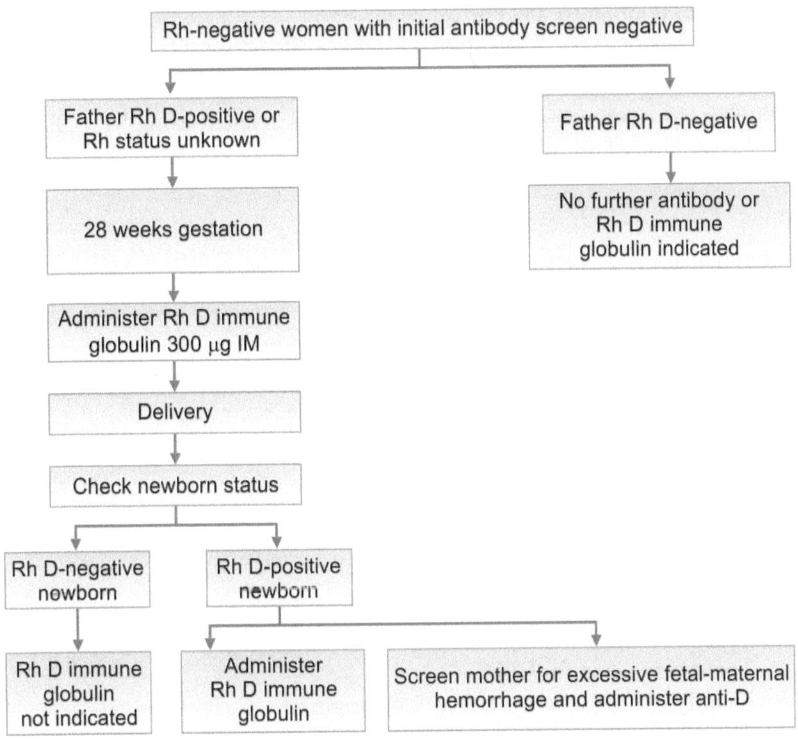

Management of Rh Isoimmunized Pregnancy

First Sensitized Pregnancy

- ICT is positive.
- Critical level 1:16.
- Safe level of anti-D antibody level is <15 IU/ml.
- Serial antibody testing used to detect the progress of disease from mild to severe.
- Minimal fetal/neonatal disease.

Flow chart 8.2: Management of Rh isoimmunization pregnancy

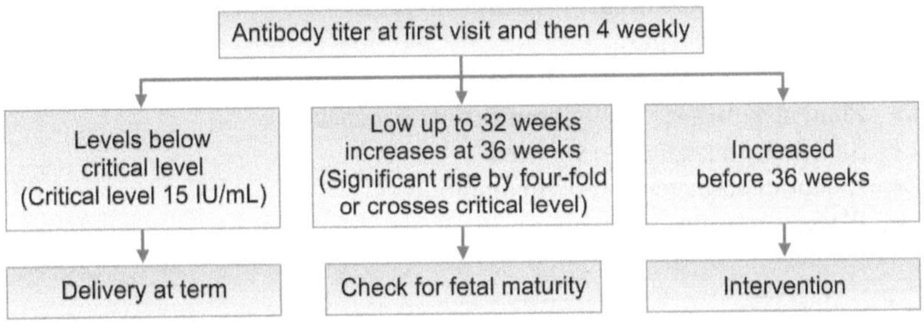

Serial Antibody Titer is not Applicable in the Following Situations

- Initial titer at or above the critical level.
- Titer reaches or exceeds the critical level any time during gestation.
- Significant rise in titer (4-fold raise) between 2 consecutive samples.

Further management will be based on fetal assessment using MCA PSV and the concentration of bilirubin in the amniotic fluid.

Management of Prior Affected Pregnancy

- Maternal antibody titer is not useful.
- Past-obstetric history is the important indicator of outcome.

Noninvasive Evaluation

1. **Serial USG Doppler-fetal MCA, peak systolic volume (PSV)**
    - Accurate non-invasive method for the diagnosis of fetal anemia.
    - Useful between 18–35 weeks.

Indications:

- Anti-body titer above the critical level (1:16).
- H/o previous fetal loss, intrauterine transfusion.
- Fetus should be resting.

Procedure:

- Transverse plane for BPD.
- Identify middle cerebral artery at its origin.
- Angle of insonation as close to zero.
- Peak systolic velocity of at least 3 waveforms.

Advantages:

- Non-invasive, simple, high index of reproducibility.
- Highly sensitive (100%) false positive rate (12%)
- PPV of 5%
- NPV of 100%
- 70% reduction in amniocentesis if used.

Disadvantages:

- Accuracy diminishes after 35 weeks and after multiple transfusions.
- Needs expertise.

2. **USG for fetal assessment: Findings include –**
    - Hepatosplenomegaly
    - Increase in portal venous diameter flow velocity (Normal velocity <5 mm)
    - Fluid in serous cavities (1st in pericardial space)
    - Subcutaneous edema—very late
    - Liquor disturbances—Polyhydramnios
    - Placentomegaly

Invasive Evaluation

3. **Amniotic fluid bilirubin concentration**
    - No longer used
    - Application requires serial invasive procedures for several weeks

- Amniotic fluid spectrometry is an indirect test for fetal anemia, less superior than maternal ICT
- Amniocentesis and OD 450 was modeled on anti-D alloimmunization, which has poor performance
- No clinical correlation between OD 450 and fetal hemoglobin <28 weeks
- Variety of extrinsic errors present

4. Fetal blood sampling

Indications

- Increased MCA-PSV (>1.5 MoM)
- Delta OD 450 in high middle zone or in zone 3
- USG shows fetal hydrops
  - Gold standard for detection of fetal anemia
  - Site: Near placental insertion of umbilical cord in umbilical vein (Percutaneous umbilical blood sampling—(PUBS)
  - Hematological parameters studied are—
    - Purity of blood sample
    - ABO and Rh typing
    - Hemoglobin and hematocrit
    - Platelet count
    - Immature erythrocytes
    - Direct agglutination test

Intrauterine Transfusion

- Indications (can be performed up to 35 weeks)
  - Fetal hematocrit <30%
  - Fetal hemoglobin <2 gm% below mean for normal
- Routes of approach
  - Intraperitoneal
  - Intravascular through umbilical vein or intrahepatic portal vein
  - Intracardiac

Intraperitoneal Transfusion

- Only used for small fetus <24 weeks with severe anemia.
- Amount of volume to be transfused is calculated as (gestation in weeks-20) x 10 ml.

Disadvantages

- Requires fetal respiration for absorption.
- Slow correction of hemoglobin deficit.
- Higher risk of trauma and obstructing cardiac return.

Intravascular Transfusion

Goal: Delivery of a healthy, non-anemic neonate at term

- Transfusions are begun when the fetal hematocrit declines below 30%
- Second transfusion
  - 24 hrs later in hydrops
  - 2 weeks later in nonhydrops
- Amount to be transfused as mentioned in the table below.

Approximate volume of 72% hematocrit blood required for intravascular transfusion after the first transfusion.

Gestation (Weeks)	Volume (ml)
≤22.5	25–40
22.5–27.49	45–65
27.5–32.49	75–90
≥32.5	100–120

Protocol for intravascular transfusion
- Infuse half estimated requirement.
- Repeat blood sampling and umbilical vein pressure measurement (UVP).
- Stop transfusion if UVP >10 mm Hg.
- If UVP acceptable: infuse remaining volume.

Follow-up: Monitor fetus until spontaneous movement resumes.

Acute non-hematologic effects of intravascular transfusion:

Cardiovascular

- Increased intravascular volume
- Decreased heart rate
- Decreased cardiac output
- Increased umbilical venous pressure
- Increased renal blood flow
- Decreased placental resistance measured by Doppler.
- Decreased aortic resistance measured by Doppler.

Biochemical

- Acidemia
- Increased oxygen-carrying capacity
- Increased viscosity
- Increased atrial natriuretic peptide
- Increased prostacyclin
- Increased prostaglandin E2
- Increased iron stores

Disadvantages

- Requires expertise
- Pregnancy loss rate of 1%
- Risk of sensitization.

Timing of Delivery

Depends upon the severity of disease and neonatal facilities. Doppler MCA-PSV used as a guide as follows:
- Steroids for lung maturity
- Deliver by 37–38 weeks.

Flow chart 8.3: Management of Rh negative pregnancy based in Doppler

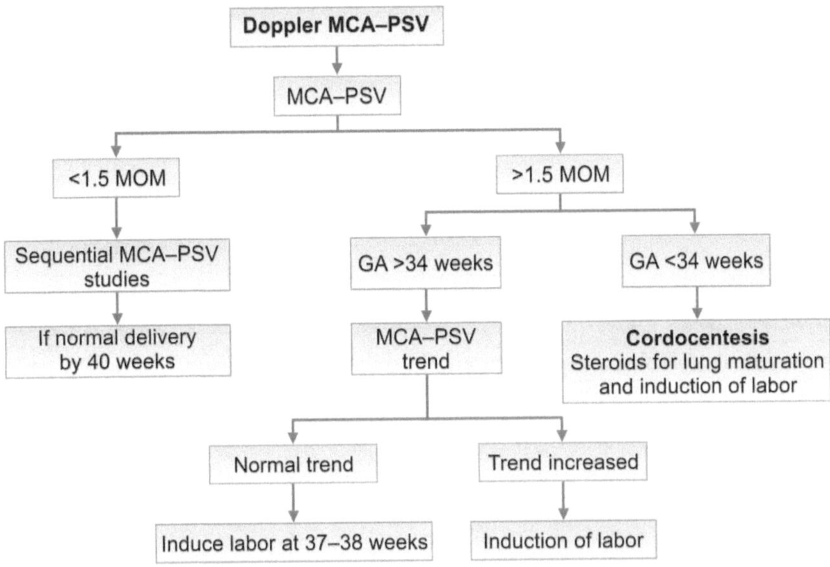

Neonatal Management

- If baby is anemic, give immediate exchange transfusion.

In Repeated Pregnancy Loss—

- IVF with embryo biopsy and transfer of only Rh-negative embryos.
- Donor insemination from Rh-negative donor.

CHAPTER

9

Oligoamnios

DEFINITION

At any gestation absence of amniotic fluid pocket, measuring less than 2 cm in vertical diameter, less than 5th percentile of the normal of that gestational age or AFI <5 cm.

CONDITIONS ASSOCIATED WITH OLIGOAMNIOS

Idiopathic

Fetal

- Chromosomal abnormalities
- Growth restriction
- Demise
- Renal agenesis
- Polycystic kidney disease
- Collecting system abnormalities or obstruction
- Rare diseases like–Tubular dysgenesis
  - Meckel-Gruber syndrome—lethal autosomal recessive disorder, anomalies of CNS (encephalocele), enlarged kidneys with cystic dysplasia, malformation of hands and feet.
  - Perlman's syndrome
- Urethral obstruction–Posterior urethral valves
  - Ureteroceles
  - Urogenital system malformations
  - Bilateral uterovesical junction
  - Pelvi ureteric junction obstruction
- GI tract conditions–gastroschisis
  - Megacystitis microcolon

Placenta

- Abruption
- Twin-twin transfusion
- Placental insufficiency

Maternal

- Premature rupture of memebranes
- Dehydration

- Hypertension
- Preeclampsia
- Diabetes insipidus
- Prolonged pregnancy

Drugs

- Prostaglandin synthase inhibitors
- Angiotensin-converting enzyme inhibitors.

TYPES

Early Onset Oligoamnios

- Onset—1st and early 2nd trimester (<22–24 weeks)
- Causes:
  Fetal
  - Chromosomal abnormality: Triploidy
  - Renal: Bilateral renal agenesis, bilateral multicystic dysplastic kidneys, renal tubular dysgenesis, complete bladder outlet obstruction
  - Congenital viral infections (CMV)

  Maternal
  - Amnion rupture sequence
  - Limb body-wall complex
  - Early ruptured membranes (PPROM)
    - Spontaneous
    - Iatrogenic: amniocentesis, cervical cerclage, fetoscopic procedures
  - NSAID administration
  - Poor placentation: IUGR.

Late Onset Oligoamnios

- Onset—late 2nd trimester and 3rd trimester (>24 weeks)
- Causes:
  - Postmaturity
  - Spontaneous rupture of membranes
  - Placental insufficiency
- Management of oligoamnios in late pregnancy depends on the clinical situation.
- In a pregnancy complicated by oligoamnios and fetal-growth restriction, close fetal surveillance.
- In cases of evidence for fetal or maternal compromise, terminate pregnancy even if preterm.
- Oligoamnios detected before 36 weeks in the presence of normal fetal anatomy and growth may be managed expectantly.

DIAGNOSIS

History

- History of leak p/v, invasive procedure
- Maternal hypertension/PET

- Maternal viral infections/exposure
- Maternal drug exposure (NSAIDs, ACE-inhibitors)
- Aneuploidy screening
- Family or previous affected pregnancies

Examination

- Uterus appears small for dates.
- Fetal parts are palpated with difficulty as uterus hugs the fetus.
- In PROM–sterile speculum examination.

Investigations

- Ultrasound
  - Degree of oligoamnios (Amniotic fluid index–4 quadrant, SDP)
  - Careful targeted fetal anatomy scan
  - Presence of growth restriction
  - Presence and appearance of fetal bladder
  - Presence and appearance of fetal kidneys
  - Fetal well-being
- Color and spectral Doppler of fetal renal artery, uterine aretry, umbilical artery, middle cerebral artery.
- Fetal karyotype in early onset oligoamnios to rule out lethal anomalies. If severe oligoamnios karyotype may be obtained by placental biopsy.
- In PROM—confirmatory tests like vaginal pH, examination of dried secretions for ferning, USG examination for AFI, cervical/placental α microglobulin-1.

Complications

- Oligoamnios sequence
- Anomalies
- Fetal distress
- Fetal death
- Pulmonary hypoplasia (If severe oligoamnios occurs in the period up to 26 weeks—canalicular phase of lung development)
- Preterm delivery
- Prematurity
- Increased perinatal mortality
- Chorioamnionitis
- Increased risk of cesarean section
- Potter's sequence (Bilateral renal agenesis)
  - Type I–autosomal recessive polycystic kidneys
  - Type II–renal dysplasia
  - Type III–autosomal dominant polycystic kidney.

Pressure effects—Talipes, dislocated hip, ankylosis of joints, intrauterine adhesions from skin to amnion causing constriction of limb or amputation.

Congenital Anomalies Associated with Oligoamnios

- Amnionic band syndrome
- Cardiac: Fallot tetralogy, septal defects

- Central nervous system: Holoprosencephaly, meningocele, encephalocoele, microcephaly
- Chromosomal abnormalities: Triploidy, trisomy 18, Turner syndrome
- Cloacal dysgenesis
- Cystic hygroma
- Diaphragmatic hernia
- Genitourinary: Renal agenesis, renal dysplasia, urethral obstruction, bladder exstrophy, Meckel-Gruber syndrome, ureteropelvic junction obstruction, Prune-belly syndrome
- Hypothyroidism
- Skeletal: Sirenomelia, sacral agenesis, absent radius, facial clefting
- TRAP (twin reverse arterial perfusion) sequence
- Twin-twin transfusion
- VACTERL (vertebral, anal, cardiac, tracheo-esophageal, renal, limb) association.

Oligoamnios Sequence

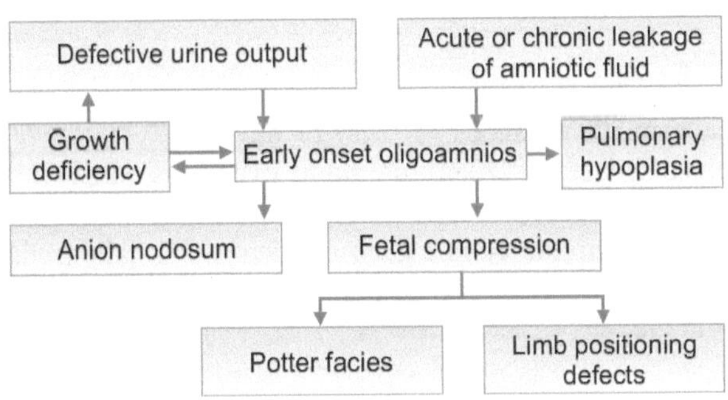

MANAGEMENT

Antepartum

- Bed rest
- Nutritious diet
- Serial USG for growth monitoring, liquor volume and wellbeing assessment every fortnightly.
- Counseling and termination of pregnancy if lethal malformation is confirmed.
- Therapeutic amnioinfusion—about 250–500 ml NS may be injected under ultrasonic control transabdominally.
- Aminoinfusion after 28 weeks.
- *Other procedures under trial are:*

  Sealing of membrane leak (amniopatch)—
  - In premature rupture of membranes.
  - Intra-amniotic infusion of platelet concentrate followed by cryoprecipitate. Autologous platelet concentrate 48×10^9 in 30 ml
  - Fibrinogen in cryoprecipitate (20 ml) 680 mg/dl
  - Amnio-platelet-cryoprecipitate

Vesicoamniotic shunting—

- In obstructive uropathies.
- Prevents pulmonary hypoplasia.
- Often renal damage has already occurred so 40% may anyway die.
- 30–50% of survivors have renal insufficiency.
- 20–30% have major growth and continence problems.

Intrapartum

- Induction of labor or elective CS when maturity is achieved.
- Oligoamnios is not a contraindication for induction of labor/trial of labor.
- Continuous electronic fetal monitoring in labor.

AMNIOINFUSION

Indication

- Severe oligoamnios
- Gestational age >28 weeks
- Congenital anomalies ruled out

Procedure

- Amino acid drip 500 ml once over 2 hrs on day 1, 3.
- IV infusions of 200 ml of 1/2 normal saline over 2 hrs on day 2, 4.
- Oral rehydration after day 5—2000 ml over 2 hrs everyday.
- Arginine sachet 3 gm mixed in 1 glass of water 1-1-1 daily (reduces maternal osmolality)
- High-protein diet.

Follow-up

- Obstetric scan for AFI once every 3 days.
- AFI and fetal weight increase within 1 week.

Transabdominal Amnioinfusion

Done for severe oligoamnios before 24 weeks.

Indication

Diagnostic:

- To improve visualization on ultrasound.
- To determine any leak by instilling indigo carmine dye (2–5 ml).
- Reaspiration of fluid for fetal karyotyping.

Therapeutic:

- To prevent pulmonary hypoplasia
- For instillation of surfactant.

Pre-requisites

- Broad spectrum antibiotics to be administered before the procedure.

- Informed consent
- Anti-D immunoglobulin administered for Rh-negative pregnancy.

Procedure

- Lignocaine is injected into the tissues overlying the selected site.
- Under ultrasound guidance 20 guage needle is advanced into the gestational sac.
- The placenta should be avoided.
- Needle is aimed for an existing fluid pocket.
- If fluid is present, fluid may be aspirated, if no fluid small amount of saline may be injected to confirm intra-amniotic needle placement.
- The needle is attached to a tubing, a 3-way valve and a 50 ml syringe.
- Warm saline is infused at the rate of 8–10 ml/min for 4–6 hrs under continuous ultrasound guidance.
- Aim is to achieve normal AFI (8).
- Observe for 24 hrs for leakage, fever and uterine contractions.

Risks

- Failed amnioinfusion–4%
- Possible PPROM–1%
- Amnionitis–4%

Transvaginal Amnioinfusion

- Described by Miyazaki and Taylor.
  It may be **therapeutic** (amnioinfusion only if fetal heart rate variable decelerations occur) or **prophylactic** (for women in labor with oligoamnios, but not fetal heart deceleration). According to Cochrane review there appears to be no advantage of prophylactic amnioinfusion over therapeutic amnioinfusion.
- Normal saline is infused via an intrauterine pressure catheter into the uterus, either by gravity or utilization of an infusion pump.
- Initial bolus of 600 ml or 10–12 ml/min for the first hour is used.
- Followed by a maintenance rate of 3 ml/min.
- Maintenance rate is continued till delivery or till variable decelerations cease.

Complications

- Amnionitis
- Uterine hyperstimulation
- Amniotic fluid embolism

CHAPTER

10

Polyhydramnios

DEFINITION

Pathological accumulation of amniotic fluid defined as AFI >25 or Single vertical pocket >8 cm at any gestational age or >95th percentile at any gestational age.

- Incidence is 1%.

CAUSES

- Idiopathic (65%)
- Maternal (15%)
  - Rh isoimmunization
  - Diabetes
- Placental (<1%)
  - Placental chorioangioma
  - Circumvallate placental syndrome
- Fetal (18%)
  - Multiple pregnancy
  - Fetal anomalies
  - CNS abnormalities–open NTD
  - GI abnormalities—esophageal atresia, annular pancreas, jejunal atresia, diaphragmatic hernia, duodenal atresia, gastrochisis, omphalocele
  - GU abnormalities—renal obstruction (partial or complete), skeletal arthrogryposis, **osteogenesis imperfecta**
- Skeletal malformations
- Fetal tumors—**sacrococcygeal** teratoma, cystic adenamatoid malformation of lung
- Cardiac anomalies—severe congenital heart disease, persistent arrhythmias
- Chromosomal abnormalities—Trisomy 13,18, 21
- Genetic syndromes—myotonia dystrophica
- Hematologic disorders—alpha thalassemia, any fetomaternal hemorrhage
- Intrauterine infections—rubella, syphilis, toxoplasmosis
- Miscellaneous—nonimmune hydrops

COMPLICATIONS

Maternal

During Pregnancy

- Preeclampsia (25%)
- Malpresentations

- PROM
- Preterm labor
- Abruption

During Labor

- Prolonged labor
- PROM
- Cord prolapse
- Uterine inertia
- Increased incidence of operative delivery
- Retained placenta
- PPH

During Puerperium

Subinvolution

Fetal

- Prematurity
- Congenital abnormality

MANAGEMENT

Investigations

- OGCT with 75 grams
- Blood group
  Ultrasound for anomalies and to rule out multiple gestation
- TORCH screening
- Fetal karyotyping by amniocentesis

Treatment

- If fetal lethal abnormality—termination irrespective of gestation
- If fetal non lethal abnormality—depending upon the patient's choice—termination or continuation
- If no fetal anomalies—
  - If maternal distress
    <32 weeks–indomethacin/sulindac, no response—serial amnioreduction
    32–37 weeks–serial amnioreduction,
    >37 weeks–amnioreduction + induction of labor if vertex presentation
  - If no maternal distress—continuation of pregnancy till 40 weeks.

Indomethacin

- NSAID
- Mechanism of action—decreases urine output due to increased renal tubular absorption by inhibiting prostaglandins.
- Orally or rectally 1.4–3 mg/kg/daily
- Common regimen: 25 mg 6 hrly till maximum dose is 200 mg/day

- AFI should be done twice weekly during this treatment.
- Treatment can be discontinued once liquor decreases to 2/3 of pretreatment
- Side effects:
  - Maternal: nausea, epigastric discomfort, rectal irritation, cholestatic jaundice
  - Fetal: Transient renal failure, premature closure of ductus arteriosus, oligoamnios
- Concomitant use of corticosteroids increases the chances of intestinal perforation
- Contraindicated in TTTS as donor twin will be severely affected.

Fetal surveillance with indomethacin:

Fetal echocardiography for the detection of ductal constriction

- Initially after 48–72 hours of therapy.
- Weekly for the duration of treatment.
- Discontinue therapy if severe constriction detected.

Amniotic fluid evaluation for the detection of oligohydramnios

- Before initiating therapy.
- After 48–72 hours of therapy.
- Twice weekly for the duration of therapy.
- Discontinue therapy if oligohydramnios detected.

Sulindac

- NSAID.
- Reduced risk of ductus arteriosus constriction

Amnioreduction

- Indications:
  - TTTS
  - Maternal distress
- Frequent removal of smaller volumes (45–90 ml/min)/aggressive amnio-reduction (fluid is removed rapidly) under ultrasound guidance (total 1.5–2 liters/day)
- It should be repeated every 1–3 weeks if needed
- No need for antibiotic prophylaxis
- Complications: 4–15%
  - PPROM
  - Infections
  - Placental abruption
  - Fetal death

During Labor

- Controlled ARM in active phase of labor.
- After rupture of membranes, do P/V to exclude cord prolapse.
- Active management of third stage to prevent PPH.

In Neonate

- Rule out congenital abnormalities (especially esophageal atresia).

CHAPTER

11

Antepartum Hemorrhage

DEFINITION

It is the bleeding from or into the genital tract after 20 weeks of gestation and before completion of 2nd stage of labor.

GENERAL MANAGEMENT

- History: Regarding amount/color of bleeding
  - Associated pain in abdomen
  - H/o hypertensive disease complicating pregnancy
  - H/o trauma/coitus
  - Confirm gestational age, information regarding placental location
  - H/o number of past bleeding episodes, ruptured membranes and past obstetric history.
- Perform a rapid evaluation of the general condition of the woman including vital signs (Temperature, Pulse, blood pressure and Respiratory rate)
  - Abdominal examination includes fundal height measurement, consistency of uterus (normal or hard), presence of tenderness, palpable uterine contractions, fetal lie, presentation and viability.
  - Vulval inspection should include an assessment of the amount of bleeding and determination of whether or not the bleeding is continuing. A speculum examination is essential to rule out local causes of bleeding (after ultrasound-ruling out placenta previa and abruptio placentae).

Do not do per-vaginal examination unless previous scan report rules out placenta previa

- Resusciate the patient if in shock.
- Ask for help.
- Insert 2 large bore IV cannulae (16 guage) and start infusion of normal saline/ Ringer's lactate.
- Collect blood for estimation of complete blood count, grouping and cross-matching, bedside clotting test before infusing fluids. Send coagulation profile if abruptio placentae is suspected. Arrange adequate blood products, a minimum of 4 units of whole blood/packed cells.
- Infuse IV fluids (crystalloids) initially at the rate of 1 liter in 15–20 minutes. Give at least 2 liters of these fluids in the first hour. Aim to replace 2–3 times the estimated blood loss.

- No oral fluids.
- If a peripheral vein cannot be cannulated, perform a venous cut down.
- Give oxygen at 6–8 liters per minute by mask or nasal cannula.
- Continue to monitor vital signs and blood loss every 15 minutes.
- Monitor intake and output chart.
- In the event of recurrent vaginal bleeding >20 weeks of gestation, anti-D Ig should be given at a minimum of 6 weekly intervals.

DIAGNOSIS

Flow chart 11.1: Diagnosis of APH

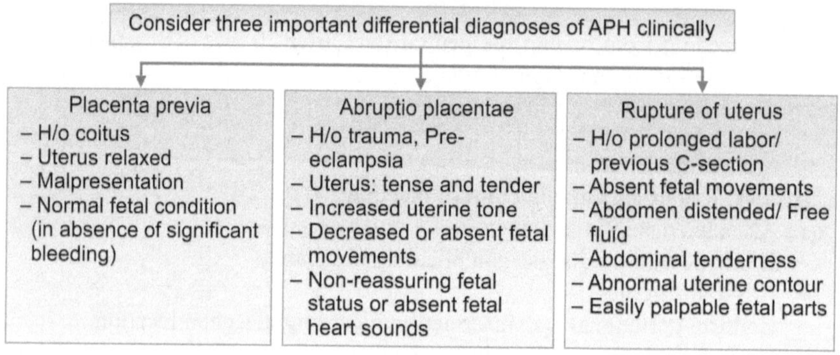

Figure 11.1: Diagnosis of APH

Confirmation of Diagnosis by Ultrasonography

- Look for the lower edge of placenta.
- Localize the internal os and measure the distance from the lower edge of placenta to the os.
- Transvaginal USG is helpful.
- Diagnose the type of placenta previa (anterior/posterior).
- Look for retroplacental clots if placenta is in upper segment for diagnosing abruptio placentae (High false negative rate).
- Look for fetal cardiac activity, liquor, average gestational age and estimated fetal weight.
- In anterior placenta previa with a previous lower segment scar, placenta accreta should be suspected, can be confirmed by the loss of the echolucent area between the uterus and placenta, multiple placental lacunae (Swiss-Cheese appearance), loss of echolucent line between uterus and bladder and presence of focal exophytic masses extending into bladder. Doppler confirms presence of retroplacental vessels invading the myometrium which obscure the bladder-serosal interface.

PLACENTA PREVIA

Placenta implanted partially or completely over the lower uterine segment (over and adjacent to the internal os after 20 weeks of gestation).

Placenta previa–When the lower margin of placenta lies below the BPD plane (5 cm from the internal os).

Risk Factors

- Black race
- Advanced maternal age
- High gravidity
- High parity
- Previous abortion: induced and spontaneous
- Prior cesarean delivery
- Cigarette smoking
- Multiple gestation

Placenta previa has traditionally been classified into four types:

1. Complete placenta previa, where the placenta completely overlies the internal os (Type IV).
2. Partial placenta previa, where the placenta partially overlies the internal os (Type III).
3. Marginal placenta previa, where the placental edge just reaches the internal os, but does not cover it (Type II). It is subdivided into type A and B, depending on whether placenta lies on the anterior or the posterior wall respectively.
4. Low-lying placenta, which reaches the lower uterine segment but does not reach the internal os, placental edge lies >2 cms from the os (Type I).
   Also classified as:
   - Major degree: if placenta lies less than 2 cm from os
   - Minor degree: if placenta lies more than 2 cm

   Ultrasound diagnosis

Flow chart 11.2: USG in placenta previa

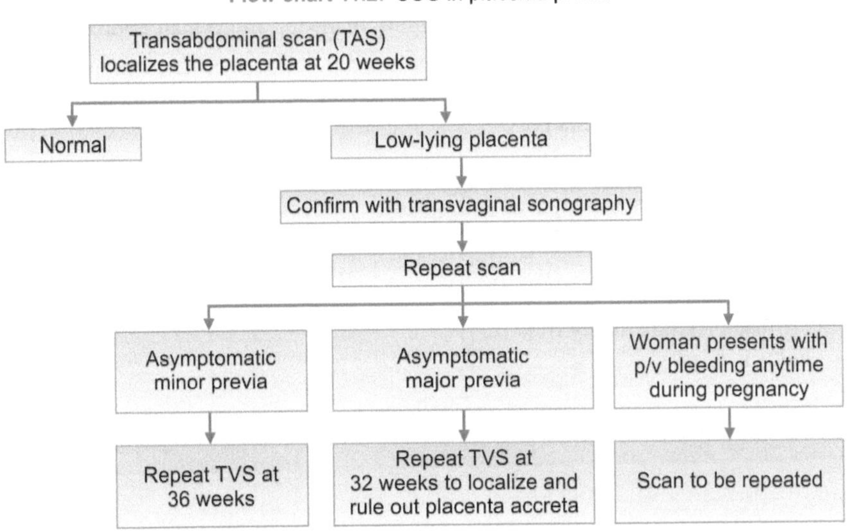

Management of Placenta Previa

- Obstetric management depends on gestational age, maternal and fetal condition and presence of active bleeding.
- In the event of recurrent vaginal bleeding >20 weeks of gestation, anti-D Ig should be given at a minimum of 6 weekly intervals.

Two options

Expectant management (Macafee and Johnson)	Active management
• Gestational age <37 weeks • No active bleeding • Maternal and fetal condition stable • Adequate cross-matched blood	• Gestational age >37 weeks • Labor pains • Excessive bleeding • FHS absent • Major fetal congenital anomaly (Incompatible with life)

Expectant Management: Can be Given on Inpatient or Outpatient Basis

- Outpatient management is offered to women who are ready to come for regular follow-up, have ready access to the hospital if there is any further bleeding, contractions, pain or discomfort.
- Inpatient management is provided to women who are non-compliant. Women with repeated episodes of bleeding especially after 34 weeks should remain in the hospital.
- In an institution with blood bank facility, 24 hrs availability of senior obstetrician, anesthesiologist and neonatologist.
- If gestational age <34 weeks–steroids.
- Catheterize the patient for 48 hrs after steroids to provide pelvic rest. If no bleeding for 24 hrs, catheter can be removed after 24 hrs.
- Pelvic rest: No intercourse, no vaginal douches or pelvic examinations.
- Avoid sternous activities such as running or lifting more than approximately 9.1 kgs (20 lbs).
- Prophylactic tocolysis and cervical encerclage are not recommended in the management of placenta previa.

Termination of Expectant Management

- 37 completed weeks of gestation
- Onset of active labor
- Fetal/Maternal jeopardy
- Profuse bleeding at any time
- Fetus is dead.

Elective delivery by cesarean section in asymptomatic women is not recommended before 38 weeks of gestation for placenta previa, or before 36–37 weeks of gestation for suspected placenta accreta.

Flow chart 11.3: Mode of termination of pregnancy in placenta previa

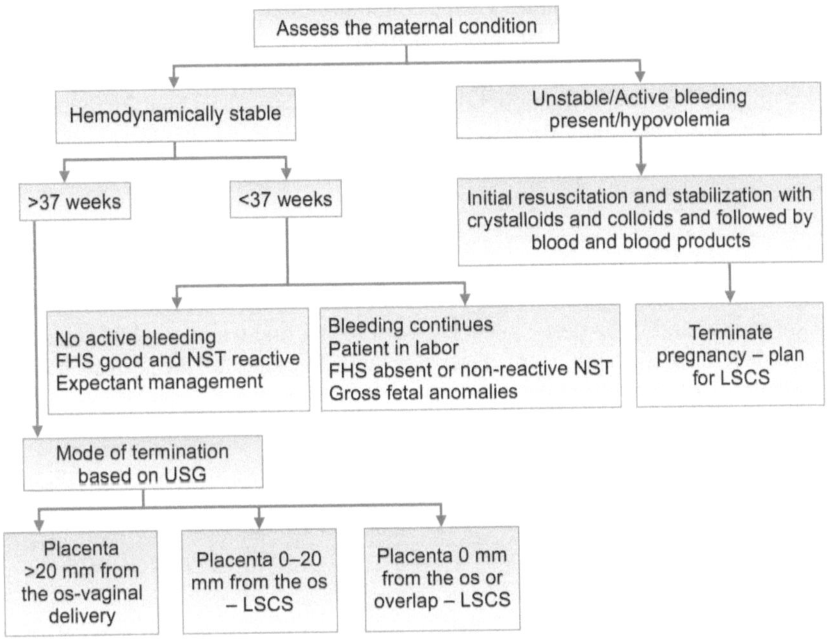

Precautions During Vaginal Delivery

- Active management of labor.
- Postpartum hemorrhage more likely.
- Morbid adherence of placenta can occur.

Precautions During Cesarean Section

- Regional anesthesia is preferred.
- Poorly formed lower uterine segment: Incision can be extended in J, U or inverted T fashion if extraction is difficult.
- Large vessels in the line of incision: can be ligated individually before incising the uterus.
- Delivery of fetus: When placenta is anterior, hand is inserted to reach the placental edge, membranes ruptured and the baby extracted. The other option is to cut through the placenta, but the extraction has to be quick because of the danger of fetal hemorrhage.
- Bleeding from the placental bed:

a. If bleeder is seen, oversewing with figure of eight sutures.
b. Pressure with hot mops for 2–3 minutes.
c. Oxytocin infusion 20 units/Prostaglandin F2α 250 microgram intramyometrial to be given.
d. Compression sutures: Hayman's, modification of B-Lynch may be tried.
e. Intrauterine tamponade: Using condom catheter or balloons like Bakri, Rusch, Sengstaken Blakemore are used.
f. Devascularization procedures: If bleeding not controlled, uterine artery ligation, stepwise ligation, bilateral internal iliac artery ligation to be done. Uterine artery embolization is done if facilities are available.
g. Total hysterectomy may be the last resort to control bleeding from the lower segment.

MORBIDLY ADHERENT PLACENTA (TOTAL PLACENTA ACCRETA)

- If a distinct cleavage plane between the placenta and the uterine wall cannot be located and if the tissue plane between the uterine wall and placenta cannot be developed through blunt dissection with the edge of the gloved hand, a diagnosis of invasive placenta should be considered.

Risk of Placenta Accreta in Previous Section

No. of sections	Percentage of placenta accreta
0	3%
1	11%
2	40%
3	61%
4	67%
5	67%

Conservative Management

- Catheterize the uterine vessels preoperatively.
- Cesarean done in the presence of interventional radiologist.
- Classical cesarean, cut the cord short and push it in, don't disturb the placenta, UAE immediately after delivering the baby.
- The woman should be warned of the risks of bleeding and infection postoperatively and prophylactic antibiotics may be helpful in the immediate postpartum period to reduce this risk. Neither methotrexate nor arterial embolization reduces these risks and neither is recommended routinely.
- Some trials show usage of Inj. Methotrexate 50 mg/m^2 x single doses postoperatively help autolysis.
- β hCG levels used for monitoring (monitored till undetectable), USG should supplement hCG.
- Evacuation of bits of placenta is done after 1–2 weeks.

Conservative management of placenta accreta when the woman is already bleeding is unlikely to be successful and risks wasting valuable time.

Surgical Management

If bleeding continues despite conservative management, the following options are used:

- Bilateral uterine artery ligation (both upper and lower)
- Ligation of internal iliac artery vessels
- Uterine artery embolization

ABRUPTIO PLACENTAE

Premature separation of normally situated placenta after 20 weeks of gestation and before delivery.

Risk Factors

- Uterine: Myomas, Uterine septum, Uterine malformations
- Demographic/Socioeconomic: High parity, Single parent, Low education, Infertility.
- Medical: Unexplained elevated MSAFP and hCG, Decreased inhibin A, Antiphospholipid syndrome, Pregestational diabetes, Hypertensive disorders of pregnancy.
- Preterm rupture of membranes with chorioamnionitis.
- Thrombophilias: Prothrombin 20210A mutation, Hyperhomocysteinemia, Factor V Leiden mutation, APCR, Protein C and S deficiency, MTHFR mutation, Dysfibrinogenemia.
- Iatrogenic: Sudden decompression of uterus (amniocentesis), External cephalic version for breech.
- Cigarette smoking
- Cocaine abuse
- Blunt trauma
- Incorrectly applied seat belt
- Intrauterine pressure catheter placement
- Heavy physical activity

Diagnosis

- It is clinical diagnosis.
- Sensitivity of ultrasound is only 50%.
- MRI can be used to visualize chronic abruption.
- USG

Role of USG in placental abruption

- To localize the placenta and to rule out placenta previa
- Fetal growth and expected fetal weight
- Fetal presentation
- Confirm IUD

USG findings in abruption

- Retroplacental collection—Sonographic appearance of retroplacental hemorrhage—depends on age and location of the bleed

Acute (48 hrs)—Hyperechoic
3–7 days—Isoechoic
1–2 weeks—Hypoechoic
>2 weeks—Anechoic

Rate of decrease in the size of clot is variable.
- Preplacental collection under the chorionic plate
- Jelly-like movement of choionic plate with fetal activity
- Marginal hematoma
- Subchorionic hematoma
- Intra-amniotic hematoma
- Increased heterogeneous placental thickness (>5 cm).

COMPLICATIONS

Maternal	Fetal
Anemia	Prematurity
Shock	IUGR
DIC	Perinatal mortality
PPH	Congenital malformations
Puerperal sepsis	Rh isoimmunization
IUD	
Renal failure	

Quick Initial Assessment and Determine the Severity of Abruption

Clinical grading of abruptio placentae (Sher's classification)
- Grade 0: Asymptomatic patient with a small retroplacental clot.
- Grade I: Vaginal bleeding; uterine tetany and tenderness may be present; no signs of maternal shock or fetal distress.
- Grade II: External vaginal bleeding possible; no signs of maternal shock; signs of fetal distress.
- Grade III: External bleeding possible; marked uterine tetany, yielding a board like consistency on palpation; persistent abdominal pain,with maternal shock and fetal demise; coagulopathy may be evident in 30% of cases.
  Grade III A: Presence of coagulopathy
  Grade III B: Absence of coagulopathy
- Monitor vitals, intake/output and chart abdominal girth and fundal height 2 hourly.

Management of Placental Abruption

Flow chart 11.4: Management of abruptio placenta

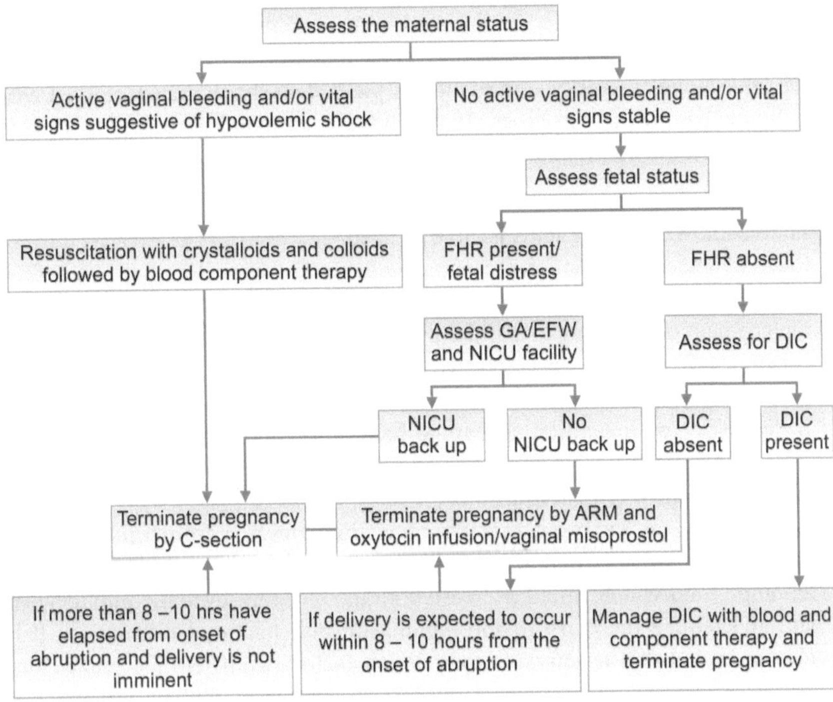

Management depends upon:
1. Severity
2. Associated complications
3. Condition of the mother and fetus
4. Gestational age

It includes:
a. General measures (common to all patients with bleeding)
b. Specific measures: Immediate delivery

Expectant management of suspected placental abruption is the exception and not the rule. The goal is to prolong pregnancy with the hope of improving fetal maturity and survival. It may be considered when the mother is stable, fetus is immature (<34 weeks) and fetal heart tracing is reassuring.

- The patient should be observed in the labor suite for 24–48 hrs to ensure that further placental separation is not occurring.
- Continuous fetal and maternal monitoring should be maintained. Sea-saw pattern of uterine contraction, sinusoidal pattern of fetal heart rate implicate an advanced grade of placental abruption.
- Administration of corticosteroids to accelerate fetal lung maturity may be a part of the plan.

- Use of tocolytics is controversial. Beta-mimetics can mask or blunt the patient's cardiovascular response and calcium channel blockers may further reduce the blood pressure, hence best avoided. $MgSO_4$ is the drug of choice.
- Once the patient is stable, the decision to manage the patient as an outpatient should be tailored and the fetus should be followed closely with CTG. Once the fetus attains maturity, termination of pregnancy should be considered with individualization of the cases. If the initial ultrasound scan shows a retro-placental clot, the clot may be monitored by serial ultrasound scans.

Immediate delivery: The need for immediate delivery depends on the severity of abruption and whether the fetus is alive or dead.

- Cases of placental abruption presenting with hemorrhage, uterine spasm or fetal distress should be treated as an acute emergency with adequate fluid and blood replacement (taking care to avoid fluid overload) and termination of pregnancy is mandated.
- If the fetus is dead, maternal resuscitation and vaginal delivery is the goal.
- If the degree of separation appears to be limiting and continuous, fetal heart tracing is reassuring, vaginal delivery should be attempted with induction, amniotomy and oxytocin infusion.
- Amniotomy, as early as feasible, has long been recommended in the management of placental abruption. The rationale behind this is escape of amniotic fluid which would decrease both the bleeding from the implantation site and reduce the entry of thromboplastin into maternal circulation. It is also proposed that it activates coagulation factors from retroplacental clots. However, in an immature fetus, its role is controversial. The intact sac is proposed to aid in cervical dilatation and labor.
- Oxytocin should be used cautiously in cases with a tonically contracted uterus, as uterine rupture may be caused by an overstimulated uterus. The progress is assessed by observing the cervical dilatation. Uterine stimulation to effect vaginal delivery provides benefits that override the risks.

Indications of Cesarean Delivery

Fetal indications:

- Fetus is in good condition, but the cervix is not favorable and in the face of progressive or severe placental separation.
- Non reassuring fetal status and where delivery is not imminent, with good NICU backup.

Maternal indications:

- Uncontrollable hemorrhage
- Rapidly expanding uterus with concealed hemorrhage with or without a live fetus
- Uterine apoplexy or refractory uterus.

Peritoneal drain and subcuticular drain are to be considered in cases of suspected DIC.

Flow chart 11.5: Management of abruptio placenta based on maternal status

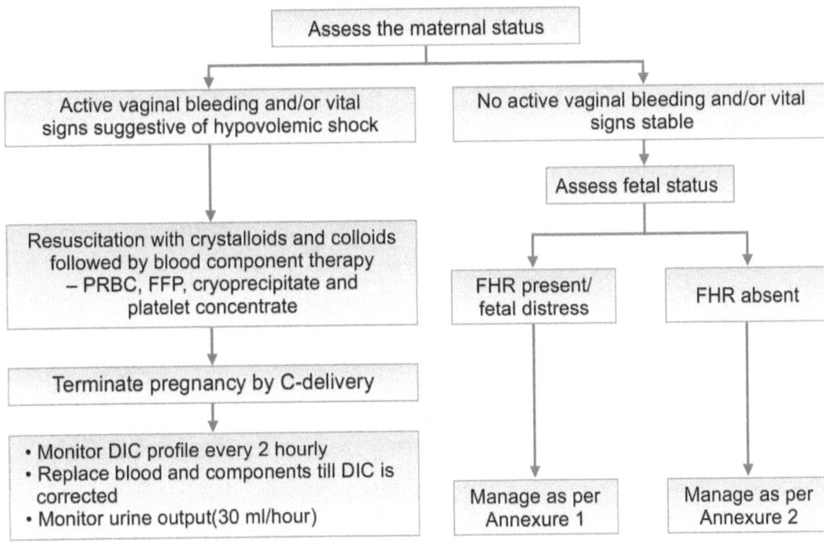

Annexure 1

Flow chart 11.6: Management of abruptio placenta based on fetal status

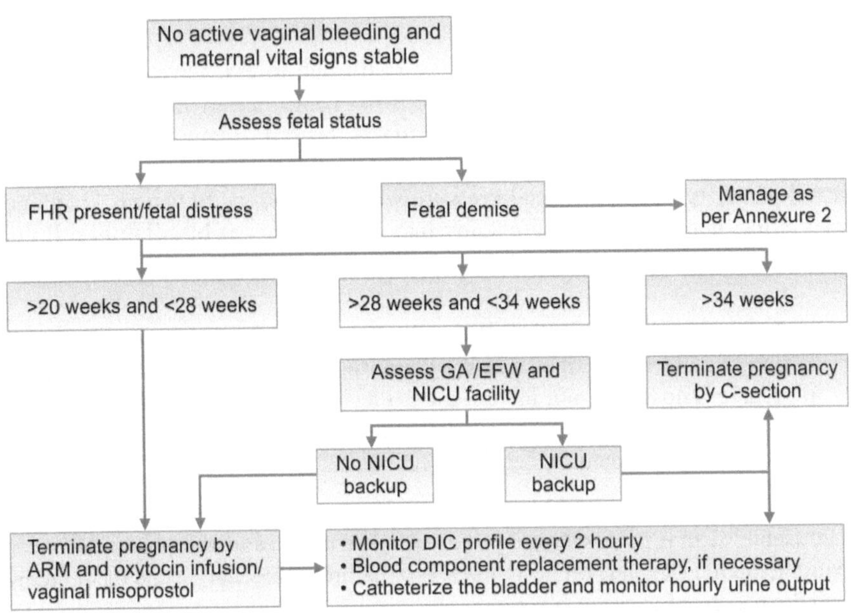

Annexure 2

Flow chart 11.7: Management of abruptio placenta with a dead fetus

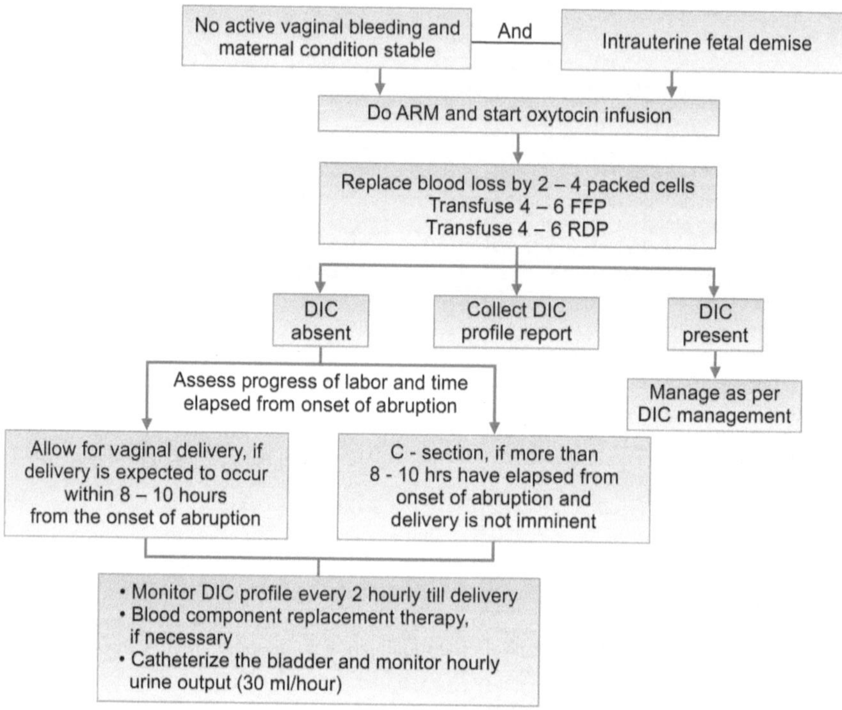

Couvelaire uterus: Uterine atony may result due to extensive infiltration of the myometrial wall with blood. If PPH is not controlled by medical methods, B-lynch sutures are used. If child-bearing is desired, bilateral uterine artery ligation should be done. If ineffective, bilateral ligation of the hypogastric arteries may reduce the arterial pressure within the uterus to venous level and may effect hemostasis. Hysterectomy may be necessary if bleeding is still not controlled.

Indeterminate/Unclassified APH

- Group of collective entities where a diagnosis of placenta previa and abruptio placentae is not made, nor there is a local lesion to account for the bleeding.
- Causes: Marginal sinus rupture, show, cervicitis, trauma, vulvovaricosities, genital tumors, hematuria, genital infections and vasa previa.

Diagnosis: It is made after placental abruption and placenta previa are excluded. Ultrasound scan is necessary to exclude placenta previa and abruption.
Management: Depends on gestational age, nature of bleeding, state of the fetus and the presumed cause of bleeding.
Before 37 weeks: If bleeding is recurrent and significant, delivery is justified. Mode of delivery depends on state of fetus, its lie, and other associated factors.

If bleeding is not significant, expectant management is chosen as mentioned above.
At or beyond 37 weeks: Delivery is the management option of choice, when bleeding is recurrent or significant or associated fetel demise. Vaginal delivery is not contraindicated if there is no fetal demise.

VASA PREVIA

Fetal vessels in the membranes cross the region of the cervical os below the presenting fetal part.
Incidence: 1 per 2500 deliveries
Type I: Occurs with single lobed placenta with velamentous insertion of cord.
Type II: Occurs when vessels join the placenta to an accessory lobe.
Clinical presentation: Typically presents with painless vaginal bleeding at the time of spontaneous or artificial rupture of membranes, followed by fetal heart rate abnormalities.
Diagnosis: Vasa previa can be accurately diagnosed with color Doppler ultrasound, often utilizing the transvaginal route. But no evidence for screening during the mid-trimester scan.

In cases of vasa previa identified in the second trimester, imaging should be repeated in the third trimester to confirm persistence.

Management

- In the presence of bleeding vasa previa, delivery should be achieved by category 1 emergency cesarean section.
- If there is either an ultrasound or clinical suspicion of vasa previa in the absence of fetal compromise, a formal systematic assessment of the region of the internal cervical os should be undertaken using transvaginal color Doppler ultrasound.
- In confirmed cases of vasa previa at term, delivery should be carried out by elective cesarean section in a timely manner.
- Laser ablation in utero may have a role in the treatment of vasa previa (Level 3 evidence).

CHAPTER

12

Intrauterine Fetal Death

DEFINITION

Antepartum death occurring beyond 28 weeks is termed as intrauterine fetal death.

DIAGNOSIS

Symptoms and Signs

- Loss of fetal movements
- Absent fetal heart sound

Sonography

- Lack of movements and cardiac activity over 10 min
- Oligoamnios
- Collapse of cranial bones (Spalding sign–7 days after death)
- Hyperflexion of spine (Ball sign)

X-ray—Gas shadows in the aorta (Robert sign–12 hrs of IUD).

Grade of maceration	Features	Duration of intrauterine demise
0	"Parboiled" reddened skin	<8 hours
I	Skin slippage and peeling	>8 hours
II	Extensive skin peeling Red serous effusions in chest and abdomen due to hemoglobin staining	2–7 days
III	Liver yellow-brown Turbid effusion May be mummified	≥8 days

Additional Dating

- Bullae in epidermis (leading to peeling): Appear at about 24 hours
- Hemoglobin staining of internal viscera (loss of normal color): 24–48 hours
- Separation of dura from calvarium bone: 5+ days

Evaluation

By evaluating both fetus and mother, the likelihood of recurrence and the possibility of prevention can be ascertained.

Flow chart 12.1: Evaluation of IUD

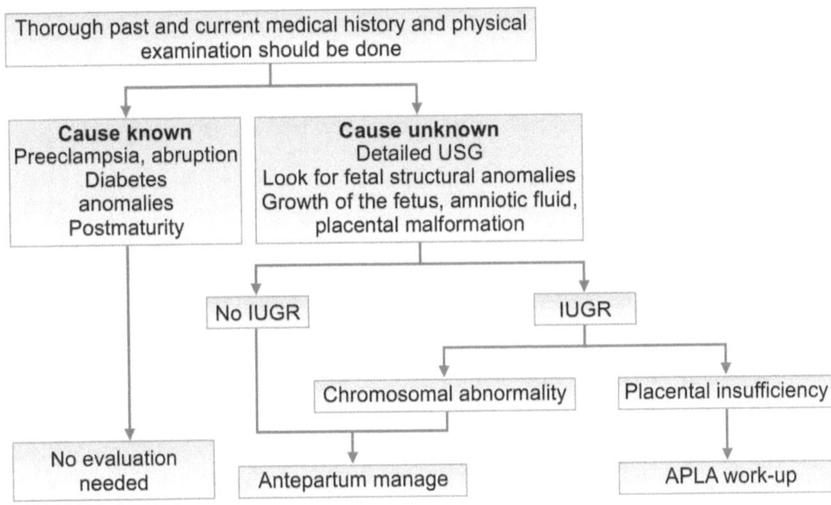

Antepartum Management

Fetal

Fetal karyotyping (subcutaneous tissue, fascia, muscle, amniocytes)

- Chromosomal abnormality in IUD (15%)
- Infection work up
- Fetal products
- Amniotic fluid (amniocytes and placental tissue can be cultured weeks after delivery. Fetal fascia, muscle and subcutaneous tissue fail to provide viable cells).

Maternal

- Complete hemogram
- HbA1C, FBS
- ICT if Rh incompatibility
- Coagulation profile (if duration >4 weeks, chance of DIC <2% if duration <4 weeks).

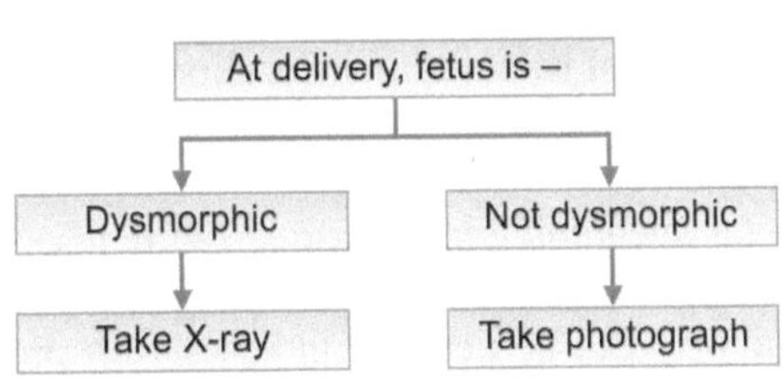

Autopsy

- Send for autopsy after taking consent.
- Gross external examination along with photography, radiology, MRI, bacterial cultures and selective use of chromosomal and histopathology studies often can aid in determining the cause of death.

Protocol for Examination of Stillborn Infants

Infant Description

- Malformations
- Skin staining
- Degree of maceration
- Color-pale, plethoric

Umbilical Cord

- Prolapse
- Entanglement—neck, arms, legs
- Hematomas or strictures
- Number of vessels
- Length
- Wharton's jelly—normal, absent

Amniotic Fluid

- Color—meconium, blood
- Consistency
- Volume

Placenta

- Weight
- Staining—meconium
- Adherent clots
- Structural abnormalities—circumvallate or accessory lobes, velamentous insertion
- Edema—hydropic changes

Membranes

- Meconium stained or cloudy
- Thickening

Indications for Karyotyping

1. Fetuses with dysmorphic features, inconsistent growth measurements, anomalies, hydrops or growth restriction.
2. Either parent is a carrier of balanced translocation.
3. History of recurrent losses or IUDs in first degree relatives.
4. Unexplained IUD.
5. If fetal or placental aneuploidy are detected (chromosomal translocation or rearrangement) parental karyotyping is indicated.
    - Full karyotype may not be possible in cases with prolonged intrauterine infection. FISH might be used to rule out numerical abnormalities or to look for certain common deletions, ex. DiGeorge syndrome.
    - 3 ml of fetal blood obtained from umbilical cord preferably or by cardiac puncture is placed in a sterile heparinized tube for cytogenetic study. If blood cannot be obtained a piece of fetal or placental tissue can be substituted if no maceration.

Tissue–Skin with attached dermal tissue or fascia from thigh, inguinal region or achilles tendon measuring 1 cm^2 washed with sterile saline and placed in saline or sterile cytogenetic medium. Do not use formalin.
Placenta–Sent for HPE.
APLA work-up–after 6 weeks.

MANAGEMENT

- 90% of women with IUD will go into spontaneous labor within 3 weeks of IUD.
- 25% of women who retain dead fetus for more than 4 weeks after 20 weeks develop chronic consumptive coagulopathy.
- If the woman is stable, membranes are intact and there is no evidence of pre-eclampsia, infection or bleeding, expectant management for 48 hours can be considered.
- Induction of labor as soon as IUD is diagnosed in order to prevent severe autolysis of the fetus and to obtain viable tissue for autopsy. It also brings an end to an emotionally painful event.
- Vaginal delivery is the preferred mode. If vaginal delivery fail, cesarean delivery. In modern obstetrics there is no role for destructive procedures.
- Oral mifepristone, followed by vaginal PGE2 or vaginal misoprostol, should usually be recommended as the first-line intervention for induction of labor.
- Mifepristone 200 mg orally followed by misoprostol 25–50 µg 4th hourly vaginally, maximum 6 doses.
    - If contractions are not adequate with first dose of 50–100 µg, give 200 µg, maximum being 600 µg/day.
    - If previous LSCS—halve the dose. Risk of rupture is 1.2–10%.
    - If contractions >2/10 min dose not to be repeated. Start oxytocin 4 hrs after the last dose.
    - If no expulsion within 24 hrs repeat the dose a second time.
    - If not expelled with second dose—surgical evacuation or expectant management.
- Vaginal misoprostol is more effective and has less side-effects than oral, when used specifically for pregnancy termination in IUD.
- Women with two previous LSCS should be counseled that in general the absolute risk of induction of labor with prostaglandin is only a little higher than for women with a single previous LSCS.
- Women undergoing VBAC should be closely monitored for features of scar rupture.
- Oxytocin augmentation can be used for VBAC, but the decision should be made by a consultant obstetrician.
- Low dose oxytocin augmentation can be used for VBAC.
- Women with sepsis should be treated with intravenous broad-spectrum antibiotic therapy (including anti-chlamydial agents).
- Routine antibiotic prophylaxis is not necessary.
- Labor has to be induced after treatment of coagulopathy and coagulopathy will resolve in 48 hours after delivery.

- If Rh -ve should be checked for isoimmunization, if isoimmunized offer immediate Kleihauer test.
- If there has been a large FMH, the dose of anti-RhD gammaglobulin should be adjusted upwards and the Kleihauer test should be repeated at 48 hours to ensure the fetal red cells have cleared.
- It is important to know the baby's blood group; if no blood sample can be obtained from the baby or cord, RhD typing should be undertaken using free fetal DNA (ffDNA) from maternal blood taken shortly after birth.

Postpartum

- Patient should be monitored after delivery because of the risk of postpartum atony and placental retention.

Parental Psychosocial Care

- Counsellors should facilitate the grevious process.
- Parent should be encouraged to view the newborn and they should be informed any bruising or facial marks are normal.
- Upon discharge should be called after 1 month, results of all studies should be performed or reviewed and all their questions should be addressed.
- If the cause of death is found, its implication to subsequent pregnancies should be discussed.

EVALUATION PRIOR TO NEXT PREGNANCY

- Actions needed should be cause specific, e.g. maternal thrombophiliapro-phylactic anticoagulation, aneuploidy (1% recurrent risk). Famililal DiGeorge (50% recurrent risk), abruption (10% recurrent risk)—CVS and amniocentesis to be done in subsequent pregnancies.
- Fortunately, recurrence of IUD is 0–8%. Practice of antenatal surveillance test is a waste of resources if the subsequent pregnancy is characterized by normal presentation.
- Antepartum fetal surveillance should begin 32 weeks or later in otherwise healthy woman with history of IUD.

Chance of IUD in Subsequent Pregnancy

- Living growth restricted term infant–2-fold increased risk of IUD.
- Living growth restricted preterm infant–5-fold increased risk of IUD.

CHAPTER

13

Preterm Labor

Preterm labor is the onset of labor with intact membranes after 28 weeks and before 37 completed weeks of gestation from first day of last menstrual period.

Risk factors associated with preterm births are classified as follows:

1. Demographic
    a. Age <18 or >35 years
    b. Race–increased incidence in blacks
    c. Low socioeconomic status
    d. Unmarried
    e. Uneducated
    f. Familial
2. Behavioral
    a. Smoking 20–30%
    b. Other substance abuse
    c. Poor nutrition
    d. Excessive physical activity
    e. Psychological stress
3. Health care
    a. Absent or inadequate prenatal care
4. Medical or obstetrical risks
    a. Prior mid-trimester pregnancy loss
    b. Uterine anomaly
    c. Cervical trauma
    d. Anemia
    e. Fibroid uterus (5 cm or more in diameter or submucous)
    f. Diethylstilbesterol exposure during pregnancy (causes uterine anomalies)

Risk of Preterm Birth According to Obstetric Outcome

First birth	Second birth	Subsequent preterm births
Term	4%	
Preterm	17%	
Term	Term	3%
Preterm	Term	6%
Term	Preterm	11%
Preterm	Preterm	28%

5. Medical disorders like–
   a. Cardiac disease
   b. Hypertension
   c. Diabetes mellitus
   d. Renal disorder
   e. Anemia
6. Current pregnancy risks
   a. Multifetal gestation >50%
   b. Assisted conception
   c. Antepartum hemorrhage
   d. Systemic infection–septicemic pyelonephritis
   e. Asymptomatic bacteriuria
   f. Recurrent urinary tract infection
   g. Chorioamnionitis
   h. Fetal anomaly
   i. Cervical incompetence
   j. Gestational hypertension
   k. Polyhydramnios
   l. Placental abnormality

SCREENING OF PRETERM LABOR

Clinical Predictors

- Risk scoring system (Pappernick's). Score >10–High risk for spontaneous preterm labor (sensitivity–25%).

Predictors at 22–24 Weeks of Spontaneous Preterm Birth Before 35 Weeks

Test	Sensitivity	Specificity	Positive predictive value	Negative predictive value
Multiple preterm birth symptoms	50%	63%	21%	86%
Uterine contractions ≥4/hr	7%	92%	25%	84%
Bishop score ≥4	32%	91%	42%	87%
Cervical length ≤25 mm	40%	89%	42.5%	89%
Fibronectin ≥50 ng/ml	18%	95%	43%	85%

Warning Symptoms of Preterm Labor

- Irregular, non rhythmical, and either painful or painless
- Low dull backache
- Pelvic pressure
- Menstrual-like cramps
- Watery vaginal discharge

Biophysical Predictor

- Uterine contractions >4/hr
- Cervical examination

Routine P/v examination to assess the cervix–only in high risk
- TVS.

Indications for Cervical Ultrasound Screening in the Second Trimester

- H/o previous deliveries between 16 and 36 weeks gestation.
- H/o conception after infertility treatment.
- H/o cervical instrumentation.
    - Cervical cone biopsy or LEEP
    - Dilation and curettage for diagnosis or therapeutic indications, including first and second trimester pregnancy terminations.
- H/o prior genital tract infections or persistently abnormal Pap smear.
- All African Americans
- Women with depression, low body mass index (<19.6), or who smoke.
- Cervical length is <3 cm on a midtrimester transabdominal ultrasound examination.
- Women with signs or symptoms of preterm delivery in the current pregnancy
- Vaginal bleeding or spotting without obvious cause
- Persistent symptoms of pelvic pressure, cramps, change in vaginal discharge after 16 weeks' gestation.

Biochemical Predictors

Cervicovaginal secretions:
- Fetal fibronectin >50 ng/ml
- IL-6, IL-8, TNF α, matrix metalloproteinases (1, 8, G)
- Estriol >2.3 ng/ml
- Phosphorylated insulin like growth factor.

Serum Markers

- Alfa fetoprotein (AFP), Alkaline phosphatase (ALP), Granulocyte Monocyte Colony Stimulating Factor (GM CSF), Defensins, Corticotropin releasing hormone (CRH).

Recommended Screening Strategies to Prevent Preterm Labor

- No current data support use of home uterine-activity monitoring or bacterial vaginosis screening.
- Screening for risk of preterm labor, other than historical risk factors, is not beneficial in general obstetrical population.
- Sonography to determine cervical length and/or fetal fibronectin level measurement may be useful in determining women at risk for preterm labor.

Investigations

- CBC
- Urine routine, culture and sensitivity
- Speculum examination—for any leak, pooled fluid, pH, cervical swab C and S.
- USG-AFI, gestational age, EFW, placental location, cervical length.

PREVENTION OF PRETERM LABOR

Preconceptional Measures

- Avoidance of heavy manual work or mental stress and specific habits like alcohol, smoking and chemical dependency.
- Weight reduction in obesity.

Antenatal Preventive Measures

- Assessment of risk
- Patient education regarding warning symptoms
- Early and regular antenatal care
- Strategies for prevention of preterm labor and preterm birth–primary prevention.

Primary Prevention

1. **Treatment of vaginal infection**
   - Bacterial vaginosis, trichomonas vaginosis, urea plasma urealyticum, mycoplasma hominis—screening and treatment of asymptomatic woman is not promising in prevention of preterm labor.
2. **Treatment of periodontal disease** is not helpful.
3. **Use of progesterone**

   Studies show some benefit in reducing preterm birth but further studies are needed as to optimal preparation, dosage, route of administration and appropriate gestational age at which to start the therapy.

   Inj. 17(OH) progesterone 250 mg every week/500 mg every 15 days IM from 16 to 36 weeks of gestation if the cervical length between 16 to 24 weeks of gestation is <2 cm.
4. **Tocolysis**

   No role for prophylactic tocolysis.
5. **Cervical cerclage**

   It is also known as tracheloplasty. A cervical stitch is placed when there is increased risk of preterm birth or cervical incompetence causing mid-trimester abortions.

Types of Cervical Encerclage

1. **History-indicated cerclage**

Indication

Women with previous obstetric history suggestive of increased risk of preterm in present pregnancy:

- Three or more previous preterm births and/or second-trimester losses.
- Previous adverse event, such as painless dilatation of the cervix or rupture of the membranes before the onset of contractions, or additional risk factors, such as cervical surgery, are not helpful in the decision to place a history-indicated cerclage.
- Prepregnancy diagnostic techniques such as assessment of cervical resistance index, hysterography or insertion of cervical dilators to assess cervical weakness are not recommended in order to take decision of history-indicated cervical encerclage.

Cerclage is done electively at 12–14 weeks of gestation after doing NT scan to rule out lethal abnormality and aneuploidy.

2. **Ultrasound-indicated cerclage**

Indications

- Women with a singleton pregnancy and a history of spontaneous mid-trimester loss or preterm birth.
  - Who have not undergone a history-indicated cerclage
  - Who are undergoing transvaginal sonographic surveillance of cervical length with length of ≤2.5 cm and before 24 weeks of gestation.

Not Recommended

- Incidental finding of cervical length ≤2.5 cm on TVS without history of previous spontaneous second trimester losses/preterm delivery.
- Solely funneling of internal os in the absence of cervical shortening to 2.5 cm or less.

Surveillance

- Serial sonographic cervical length measurement from 14–24 weeks gestation by TVS is indicated.
- Women should be counseled that expectant management is a reasonable alternative since there is a lack of direct evidence to support serial sonographic surveillance over expectant management.
- Placement of an ultrasound-indicated cerclage in the presence of cervical length shortening cannot be recommended as compared with expectant management, it may be associated with an increase in both pregnancy loss and delivery before 35 weeks of gestation.

Cerclage is done electively when cervical length becomes ≤2.5 cm before 24 weeks after ruling out anomalies.

Special Cases

- The insertion of a history or ultrasound-indicated cerclage is not recommended in–
  - Women with multiple pregnancies
  - Other high-risk groups such as women with Mullerian anomalies, previous cervical surgery (cone biopsy, large loop excision of the transformation zone or destructive procedures such as laser ablation or diathermy) or multiple dilatation and evacuation.
- The decision to place a concomitant cerclage at radical trachelectomy should be individualized.

3. **Rescue cerclage:**

- Insertion of cerclage as a salvage measure in the case of premature cervical dilation with exposed fetal membranes in the vagina.
- The decision to place a rescue cerclage following an elective or ultrasound-indicated cerclage should be made on an individual basis, taking into account the clinical circumstances.
- It may delay delivery by a further 5 weeks on average compared with expectant management/bed rest alone.

- A two-fold reduction in the chance of delivery before 34 weeks of gestation.
- Advanced dilatation of the cervix (more than 4 cm) or membrane prolapse beyond the external os appears to be associated with a high chance of cerclage failure.

Contraindications for Cerclage

- Active preterm labor
- Clinical evidence of chorioamnionitis
- Continuing vaginal bleeding
- PPROM
- Evidence of fetal compromise
- Lethal fetal defect
- Fetal death

Routes of Cerclage

1. **Transabdominal cerclage (Benson and Durfee):**
   Suture is placed at the uterine isthmus through abdominal route. It is performed in preconceptional or in early pregnancy, but this procedure may be associated with increased maternal morbidity.
   Indications:
   - Women with a previous failed transvaginal cerclage.
   - Traumatic or surgical damage making a vaginal approach difficult.

There is lack of evidence for laparoscopic approach of transabdominal cerclage. All women with a transabdominal cerclage require delivery by cesarean section, and the abdominal suture may be left in place following delivery.

Management Decisions in Cases of Delayed Miscarriage or Fetal Death in Women with an Abdominal Cerclage

- Successful evacuation through the stitch by suction curettage or by dilatation and evacuation (up to 18 weeks of gestation).
- Alternatively, the suture may be cut, usually via a posterior colpotomy. Failing this, a hysterotomy may be required or cesarean section may be necessary.

2. **Transvaginal cerclage (McDonald)**
- A transvaginal purse-string suture placed at the cervicovaginal junction, without bladder mobilization.
- Knot tied anteriorly, as pregnancy progresses uterus anteverts making the access to posterior aspect difficult.

3. **High transvaginal cerclage (Shirodkar)**
   - A transvaginal purse-string suture placed following bladder mobilization, to allow insertion above the level of the cardinal ligaments.
   - Knot tied posteriorly to decrease bladder irritation.
4. **Occlusion cerclage (Wurm stitch)**
   Occlusion of the external os by placement of continuous non-absorbable suture. The theory behind the potential benefit of occlusion cerclage is retention of the mucus plug.

Counseling Before the Procedure

- Cerclage insertion is associated with doubling in risk of maternal pyrexia but no apparent increase in chorioamnionitis.
- Cerclage insertion is not associated with an increased risk of PPROM, induction of labor or cesarean section.
- The insertion of a cervical suture is not associated with an increased risk of preterm delivery or second-trimester loss.
- There is a small risk of intraoperative bladder damage, cervical trauma, membrane rupture and bleeding during insertion of cervical cerclage.
- Shirodkar cerclage usually requires anesthesia for removal, and therefore, carries the risk of an additional anesthetic.
- Cervical cerclage may be associated with a risk of cervical laceration/trauma if there is spontaneous labor with the suture in place.

Preoperative Care

- First-trimester ultrasound scan and screening for aneuploidy before the insertion to ensure both viability and the absence of lethal/major fetal abnormality.
- Investigations for subclinical chorioamnionitis are not recommended. In case of clinical suspicion maternal white cell count and C-reactive protein may be performed.
- There is insufficient evidence to recommend routine amniocentesis before rescue or ultrasound indicated cerclage. In selected cases where there is suspicion of intra-amniotic infection, amniocentesis may be performed to aid the decision about rescue cerclage, as the presence of infection is associated with a poor prognosis.
- Amniocentesis before rescue cerclage does not appear to increase the risk of preterm delivery before 28 weeks of gestation.
- No evidence to support amnioreduction before insertion of rescue cerclage.
- Routine genital infection screening is not recommended. If genital swab is culture positive, a complete course of sensitive antimicrobial eradication therapy before cerclage insertion would be recommended.
- Perioperative tocolysis is not recommended.
- Antibiotics, type of anesthesia and suture material are operative surgeon's choice, should be individualized.

Antibiotics

- The use of antibiotics prior or after the cerclage is controversial.
  In elective cerclage, prophylactic antibiotics are not used.
- In urgent or emergency cerclage, the membranes have been exposed to the vaginal flora, and hence the pregnancy and the mother are both at risk of infection. In these cases, antibiotics may be used to provide broad coverage.
  Inj. Cefixime 1 g IV after test dose half an hour before the procedure followed by oral Cefixime 200 mg BD for 5 days.

Anesthesia–General anesthesia

Suture material–No. 2 black silk

- There is no current evidence to support the placement of two purse-string sutures over a single suture.
- There is no current evidence to support the placement of a cervical occlusion suture in addition to the primary cerclage.

Postoperative Care

- Elective transvaginal cerclage can safely be performed as a day care procedure.
- Women undergoing ultrasound-indicated or rescue cerclage, given the higher risk of complications such as PPROM, early preterm delivery, miscarriage and infection, may benefit from at least a 24-hour postoperative period of observation in hospital. Cases should be managed on an individual basis.
- In women undergoing insertion of transabdominal cerclage via laparotomy, an inpatient stay of at least 48 hours is recommended.
- Supplementary progesterones are not recommended routinely postoperatively.
- No routine recommendation of bed rest and abstinence.
- Routine serial sonographic measurement of the cervix is not recommended, it may be useful in individual cases following ultrasound-indicated cerclage to offer timely administration of steroids or in utero transfer.
- Routine fetal fibronectin testing is not recommended post-cerclage.

Removal of Stitch

- Should be removed before labor, usually between 36+1 and 37 weeks of gestation, unless delivery is by elective cesarean section, in which case suture removal could be delayed until this time.
- In women presenting in established preterm labor, the cerclage should be removed to minimize potential trauma to the cervix.
- Delayed suture removal until labor or delivery is associated with an increased risk of maternal/fetal sepsis and is not recommended.
- Given the risk of neonatal and/or maternal sepsis and the minimal benefit of 48 hours of latency in pregnancies with PPROM before 23 and after 34 weeks of gestation, delayed suture removal is unlikely to be advantageous in this situation.

Complications

- **Intraoperative**
  Rupture of membranes, hemorrhage.
- **Immediate postoperative**
  Preterm labor, sepsis.
- **Delayed postoperative**
  Bucket handle tear of cervix, uterine rupture, cervical dystocia, ischemic necrosis of cervix, stillbirth due to obstructed labor.

Diagnosis of Preterm Labor

- ACOG criteria for diagnosing preterm labor.
  1. Regular uterine contractions occur at 4/20 min. or 8/60 min with progressive change in the cervix.
  2. Cervical dilatation >1 cm
  3. Effacement >80

Flow chart 13.1: Diagnosis of pre-term labor

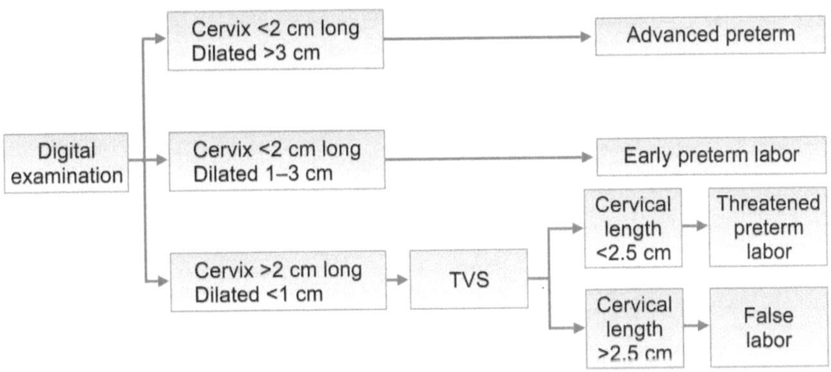

Management of Preterm Labor

- Traditional first steps
  - Bed rest
  - Not proven beneficial
  - Hydration
- Treat underlying conditions

Flow chart 13.2: Management of pre-term labor

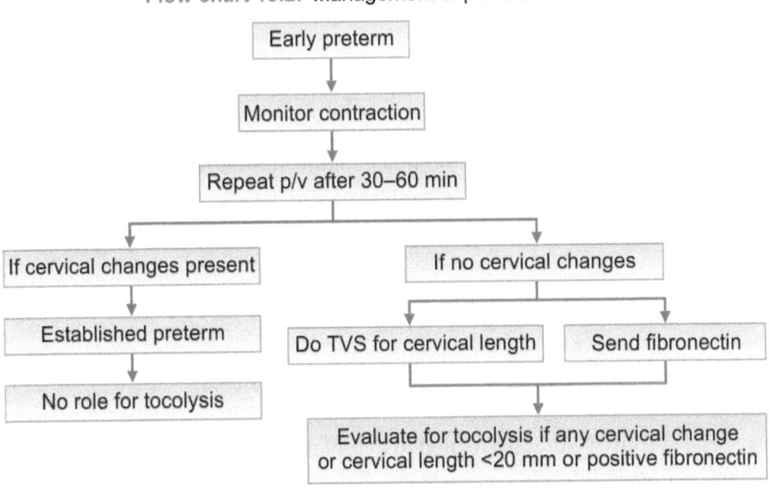

Flow chart 13.3: Management of threatened pre-term

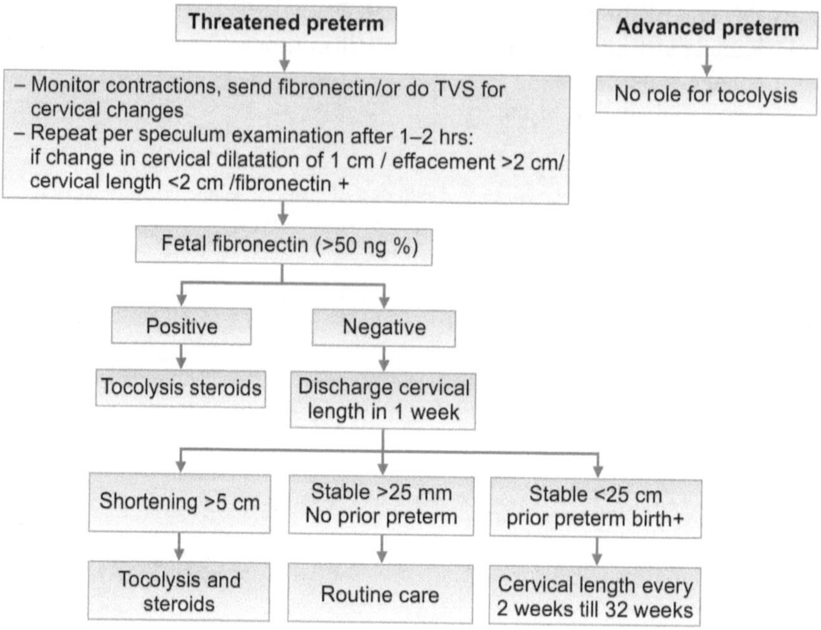

Tocolysis

Candidates for Tocolysis

- Gestational age between 24–34 weeks
- Cervical dilatation <4 cm
- No contraindications to drugs
- Fetus alive
- Clear diagnosis of preterm labor

RCOG Recommendation for Tocolysis

- It is reasonable not to use tocolytic drugs, as there is no clear evidence that they improve outcome. However, tocolysis should be considered if the few days gained would be put to good use, such as completing a course of corticosteroids, or *in utero* transfer.

TOCOLYTICS

Calcium Channel Blockers

Mechanism of Action

Myometrial activity is directly related to cytoplasmic free calcium, and a reduction in its concentration inhibits contractions. Calcium-channel blockers act to inhibit by a variety of mechanisms, the entry of calcium through channels in the cell membrane.

Nifedipine

- 30 mg initial followed by 20 mg 8 hrly for 48 hrs.
- Withhold if BP <90/60 and pulse rate 110 beats per minute.

Side effects:
- Hypotension-Headache (20%) flushing, dizziness, nausea, peripheral edema.
- MI rare.

Contraindications:
- Hypotension, aortic stenosis, CCF.

Betamimetics

Mechanism of Action

β-Adrenergic agents stimulate the β-adrenergic receptors of the sympathetic nervous system. Interactions with the receptor sites cause an increase in intra-cellular production of cyclic adenosine monophosphate. This phenomenon results in the reduction of intracellular calcium concentration in the smooth muscle. The lower level of calcium inhibits activation of the contractile proteins actin and myosin, which in turn, results in relaxation of the myometrium.

Two types of β-receptors exist-β1 and β2. Uterine musculature contains β2 receptors, because terbutaline possesses β2-specific properties, it is the drug of choice when uterine relaxation is desired.

Ritodrine

- Initial IV infusion at 100 μg/min, increase every 10 min by 50 μg/min until contractions cease or pulse rate exceeds 120 bpm or toxicity appears or till maximum rate of 350 μg/min.
  Sustain this for 12 hrs after contractions cease. IV infusion should not be followed by oral therapy.

Terbutaline

Intravenous
- Initial IV infusion at 10 μg/min, increase every 10 min 5 μg/min until contractions cease or pulse rate exceeds 120 bpm or toxicity appears or till maximum rate of 50 μg/min. Sustain this for 12 hrs after contractions cease. IV infusion should not be followed by oral therapy.

Subcutaneous
- 250 g subcutaneous, every 3–4 hrs
- Uterine quiescence should be maintained for 12 hrs and pulse rate to be maintained at 100–120 beats/min.

Side Effects

Palpitations, chest pain, breathlessness, pulmonary edema, MI, hypokalemia, arrhythmias, headache, tremor.

Contraindications:

PIH, IDDM, hyperthyroidism, sickle cell disease, cardiac conduction defects, ventricular outflow obstruction, bleeding, gestation >37 weeks, chorioamnionitis.

Magnesium Sulfate

Mechanism of Action

Although the exact method is unknown, it is generally believed that the major action of magnesium sulfate relates to its inhibitory effect on calcium uptake and distribution. It seems that magnesium inhibits smooth muscle contractions by its direct effect on calcium activity. Magnesium modulates calcium uptake by reducing calcium binding and distribution in the myometrium. Elevated magnesium levels inhibit calcium influx at cellular membranes by competing for calcium binding sites. High titers of magnesium also increase the level of intracellular cyclic adenosine monophosphate and consequently reduce intracellular calcium.

Dosage

High: 6 g loading dose over 15–30 minutes followed by 2–6 g an hour for 12–24 hrs.
Low: 4 g loading dose over 15–30 minutes followed by 2 g an hour for 12–24 hrs.

Therapeutic level-Serum levels between 5 and 8 ng/dL of magnesium are needed to attain myometrium inhibition.

Toxic Levels

Loss of patellar reflexes at 10 mEq/liter
Respiratory depression at 12 to 15 mEq/liter
Cardiac arrest >15 mEq/liter

Toxicity reversed by Inj Calcium gluconate (10 ml of 10% calcium gluconate 1 gm IV).

Side Effects

Maternal		
Short-term	*Long-term*	*Toxicity*
Lethargy	Osteoporosis	Absent deep tendon reflexes
Nausea	Tetany	Respiratory depression
Vomiting	Paralytic ileus	Cardiac arrhythmia
Flushed	Pulmonary edema	Cardiac arrest
Hot feeling	Hypothermia	Death
Headaches	Renal stones	
Constipation	Rhabdomyolysis	
Dry mouth		
Hypocalcemia		

Contd...

Contd...

Fetal		
Short-term	*Long-term*	*Toxicity*
Decreased fetal movement	Decalcification of bones	
Absent fetal breathing		
Decreased short-term variability of fetal heart		
Altered uterine blood flow		
Blunted fetal response		
Neonatal		
Short-term	*Long-term*	*Toxicity*
Hypermagnesemia	Neonatal death?	Neuroprotective
Hypocalcemia		
Lethargy		
Depressed apgars		
Hypotonia		
Decalcification of bones		

Contraindications

Myasthenia gravis, heart blocks.

PG Synthesis Inhibitors

Mechanism of Action

Antiprostaglandin agents arrest labor through the inhibition of the enzyme prostaglandin synthetase or cyclooxygenase (COX). This enzyme is responsible for the conversion of arachidonic acid to an intermediate endoperoxide and finally resulting in the formation of a prostaglandin. Prostaglandins are facilitators of myometrial contractions by increase in calcium within myometrial cells leading to increased activity of myosin light chain kinase, a protein directly tied to myometrial contraction. They also coordinate uterine contractions by increasing gap junctions. Also play a vital role in production of collagenases and proteases that promote ripening of the cervix.

An ideal tocolytic therapy would target the prostaglandin-mediated mechanism of labor activation while not interfering with fetal development or causing undue maternal symptomatology.

Indomethacin

Both COX1 and COX 2 inhibitor.

Dosage

50 to 100 mg loading dose usually by rectal suppository, followed by 25 mg orally every 6 to 8 hours for 48 hrs.

Precautions

- Restrict usage to <32 weeks gestation.
- Limit duration of therapy to less than 72 hours if possible.
- Avoid treatment with growth-restricted fetuses.
- Avoid therapy in the setting of oligohydramnios.

Side Effects

Headache, dizziness, gastritis, vomiting, diarrhea fetal-ductus arteriosis constriction, oligohydramnios pulmonary HTN.

Contraindications

APD, hepatic failure, renal failure, HTN, asthma.

Oxytocin Antagonist

Atosiban

Mechanism of Action

This nonapeptide oxytocin analogue is a competitive antagonist of oxytocin-induced contractions.

Dosage: IV 6.75 mg bolus, followed by infusion 18 mg/hr for 3 hrs then 6 mg/hr for 45 hrs.

Side Effects

Dyspnea, chest pain.

Contraindications

Hepatic and renal failure.

Vasodilator

Mechanism of action: These potent smooth-muscle relaxants affect the vasculature, gut, and uterus.

Nitroglycerin

- Dermal patch–5 to 10 mg patch over gluteal region, if contraction persists after 1 hr patch can be repeated.
- Patch to be repeated after 24 hrs, can be kept for 48 hrs.

Side Effects

Transient headache.

Management of Persistent Contractions Despite 12–24 hrs of Tocolysis

If infections, abruption, fetal compromise can be excluded, stop tocolysis for 24 hrs and observe, most patients will stop contractions spontaneously. There is no role for second or combined tocolysis.

STEROIDS

ACOG (February 2011) recommends a single course of corticosteroids for pregnant women between 24–34 weeks who are at risk of preterm delivery within 7 days.

RCOG (October 2010) recommends antenatal corticosteroids should be given to all women.

- At risk of iatrogenic or spontaneous preterm birth up to 34 + 6 weeks of gestation.
- For whom an elective cesarean section is planned prior to 38 + 6 weeks of gestation.
- With multiple pregnancy at risk of imminent iatrogenic or spontaneous preterm delivery between 24 weeks and 34 weeks 6 days of gestation.

Dosage: Betamethasone 12 mg IM 24 hrs apart–2 doses

Dexamethasone 6 mg IM 12 hrs apart–4 doses

Antenatal corticosteroids are most effective in–

- Reducing RDS in pregnancies that deliver 24 hours after and up to 7 days after administration of the second dose of antenatal corticosteroids.
- Reduces neonatal death within the first 24 hours, and therefore, should still be given even if delivery is expected within this time.

Special Situations

- Senior opinion should be sought when contemplating delaying delivery for steroid prophylaxis in cases of overt chorioamnionitis.
- Diabetes mellitus is not a contraindication to antenatal corticosteroid treatment for fetal lung maturation.
- Women with impaired glucose tolerance or diabetes who are receiving fetal steroids should have additional insulin according to an agreed protocol and be closely monitored.
- Pregnancies affected by fetal growth restriction between 24 + 0 and 35 + 6 weeks of gestation at risk of delivery should receive a single course of antenatal corticosteroids.
- Contraindicated in active maternal tuberculosis.

Advantage

Reduce risk of–

- Respiratory distress syndrome
- Intraventricular hemorrhage
- Necrotizing enterocolitis

Betamethasone versus Dexamethasone

- Both cross the placenta in their active form and have nearly identical biological activity.
- Both lack mineralocorticoid activity and have relatively weak immunosuppressive activity with short term use.

- Betamethasone has a longer half-life.
- According to Cochrane review, there was decreased incidence of intraventricular hemorrhage with dexamethasone.
- The Cochrane review on antenatal corticosteroids for accelerating fetal lung maturation for women at risk of preterm birth suggests that betamethasone treatment causes a larger reduction in RDS than dexamethasone.
- Less frequent adverse neurological outcome at 18–22 months after betamethasone exposure.
- A large nonrandomised retrospective study has suggested that infants exposed to antenatal betamethasone have less neonatal cystic periventricular leukomalacia than infants exposed to antenatal dexamethasone.
- Dexamethasone is associated with complete fetal heart block.

Due to inconsistent and limited data it is not possible to recommend one steroid regimen over the other.

Multiple Courses Versus Single Course

- There is no recommendation for multiple course of steroids. In fact, it is associated with various adverse effects:

  Fetal effects
  - Growth delay
  - Profound suppression of fetal breathing and movement
  - Impaired myelination
  - Cerebral palsy
  - Microcephaly
  - Lung development problems
  - Reduction in birth weight
  - Necrotizing enterocolitis
  - Placental infarction
  - Adrenal gland insufficiency

  Maternal effects
  - Increased risk of infection
  - Suppression of hypothalamopituitary–adrenal axis.

A rescue course of two doses of 12 mg betamethasone or four doses of 6 mg dexamethasone should only be considered with caution in those pregnancies where the first course was given at less than 26 + 0 weeks of gestation and another obstetric indication arises later in pregnancy.

Side Effects of Steroids

- Maternal infection [PROM]
- Abnormal glucose tolerance test–worsen existing DM
- Pulmonary edema when given with a tocolytic agent in the setting of an underlying infection.

ANTIBIOTICS

Indications and non-indications for intrapartum antibiotic prophylaxis to prevent early onset group B streptococcal (GBS) disease.

Indications	Nonindications
• Previous infant with invasive GBS disease • GBS bacteriuria during any trimester of the current pregnancy	• Colonization with GBS during the previous pregnancy • GBS bacteriuria during previous pregnancy
• Positive GBS screening culture during current pregnancy (unless a cesarean delivery is performed before onset of labor on a woman with intact amniotic membranes) • Unknown GBS status at the onset of labor (culture not done, incomplete or results unknown) and any of the following: –Delivery at <37 weeks of gestation –Amniotic membrane rupture ≥18 hrs –Intrapartum temperature ≥100.4°F (38°C) –Intrapartum nucleic acid amplification Test (optional) positive for GBS	• Cesarean delivery performed before onset of labor on a woman with intact amniotic membranes, regardless of GBS colonization status or gestational age • Negative vaginal and rectal GBS screening culture result in late gestation (35–37 weeks) during the current pregnancy regardless of intrapartum risk factors

What we follow is risk-based approach, with this approach, we will be able to prevent early onset neonatal disease by 69% vs 86% by universal screening approach.

Treatment of GBS carrier before pregnancy has no benefit. Immunization satrategies are currently being evaluated.

Treat symptomatic bacteriuria during prenatal period.

Intrapartum prophylaxis is for 48 hrs or until delivery occurs whichever is earlier. Antibiotic prophylaxis need not be continued after delivery.

Flow chart 13.4: Antibiotic prophylaxis

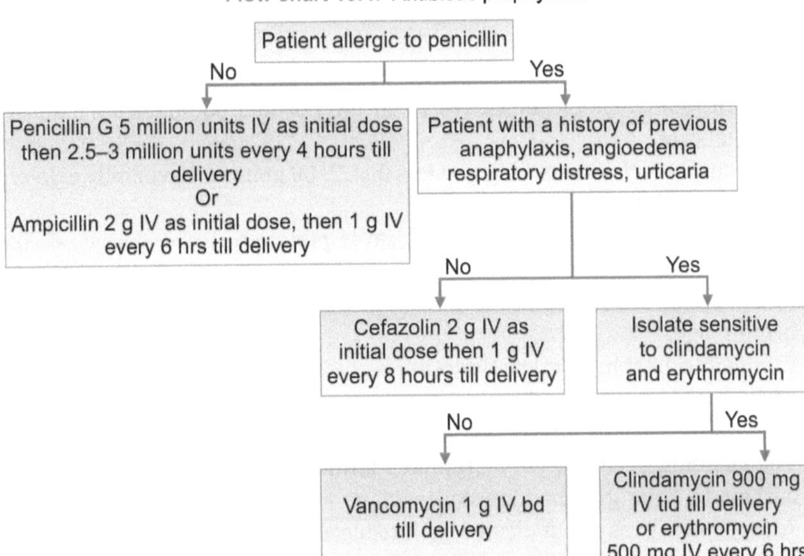

ADJUNCTIVE PROPHYLACTIC ANTIBIOTIC THERAPY

ORACLE 2 for Spontaneous Preterm

- In the absence of overt infections, use of antibiotics in preterm labor with intact membranes does not contribute positively to the neonatal outcome.
- Also showed increased risk of cerebral palsy with erythromycin or co-amoxiclav.
- Only GBS prophylaxis is recommended.

So adjunctive prophylactic antibiotic therapy in threatened or actual preterm labor, for the purpose of preventing preterm delivery and maternal and fetal infectious morbidity is not indicated.

ORACLE 1 for PPROM

- Erythromycin 250 mg 6th hourly for 10 days or until delivery whichever is earlier has been found to be effective in preventing infectious morbidity but ORACLE children study 1 showed it did not make a substantial difference to the children's health and development.
- Co-amoxiclav was associated with an increase in risk of NEC.

In the presence of signs of intrauterine infections (e.g. maternal pyrexia, maternal tachycardia, fetal tachycardia, persistent uterine tenderness, offensive vaginal discharge with increased white cell count and CRP) in spontaneous pretem, PROM and PPROM following regimen is used:

- Inj. Ampicillin 2 g IV stat followed by 1 g IV 6th hrly, inj gentamicin 160 mg IV/IM daily and inj metronidazole 500 mg IV tid till delivery followed by cap. ampicillin 500 mg 6th hrly for 5 days.

Emergency Cesarean delivery spontaneous pretem, PROM and PPROM-GBS prophylaxis + inj gentamicin 160 mg IV single dose + inj metronidazole 500 mg IV 4 doses followed by oral ampicillin 500 mg qid for 5 days.

MANAGEMENT OF LABOR

- Preterm infants should be delivered in the hospital equipped for intensive neonatal care.
- Premature breech infants weighing less than 2500 grams are generally delivered by cesarean delivery.
- If presentation is cephalic, vaginal birth is preferred in the absence of fetal distress.
- Every effort should be made to avoid fetal hypoxia and intraventricular hemorrhage.
- Continuous fetal heart rate monitoring is preferred.
- Birth should be gentle and slow to avoid rapid compression and decompression of the head.
- The membranes should not be ruptured artificially. The amniotic fluid acts as cushion for the soft premature skull with its widely separated sutures.
- An episiotomy may be indicated, as it reduces pressure on the fetal head.

- Spontaneous delivery is preferred when possible, low forceps, however, may be needed occasionally to guide the head over the perineum. The forceps acts like a protective cage. Ventouse delivery is contraindicated before 34 weeks of gestation.
- Delayed cord clamping confers an advantage to the neonate (Reduction in the need for infant transfusion anemia and a reduction in IVH).
- Breech presentation poses special problems. The preterm breech is at risk for prolapse of umbilical cord and entrapment of the head. For these reasons, cesarean should be considered for any infant in breech presentation whose weight is estimated at less than 2500 grams.
- Precipitous and unattended births are dangerous for preterm infant.
- Every effort should be made to have an appropriate resuscitative team and senior pediatrician.
- If delivery is not imminent, transport of the mother to an appropriate center staffed and equipped for high-risk infants, offers the best prognosis for these infants.

NEONATAL COMPLICATIONS

Organ or System	Short-term problems	Long-term problems
Pulmonary	Respiratory distress syndrome, air leak, bronchopulmonary dysplasia, apnoea of prematurity	Bronchopulmonary dysplasia, reactive airway disease, asthma
Gastrointestinal or nutritional	Hyperbilirubinemia, feeding intolerance, necrotizing enterocolitis, growth failure	Failure to thrive, short-bowel syndrome, cholestasis
Immunological	Hospital-acquired infection, immune deficiency, perinatal infection	Respiratory syncytial virus infection, bronchiolitis
Central nervous system	Intraventricular hemorrhage, periventricular leukomalacia, hydrocephalus	Cerebral palsy, hydrocephalus, cerebral atrophy, neurodevelop-mental delay, hearing loss
Ophthalmological	Retinopathy of prematurity	Blindness, retinal detachment, myopia, strabismus
Cardiovascular	Hypotension, patent ductus arteriosus, pulmonary hypertension	Pulmonary hypertension, hypertension in adulthood
Renal	Water and electrolyte imbalance, acid-base disturbances	Hypertension in adulthood
Hematological	Iatrogenic anemia, polycythemia, need for frequent transfusions, anemia of prematurity	
Endocrinological	Hypoglycemia, transiently low thyroxine levels, cortisol deficiency, hypothermia	Impaired glucose regulation, increased insulin resistance

CHAPTER

14

Premature Rupture of Membranes

DEFINITION

Rupture of fetal membranes before the onset of uterine contractions.
Incidence: 10%

- 80% of term PROM go into labor in 24 hrs.
- 95% within 72 hrs.

Risk factors:

- Uterine overdistension (multiple gestation, polyhydramnios)
- Genital tract infections
- Cervical insufficiency
- Amniocentesis
- Malpresentations and malpositions
- Coitus
- Maternal smoking, cocaine abuse

MANAGEMENT

Confirm the diagnosis.

- History
- Sterile speculum examination
- Pad for observation

CLINICAL EXAMINATION

1. General condition: See for evidence of infection such as maternal tachycardia, febrile morbidity, uterine tenderness, presence of purulent discharge, fetal tachycardia.
2. Abdominal examination: Symphysis fundal height, adequacy of liquor, EFW.
3. Per-speculum examination—leak, cervical length, any purulent discharge, evidence of bleeding (associated risk of abruption), any cord events.
4. Pad for observation if diagnosis of leak is inconclusive and to be observed for 48 hrs. Repeated dry pads and normal AFI on scan makes the diagnosis of PROM unlikely.

Investigations

- CBC, blood grouping and typing.
- C-reactive protein (unreliable).
- Urine routine and culture sensitivity.
- Swabs—high vaginal, endocervical, rectal.
- HIV, HBSAg, VDRL, Blood grouping.
- Obstetric scan for AFI (obvious only if substantial loss), cervical length, EFW, placental location, also associated anomalies can be ruled out.
    - Special tests for amniotic fluid are nitrazine test (sensitivity–90%, false positive rate–17%), ferning test, nile blue sulfate test, indigo carmine dye injection test (not routinely recommended unless diagnosis is inconclusive).
    - Fetal fibronectin if positive—confirmatory test (specificity–97%, sensitivity–94%)
    - Insulin-like growth factor binding protein (specificity–97%, sensitivity– 75%).
    - Biophysical testing–NST
    - Avoid digital examination during expectant management as it prevents infection and increases delivery period.

Flow chart 14.1: Management of PROM

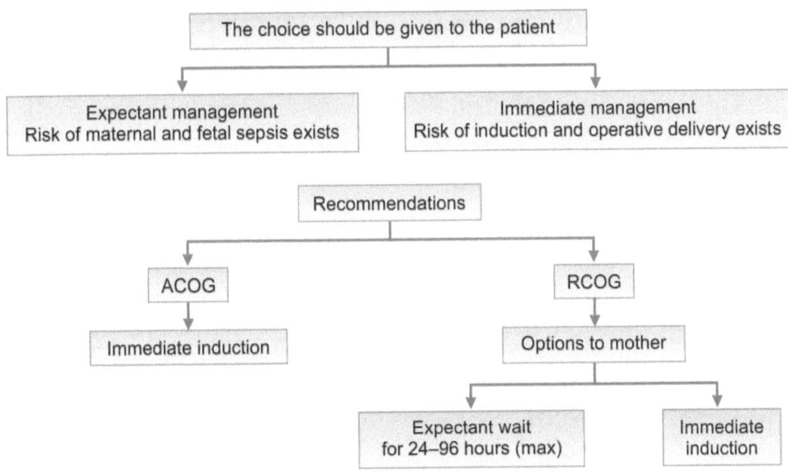

80% will go into labor in 24 hrs, if not after 18 hrs.

- Start on prophylactic antibiotics in expectant management.
- Ideally wait for not more than 6 hrs in our set-up from the time of active leak (increased chances of infection with increasing duration after 6 hrs).
- Induction is recommended after 6 hrs of leak.
- Induction agents: PGE2 gel to be avoided because of leakage of fluid and chance of infection and oxytocin (bishop score decides).
- During labor monitoring for the evidence of infection, fetal status with cardiotocography (CTG).

Antibiotics: Same as preterm

Flow chart 14.2: Management of term PROM

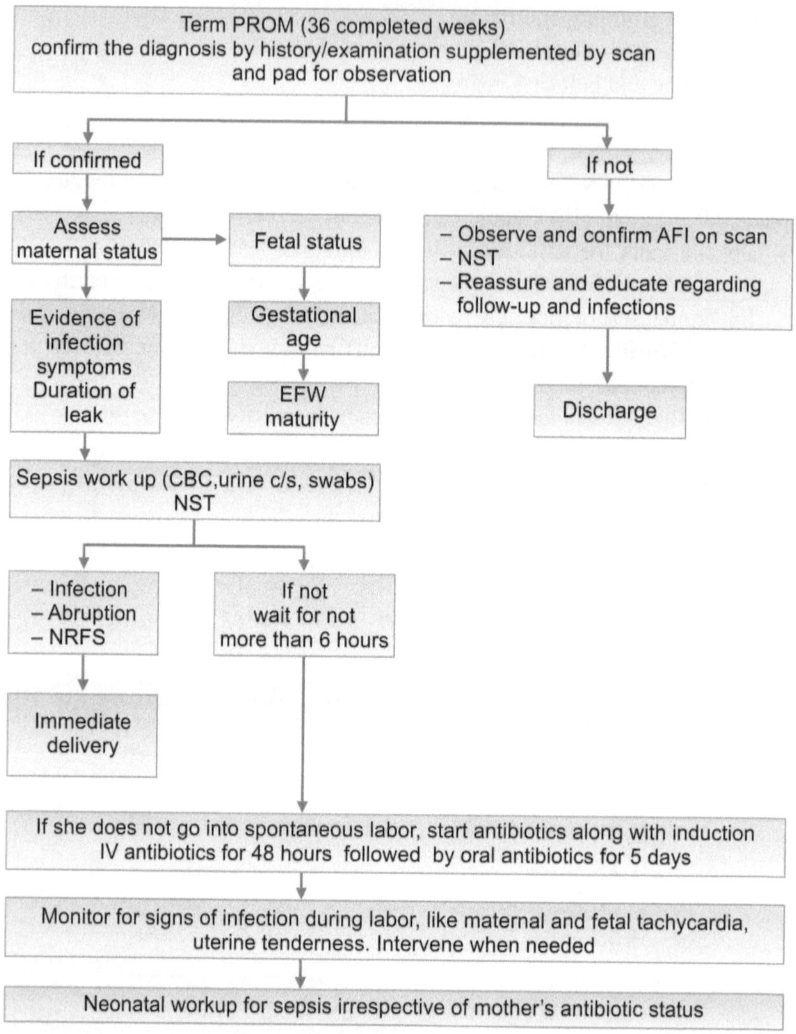

PROM AFTER 35 COMPLETED WEEKS

- The woman should be given the choice of either expectant management or immediate induction of labor.
- Expectant management of women with prelabor rupture of the membranes at term should not exceed 96 hours following membrane rupture, however, it is recommended that induction should commence after 36 hours.
- Prostaglandins or oxytocin can be used when induction of labor is undertaken in either nulliparous or multiparous women with ruptured membranes, regardless of their cervical status, as they are equally effective.

- Currently there is no indication that women with PROM require antibiotic prophylaxis if they are at term.
- A lower vaginal swab should be taken at the time of admission with PROM to exclude Group B streptococcus.

Maternal Risks Due to PROM

- Acute chorioamnionitis
- Subacute chorioamnionitis
- Abruption
- Postpartum endometritis
- Sepsis
- Death

Diagnosis of Chorioamnionitis

- Fever >100°F
  and
  Two or more of the following:
- Maternal tachycardia (>100 b/min)
- Fetal tachycardia (>160 b/min)
- Uterine tenderness
- Maternal leukocytosis (>15,000/mm^3)
- Foul smelling vaginal discharge
- C-reactive protein >2.7 mg/dl

CHAPTER

15

Preterm Premature Rupture of Membranes

When membrane rupture occurs before 37 weeks' gestation, it is known as preterm PROM.

DIAGNOSIS AND MANAGEMENT OF PRETERM PROM (PPROM)

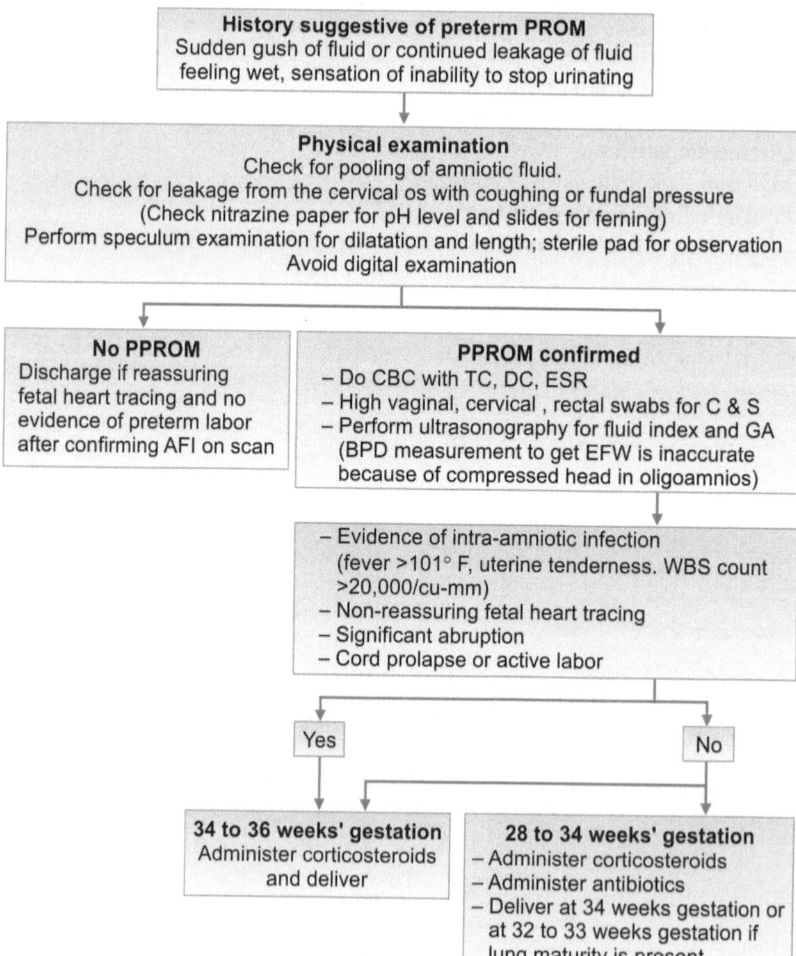

EXPECTANT LINE OF MANAGEMENT

Clinical Surveillance

Maternal FHR, contractions, uterine tenderness, fever ≥38°C
BPP/NST for variable decelerations, fetal tachycardia and absent movements.

Laboratory Tests

WBC >20,000/cu-mm (sensitivity 23–80%, specificity 60–95%, PPV 50–75%, NPV 40–90%).

Antibiotics

Antibiotics. Improve neonatal outcome

- Prevent infectious morbidity
- Prolong latency

Cochrane review—reduction in maternal infection, delay in delivery, neonatal infection, surfactant requirement.

GBS Prophylaxis

Pencillin G 5 million units IV stat followed by 2.5 million units IV 4th hrly.

or

Ampicillin 2 g IV stat followed by 1 g IV 4th hrly.

or

Cefazolin 2 g IV followed by 1 g 8th hrly.

Erythromycin (250 mg orally 6 hrly) should be given for 10 days following the diagnosis of PPROM.

- Co-amoxiclav is not recommended for women with PPROM because of concerns about necrotizing enterocolitis.
- But we follow inj. ampicillin 2 g IV stat followed by 1 g IV 6 hrly then cap. ampicillin 500 mg 6th hrly for 5 days.

Management During Labor

- If the GBS status of the patient is unknown, appropriate parenteral antibiotics (IV ampicillin 2 g IV stat and 1 g IV every 6 hours, gentamycin 160 mg IM daily and metronidazole IV 500 mg every 12 hours) should be administered during labor.

Steroids

Steroids before 34 weeks—fetal lung maturity.

Betamethasone 12 mg IM 24 hrs apart 2 doses or dexamethasone 6 mg IM every 12 hrs–4 doses

(Betamethasone is preferred because chance of periventricular leukomalacia is less with betemethasone).

Tocolytics

- No role of prophylactic tocolysis
- Therapeutic tocolysis to achieve lung maturity

CHAPTER

16

Prolonged Pregnancy

DEFINITION

Prolonged pregnancy is defined as pregnancy lasting 42 completed weeks (294 days) or more from the first day of the last menstrual period.

DIAGNOSIS

- Based on gestational age (294 days from LMP) in a woman with regular menstrual cycles and is sure of her dates.
- Early pregnancy ultrasound scan (up to 24 weeks), if cycles irregular or woman not sure of dates.

PREVENTION OF PROLONGED PREGNANCY

- Membrane stripping weekly from 38 completed weeks/every 72 hours if she comes at 40 weeks of gestation.

MANAGEMENT

Complicated: Pregnancy is not allowed beyond 40 weeks, early delivery may be indicated depending on the condition.

Uncomplicated: Fetal monitoring is started after 40 weeks, to identify onset of uteroplacental insufficiency and fetal hypoxia. The methods recommended are:

- Daily fetal movement score
- Nonstress test/Modified manning—Frequency of testing to be individualized according to the case.
- Amniotic fluid index
- Biophysical profile—When modified manning score is abnormal.

Management Options

Expectant Management

Done when fetal surveillance is normal till gestational age up to 41 weeks

Induction of Labor

Indicated when benefits of delivery outweigh the risk of continuing the pregnancy to the mother or fetus.

- Gestational age >41 weeks (Policy of induction after 41 weeks of gestation slightly reduces the risk of perinatal death and incidence of cesarean delivery).
- Gestational age <41 weeks, if fetus is compromised on antenatal fetal survillence (either clinical or sonographic methods).

Induction in Prolonged Pregnancy

If cervix is favorable (Modified Bishop score >6):

- Misoprostol 50 μgm orally/25 μgm vaginally every 4 hours for maximum 6 doses.
- Low/High dose oxytocin regimen and amniotomy.

If cervix is unfavorable (Modified Bishop score <6):

- Prostaglandin E2 gel 0.5 g intracervical, maximum 3 doses 6 hours apart.
- Foley's bulb: Catheter no. 12F introduced intracervically, the bulb lying above the internal os and inflated with 30 ml of normal saline. Retained for maximum of 12 hours.
- No oxytocin should be started within 4 hours of vaginal prostaglandins, 2 hours of oral prostaglandins and 1 hour of ARM.
- Amniotomy should be tried first before considering oxytocin augmentation for inadequate uterine action.
- Prostaglandins should not be used for augmentation of labor unless uterine contractions are <2 contractions lasting for <20 sec, where the cervix is not well-effaced.

Intrapartum Management

- Monitor progress of labor, use partograph.
- Early amniotomy in early active labor to diagnose thick meconium-stained liquor.
- Careful monitoring of fetal heart in cases of induced labor/oligoamnios.

Complications

Intrapartum

- Fetal asphyxia due to uteroplacental insufficiency
- Cord compression due to oligoamnios
- Meconium passage
- Shoulder dystocia in macrosomic baby (10% of prolonged pregnancy)

Neonatal

- Neonatal depression with asphyxia
- Meconium aspiration
- Birth injuries
- Hypoglycemia
- Polycythemia
- Hypothermia

Indications of Cesarean Delivery

- Failed induction of labor (failure to enter active labor with maximum dose of inducing/ripening agent, surgical method to be tried before labeling as failed induction).

- Nonreassuring fetal heart status.
- Cephalo-pelvic disproportion.

Flow chart 16.1: Management of prolonged pregnancy

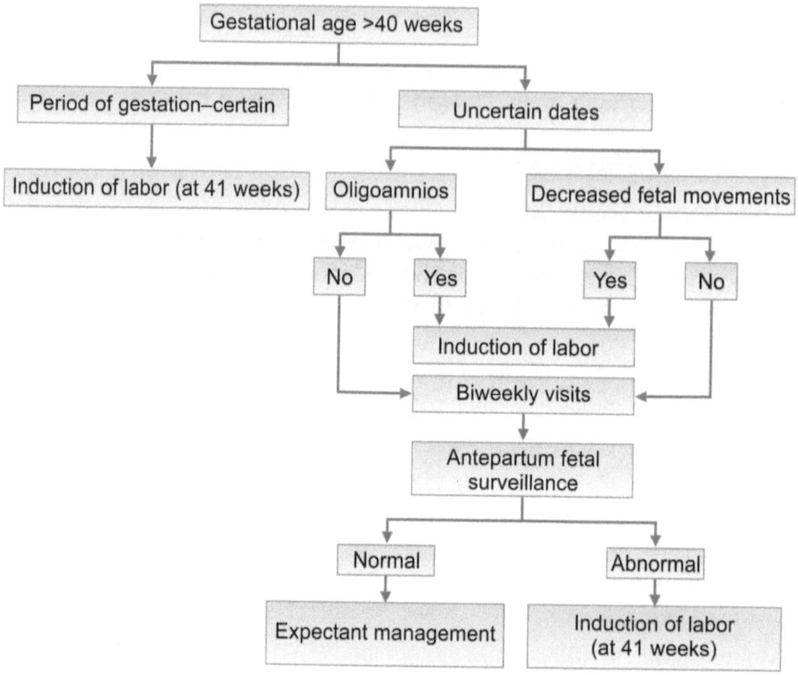

Features of Postmaturity Syndrome

- Wrinkled (sometimes peeling) skin
- Meconium-stained skin and nails
- Long nails
- Calcified skull
- Thin body due to wasting of subcutaneous fat
- Little or no vernix
- No lanugo
- Alert look.

Reliability of the EDD

Excellent Dates

1. Adequate clinical information (known LMP: 28–30 days cycle: no use of hormonal contraception in the past 3 months: uterine size in agreement with dates) PLUS ultrasound examination between 16 and 24 weeks in agreement with the clinical estimation of gestational age.

2. Inadequate clinical information but with two ultrasound examinations between 16 and 24 weeks showing linear fetal growth and similar EDD.

Good Dates

1. Adequate clinical information and one confirming ultrasound examination obtained after 24 weeks of gestation.
2. Inadequate clinical information and two or more ultrasound examinations showing adequate growth and similar EDD.

Poor Dates

Any clinical situation different from those listed above.

CHAPTER

17

Previous LSCS (Vaginal Birth after Cesarean Delivery)

DEFINITION OF TERMS

Planned VBAC

Planned VBAC (vaginal birth after cesarean) refers to any woman who has experienced a prior cesarean birth who plans to deliver vaginally rather than by ERCS (elective repeat cesarean section).

Successful and Unsuccessful Planned VBAC

A vaginal birth (spontaneous or assisted) in a woman undergoing planned VBAC indicates a successful VBAC.

Birth by emergency cesarean section during the labor indicates an unsuccessful VBAC.

Maternal Outcomes

- Uterine rupture is defined as a disruption of the uterine muscle extending to and involving the uterine serosa or disruption of the uterine muscle with extension to the bladder or broad ligament.
- Uterine dehiscence is defined as disruption of the uterine muscle with intact uterine serosa.

Risk factors for uterine rupture during atrial of labor after cesarean delivery:

1. **Type of scar**

   Spontaneous rupture of an UNSCARRED uterus-1/15,000

   The rate of uterine rupture with–

   - One low transverse: 0.36–0.85% (0.68%)
   - Two low transverse: 0.92%
   - Classical cesarean: 4–9% (12%)
   - Inverted T/J shaped scar: 1.9%
   - Low vertical: 1–7% (2%)

   Inadvertent uterine extension at the time of primary cesarean is associated with an increased risk (6% vs. 0.7%) of uterine rupture when compared with no prior extension, and this factor should be considered at least as a caution, if not contraindication, for planned VBAC.

   Women who have undergone abdominal myomectomy where the intrauterine cavity had been breached are also at increased risk of uterine rupture (but unable to quantify); there is a consensus opinion that the degree of myometrial disruption would warrant cesarean delivery.

2. **Number of previous cesareans**
No major differences between the rates of VBAC success (75% vs. 70%), uterine rupture (0.7% vs. 1.6%) and hysterectomy (0.2% vs. 0.5%) between women with one previous cesarean compared to two previous cesarean deliveries. Hence, planned VBAC is considered safe and appropriate for most women who have had a single prior cesarean delivery and for some women who have had two previous cesareans provided they have factors prognostic for successful VBAC.
Previous uterine rupture: This is an absolute contraindication.
3. **Previous vaginal delivery**
Previous vaginal delivery protects against uterine rupture
The risk for a uterine scar separation is lower with each additional sucessful VBAC.
    - TOL (trial of labor) success rate should be: 60–80%
    - VBAC rate = #VBACs/# pts with prior CDs × 100 (CD-cesarean delivery)
    - VBAC success rate = #VBACs/# pts who had TOL after CD × 100
    - Overall success rate is–75%
    - Success rate with history of CD for breech–90%
    - Success rate with history of CD for fetal distress–80%
    - Success rate with history of CD for dystocia–70%
    - Previous vaginal delivery lowered the uterine rupture rate–60%.
4. **Inter-delivery interval**
For women with inter-delivery interval of 12 months or less, the rate of uterine rupture is 2.8% compared to 1% for women with longer interdelivery intervals. A short inter-delivery interval increases risks of both placenta previa and placental abruption.
5. **Postpartum fever after CS**
Febrile morbidity at the time of CS might predispose to poor wound healing and fever after the previous CS is a contraindication to TOLAC.
6. **Maternal age**
>30 years may be associated with a higher risk of rupture.
7. **Uterine anomalies**
The rate of uterine rupture is 8% in women with known Mullerian duct anomalies compared to 0.6% for women without these anomalies.

Table 17.1: Risks of planned VBAC labors from NICHD study (N = 17, 898 planned VBACs)

	Induced	Augmented	Spontaneous	Overall (all planned VBACs)
Uterine rupture	Overall	87 per 10,000	36 per 10,000	69 per 10,000
	102 per 10,000 (1.0%)	0.9%	0.4%	0.7%
	PG method			
	104 per 10,000 (1.4%)			
	Non-PG method			
	89 per 10,000 (0.9%)			
Unsuccessful VBAC (cesarean)	33%	26%	19%	27%
Successful VBAC	67%	74%	81%	73%

PLANNED VBAC IN SPECIAL CIRCUMSTANCES

1. **Macrosomia**
   Significantly decreased likelihood of successful trial of VBAC for pregnancies with infants weighing 4000 g or more (55–67%) compared to smaller infants (75–83%).
2. **Gestation beyond the estimated date of delivery (>41 wks)**
   Induction of labor compared to spontaneous labor is associated with increased risks of emergency cesarean section (by 1.5-fold) and uterine scar rupture (by 2–3 fold).
   Schedule a 'provisional ERCS' at around 40 + 10 days and converting to induction of labor depending on the clinical review at 40 + 10.
   This review should assess: Her likelihood of successful VBAC (e.g. favorable cervix, previous vaginal birth, absence of any obstetric or fetal complications); the priority attached to achieving vaginal birth (such as her plans for many future pregnancies); her understanding of the increased maternal and perinatal risks if induction is chosen; her preference for membrane sweep, spontaneous VBAC, induced (amniotomy or PG) VBAC or ERCS.
3. **Thickness of LUS**
   Ultrasound examination of the uterus might be a useful tool for identification of women at high risk for uterine rupture. The risk was 0% with LUS more than 4.5 mm, 0.6% with LUS 3.6 to 4.5 mm thick, 6.6% with LUS 2.6 to 3.5 mm thick and 9.8% with LUS less than 2.5 mm thick.
4. **More than one previous cesarean delivery**
   It is reasonable to consider women with two previous low transverse cesarean deliveries to be candidates for TOLAC.
5. **Previous low vertical incision**
   They have similar rates of successful vaginal delivery compared with women with a previous low transverse uterine incision.
6. **Unknown type of previous uterine incision**
   TOLAC is not contraindicated for women with one previous cesarean delivery with an unknown uterine scar type unless there is a high clinical suspicion of a previous classical uterine incision.
7. **Twin gestation**
   The similar successful rates of VBAC in twin pregnancies to that in singleton pregnancies (65–84%). No longer twin pregnancy is a contraindication to VBAC.
8. **Preterm birth**
   Planned VBAC success rates for preterm and term pregnancies were similar (72.8% vs. 73.3%), however, the rates of uterine rupture (34 per 10,000 vs. 74 per 10,000, respectively) and dehiscence (26 per 10,000 vs. 67 per 10,000 respectively) are significantly lower in preterm compared with term VBAC. Perinatal outcomes were similar with preterm VBAC and preterm ERCS–74%) but with a lower risk of uterine rupture.

PLANNED VBAC ADVERSE MATERNAL OUTCOMES

Maternal morbidity is increased in planned VBAC compared to ERCS–

- Increased the risk of uterine rupture (0.5% vs. 0.02%)

- Blood transfusion (1.7% vs. 1.0%)
- Endometritis (2.9% vs. 1.8%).

Unsuccessful compared to successful VBAC
- Increased the risk of uterine rupture (2.3% vs. 0.11%)
- Uterine dehiscence (2.1% vs. 0.15%)
- Hysterectomy (0.5% vs. 0.15%)
- Transfusion (3.2% vs. 1.2%)
- Endometritis (7.7% vs. 1.2%).

Planned VBAC Adverse Perinatal Outcome Includes—

- 10 per 10,000 prospective risk of antepartum stillbirth beyond 39 weeks whilst awaiting spontaneous labor.
- 8 per 10,000 risk of hypoxic ischemic encephalopathy, HIE (approximately half of the increased risk of HIE is related to uterine rupture and is 4.6 per 10,000).
- 4 per 10,000 risk of term delivery-related perinatal death (compared to 1 per 10,000 risk with ERCS).

PLANNED ERCS AND ADVERSE PERINATAL OUTCOME

- Increased the risks of transient tachypnea of the newborn (TTN) (5% vs. 2%) and respiratory distress syndrome (RDS) (0.5% vs.<0.05%).
- Increased the risk of maternal mortality (13 per 100,000 vs. 4 per 100,000).

3-fold increase (0.38% vs. 0.13%; OR 2.90 [95% CI 1.74–4.81]) for one or more serious adverse perinatal outcomes (antepartum stillbirth, term delivery-related perinatal death or HIE) for planned VBAC at term compared to ERCS. Hence, it is estimated that planned VBAC exposes the woman to a very low additional 0.25% risk (or 1 in 400) for experiencing an adverse perinatal outcome compared to opting for ERCS at 39 + 0 weeks' gestation.

In a hypothetical group of 100,000 women of any gestational age, planned VBAC compared to ERCS is associated with: lower (4 vs. 13) maternal death, higher (325 vs. 26) uterine rupture and higher (130 vs. 50) perinatal death.

The risk of uterine rupture is 50 per 10,000 for planned VBAC and 2 per 10,000 for ERCS.

Table 17.2: Risks and benefits of opting for VBAC vs ERCS at 39 + 0 weeks gestation

	Planned VBAC	ERCS at 39+0 weeks
Mother benefits	72–76% chance of successful VBAC: if successful, shorter hospital stay and recovery. Increases likelihood of future vaginal birth.	Able to plan to know delivery date. Less risk of blood transfusion (1%) and endometritis (1.8%)[a]. Extremely low-risk of uterine scar rupture (<0.02%). Protects pelvic floor, reduction of urinary incontinence. Option for sterilization if fertility complete.

Contd...

Contd...

Mother risks	0.5% risk of uterine scan rupture-if occurs associated with maternal morbidity and fetal morbidity/mortality. 24–28% chance of emergency cesarean. 10–15% chance of instrumental delivery and perineal tear/episiotomy. Higher risk of blood transfusion (1.7%) and endometritis (2.9%)[a].	0.1–2% risk of surgical complications. Longer recovery. Future pregnancies: likely to require cesarean delivery, increased risk of placenta previa/accreta and adhesions with successive cesarean deliveries. Increased risk of maternal death (13 per 100,000 vs. 4 per 100,000) compared with planned VBAC (at any gestation); although absolute risks are extremely low.
Infant benefits	Reduced (1%) risk of transient respiratory morbidity.	Avoids 10 per 10,000 risk of stillbirth beyond 39+0 weeks. Virtually 0 (≤1 per 10,000) risk of delivery-related perinatal death or hypoxic ischemic encephalopathy (HIE).
Infant risks	10 per 10,000 prospective risk of antepartum stillbirth beyond 39+0 weeks whilst awaiting spontaneous labor.[b] 8 per 10,000 (0.08%) risk of hypoxic ischemic encephalopathy (HIE). 4 per 10,000 (0.04%) risk of delivery-related perinatal death.	Marginally higher (2–3%) risk of transient respiratory morbidity [6% risk if delivery performed at 38 instead of 39 weeks, but additional risk minimized if antenatal corticosteroids administered].

The estimates of risk for adverse maternal or fetal events in VBAC are based on women receiving continuous electronic monitoring during their labor.
[a]In the NICHD study there was no statistically significant difference between planned VBAC and ERCS groups in relation to hysterectomy (23 per 10,000 vs. 30 per 10,000), thromboembolic disease (4 per 10,000 vs. 6 per 10,000).
[b]A retrospective cohort study in Scotland showed that the risk of unexplained stillbirth associated with previous cesarean differed with gestational age; the excess risk was apparent from 34 weeks' gestation at a hazard ratio of 2.23 (95% CI 1.48–3.36).

How should Future Pregnancies be Managed after Uterine Rupture?

Rate of repeat rupture is 6% when the ruptured scar is confined to lower segment and 32% when it includes the upper segment of uterus. So women who have had previous uterine rupture should undergo elective section at 37 completed weeks.

How should Second Trimester Delivery or Delivery of an Intrauterine Fetal Demise be Accomplished in Women with a Previous Cesarean Delivery?

Second trimester abortion: Dilatation and evacuation as well as induction of abortion with prostaglandins are reasonable options (scar rupture is 1%).

In patients after 28 weeks of gestation with an intrauterine fetal demise and a prior cesarean scar, cervical ripening with a transcervical Foley catheter has been associated with uterine rupture rates comparable with spontaneous labor.

Candidates for VBAC

The following recommendations are based on good and consistent scientific evidence (Level A):

- One previous cesarean delivery with a low transverse scar.

The following recommendations are based on limited or inconsistent scientific evidence (Level B):

- Two previous low transverse cesarean.
- Multiple gestation with one previous low transverse cesarean delivery.
- External cephalic version for breech presentation is not contraindicated in women with a prior low transverse uterine incision.
- Previous cesarean delivery with an unknown uterine scar.

Contraindications for VBAC

- Previous classical or inverted T-shaped uterine scar.
- Previous 3 or more cesarean deliveries.
- Previous hysterotomy or myomectomy.
- Previous uterine scar.
- Presence of a condition which is contraindicated to vaginal deliveries such as placenta previa or malpresentation.

Risk Factors for Unsuccessful VBAC

- Induced labor
- No previous vaginal birth
- BMI >30
- Previous cesarean for dystocia.

When all these risk factors are present, success rate is achieved in only 40% of cases.

Successful VBAC

- Previous vaginal birth particularly previous VBAC is the single best predictor for successful VBAC and is associated with 87–90% success. Prior vaginal delivery is also independently associated with a reduced risk of uterine rupture.
- Greater maternal height
- Maternal age <40 years
- BMI <30
- Gestation <40 weeks
- Infant birth weight <4 kg
- Spontaneous onset of labor
- Vertex position
- Fetal head engagement or a lower station
- Higher admission Bishop score

Table 17.3: Risk factors prognostic of successful or unsuccessful VBAC

Successful VBAC	Unsuccessful VBAC
Previous vaginal delivery	No previous vaginal delivery
Spontaneous labor	Induced or augmented labor
Admission cervical dilatation	Admission cervical dilatation
>4 cm	<4 cm
Previous cesarean delivery for fetal malpresentation or non-reassuring fetal well-being	Previous cesarean delivery for cephalopelvic disproportion or failure to progress Previous preterm cesarean delivery

Contd...

Contd...

>18 months from previous	<18 months from previous
Cesarean delivery	Cesarean delivery
BMI <30	BMI >30
Birthweight <4000 g	Birth weight >4000 g Second pregnancy birth weight exceeds the first by >500 g and the prior Cesarean indication was dystocia Post dates (at or after 41 weeks gestation)
Epidural analgesia	No epidural analgesia
Non-advanced maternal age	Advanced maternal age
(<40 years)	(>40 years)
Caucasian ethnicity	Non-Caucasian ethnicity
Maternal stature not short	Short maternal stature
(>150 cm)	(<150 cm)
Female infant	Male infant

VBAC, Vaginal birth after Cesarean.

ANTENATAL COUNSELING

How should Women be Counseled in the Antenatal Period?

They should be informed that, overall, the chances of successful planned VBAC are 72–76%.

After counseling, the ultimate decision to undergo TOLAC or a repeat cesarean delivery should be made by the patient in consultation with her health care provider. The potential risks and benefits of both TOLAC and ERCD should be discussed. Documentation of counseling and the management plan should be included in the medical record.

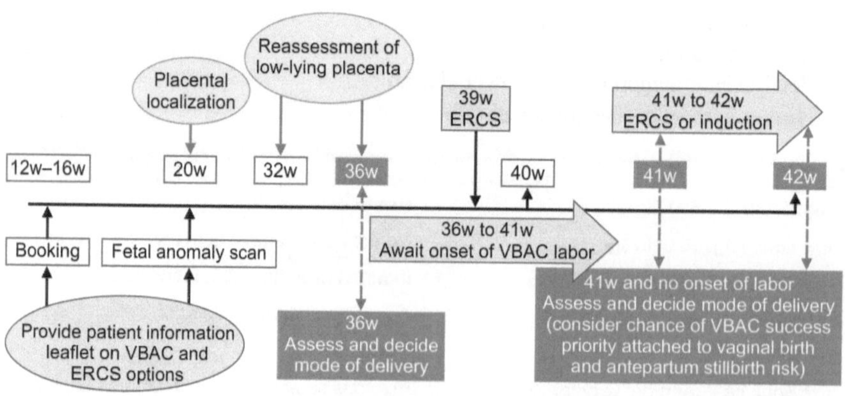

Figure 17.1: Plan of case for singleton uncomplicated pregnancy with previous cesarean delivery. (VBAC, Vaginal birth after cesarean; ERCS, elective repeat cesarean section)

Table 17.4: Items to be discussed during antenatal counseling

Items	Special considerations
1. Review of previous cesarean delivery	Identify indication, uterine incision used and any peri-operative complications.
2. Suitability for VBAC	Any contraindications to VBAC.
3. The maternal and perinatal risks and benefits of VBAC compared with ERCS	Particularly the patient's attitude towards the risks of rare but serious adverse outcomes and how she values them.
4. The likelihood of a successful VBAC	This should be individualized. For example, if patient has had a previous vaginal birth, then VBAC is likely to be successful.
5. Plans for future pregnancies	If a large family is desired, then achieving VBAC may have greater importance as subsequent births would avoid the risks associated with repeated cesarean delivery.
6. Personal preference for mode of delivery	This should be respected

VBAC, vaginal birth after Cesarean; ERCS, elective repeat Cesarean section.

Timing of ERCS

Women considering ERCS should be counseled that delaying delivery by 1 week from 38 to 39 weeks enables around a 5% reduction (6% vs. 1%) in the incidence of respiratory morbidity (particularly reducing the incidence of TTN), but this delay may be associated with a 5 per 10,000 increase in the risk of antepartum stillbirth. Should there be a need to perform ERCS prior to 39 weeks, then prophylactic betamethasone should be administered at least 48 h prior to delivery.

INDUCTION AND AUGMENTATION OF LABOR

How should Women with a Previous Cesarean Birth be Advised in Relation to Induction of Labor or Augmentation?

- Induction (particularly women with an unfavorable cervix or by prostaglandin method) or augmentation of VBAC labor are associated with a 2–3-fold increased risk of uterine rupture and around 1.5-fold increased risk of cesarean section compared to spontaneous VBAC labor.
- The decision to induce the method chosen, the decision to augment with oxytocin, the time intervals for serial vaginal examination and the selected parameters of progress that would necessitate and advise on discontinuing VBAC should be discussed with the woman by a consultant obstetrician.

Induction of Labor

For candidates with an unfavorable cervix:
- Transcervical catheters: Preferable option as there is less chance of rupture.
- Prostaglandin E2: Data are limited. There is increase in uterine rupture only when oxytocin was used after cervical ripening with prostaglandins.

- Misoprostol should not be used for third trimester cervical ripening or labor induction in patients who have had a cesarean delivery or major uterine surgery.
- Risk of uterine rupture–1.02%, 0.87% and 0.36% (2–3 fold increased risk) for induced, augmented, spontaneous labor VBAC respectively.
- Risk of emergency cesarean–33%, 26% and 19% for induced, augmented, and spontaneous labor groups respectively.
- Risk of uterine rupture for prostaglandin and nonprostaglandin induced labor–87 per 10,000 vs. 29 per 10,000) and a higher risk of perinatal death due to uterine rupture (11.2 per 10,000 vs. 4.5 per 10,000).

Augmented VBAC Means that–

- Augmentation is not contraindicated. Oxytocin augmentation should be titrated such that it should not exceed the maximum rate of contractions of 4 in 10 minutes; the ideal contraction frequency would be three to four in 10 minutes.
- Careful serial cervical assessments, preferably by the same person, are necessary to show adequate cervicometric progress, thereby allowing augmentation to continue (>0.5 cm/hr).

Management of Augmentation in Established VBAC Labor

Clinical Management Issues

- The decision for augmentation should follow careful obstetric assessment, maternal counseling and be consultant-led.
- Oxytocin augmentation should be titrated such that it should not exceed the maximum rate of contractions of 4 in 10 min. Particular caution is necessary when using high oxytocin augmentation dose as there is a "dose response" for maximum oxytocin amount and uterine rupture.
- Careful serial cervical assessments, preferably by the same person, are necessary to show adequate cerviocometric progress, thereby allowing augmentation to continue. These intervals should not exceed 4 h.
- If there was less than 2 cm progress after 4 h of oxytocin then cesarean section should be considered. A more conservative threshold of inadequate progress after 2 h of augmentation may also justify consideration for cesarean section depending on the woman's individual circumstances.
- If there was 2 cm or more progress, augmentation should be continued and vaginal examinations performed 4 hourly.

MANAGEMENT OF LABOR

Where and How should VBAC be Conducted?

Should be conducted in tertiary care center where facility for immediate cesarean section and advanced neonatal resuscitation is available.

Analgesia: Epidural analgesia for labor may be used as part of TOLAC.

- Women should be advised to have continuous electronic fetal monitoring.
- Continuous intrapartum care is necessary to enable prompt identification and management of uterine scar rupture.

Early diagnosis of **uterine scar rupture** followed by expeditious laparotomy and resuscitation is essential to reduce associated morbidity and mortality in mother and infant.

Table 17.5: Clinical features associated with uterine rupture in women with previous Cesarean delivery

Risk factors	Symptoms	Signs
Induction (prostaglandin, amniotomy, intracervical Foley catheter)	Severe abdominal pain, especially if persists in between uterine contractions	Abnormal CTG (decelerations, tachycardia, bradycardia)
Augmentation with oxytocin	Acute onset of lower abdominal pain	Loss of station of the presenting part
Abnormal labor progress (prolonged latent phase, dysfunctional or secondary arrest)	Cessation of previously efficient uterine activity Hematuria	Acute onset scar or lower abdominal tenderness
More than one prior Cesarean delivery	Abnormal excessive vaginal bleeding	Maternal tachycardia, hypotension, shock
Previous myomectomy	Post-delivery maternal collapse	
Multiparity*		
Previous uterine perforation at surgery		
Short inter-delivery interval (<18 months) from previous Cesarean		

CTG, cardiotocograph.
*Multiparity is an independent risk factor for uterine rupture. However, prior vaginal delivery appears to be protective against uterine rupture in planned vaginal birth after Cesarean (VBAC). Hence, multiparity may or may not behave as a risk factor for uterine rupture during VBAC labor.

Signs of Uterine Scar Rupture

- Abnormal cardiotocograph (CTG): It is the most consistent finding in uterine rupture and is seen in 55–87% of cases, viable decelerations, fetal tachycardia followed by bradycardia.
- The routine use of intrauterine pressure catheters in the early detection of uterine scar rupture is not recommended.

The diagnosis is ultimately confirmed at emergency cesarean section or postpartum laparotomy.The decision to delivery interval should be 15 minutes to reduce the morbidity and mortality.

Problems Encountered in Repeat Cesarean Delivery

- No proper starvation of patient and hence risk of aspiration during GA.
- Patient is already exhausted, has tachycardia, and a higher risk of infection if she has been leaking for few hours.
- Abdominal scar excision facilitates better healing of the wound later.

- All cases of previous LSCS can have intra-abdominal adhesions, bladder may be drawn up and great care has to be taken while opening the parietal peritoneum so as not to injure the bladder. Also the UV fold has to be opened and pushed down well in order to avoid injury. Sharp dissection is better. Where adhesions are very dense, lateral approach is better for bladder dissection.
- The delivery of head may be difficult if it is deeply engaged and can result in tears of LUS extending upto cervix or extension of incision into broad ligament.
- The thinned out LUS may be hard to suture, and sutures cut through easily.
- Higher risk of atonic uterus and PPH.
- Patients with previous LSCS have a much higher rate of placenta previa and placenta accreta. The management of the same has been discussed in PPH chapter.

Vaginal Delivery

Cut short the second stage of labor with the help of ventouse preferably as it occupies less space compared to obstetric forceps. Manual uterine exploration after VBAC and subsequent repair of asymptomatic scar dehiscence is not recommended. Excessive vaginal bleeding or signs of hypovolemia are potential signs of uterine rupture and should prompt complete evaluation of the genital tract and emergency laparotomy.

Management of Pregnancy after Uterine Rupture

- If the site of ruptured scar is confined to the lower segment of the uterus, rate of repeat rupture or dehiscence in labor is 6%.
- If scar involves upper segment–repeat rupture rate is 32%.
- It is recommended that women with previous uterine rupture should give birth by cesarean delivery at 37 completed weeks.

Second Trimester Abortion or Delivery of IUD in Women with Previous Cesarean Delivery

- Induction of labor with prostaglandins—outcome similar to nonscarred uterus.
- Frequency of rupture: <1%.

CHAPTER

18

Resuscitation in Pregnancy and Puerperium

RESUSCITATION IN PREGNANCY AND PUERPERIUM

- Factors peculiar to pregnancy that weigh the balance against survival include: **Anatomical changes:** Difficult to maintain a clear airway and perform intubation, **Pathological changes:** Laryngeal edema
  Physiological changes: Increased oxygen consumption, increased likelihood of pulmonary aspiration.

In the third trimester the most important factor is compression of the inferior vena cava and impairment of venous return by the gravid uterus when the woman lies supine.

- These difficulties may be exaggerated by obesity.
  Physiological changes in late pregnancy affecting cardiopulmonary resuscitation:

	Changes in pregnancy	Impact on resuscitation
Cardiovascular system		
Plasma volume	Increased by up to 50%	Dilutional anemia Reduced oxygen-carrying capacity
Heart rate	Increased by 15–20 bpm	Increased CPR circulation demands
Cardiac output	Increased by 40% Significantly reduced by pressure of gravid uterus on IVC	Increased CPR circulation demands
Uterine blood flow	10% of cardiac output at term	Potential for rapid massive hemorrhage
Systemic vascular resistance	Decreased	Sequesters blood during CPR
Arterial blood pressure	Decreased by 10–15 mmHg	Decreased reserve
Venous return	Decreased by pressure of gavid uterus on IVC	Increased CPR circulation demands Decreased reserve
Respiratory system		
Respiratory rate	Increased	Decreased buffering capacity, acidosis more likely

Contd...

Contd...

Oxygen consumption	Increased by 20%	Hypoxia develops more quickly
Residual capacity	Decreased by 25%	Decreased buffering capacity, acidosis more likely
Arterial PCO_2	Decreased	Decreased buffering capacity, acidosis more likely
Laryngeal edema	Increased	Difficult intubation
Other changes		
Gastric motility	Decreased	Increased risk of aspiration
Lower esophageal sphincter	Relaxed	Increased risk of aspiration
Uterus	Enlarged	Diaphragmatic splinting reduces residual capacity and makes ventilation more difficult
		Aortocaval compression causes supine hypotension, reduces venous return and significantly impairs CPR
Weight	Increased	Large breasts may interfere with intubation Makes ventilation more difficult

CPR, cardiopulmonary resuscitation; IVC, inferior vena cava; PCO_2, partial pressure of carbon dioxide

Specific Difficulties in Pregnant Patients

- Airway
  - Patient needs to be inclined laterally for:
  - Suction or aspiration
  - Removing dentures or foreign bodies
  - Inserting airways
- Breathing
  - Greater oxygen requirement
  - Reduced chest compliance
  - More difficult to see rise and fall of chest
  - More risk of regurgitation and aspiration
- Circulation

  External chest compression difficult because:
  - Ribs flared
  - Diaphragm raised
  - Patient obese
  - Breasts hypertrophied
  - Supine position causes inferior vena cava compression by the gravid uterus
- DOs
  - A speedy response is essential.
  - Once respiratory or cardiac arrest has been diagnosed, the patient must be positioned appropriately and basic life support started immediately.
  - This must be continued while venous access is secured.
  - Any obvious causal factors are corrected (for example, hypovolemia), and the necessary equipment, drugs, and staff are assembled.

- Aortocaval compression significantly reduces cardiac output from 20 weeks of gestation onwards. Aortocaval compression significantly reduces the efficacy of chest compressions during resuscitation.
- Changes in lung function, diaphragmatic splinting and increased oxygen consumption make the pregnant woman become hypoxic more readily and make ventilation more difficult.
- Difficult intubation is more likely in pregnancy.
- Pregnant women are at an increased risk of aspiration.
- From 20 weeks of gestation onwards, the pressure of the gravid uterus must be relieved from the inferior vena cava and aorta.
- A left lateral tilt of 15° on a firm surface will relieve aortocaval compression in the majority of pregnant women and still allow effective chest compressions to be performed.
- The airway should be protected as soon as possible by intubation with a cuffed endotracheal tube.
- Supplemental oxygen should be administered as soon as possible.
- Bag and mask ventilation should be undertaken until intubation can be achieved.
- In the absence of breathing, despite a clear airway, chest compressions should be commenced immediately.
- Two wide-bore cannulae should be inserted as soon as possible.
- There should be an aggressive approach to volume.
- Abdominal ultrasound by a skilled operator can assist in the diagnosis of concealed hemorrhage.
- The same defibrillation energy levels should be used as in the nonpregnant patient.
- There should normally be no alteration in algorithm drugs or doses.
- Common, reversible causes of maternal cardiopulmonary arrest should be considered throughout the resuscitation process.
- Resuscitation efforts should be continued until a decision is taken by the consultant obstetrician, and consultant anesthetist in consensus with the cardiac arrest team.
- **4 Minute Rule:** Maternal CPR for 4 minutes, infant should be delivered by the 5th minute.
- Perimortem cesarean section should not be delayed by moving the woman—it should be performed where resuscitation is taking place.
- Senior staff with appropriate experience should be involved at an early stage.
- Transfer should be supervised by an adequately skilled team with appropriate equipment.
- In the case of maternal collapse secondary to antepartum hemorrhage, the fetus and placenta should be delivered promptly to allow control of the hemorrhage.
- In the case of massive placental abruption, cesarean section may occasionally be indicated even if the fetus is dead to allow rapid control of the hemorrhage.
- The management of AFE is supportive rather than specific, as there is no proven effective therapy.
- Early involvement of senior experienced staff, including obstetrician, anesthetist, hematologist and intensivist, is essential to optimize the outcome.

- Coagulopathy needs early, aggressive treatment, including aggressive use of fresh frozen plasma.
- After successful resuscitation, cardiac cases should be managed by an expert cardiology team.

BASIC LIFE SUPPORT

Airway

1. Clearly established with—
   a. Head tilt, jaw thrust.
   b. Head tilt, with chin lift maneuver.
2. Suction to be done to aspirate vomiting.
3. Badly filling dentures and other foreign bodies to be removed.
4. Airway should be maintained.
5. These procedures should be performed with patient inclined laterally/supine and uterus displaced.

Breathing

- Intermittent positive pressure ventilation—to be started once the airway is cleared.
  - Mouth to mouth
  - Mouth to nose
  - Mouth to airway
- Ventilation should be carried out until self-inflating bag and mask are available. Ventilation should be continued with 100% oxygen and a reservoir bag.
- Cricoid pressure: It should be applied until airway has been protected by a cuffed endotracheal tube.

Circulation

- Circulatory arrest is diagnosed by the absence of a palpable pulse in a large artery (carotid or femoral).
- Chest compressions are given at the standard rate and ratio of 30:2.

Methods to overcome difficulties:

- Lateral displacement of the uterus: Effective forces for chest compression can be generated with patients inclined at angles of up to 30°.
- The Cardiff resuscitation wedge: It is not commercially available, so other techniques need to be used.

Goal 1 – save the mother
Goal 2 – save the fetus

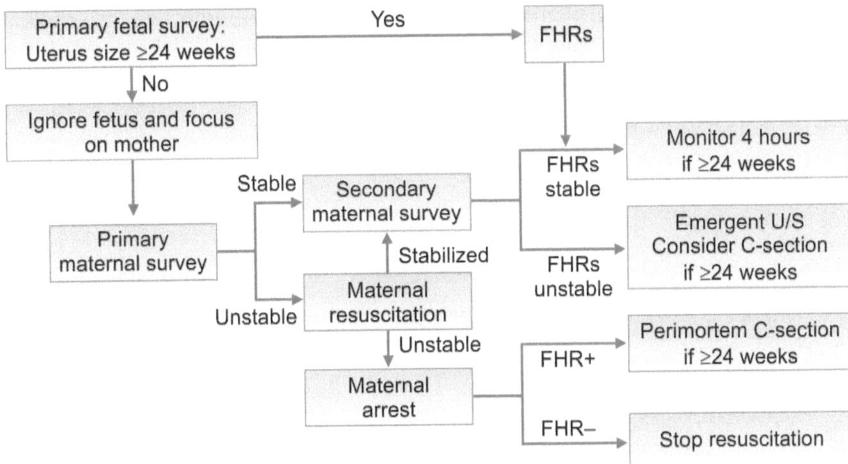

ADVANCED LIFE SUPPORT

Intubation

a. Tracheal intubation should be carried out as soon as facilities and skills are available.
   Difficulties:
   - Short obese neck
   - Full breasts due to pregnancy
b. Mouth to mouth or bag and mask ventilation is best done without pillows under the head and with the head and neck fully extended.
c. In the event of failure to intubate the trachea or ventilate the patient's lungs with a bag and mask, insertion of a laryngeal mask airway should be attempted.
d. Cricoid pressure must be temporarily removed in order to place the laryngeal mask airway successfully. Once the airway is in place, cricoid pressure should be reapplied.

Defibrillation and Drugs

- Defibrillation and drug administration is in accordance with advanced life support recommendations.
- On a practical note, it is difficult to apply an apical defibrillator paddle with the patient inclined laterally, and great care must be taken to ensure that the dependent breast does not come into contact with the hand holding the paddle. This problem is avoided if adhesive electrodes are used.

Cesarean Delivery

- Many successful resuscitations have occurred after prompt surgical intervention.
- The probable mechanism for the favorable outcome is that occlusion of the inferior vena cava is relieved completely by emptying the uterus, whereas it is only partially relieved by manual uterine displacement or an inclined position.

- Delivery also improves thoracic compliance, which will improve the efficacy of chest compressions and the ability to ventilate the lungs.
- <23 weeks gestation survival chance ~ 0%.
- Maternal CPR >20 minutes, fetal survival unlikely.

Resuscitation in Cardiac Arrest

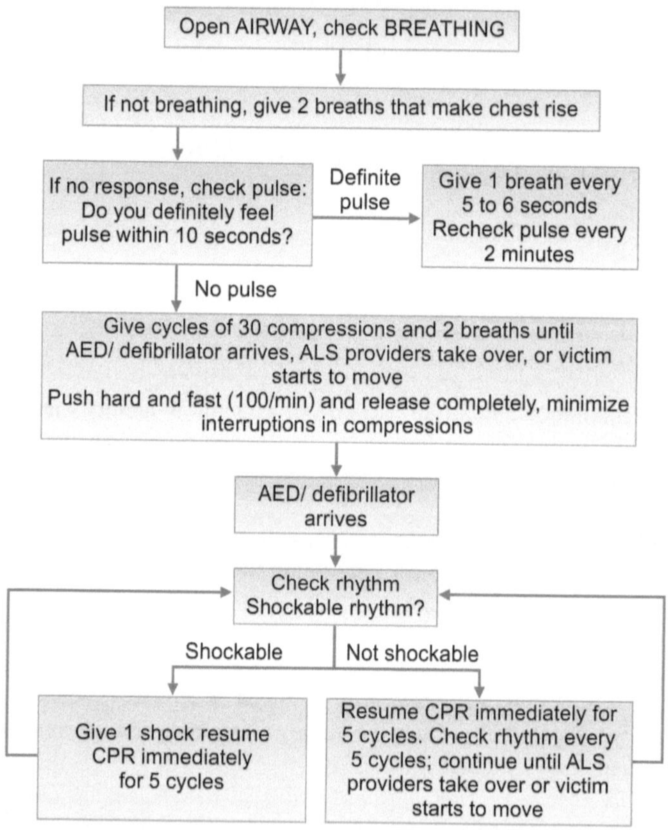

Circulation

Palpation of carotid pulse for at least 5 sec, but not more than 10 sec. If no definite pulse is palpated, then chest compressions are begun at a rate of 100 compressions/ min, alternating with ventilation in 30:2 ratio. Compressions continue at 100/min without stopping ventilation at 10–12 breaths/min.

Return of spontaneous circulatory flow should be re-evaluated, after every 5 cycles or 2 min. After successful return to a perfusing rhythm continue for additional 2 min.

Breathing

In the absence of adequate ventilation, the rescuer will initiate 2 breaths via bag and mask ventilation with 100% oxygen. Breaths should be evaluated and maintained at 10–12 breaths/min.

Airway

Airway patency should be assessed with a head tilt-chin lift maneuver. The patient should be evaluated for spontaneous ventilation, by looking for rise and fall of chest, listening for exhalation and feeling for airflow. A definitive airway may be placed but only by an experienced person. Proper placement of ET tube is confirmed by auscultation and end tidal CO_2 measurement.

At the earliest safe opportunity call for help for assistance.

Advanced Life Support

Intubation

With a cuffed endotracheal tube of 7.5 should be carried out.

Vasopressors

May be used to maintain circulation. Dopamine and norepinephrine may be used.

Defibrillation

Can be used at standard doses.

SECTION 2

LABOR

- Normal Labor
- Malpresentation and Malposition
  - Occipito-Posterior Position
  - Breech Presentation
  - Face Presentation
  - Brow Presentation
  - Transverse Lie
  - Cord Prolapse
  - Shoulder Dystocia
  - Version
- Episiotomy
- Active Management of Third Stage of Labor
- Nutrition in Labor
- Induction of Labor
- Labor Analgesia
- Prolonged Labor
- Obstructed Labor
- Instrumental Delivery
- Cesarean Delivery

CHAPTER

19

Normal Labor

DEFINITION

Labor

It is defined as the series of events that take place in the genital organs in an effort to expel the viable products of conception out of the womb through the vagina to the exterior world.

Normal Labor

WHO defines normal labor as spontaneous in onset, low risk at start and remaining so throughout labor and delivery. The infant is born spontaneously by vertex presentation, at term, and the mother and infant are in good condition after birth.

DIAGNOSIS

- Painful uterine contractions at regular intervals with increasing intensity and frequency
- Cervical dilatation and effacement
- Formation of bag of membranes
- Show

Differences Between True and False Labor

True labor	False labor
1. Contractions occur at regular intervals	Contractions occur at irregular intervals
2. Interval gradually shortens	Interval remains irregular
3. Intensity of pain gradually increases	Intensity of pain remains the same
4. Duration of contractions increases	Duration of contractions varies and tends to become less
5. Progressive cervical effacement and dilatation	No progress in cervical effacement and dilatation
6. Progress of labor not stopped by sedation	Painful contractions are relieved by sedation and there is no progress in labor

STAGES OF LABOR

Stages of labor		Definition	Duration	
			Nullipara	Multipara
First stage	Latent phase	Cervical dilatation <4 cm	12 hr	8 hr
	Active phase	Cervical dilatation >4 cm	6–8 hr or rate of cervical dilatation 1 cm/hr	4–6 hr or rate of cervical dilatation 1.5 cm/hr
Second stage		Full dilatation of cervix to expulsion of fetus	2–3 hrs	1–2 hrs
Third stage		From expulsion of fetus to the delivery of placenta	30 min	30 min

MANAGEMENT OF LABOR

Risk Category

Common Risk Factors

Maternal factors	Past reproductive history	Present pregnancy	Associated medical/surgical problems
• Age: <16 yrs >35 yrs • Parity: 0 stillbirth >5 • Obesity • Height <140 cm	• >1 abortion • Previous stillbirth • Previous cesarean section • Previous PPH/ MRP disorder • Hypertensive disorder complicating pregnancy • IUGR • Congenital anomaly • Previous early neonatal death	• Bleeding in pregnancy • Prematurity, PROM • Postmaturity • Hypertensive disorder complicating pregnancy • IUGR • Multiple pregnancy • Malpresentation • Malposition	• Heart disease • Diabetes • Anemia • Jaundice • Hypertensive • Renal disease • Thyroid disease • Epilepsy • Asthma

History

- Booked or unbooked.
- History of present pregnancy, presenting complaints and any risk factors.
- Obstetric history: Obstetric score and significant history of previous pregnancies.
- Menstrual history—gestational age according to Naegele's rule if cycles are regular of 28 days duration without usage of hormonal contraception in the past 3 months, according to scan if cycles are irregular.
- Past medical and surgical illness and family history.
- If booked case, check previous records.

General Examination

- Height and weight
- Pallor, pedal edema, jaundice and cyanosis
- Vitals and CVS, RS
- Examine breasts, thyroid and spine

Per-abdominal Examination

- Height of the uterus (whether corresponding to gestational age)
- Features of obstructed labor and contour of the uterus
- Presentation, attitude, fetal head (rule of fifths)
- Uterine contractions–+/-, intensity, duration and frequency per 10 minutes
- Amount of liquor
- Size of the baby/estimated baby weight (By Johnson's formula in cephalic presentation, clinically in breech presentation)
- Fetal heart sounds

Per-vaginal Examination

Aseptic precautions—handwashing and sterile gloves.
- Cervical dilatation and effacement
- Presentation and station of presenting part
- Position and degree of flexion (sutures and fontanelle)
- Status of membranes and if leak present, color of liquor
- Cord prolapse or presentation to be ruled out
- Pelvic adequacy and rule out CPD

INVESTIGATIONS

- Hemoglobin, urine routine, blood grouping
- HIV, HbSAg, VDRL
- Admission CTG

CTG

Key Recommendations

1. Fetal heart monitoring is recommended for all women in labor. Intermittent auscultation may be used for low-risk women and electronic fetal monitoring (EFM) for women when an increase in risk has been identified.
2. Cardiotocographs (CTGs) should be labelled with the woman's name, hospital number, date and time of commencement and the woman's heart rate.
3. The current evidence base does not support the use of the admission CTG in low-risk pregnancies and is, therefore, not recommended as a routine.
4. Communication between staff should convey the clinical context and use consistent terminology to describe the features of the CTG, the level of concern and the urgency of the situation. CTGs can be classified as normal, suspicious or pathological.
5. Ideally, intrapartum fetal blood sampling should be available to assess fetal wellbeing in selected cases where the CTG is considered abnormal.

6. Fetal blood sampling is not possible, the baby should be delivered as soon as possible based on the clinical circumstances of the CTG.
7. The oxytocin infusion rate should be reduced if contractions occur more frequently than five contractions in 10 minutes.
8. If the fetal heart rate trace is classified as pathological, the oxytocin infusion should be stopped and a full assessment of the fetal condition should be undertaken by an experienced obstetrician before the oxytocin is recommended.
9. Women using an epidural for pain relief in labor should be on continuous EFM.
10. Each maternity unit should ensure that both obstetric and midwifery staff are trained in the interpretation of CTGs.

Standardization of Fetal Heart Rate Monitoring

Fetal heart rate monitoring, whether by intermittent auscultation (IA) or electronic fetal monitoring (EFM), should be recommended to all women in labor. Risk factors should be identified and recorded. These factors may evolve through the course of labor.

Intermittent Auscultation (IA)

For a woman who is healthy and has an uncomplicated pregnancy (low risk), intermittent auscultation should be offered and recommended in labor using either a Doppler ultrasound or a Pinard stethoscope. The maternal heart rate should also be recorded hourly during fetal heart rate monitoring.

- First stage of labor: IA should occur at least every 15 minutes after a contraction and for a minimum of 60 seconds.
- Second stage of labor: IA should occur every 5 minutes after a contraction and for a minimum of 60 seconds.
- Intrapartum events that may affect the FHR, for example, the sitting of an epidural or the commencement of oxytocin should be noted comprehensively in the maternal notes, signed, dated and timed.

Electronic Fetal Monitoring (EFM) Settings

- Settings on a CTG machine should be standardized to enable a consistent approach to teaching and interpretation of EFM traces.
- Paper speed of 1 cm per minute should be adopted.
- Date and time settings on CTG machines should be validated at commencement of every CTG.
- CTGs should be labelled with mother's name, hospital number, date and time of commencement.
- Maternal heart rate should be recorded and noted on CTG.
- Following birth, the midwife should sign and note the date, time and mode of delivery on the CTG.
- The CTG should be stored securely with the woman's notes.
- Tracer systems should be available for all CTGs if stored separately from the woman's notes.

Continuous EFM should be Offered and Recommended When–

- Antepartum risk factors exist at the onset of labor.
- Intrapartum risk factors exist at the onset of labor or develop during labor.
- A FHR <110 bpm or >160 bpm is heard during IA.
- Any decelerations are heard after a contraction.

Risk Factors Requiring Electronic Fetal Monitoring (EFM)

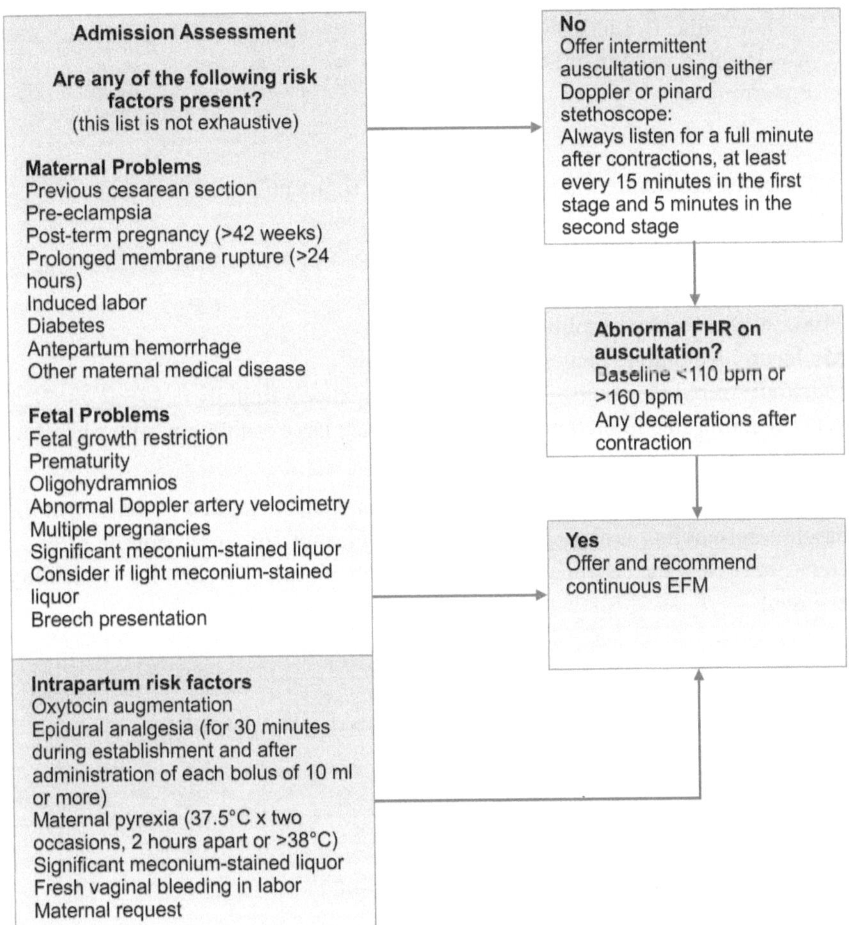

Note: Individual units may choose to adapt these indications for EFM

Appendix 1: Adapted from admission assessment and options for fetal monitoring in labor (based on NICE guidelines 2001–2007)

Features of CTG

1. Baseline heart rate
2. Baseline variability (BLV)
3. Accelerations
4. Decelerations

NICHD 2008 Workshop on Electronic Fetal Monitoring

Baseline Heart Rate

- Mean FHR in increments of 5 bpm during 10 min tracing segment, excluding:
  - Periodic/Episodic changes.
  - Periods of marked FHR variability
  - Baseline that differs >25 bpm

  Bradycardia: Borderline-100–109 bpm
  Abnormal-<100 bpm
  Tachycardia: Borderline-161–180 bpm
  Abnormal term fetus->180 bpm
  Preterm fetus->190 bpm

Variability

- Baseline–minimum of 2 min in any 10 min segment.
- Fluctuations in the FHR 2 cycles per min/greater.
- Variability is visually quantified as amplitude of peak to trough in bpm.

Absent: Undetectable amplitude range
Minimal: Detectable amplitude range <5 bpm
Moderate: Amplitude range 6–25 bpm {Normal}
Marked: Amplitude range >25 bpm (Saltatory pattern–Rapidly recurring couplets of acceleration and deceleration causing relatively large oscillations of the baseline fetal heart rate–It is not abnormal).

Sinusoidal pattern differs from variability. It is seen as a regular oscillation of the baseline resembling a sine wave with 3–5 cycles/mt and an amplitude of 5–15 above and below the baseline, lasting at least ten minutes. The baseline variability is absent.

Etiology of Sinusoidal Pattern

- Anemia (rhesus disease, hemoglobinopathies, FMH, vasaprevia)
- Cord compression
- Hypovolemia
- Idiopathic (thumb sucking)
- Drugs
- Abruption

Accelerations

- Visually apparent increase: Onset to peak <30 sec in the FHR from the most recently calculated baseline.
- Duration: Time from initial change in FHR from baseline to the return of the FHR to the baseline.
  <32 weeks: >10 bpm, >10 sec,<2 min
  >32 weeks: >15 bpm, >15 sec,<2 min
  Prolonged acceleration >2 min, <10 min
  If it lasts for >10 min, it is baseline change/shift.

Decelerations

Early Deceleration

- With uterine contraction, a visually apparent, usually symmetrical, gradual onset to nadir >30 sec—decrease in FHR of 15 bpm with return to baseline before end of contraction.
- Nadir of deceleration occurs at the same time as peak of contraction.

Late Deceleration

- With a uterine contraction, a visually apparent, gradual onset to nadir >30 sec decrease in FHR of 15 bpm with return to baseline.
- Onset, nadir and recovery of the deceleration occur after the beginning, peak, and end of the contraction, respectively.
- Shallow deceleration <15 bpm is detrimental when associated with reduced baseline variability.

Variable Deceleration

- An abrupt onset to nadir <30 sec, visually apparent decrease in the FHR below the baseline.
- The decrease in FHR is >15 bpm, with a duration of >15 sec but <2 min.

Shouldering—suggestive of well-compensated fetus.

Atypical Variable Deceleration

- Deceleration to <70 bpm lasting >60 sec
- Loss of variability in the baseline FHR and in the trough of the deceleration
- Biphasic decelerations
- Prolonged secondary acceleration (post-deceleration overshoot of >20 bpm and/or lasting 20 sec)
- Slow return to baseline
- Continuation of the baseline at a lower level after the deceleration
- Associated fetal tachycardia

Prolonged Deceleration

- Visually apparent decrease in the FHR below the baseline.
- Deceleration is >15 bpm , lasting >2 min but <10 min from onset to return to baseline.

Categorization of Features

Category	Definition
Normal	A FHR trace in which all four features are classified as reassuring
Suspicious	A FHR trace with one feature classified as non-reassuring and the remaining features classified as reassuring
Pathological	A FHR trace with two or more features classified as non-reassuring or one or more classified as abnormal

Classification of Cardiotocographs

Feature	Baseline (BPM)	Variability (BPM)	Decelerations	Accelerations
Reassuring	110–160	>5	None	Present
Non-reassuring	100–109 161–180	<5 for 40–90 minutes	Typical variable decelerations with over 50% of contractions occurring for over 90 minutes. Single prolonged deceleration for more than 3 minutes.	The absence of accelerations with otherwise normal trace is of uncertain significance
Abnormal	<100 >180 Sinusoidal pattern >10 minutes	<5 for 90 minutes	Either atypical variable decelerations with over 50% of contractions or late decelerations, both for over 30 minutes. Single prolonged deceleration for more than 3 minutes.	

The Trace should be Read by the Mnemonic
DR. C BRAVADO

DR-Define Risk-? Pre-eclampsia, diabetes, IUGR, smoker, etc.
C-Contractions–in the 2nd stage of labor–ideally <5 contractions in 10 minutes
BRA-Baseline rate-10–160 bpm
V-Variability-5–25 beats
A-Accelerations-2 in 20 minutes
D-Decelerations–abnormal
O-Overall risk

Suspicious CTG

↓

Ensure adequate quality recording of both fetal heart rate and contraction pattern

Inadequate quality CTG?
Check maternal pulse
Poor contact from external transducer?
- Check position of electrode
- Consider applying fetal scalp electrode (FSE)

FSE not working
- Check position of electrode
- Confirm fetal heart with Pinard stethoscope and/or ultrasound)

Uterine hypercontractility?
Is the mother receiving oxytocin?
- Reduce/stop infusion

Has the mother recently received vaginal prostaglandins?
Has the mother recently received vaginal prostaglandins?
- Consider tocolysis with subcutaneous terbutaline 0.25 mg

Maternal tachycardia/Pyrexia
Is there a maternal infection?
- Check on temperature. If 37.5°C on two occasions, 2 hours apart or 38.0°C or higher, consider screening and treatment

Is mother dehydrated?
- Check blood pressure and give 500 ml crystalloid (IV) if appropriate

Is mother receiving tocolytic infusion?
- If maternal pulse >140 bpm reduce infusion

Other maternal factors
What is the mother's position?
- Encourage mother to adopt left-lateral position

Consider
- Is mother hypotensive?
- Has a vaginal examination just been performed?
- Has mother been vomiting or has a vasovagal episode?
- Has mother just had epidural sited?

Check blood pressure and give 500 ml crystalloid (IV) if appropriate

If CTG remains suspicious, continue to observe for further non-reassuring or abnormal features and always consider in context with clinical circumstances.
If CTG becomes pathological, see actions for pathological CTG

Pathological CTG

Fetal blood sampling (FBS) possible and/or appropriate?
Encourage mother to adopt left lateral position. Check blood pressure and give 500 ml crystalloid (IV) appropriate.

FBS result (pH)	Recommended action
Normal 7.25 or above	• FBS should be repeated in 1 hour if FHR abnormality persists or sooner if there are further abnormalities • If result remains stable after second test, a third/further sample may be deferred unless there are further abnormalities of the CTG
Borderline 7.21 – 7.24	• Repeat FBS within 30 minutes if the FHR remains pathological or sooner if there are further abnormalities (consideration should be given to the time taken to perform FBS when planning repeat samples) • If the third sample is indicated, a consultant obstetric opinion should be sought
Abnormal 7.20 or less	• Consultant obstetric advice should be sought • Urgent delivery within 30 minutes
All FBS results should be interpreted taking into account the previous pH measurement, the rate of progress in labor and the clinical features of mother and fetus.	

Fetal blood sampling not possible/inappropriate?
- Encourage mother to adopt left lateral position. Check blood pressure and give 500 ml crystalloid (IV) if appropriate.

Expedite delivery
- The urgency and mode of delivery should take into account the severity of the fetal heart rate and the clinical circumstances.
- The accepted standard is that delivery should be accomplished within 30 minutes.

If fetal blood sampling is not possible, the baby should be delivered as soon as possible based on the clinical circumstances of the CTG.

Continuous EFM in the Presence of Oxytocin

Oxytocin to augment labor is usually used to treat inefficient uterine action, particularly, in first-time mothers.

- If the fetal heart rate is normal, an oxytocin infusion may be increased until the woman is experiencing four to five contractions every 10 minutes. The oxytocin infusion rate should be reduced by10 dpm per minute (10 IU in 1L normal saline) initially if contractions occur more frequently than five contractions in 10 minutes.
- If the fetal heart rate trace is classified as suspicious when an oxytocin infusion is in progress, a review by an experienced obstetrician should be requested.

Once reviewed, the obstetrician may recommend that the oxytocin continues to be increased but only to a dose which achieves four to five contractions in 10 minutes.

- If the fetal heart rate trace is classified as pathological, the oxytocin infusion should be stopped and clinical reassessment undertaken before the oxytocin is recommenced.

Fetal Blood Sampling (FBS)

- If FBS is not available, or is inappropriate, decisions regarding delivery should take into account the severity of the FHR abnormality and the clinical circumstances.
- Fetal blood sampling not possible or inappropriate.
- Encourage the woman to adopt left lateral position. Check blood pressure and give 500 ml crystalloid (IV), if appropriate.

Expedite Delivery

The urgency and mode of delivery should take into account the severity of the fetal heart rate and the clinical circumstances.

Ideally, delivery should occur within 30 minutes.

Delivery should be expedited where –

- Significant fetal acidosis is suspected
- There is clear evidence of serious fetal compromise (FBS not appropriate)
- CTG abnormalities require further assessment but FBS is considered clinically inappropriate or not feasible.

Contraindications for FBS

- Clear evidence of severe fetal compromise
- Fetal bleeding disorders
- Maternal infection (Herpes, HIV, Hepatitis, etc.)
- <34 weeks gestation
- Face presentation

Newborn Assessment

- Both clinical and biochemical information is required to identify an hypoxic infant. Therefore, the following should be recorded.
  - Apgar scores.
  - Need for intubation.
  - Abnormal behavior.
  - Paired samples for umbilical artery and umbilical vein blood gas analysis.
- This should be considered in the following circumstances:
  - Emergency cesarean section for fetal distress
  - Instrumental delivery for fetal distress
  - FBS has been performed in labor
  - Poor neonatal condition at birth
  - Apgar <7 at 5 minutes

GRADUALLY DEVELOPING HYPOXIA

Disappearance of accelerations

↓

Tachycardia

↓

The fetus responds to decreased oxygen by increasing cardiac output which results in tachycardia – mediated by sympathetic system

↓ Stress to distress interval

Decrease in baseline variability <5 b/min (silent pattern or flat baseline variability)
This occurs due to parasympathetic system antagonizing parasympathetic system
This indicates that fetus may be hypoxemic, acidemic or going to become acidemic soon. When FHR reaches maximum and BLV < 5 bpm – distress period.
At this point onset of acidosis cannot be predicted by observing FHR pattern.

↓

FHR drops
Staircase like drop in FHR pattern to the point the fetus point – distress to death interval
Baby should be delivered within 20–60 min

Stress pattern–Presence of decelerations in the absence with rise in baseline heart rate or reduction in baseline variability in a FHR trace which was reactive.

Chronic Hypoxia

A fetus with chronic hypoxia prior to onset of labor—non-reactive trace with BLV <5 bpm, and exhibit shallow decelerations with onset of uterine contractions.

Some fetuses may have normal baseline FHR with all other features being abnormal and may not gradually increase the baseline FHR.

There may be sudden bradycardia. **So delivery should occur within 1–2 hrs.**

FHR trace with abnormal features without repeated decelerations.

Causes are: chronic hypoxia, medications, fetal infections, injury, anomaly or arrhythmia.

Acute Hypoxia

Causes

Non-reversible abruption, cord prolapsed, scar dehiscence.

Reversible–epidural top up, vaginal examination, uterine hyperstimulation.

Hypoxia and acidosis will result if the bradycardia continues for more than 10 min.

Corrective measures–Left lateral position, stop oxytocin, hydration

Early action in those with suspicious fetal heart rate pattern prior to episode of bradycardia is indicated in:

1. Prolonged pregnancy
2. IUGR
3. Oligoamnios
4. Thick meconium stained liquor

First Stage of Labor

Principles of Care

- Initial assessment
- Observation and intervention if labor becomes abnormal
- Close monitoring of the fetal and maternal condition
- Adequate pain relief
- Emotional support
- Adequate hydration

Supportive Care

- Inform the parturient about her status
- Clip long pubic hair
- No routine enema unless rectum is loaded
- Loose clothing
- Mobilize patient except if PROM, breech, antepartum hemorrhage, heart diseases, anemia, hypertensive disease complicating pregnancy, preterm labor
- Frequent emptying of bladder

Nutrition

- Low-risk patient: Soft diet in latent phase, liquid diet in active phase and plenty of fluids.
- If cesarean delivery–Clear fluids only
- IV line not mandatory in latent phase
    - IV line indications—fluid infusion in dehydration, vomiting with increased risk of repeated drug administration, and patients kept nil orally due to high risk of operative delivery.
- Secure IV line in active phase
    - Fluid requirement during labor–60 to 120 ml/hr.

Pain relief: Only in active labor, if required.
- Epidural analgesia is better.

Parenteral Analgesia

- Inj. Fortwin 6 mg + Inj. Diazepam 2 mg diluted in 10 ml water IV every 2 hrs
- If not relieved Inj. Tramadol 50 mg + Inj Anafortan/ Inj. Buscopan IV
- Inj Ketamine 0.5 mg/kg BW IV loading dose followed by 0.25 mg/kg body weight maintenance dose every 20–30 min not more than two top ups
  OR
- Inj. Tramadol 100 mg IM is preferred, causes less respiratory depression, can be repeated after 6 hrs.
  OR
- Inj. Pethidine 50 mg (max 100 mg) + Inj. Phenergan 25 mg IM can be administered, can be repeated after 6 hrs.

Note: In advanced labor, PV should be done and administration with held if cervix is 6 cms or more dilated.

- Inj. Nalorphine, a potent antagonist administered to the mother in a dose of 5–10 mg IV 5 minutes before the expected time of delivery.
- Neonate: 0.1–0.2 mg/kg through umbilical vein if a baby is depressed at birth.

Antibiotics: No routine antibiotics.
Indications for antibiotics:
- Rupture of membranes for >24 hr
- Referred cases
- Any evidence of infection
- Heart disease
- Diabetes

Augmentation of Labor

- Uterine contractions are said to be effective if there is good progress of cervical dilatation and descent of head.
- Augmentation of labor should be governed by the rate of cervical dilatation based on the partogram, after the exclusion of gross disproportion or malpresentation. Minor degrees of disproportion due to malposition and poor flexion of the head may be overcome by oxytocin infusion.

Use of Oxytocin

Oxytocin is started in a low dose in normal saline/RL in 500 ml and the rate doubled every 30 min with monitoring and preferably after amniotomy.

Oxytocin regimens for stimulation of labor

Regimen	Starting dose (mIU/min)	Incremental increase (mIU/min)	Dosage interval (min)	Maximum dose (mIU/min)
Low-dose	3	3 (4 drops)	30	20
High-dose	6	6,3 (9,4 drops)	30	40

The incremental increase is halved to 3 mIU/min in the presence of recurrent hyperstimulation.

High-dose Regimen

- Add 5 units of oxytocin to 500 ml RL/5% dextrose containing fluid. Start at the rate of 9 drops/min (6 mIU/min). Increase by 9 drops (6 mIU/min) every 30 min till adequate contractions are achieved (3–4 C/45–50 sec/10 min).
- Monitor the contractions and fetal heart sounds. In case of hyperstimulation, stop the infusion and restart at lower dose (after the fetal heart sounds become normal) to prevent hyperstimulation.

Low-dose Regimen

- Add 5 units of oxytocin to 500 ml RL/5% dextrose containing fluid. Start at the rate of 4 drops/min (3 mIU/min). Increase by 4 drops (3 mIU/min) every 30 min till adequate contractions are achieved (3–4 C/45–50 sec/10 min).
- Used in grand multigravida, vaginal birth after cesarean, in mothers with IUGR fetuses.

Escalating Dose Regimen

Dilution: 10 U (2 ml) oxytocin in 8 ml distilled water
3U oxytocin in 500 ml of RL @ 16 drops/min (6 mU)

↓ 40 min

1.8U in 460 ml (12.08 mU)

↓ 40 min

2.2 U in 380 ml (23.80 mU)

↓ 40 min

2.0 U in 340 ml (28.09 mU)

↓ 40 min

1.8 U in 300 ml (33.39 mU)

↓ 40 min

1.6 U in 260 ml (40 mU)

This method prevents changing of IV fluid bottles with increment in dosage of oxytocin.

Other Drugs Used in Labor

- Drotaverine: To be given when cervix is 4 cms dilated, 40 mg slow IV, maximum 3 doses 2 hours apart.
- Valethamate bromide: To be given when cervix is 6–7 cms dilated, 4 mg slow IV, maximum 5 doses half an hour apart.

Monitoring during Labor

Partograph: Recommended for all patients

Record of the parturient should be meticulously maintained.

Using the Partograph

- Complete details of the parturient on the partograph.
- Start only in active labor and if does not have complication which needs immediate delivery.
- Record observations in all sections of partograph.
- The dilatation of cervix is plotted with 'X'.
- The level of head (5th of head felt above brim by abdominal palpation is plotted) is plotted with 'O'.
- When the patient is admitted in active phase of labor, the dilatation of cervix is plotted on alert line and the clock time written directly under the 'X' in space for time.
- Vaginal examination should be done every 4 hrs in latent labor, 2 hrs in active labor unless specifically indicated, e.g.: at rupture of membranes, fetal heart rate abnormalities.
- If partograph moves to the right of alert line, it indicates prolonged labor and the patient should be reassessed.

- At action line, the woman must be carefully reassessed for reason of lack of progress and decision should be made on further management.
- The time of fetal heart abnormality and rupture of membranes, ARM, if done, indication should be mentioned—note color of liquor using the following abbreviations:

I–Intact membranes
C–Membranes ruptured, clear fluid
M–Meconium stained liquor
B–Blood stained liquor

Moulding is graded as follows:
Grade 1–Sutures apposed
Grade 2–Sutures overlapped but reducible
Grade 3–Sutures overlapped and not reducible.

- Complete all the columns of partograph
- Highlight the high-risk factor.
- Chart PR every half hourly, BP 4 hrly and temperature 12 hrly (more frequently if abnormal).
- Contractions are recorded every half hourly—frequently (contractions per 10 min), intensity and duration. [Shading: Less than 20 seconds, between 20–40 seconds. More than 40 seconds.]

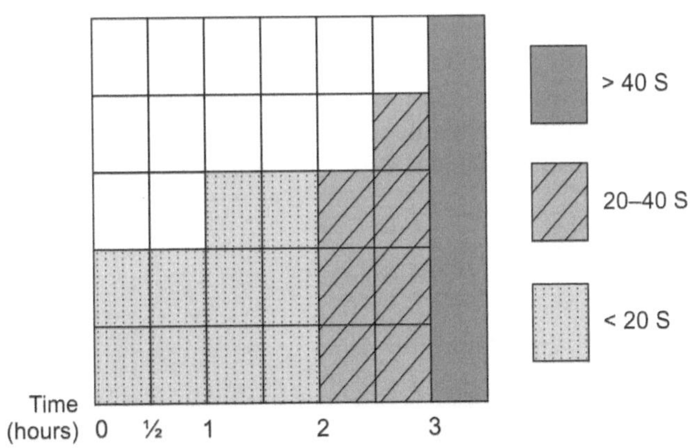

Figure 19.1: Plotting contractions on partogram

- Oxytocin if used, record the amount of oxytocin in mIU/min.
- Drugs and IV fluids if administered are recorded.
- I/O chart is maintained.
- Fetal heart monitoring

Intermittent Auscultation

- It is acceptable method of fetal monitoring in all pregnancies (both low and high risk).
- FHR should be counted for 60 seconds following a contraction (Normal FHR is 110–160 beats per minute).
- Frequency of FHR recording–

Risk situation	Ist stage	2nd stage
Low risk	Every 30 min	Every 15 min Every 5 min during pushing
High risk	Every 15 min	Every 5 min

Second Stage of Labor

- Shift the woman to labor room.
- Inform the pediatrician.
- Put her in dorsal position
- Observe universal precautions
- Clean and drape the parts
- Infiltrate the perineum with local anesthetic if episiotomy is needed
- Encourage the woman to bear down
- Episiotomy is given if needed at the time of crowning
- To control delivery of head, keep baby's head flexed and support the perineum as the head delivers. Check for cord around the neck. If loose loop is present, slip it and if tight, apply two clamps on the cord and cut between the clamps.
- After external rotation, deliver the posterior shoulder followed by the anterior and then the rest of the body.
- Clamp and cut the umbilical cord. Delayed clamping of the cord if fetus is healthy. Clamp cord early if birth asphyxiated, IUGR, thick meconium stained liquor, preterm, Rh negative pregnancy, monochorionic twin, infectious diseases of the mother.
- Hand over the baby to pediatrician.
- Practice active management of third stage of labor.
- Examine for any tears and suture if any. Suture the episiotomy if given.
- Observe the woman for 2 hours. Check every half hourly.
    - Pulse
    - Blood pressure
    - Uterus–if contracted and retracted
    - Per-vaginal bleeding
    - Make sure she passes urine.

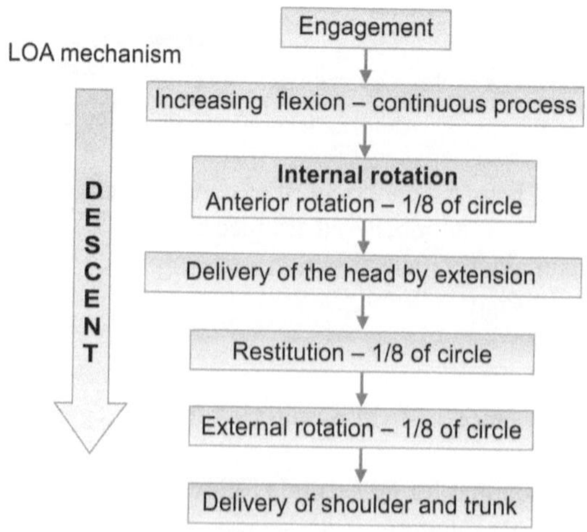

Figure 19.2: Mechanism of labor in LOA

A careful evaluation of the fetal status, descent, quality of contractions and maternal condition are more important than arbitrary time limits.

Position in the Second Stage

- Allow the woman to adopt a position that is comfortable for her. Appropriate positions may include:
    - All fours
    - Sitting up
    - Standing
    - Squatting

Method of Pushing

- If all is progressing well, then pushing should be non-directed:
    - Short periods of breath-holding
    - Short inspirations
    - Expiratory grunts
- Directive pushing should be considered when there is inadequate progress or evidence of fetal compromise where progress is not adequate with non-directive pushing.
- Directive pushing is associated with:
    - Decreased placental perfusion
    - Fetal hypoxia
    - Maternal exhaustion
    - Increased operative vaginal delivery rate
    - Need for episiotomy

Monitoring in the Second Stage

- In low-risk women, intermittent auscultation should be performed for one minute following each contraction.
- In high-risk women, continuous electronic monitoring should be maintained
- *Note:*
    - Variable decelerations may occur in up to 80% of second stages
    - FBS may be performed but the pH will drop faster in the second stage and results should be interpreted with caution.

Length of the Second Stage

- Second stage can be divided into the passive and active stages.

Passive Second Stage

This is the period between diagnosis of full dilatation and the commencement of active pushing.

- A passive stage of up to 2 hours is permissible.
- It is advisable if the woman doesn't have an urge to push especially when an epidural is in place or when the presenting part remains high especially with an OP or OT position.

Active Second Stage

- This commences when pushing commences
- The likelihood of a normal delivery decreases after 1 hour in a primi and after 30 minutes in a multigravida.

- However so long as progress is being made and the fetal and maternal conditions are reassuring then an active stage of 2 hours in a primi and 1½ hours in a multigravida is permissible.
- If at any point concerns over fetal or maternal well-being occur, then consideration of the need for an operative vaginal delivery should be made.
- If after thirty minutes there is no evidence of descent, then assessment should be done.
- If at any point after one hour if progress stops, then consideration of the need for operative delivery should be made.
- The total maximum length of the second stage should be no more than 4 hours. If delivery has not occurred within this timeframe, then a plan for operative delivery should be made unless delivery is thought to be imminent.
- The use of syntocinon in the second stage has been shown to produce effective uterine activity in the presence of an epidural but must be used with caution in multiparae.
- Any multi-syntocinon should only be used if the contractions are deemed inadequate and after full assessment.
- When commencing syntocinon in the second stage, consider commencing at 4 ml/hr in primips and 2 ml/hr in multips and increasing at 15 minute intervals rather than 30 minute intervals.
- Intervention should be based on the rate of progress rather than time elapsed.
- When delay has occurred in the second stage whether the delivery is normal or operative, problems should be anticipated. There is an increased risk of shoulder dystocia with a vaginal delivery and postpartum hemorrhage.
- The use of a prophylactic 40 IU syntocinon infusion should always be considered after a delayed second stage to help prevent a significant PPH.

KEY PRINCIPLE

If there is no progress, early intervention is essential, however, when progress is maintained, allow time to progress to a normal delivery.

MECONIUM ASPIRATION SYNDROME

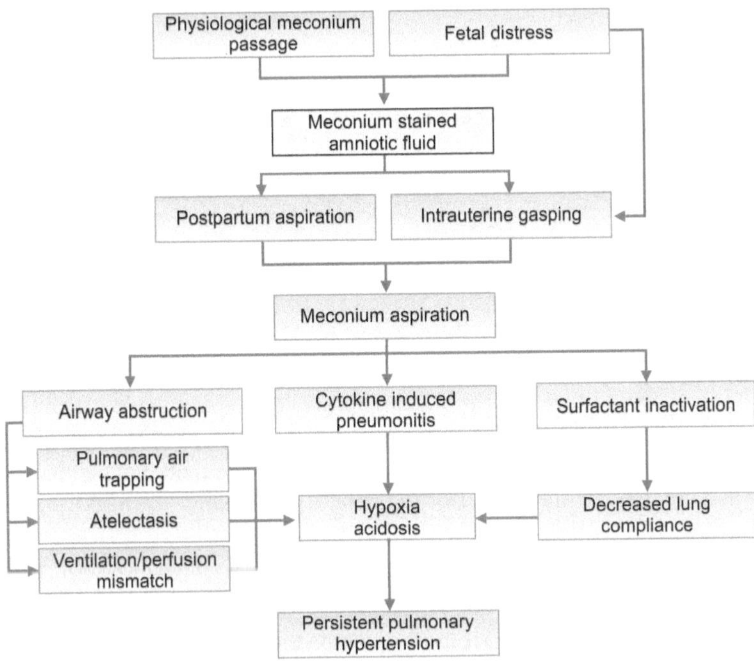

Standard grading system for meconium thickness	
Grade 1 (thin)	Refers to light green or flecking of otherwise clear amniotic fluid
Grade 2	Brown but thin uniform staining of the amniotic fluid
Grade 3 (thick)	Bright green or brown thick uniform staining of the amniotic fluid

CHAPTER

20

Malpresentation and Malposition

OCCIPITO-POSTERIOR POSITION

DEFINITION

It is a vertex presentation with fetal back directed posteriorly. The occiput and the small posterior fontanelle are in the rear segment of the maternal pelvis, and the brow and bregma are in the anterior segment.

INCIDENCE

15–30% at onset of labor.

Right occipito-posterior (ROP) is more common than left occipito-posterior (LOP) because:

- The left oblique diameter is reduced by the presence of sigmoid colon.
- The right oblique diameter is slightly longer than the left one.
- Dextro-rotation of the uterus favors occipito-posterior.

ETIOLOGY

- Anthropoid and android pelvis due to narrow fore-pelvis.
- Maternal kyphosis: The convexity of the fetal back fits with the concavity of the lumbar kyphosis.
- Anterior insertion of the placenta: The fetus usually faces the placenta (doubtful).
- Cephalopelvic disproportion
- Other causes of malpresentations:
  - Placenta previa
  - Pelvic tumors
  - Pendulous abdomen
  - Polyhydramnios
  - Multiple pregnancy

DIAGNOSIS

During Pregnancy

Symptoms

- Premature bearing down sensation
- Frequent filling of bladder

P/A

- The abdomen looks flattened below the umbilicus due to absence of round contour of the fetal back.
- A groove may be seen below the umbilicus corresponding to the neck.
- Fetal movement may be detected near the midline.
- Umbilical grip:
    - The back felt with difficulty in the flank away from the midline.
    - The anterior shoulder is at least 3 inches from the midline.
    - The limbs are easily felt anteriorly on both sides of the midline.
- First pelvic grip:
    - The head is usually not engaged due to deflexion.
    - The head is felt smaller as we catch the bitemporal diameter.
- Second pelvic grip: The head is usually deflexed.
    - FHS is heard in the flank away from the middle line on the same side as baby's back.
    - In major degree of deflexion, the FHS may be heard in middle line.
- Vaginal examination:
    - The sagittal suture is in the right oblique diameter of the pelvis.
    - The small posterior fontanelle is in the right posterior segment of the pelvis.
    - The bregma is anterior and to the left of the symphysis pubis, easily felt.
    - Since flexion is incomplete both fontanelles felt at the same level.
    - Pinna of the ear points to direction of occiput.

Mechanism of Labor in Right Occipitoposterior Position

ROP more common than LOP.

Transverse diameter-biparietal diameter 9.5 cm in the left oblique diameter of the pelvic inlet.

AP diameter—occipitofrontal in fully deflexed head 11.5 cm
—sub-occipitofrontal in partially deflexed head 10 cm.

Flow chart 20.1: Mechanism of labor in ROP

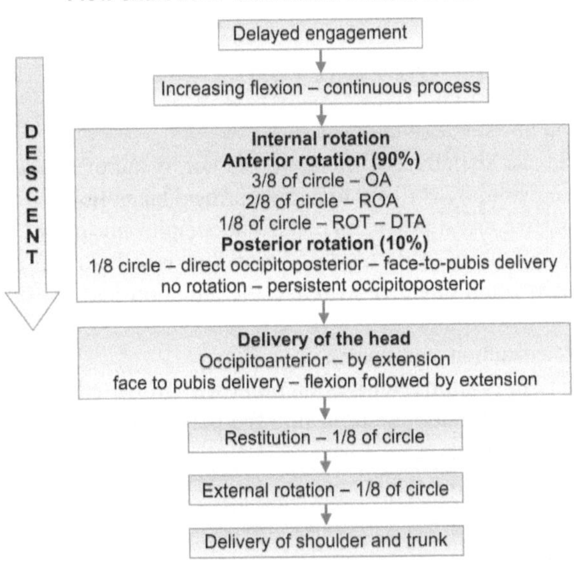

MANAGEMENT OF LABOR

First Stage

- Exclude contracted pelvis
- Exclude presentation or prolapse of cord
- Augmentation of the labor
- Adequate labor analgesia
- Avoid premature rupture of membranes by:
  - Rest in bed
  - No straining
  - Avoid high enema
  - Minimize vaginal examination
- Plot partogram from active phase. If it crosses action line, reassess progress and appropriate action must be taken.

Second Stage

Wait for 60–90 minutes.
During this period:
- Observe the mother and fetus carefully for signs of distress.
- Combat inertia by oxytocin unless it is contraindicated.

Contraindications for Oxytocin

- Cephalopelvic disproportion

Use carefully in:
1. Incoordinate uterine action
2. Uterine scar, e.g. previous CS, hysterotomy, myomectomy, metroplasty or previous perforation
3. Grand multipara
4. Fetal distress

One of the following will occur:

I. Long internal rotation 3/8 circle: It occurs in about 90% of cases and delivery is completed as in normal labor.

II. Direct occipito-posterior (face to pubis):
  - Occurs in about 6% of cases
  - The head can be delivered spontaneously or by aid of outlet forceps.
  - Liberal episiotomy is given to avoid perineal laceration.

III. Deep transverse arrest (1%) and persistent occipito-posterior (3%):
Arrest of progress in 2nd stage of labor that is 2 hours in a primigravida and 1 hour in a multipara re-evaluate the situation and consider one of the following:

A. Vacuum extraction (ventouse):
  i. Proper application over-flexion point will promote flexion of the head.
  ii. Traction will guide the head into the pelvis till it meets the pelvic floor where it will rotate.
  iii. To be applied only if all pre-requisites for vaccum application are fulfilled.

B. i. Manual rotation and extraction by forceps: Done under general anesthesia
   ii. Rotational/midcavity forceps (Kieland forceps).

Both are not done in modern obstetrics

C. Cesarean section indicated in:
   i. Failure of the above methods
   ii. Fetal distress, maternal distress
   iii. Other indications for CS as–
   - Contracted pelvis
   - Placenta previa
   - Prolapsed pulsating cord before full cervical dilatation
   - Elderly primigravida.

E. Craniotomy: If the fetus is dead.

Flow chart 20.2: Management of occipitoposterior

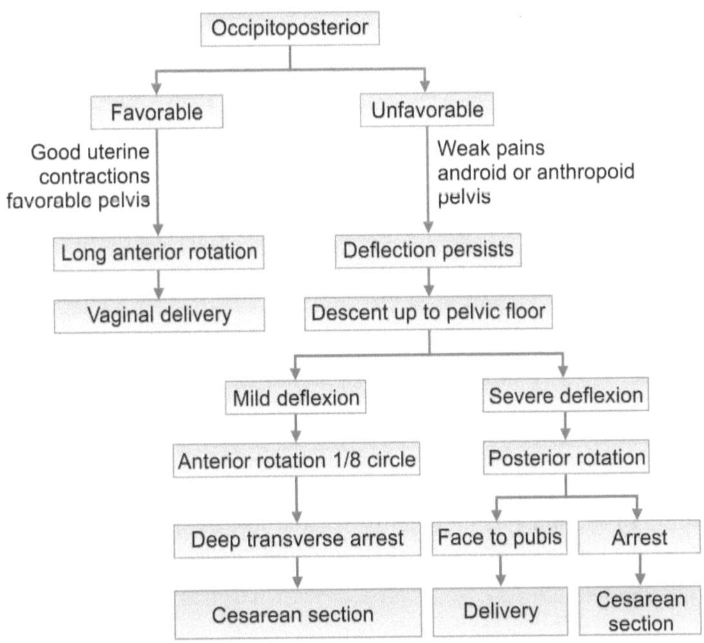

BREECH PRESENTATION

- The term "breech presentation" is used when podalic pole presents in the lower pole of the uterus.
- It is the commonest malpresentation (3–4% of all fetuses).

TYPES OF BREECH PRESENTATION

- Complete breech presentation (flexed breech):
  - The normal attitude of full flexion is maintained
  - The thighs are flexed at the hips and legs at the knees
  - Commonly present in multiparous women.
- **Incomplete breech presentation:** There are three varieties of incomplete breech.

Frank Breech

- The thighs are flexed on the trunk and the legs are extended at the knee joints.
- It is commonly present in primigravida.

Footling Presentation

- Both the thighs and legs are partially extended bringing feet to present at the brim.

Knee Presentation

- The thighs are extended, but the knees are flexed, bringing the knee down to present at the brim.

ETIOLOGICAL FACTORS

- Prematurity
- Congenital fetal malformations
- Contracted pelvis
- Pelvic tumors
- Hydramnios
- Placenta previa
- Multiple pregnancy
- Fetal growth restriction
- Mullerian anomalies
- Multiparous
- Oligohydramnios
- Cornu-fundal placenta

DIAGNOSIS

Complete Breech Presentation

Per-abdomen

- FHS: Located at higher level around the umbilicus.

Per-vaginal Examination

- Palpation of sacrum, ischial tuberosities and feet by the sides of the buttocks (Feet are identified by prominence of heel and lesser mobility of great toe).

Frank Breech Presentation

Per-abdomen Examination

- Fundal grip: Head is suggested by hard, globular mass which is not independently ballotable due to splinting action of feet. Irregular small parts of the feet may be felt by the side of the head.
- Lateral grips: Fetal back is on one side .
- Pelvic grip: Soft, broad, conical mass is felt, usually engaged.
- FHS: Heard in the midline/one of the spinoumbilical lines due to early engagement of breech.

Per-vaginal Examination

- Palpation of sacrum (can be mistaken for the head).
- Palpation of ischial tuberosities, sacrum and anus; the anus and ischial tuberosities lying in one line. (Anus is identified by absence of suckling action

of the mouth and meconium staining of the fingers—to differentiate from face presentation).

COMPLICATIONS

Maternal: Increased operative interference.

Fetal

- Perinatal morbidity—Birth asphyxia, birth trauma
- Perinatal mortality.

INVESTIGATIONS

- USG level II should preferably be performed for all cases of breech presentation antenatally to observe the following:
  - Confirm presentation
  - Amount of liquor
  - Placental position
  - Gross congenital anomaly
  - Type of breech
  - Hyperextension of neck
  - Fetal maturity
  - Estimated fetal weight

INDUCTION/AUGMENTATION OF LABOR

- Induction of labor is not generally recommended in the breech presentation. If external cephalic version is unsuccessful, declined or contraindicated, and the woman chooses not to have an elective cesarean section, induction of labor should be offered, if delivery is indicated, after discussing the associated risks with the woman.
- Labor augmentation can be done judiciously.

METHODS OF VAGINAL DELIVERY

There are three general methods of breech delivery through the vagina:

1. **Spontaneous breech delivery**: The fetus is expelled entirely spontaneously without any traction or manipulation other than support of the newborn.
2. **Assisted breech delivery**: The fetus is delivered spontaneously as far as the umbilicus, but the remainder of the body is extracted or delivered with operator traction and assisted maneuvers, with or without maternal expulsive efforts.
3. **Total breech extraction**: The entire body of the fetus is extracted by the obstetrician.

INDICATIONS FOR CESAREAN SECTION

- **Elective** (in case of live fetus after ruling out major congenital malformations)
- A large fetus (Estimated baby weight >3.5 kg)

- Fetopelvic disproportion:
  - Clinical pelvimetry should be performed.
  - No trial of labor in mild degree disproportion with breech presentation.
- Associated maternal complicating factors (case to be individualized)
- A hyperextended head
- When delivery is indicated in the absence of spontaneous labor
- Incomplete or footling breech presentation
- An apparently healthy and viable preterm fetus with the mother in either active labor or in whom delivery is indicated
- Severe fetal-growth restriction
- Previous perinatal death or children suffering from birth trauma.

PREREQUISITES FOR VAGINAL DELIVERY

- Vaginal delivery should be allowed if the woman is willing to take breech risk
- Breech risk (approximately 3–5% for term baby) should be explained keeping in mind the following factors:
  - Parity (previous obstetric performance)
  - Gestational age
  - Estimated fetal weight
  - Pelvic adequacy

To objectify breech risk, the following scoring system can be utilized (at the onset of labor):

Zatuchni and Andros Scoring System

Previous breech	Parity	Gest. age	EFW (kg)	Cervical dilatation	Station
0	0	>39 wk	>3.6	3 cms	–3
1	1	38–39 wk	3.1–3.6	2 cms	–2
2	2	<37 wk	<3.1	1 cms	–1

Score <3–high chances of complications with vaginal delivery. Score 0–4 cesarean section is indicated (This system does not include pelvic assessment, which is a disadvantage).

INTRAPARTUM MANAGEMENT

First Stage

- Informed consent for breech vaginal delivery should be taken.
- Parturient to lie in left lateral position.
- To avoid early bearing down.
- Do P/V examination in rupture of membranes to exclude cord prolapse.
- Ensure good uterine contractions—augmentation can be done if necessary.
- Early decision for LSCS if progress of labor is slow.

Second Stage

- Following should be kept ready:
  - Skilled obstetrician
  - Staff nurse
  - Pediatrician
  - Breech towel
  - Forceps (Piper or mid-cavity) for delivery of head
  - Instruments for episiotomy
  - Equipment for neonatal resuscitation
- Ensure good uterine contractions
- The fetus is delivered with the assistance of the obstetricians (assisted breech delivery). It should be encouraged in all cases.

Assisted Breech Delivery

- When the breech distends the perineum, the woman should be put in dorsal position.
- Liberal episiotomy should be given when the buttocks distend the perineum after appropriate analgesia.
- No touch technique till delivery of trunk up to the level of umbilicus.
- A loop of cord should be pulled down and placed to one side away from pressure by presenting part. Time should be noted.
- Baby to be wrapped in breech towel.
- Always keep the back of the baby anterior to avoid extension at head.
- Baby is supported by pelvic femoral grip.
- When the angle of the scapula is visible, the obstetrician should check for the arms which are usually in front of the chest.
- If they do not deliver spontaneously, these are hooked out.

Delivery of Head

- Do not be in haste (3–5 min between delivery of cord and head)
- Allow the baby to hang by its own weight till the nape of the neck, i.e. hair line is visible.
- Give suprapubic pressure (Kristeller maneuver)
- One of the following methods can be used:

Burns-Marshall technique | Mauriceau-Smellie-Veit technique | Forceps application

Burns-Marshall technique: When the hair line is seen–

- Suprapubic pressure—Body is lowered—nape of neck pivots and flexion is maintained.
- Body raised—Slight extension at neck—further suprapubic pressure (Kristeller maneuver)—head delivered by flexion.

Mauriceau-Smellie-Veit technique: When the hair line is not seen, body of the baby is placed on operator's hand; one finger in baby's mouth and two on malar bones, other hand exerts shoulder traction.

Forceps application for delivery after coming head.

Procedure

- Feet are grasped and body is lifted using towel (Savage).
- Left blade followed by right-occipitomental diameter.
- Traction directly on head—avoids damage to structures in neck.

Advantages

- Delivery can be controlled by giving pull directly on the head and the force is not transmitted through the neck.
- Flexion is better maintained.
- Baby will have space to breathe.

Arrest of Aftercoming Head

Common Causes

1. Deflexed head
2. Incomplete dilatation of cervix
3. Undiagnosed hydrocephalus
4. Fetopelvic disproportion

Management

Do PV examination: Incomplete dilatation of cervix - Duhrssen incision
Cut short 2 o'clock, which is followed by a second incision at 10 o'clock.
Infrequently, an additional incision is required at 6 o'clock.

Assess Size of Head

Suspicion of hydrocephalus → Confirm by USG → Cephalocentesis.
Pediatrician to attend the delivery and resuscitate if necessary.
Extended arms
One or both arms are fully stretched along the side of head.

- If arms are extended, either Lovset's maneuver/classical method is used.
  - For Lovset's maneuver, general anesthesia is not needed.
  - Classical method needs intrauterine manipulation while the patient is under general anesthesia.

Lovset's Maneuver

The maneuver is done when the inferior angle of the anterior scapula is visible underneath the pubic arch.

- Rotate baby through 180 degrees in the direction of thumb.
- When the posterior arm emerges under pubic arch, it is hooked out.
- The trunk is rotated in opposite direction and anterior shoulder delivered.

Classical Method

When inferior angle of the scapula is also not seen. Under general anesthesia.

Procedure

- Keep the back anterior
- Give traction to make scapula visible

- Rotate the baby by shortest distance to make one of the shoulders posterior.
- Lift the baby up and introduce hand into pelvis, deliver posterior arm followed by anterior arm.

Nuchal Arms

- Extension at the shoulder and flexion at the elbow so that forearm is trapped behind fetal head.
- Lovset's maneuver should be done.

Back Posterior

The basic rule of breech delivery is to keep back anterior. When the back is posterior, the following maneuvers can be attempted: Chin to pubis rotation, Prague's maneuver.

Chin to Pubis Rotation

Anterior rotation of chin occurs when it is not possible to rotate the back anteriorly.

- Institute deep anesthesia
- Cease all traction
- Dislodge the chin from behind the pelvis
- Rotate the face posteriorly and back anteriorly
- Flex the chin
- Effect engagement by suprapubic pressure
- Deliver head with Piper forceps

Prague's Maneuver

- Under anesthesia.
- Place fingers of left hand over shoulders and exert outward and upward traction.
- Grasp legs with right hand and swing body over mother's abdomen.
- Deliver the occiput over the perineum.

Failure of Descent of Breech

If within 30 min of full dilatation of cervix, the breech does not descend and distend the perineum, reassess the pelvis. If fetopelvic disproportion, shift for emergency LSCS.

Decomposition

Flexed breech–Reduce the bulk of the breech by converting to footling presentation.

- Hand placed inside the uterus
- Membranes ruptured
- A foot is grasped and brought out.

Frank breech–Pinnard's maneuver under GA as part of breech extraction.

- Hand in the uterus
- Membranes ruptured
- Pressure is made by fingers against the popliteal fossa in a backward and outward direction.
- This causes flexion and foot is grasped and brought out.

Third Stage

- Practice AMTSL
- Check for cervical tears if suspected
- Suture episiotomy

ROLE OF EXTERNAL CEPHALIC VERSION (ECV) DURING LABOR

If the patient is in early labor and criteria are fulfilled, ECV can be attempted (See protocol: Version).

Preterm breech infant: The greater disparity between head and abdomen dimensions results in a significant disadvantage to the preterm fetus in negotiating the pelvis, making vaginal delivery inherently riskier than for the term fetus. Most premature breech fetuses are delivered by a cesarean.

FACE PRESENTATION

DEFINITION

The lie is longitudinal, the presentation is cephalic, the presenting part is face, the attitude is of complete extension, chin (mentum) is the denominator and the presenting diameter is submentobregmatic of 9.5 cm.

Incidence: About 1:300 labors.

ETIOLOGY

A. Primary face:
- It is less common, present before onset of labor.
- It is usually due to fetal causes which may be:
  - Anencephaly: Due to absence of the bony vault of the skull.
  - Loops of cord around the neck.
  - Tumors of the fetal neck, e.g. congenital goiter.
  - Hypertonicity of the extensor muscles of the neck.
  - Dolichocephaly: Long antero-posterior diameter of the head, so as the breadth is less than 4/5 of the length.
  - Dead or premature fetus.
  - Idiopathic.

B. Secondary face:
- It is more common, occurs during labor.
- It may be due to:
  - Contracted pelvis, particularly, flat pelvis which allows descent of the bitemporal but not the biparietal diameter leads to extension of the head.
  - Pendulous abdomen or marked lateral obliquity of the uterus.
  - Deflexion of brow or occipitoposterior positions.
  - Causes of malpresentations as polyhydramnios and placenta previa.

Positions

- Right mento-posterior (RMP).
- Left mento-posterior (LMP).
- Left mento-anterior (LMA).
- Right mento-anterior (RMA), are the more common positions.

DIAGNOSIS

Left Mentoanterior

Abdominal Examination

- The long axes of the fetus and mother are parallel.
- The head is at the pelvis. Early in labor, the head is not engaged.
- The back is on the right side of the mother's abdomen, but since it is posterior, it is often felt indistinctly. The small parts are on the left and anterior. Extension of the spine causes the chest to be thrown out and the back to be hollowed. [In LMP, the back is anterior and to the right. The small parts are on the left and posterior].
- The breech is in the fundus.
- The cephalic prominence (occiput) is on the right. An important diagnostic sign of extension attitude is that the back and the cephalic prominence are on the same side.
- The fetal heart sounds are heard loudest in the left lower quadrant of the mother's abdomen.

Vaginal Examination

- The clue to diagnosis is a negative finding, i.e. absence of round, even, hard vertex. In place of the dome of the skull with its identifying suture lines and fontanelles, there is softer and irregular presenting part. One suspects face or breech. Identification of the various parts of the face clinches the diagnosis. After prolonged labor marked edema may confuse the picture.
- The long axis of the face is in the right oblique diameter of the pelvis. [In LMP, the long diameter of the face is in the left oblique diameter of the pelvis].
- The chin is in the left anterior quadrant of the maternal pelvis. In LMP, chin is in the left posterior quadrant of pelvis and forehead is in the right anterior quadrant
- Late in labor, the face becomes edematous (tumefaction) so it can be misdiagnosed as a buttock (breech presentation) where the two cheeks are mistaken with buttocks and the mouth with anus and the malar processes with the ischial tuberosities. The following points can differentiate in between (Beck's sign).
- **Face presentation**:The fetal mouth and malar processes form the apex of a triangle. The gum is felt hard through the mouth. The examining finger may be sucked by the fetal mouth during vaginal examination.
- **Breech presentation**: The presenting part is soft and irregular. The anal orifice and the ischial tuberosities are in straight line. No hard object is felt through the anus. The anus does not suck the finger.

MANAGEMENT OF LABOR

Assess–

- Pelvic adequacy
- Size of the baby
- Assosciated complicating factors–elderly primigravida, medical disorders of pregnancy, post-cesarean section, postmaturity
- Position of the mentum
- Congenital fetal malformation

A. Mento-anterior:

First Stage

Wait and watch policy, monitor maternal and fetal condition and progress of labor.

Second Stage

- Spontaneous delivery usually occurs.
- Episiotomy is necessary because of overdistension of the vulva.
- Forceps delivery may be indicated in prolonged 2nd stage.

B. Mento-posterior:

First Stage

As mento-anterior

Second Stage

- If anterior rotation of the chin occurs, spontaneous or forceps delivery is done.
- Failure of long anterior rotation by 3/8 circle or development of fetal or maternal distress at any time, cesarean section should be done.

Diagnosis of position: Left mento-transverse

Abdominal Examination

- The long axis of the fetus is parallel to that of the mother.
- The head is at the pelvis.
- The back is on the right, towards the maternal flank. The small parts are on the left side.
- The breech is in the fundus.
- The cephalic prominence is on the right, the same side as the back.

Vaginal Examination

- The long axis of the face is in the transverse diameter of the pelvis.
- The chin is to the left, at 3 o'clock.
- The forehead is to the right, at 9 o'clock.

MECHANISM OF LABOR IN LEFT MENTOANTERIOR POSITION

LMA more common than RMA.

Transverse diameter—biparietal diameter 9.5 cm in the left oblique diameter of the pelvic inlet.

AP diameter—Sub-mentobregmatic in fully extended head 9.5 cm sub-mento-vertical in incomplete extension of head 11.5 cm.

Flow chart 20.3: Mechanism of labor in left mento-anterior position

DESCENT

Delayed engagement
↓
Increasing extension – continuous process
↓
Internal rotation
Anterior rotation – 1/8 of circle
↓
Delivery of the head by flexion
↓
Restitution – 1/8 of circle
↓
External rotation – 1/8 of circle
↓
Delivery of shoulder and trunk

Management

a. Anterior rotation takes place in the majority of cases, LMT to LMA to MA. The treatment is the same as LMA. Delivery is spontaneous or assisted by low forceps.
b. Arrest as LMT low in the pelvis.
Cesarean section is performed.
c. Arrest as LMT high in the pelvis, cesarean section is performed.
PS: The face of the baby is edematous after delivery so the mother is assured that this will be spontaneously relieved within a few days.

BROW PRESENTATION

DEFINITION

Brow presentation is an attitude of partial extension, in contrast to face presentation in which extension is complete. The presenting part is the area between orbital ridges and the bregma.

INCIDENCE

About 1:3000 to 1:1000. Primary (those which occur before onset of labor) are rare, secondary (those which occur after onset of labor) are more common.

ETIOLOGY

It is usually due to fetal causes which may be:
- Cephalopelvic disproportion
- Increased fetal mobility:
    - Polyhydraminos
    - Premature baby

- Some fetal conditions prevent flexion:
  - Tumors of the neck, e.g. congenital goiter
  - Loops of cord around the neck
  - Fetal anomalies
- PROM
- Abnormal placental implantation: Placenta previa
- Uterine abnormalities: Bicornuate uterus, neoplasm of lower segment
- Idiopathic.
- Iatrogenic-external version

DIAGNOSIS

Abdominal Examination

- The lie is longitudinal.
- The head is above the pelvic brim, not engaged.
- The back is on the mother's right and posterior; it may be difficult to palpate. The small parts are on the left and anterior:
- The breech is in the fundus of the uterus.
- The occiput and back are on the same side.

Fetal heart–Heard best in the left lower quadrant of the maternal abdomen.

Vaginal Examination

- The AP diameter of the head is in the right oblique diameter of pelvis.
- The brow presents and is felt in the left anterior quadrant of the pelvis.
- The vertex is in the right posterior quadrant.
- The bregma is palpated easily.
- The frontal suture is felt, but sagittal suture is out of reach.
- Identification of supraorbital ridges.

MECHANISM OF LABOR

Presenting diameter is mentovertical–13.5 cm. It is the longest anteroposterior diameter of the head. Hence there is **no mechanism of labor.**

If engagement does occur, there will be extensive moulding and progress is slow. If baby is very small, pelvis is roomy and uterine contractions are strong, delivery can occur in anterior brow positions. Delivery occurs by a process of flexion followed by extension. The face hinges under the pubis, bregma, vertex, occiput are born by flexion. Nose, mouth, chin are born by extension.

Posterior brow positions–no mechanism of labor.

MANAGEMENT OF LABOR

A. Early in the first stage:
   - Exclude contracted pelvis, if present, do cesarean section.
   - Trial of labor–The case is considered as transient brow, observed carefully and given a chance for spontaneous conversion into either face or vertex. Conversion into face is more common.

B. In the second stage:
The case is considered as persistent brow so, cesarean section is done.
If labor becomes obstructed and baby is dead, craniotomy is done after ruling out rupture of uterus.

TRANSVERSE LIE

DEFINITION

Transverse lie is the term used when long axis of the fetus is perpendicular to the maternal spine or centralized uterine axis. Denominator is the scapula.
Incidence: 1 in 500.

POSITIONS

To be determined by the position of the back–
- Dorsoanterior–commonest. The anterior surface of fetus is better adapted to the convexity of maternal spine.
- Dorsoposterior–the chances of hand prolapse are more
- Dorsosuperior
- Dorsoinferior

ETIOLOGY

- Multiparity
- Prematurity
- Twins—more common in 2nd twin
- Hydramnios
- Contracted pelvis
- Placenta previa
- Pelvic tumors
- Congenital malformations of the uterus—arcuate and subseptate
- Intrauterine death

DURING ANTENATAL PERIOD

Diagnosis

Abdominal Examination

Inspection: The abdomen is transversely stretched and assymetrical.

Palpation

- Fundal height—less than the period of amenorrhea.
- Fundal grip—fetal pole (breech or head) is not palpable.
- Lateral grip—soft, broad irregular breech is felt to one side of the midline and smooth, hard and globular head on the other side. Head is placed at a lower level on one iliac fossa.

- Back is felt anteriorly across the long axis—dorso-anterior.
- Pelvic grip—the lower pole of the uterus is found empty.

Auscultation: FHS is heard easily below the umbilicus.

Vaginal examination—Neither the head nor the breech is felt. Presenting part is high up.

Investigations

A USG examination should preferably be performed in every case of transverse lie to determine:

- Position of back
- Fetal maturity
- Liquor
- Position of placenta
- Gross congenital anomaly of fetus

Mechanism of Labor

A persistent transverse lie cannot deliver spontaneously, and if uncorrected, impaction can take place.

Spontaneous Version

It takes place with oblique lie than with transverse lie. Before or shortly after onset of labor there is a change to longitudinal lie (breech or cephalic).

Neglected Transverse Lie

It results from misdiagnosis and improper treatment. Because of ineffective contractions the cervix dilates slowly. Due to irregularity of presenting part, the membranes rupture early. As labor pains become stronger, the fetal shoulder is forced into the pelvis uterus, molds itself around the baby and progress is halted. This results in one of the 2 outcomes:

- Uterine rupture—more common in multigravida. It occurs in the line of the retraction ring.
- Uterine inertia—more common in primigravida.

Conduplicato Corpore

If fetus is very small (<800 gm), and pelvis is roomy, the fetus is compressed with the head forced against its abdomen. A portion of the thoracic wall below the shoulder thus becomes the most dependent part, appearing at the vulva. The head and thorax then pass through the pelvic cavity at the same time. The fetus is doubled upon itself and born.

Management of Patients not in Labor

- Patients with transverse lie at 37 weeks or more should be hospitalized because the chances of early rupture of membranes and cord/hand prolapsed are very high.

- ECV can be tried in case of transverse lie at 37 weeks and beyond, provided the liquor is adequate, baby average size, uterus relaxed and there is no CPD/any other contraindication for ECV. Special care must be taken to exclude placenta previa and congenital uterine malformation as these are common causes of transverse lie, especially in primigravida.
- Patients in whom ECV fails or those who are not willing for ECV, should have elective LSCS done at 38 completed weeks.

DURING LABOR

Diagnosis

In early labor, it is similar to that in antenatal period.
Do P/A and P/V examination (before PV examination, possibility of asymptomatic placenta previa should be kept in mind, and USG if not already done, should be performed to exclude placenta previa).

Per-abdominal Examination

- Both fundal and pelvic grip are empty, and
- Ballotable head is felt on one side in lateral pelvic grip.

Per-vaginal Examination

- Cervix is generally hanging loose.
- Presenting part is high.
- Long conical bag of membranes, if ruptured, the shoulder is identified by palpating acromion process, the scapula, the clavicle and axilla. The characteristic landmarks are identification of ribs and intercostals spaces.
- Sometimes arm/cord can be found prolapsed in the vagina.

Management

- **ECV** should be attempted in early labor only when (see protocol on version):
  - Liquor is adequate.
  - Baby size is average.
  - Uterus is relaxed.
  - Bag of membranes is intact.
  - Pelvis is adequate.
  - No other contraindication for ECV is present.
- **LSCS**: Patients who are in an advanced labor and in those patients in whom ECV is not tried/failed should be taken up for emergency cesarean section. CS for transverse lie could, sometimes, pose problems.
- Problems anticipated–
  - LUS not formed–give liberal incision, J-shaped incision may be required.
  - Uterus tonically contracted over baby–uterine relaxants/halothane anesthesia may be given or inverted T-incision may be required.
- Look for uterine anomalies.
  Internal Podalic Version (IPV) (see protocol: Version)

Few indications for IPV are:
- 2nd twin with transverse lie
- When IPV is not possible, as it happens when the membranes are ruptured and liquor is drained out–Patvardhan technique–preferably under GA-J shaped uterine incision.
- **Destructive operations:** Decapitation and evisceration are rarely performed in modern obstetrics but can be considered in selected cases with dead baby if expertise is available and prerequisites are fulfilled.

Unfavorable Events

Hand prolapse: In case of neglected labor, the arm of the fetus prolapses and shoulder gets impacted into the pelvis with appearance of features of obstructed labor.

In such cases, baby is usually dead but even then cesarean section is recommended in maternal interest.

CORD PROLAPSE

INCIDENCE

- Vertex presentation—0.1–0.4%
- Extended breech—0.5%
- Flexed breech—6%
- Footling breech—12%

Occult Cord Prolapse

- Cord is placed by the side of the presenting part and is not felt by the fingers on internal examination.
- Suspected if there is persistence of variable deceleration of FHR pattern detected on continuous electronic fetal monitoring.

Cord Presentation

- Occurs when umbilical cord lies in front of the presenting part, with fetal membranes still intact.
- Diagnosed on vaginal examination when the pulsation of cord is felt behind intact membranes (Rarely detected).
- Reduce vaginal examination in order to reduce risk of rupturing the membranes.
- Continuous FHR monitoring.

Frank Cord Prolapse

- Cord lies in front of the presenting part following rupture of membranes.

Predisposing Factors

- Malpresentations
- Contracted pelvis
- Multiple pregnancy
- Polyhydramnios
- Placental factors (Battledore placenta or velamentous insertion of cord)
- Unduly long cord
- Multiparity
- Prematurity
- High presenting part
- Iatrogenic.

Anticipation

- Whenever there are factors that predispose to cord prolapse, a vaginal examination should be done immediately on spontaneous rupture of membranes.
- Vaginal examination is also done when membranes rupture prematurely or during labor in all cases of malpresentations, twins, hydramnios or cephalic presentation with unengaged head.
- ARM should preferably be done keeping everything ready for cesarean in above conditions.
- One should exclude cord presentation/occult cord prolapse in unexplained fetal distress during labor.

MANAGEMENT

Principles

- To relieve pressure
- Fetal condition

Relieve Pressure

a. **Immediate:** Gloved hand is introduced, cord is replaced in vagina and presenting part is lifted. Cord pulsations are felt and dilatation assessed.
b. **Position:** To lessen the pressure–
   - Knee elbow position
   - Exaggerated Sim's and Trendelenburg
   - Sim's lateral position
c. **Full bladder:** With 500–750 ml of normal saline. This keeps the presenting part high (Vago).
d. **Vulval pad:** To prevent exposure of cord

Flow chart 20.4: Management of cord prolapse

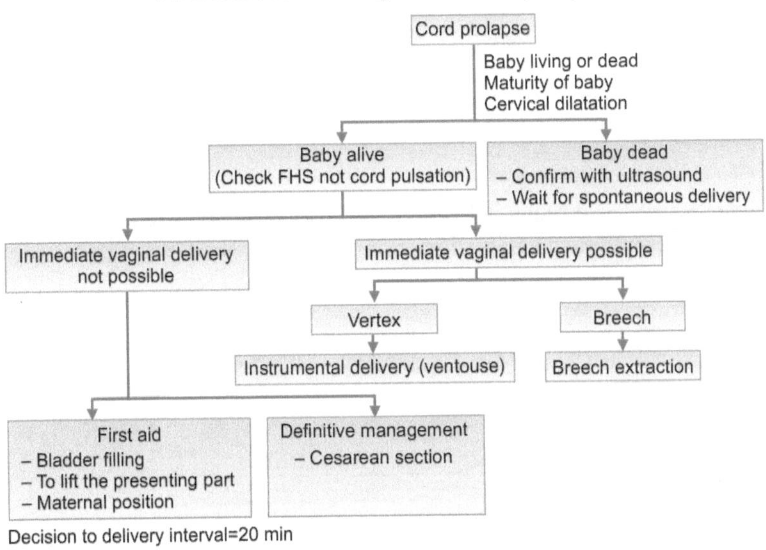

RCOG Green Top Guidelines No. 50

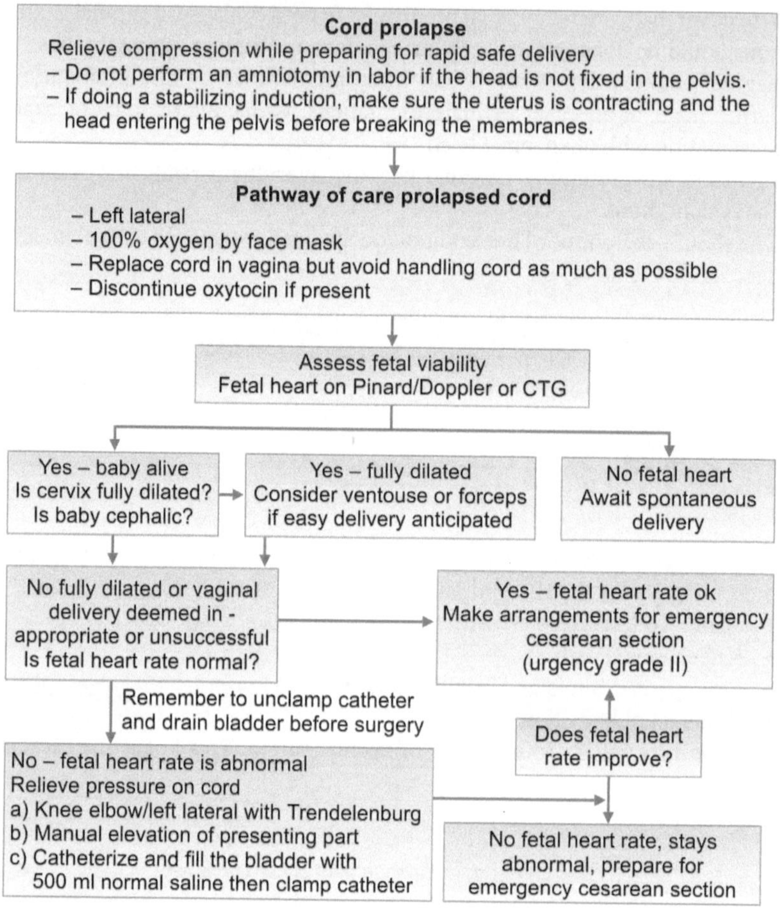

SHOULDER DYSTOCIA

DEFINITION

Shoulder dystocia is difficult delivery of the baby's shoulders requiring additional maneuvers after gentle downward traction of the fetal head.

Time delay between head and shoulder delivery >60 seconds.

FACTORS ASSOCIATED WITH SHOULDER DYSTOCIA

Antenatal

- Prolonged pregnancy
- Gestational diabetes

- Maternal BMI >30 kg/m^2
- Fetal macrosomia–Non-diabetic >4 kg
- GDM >3.5 kg
- Previous shoulder dystocia
- Induction of labor

Intrapartum

- Prolonged labor
- Secondary arrest of descent
- Oxytocin augmentation
- Operative vaginal delivery

Conditions where shoulder dystocia to be anticipated:
- Diabetes
- Obesity
- Post-term
- Anencephaly

Suspect Shoulder Dystocia

- When there is a difficulty in delivery of the face and chin.
- Head remains tightly applied to the vulva and even on extraction (Turtle sign) remains the same.
- Failure of restitution of the fetal head.
- Failure of shoulders to descend

Don'ts

- Panic
- Give excessive traction over fetal head
- Apply fundal pressure
- Clamp and cut the cord

Do's

- Call for help [senior obstetrician, pediatrician, nurses, anesthesiologist]
- Clear neonate's mouth and nose
- Perform a liberal episiotomy
- Drain the bladder if distended
- Adequate analgesia, ketamine is ideal.

Threshold between delivery of fetal head and trunk maximum 7 min.

Delivery of Shoulders in Shoulder Dystocia

Cause:
Anterior shoulder of the baby is wedged above the public symphysis
Posterior shoulder is usually in the pelvis
Diagnosis: Failure of head to restitute
Turtle's sign
If still unrecognized, then difficulty in delivering the shoulders ensues

Anticipated difficulty with shoulders after recognizing risk factors
- Macrosomia
- Maternal diabetes/obesity/excess weight gain
- Post-date's pregnancy
- Dystocia (especially with no malposition in first stage labor)
- Prolonged second stage
- Need for operative vaginal delivery

↓

Deliver in a well-staffed unit with staff well-rehearsed in shoulder dystocia drills
Have the obstetric specialist registrar in attendance
Have the neonatologist and anesthetist immediately to handle if need arises
Prepare for an active third stage (vs PPG)

↓

- Once recognized (preferably before any traction applied)
- Call for help
- Fell for anterior shoulder

↓

Anterior shoulder not in pelvis but wedged above symphysis pubis-notice time: Do not pull or apply fundal pressure
Check posterior shoulder is in sacral hollow

Anterior shoulder not in pelvis:
Encourage mother to bear down with contraction and apply moderate traction to deliver the baby

↓

No – posterior shoulder has not entered pelvis:
Cesarean section

Yes – posterior in sacral hollow, continue with maneuvers to get anterior shoulder into pelvis

Stop downward traction
↓
Summon assistance
↓
Episiotomy
↓
McRoberts maneuver
(Suprapubic pressure behind fetal shoulder to oblique with vaginal hand)
↓
Woods screw maneuver | Delivery of posterior shoulder | All fours maneuver
↓
Faiure to delivery
↓
Cephalic replacement | Abdominal rescue | Symphysiotomy
↓
If fetus is dead
↓
Cleidotomy or destructive procedure

↓

Be prepared for postpartum hemorrhage and actively manage the thrid stage.

ALARMER

A: Ask for assistance
- Mother, senior, 2 assistants, pediatrician, anesthetist.
- Explain to the mother that there is a problem in delivery and her cooperation is required.
- Send word to your senior, shout out to assistants and get them to help a trained neonatal resuscitator, anesthetist—you need their help for manual removal of posterior arm.

L: Lift the buttocks, legs **(McRoberts maneuver)**
- This procedure involves flexing and abducting the maternal hips, positioning the maternal thighs up onto the maternal abdomen.
- This position flattens the sacral promontory and results in cephalad rotation of the pubic symphysis.

A: Anterior disimpaction of the shoulder–suprapubic or vaginal.

Suprapubic Pressure (Mazzanti Technique)

- Done by assistance
- The hand of an assistant should be placed suprapubically over the fetal anterior shoulder, applying pressure in a cardiopulmonary resuscitation style with a downward and lateral motion on the posterior aspect of the fetal shoulder.
- This maneuver should be attempted while continuing downward tractions.
- Pressure should be applied from the side of the mother.
- Do not apply fundal pressure.
- With the heel of the assistant's hands moving in a downward and lateral motion on the posterior aspect of the fetal impacted shoulder.
- Initially the pressure can be continuous, but if delivery is not accomplished, a rocky motion is recommended to dislodge the shoulder from behind the pubic symphysis.

Vaginal: Rubin

- Done by the physician, RUBIN, it consists of inserting the fingers of one hand vaginally behind the posterior aspect of the anterior shoulder of the fetus and rotating shoulder towards the fetal chest.
- This motion will adduct the fetal shoulder girdle reducing its diameter.

R-Rotation of the posterior shoulder-**Woods Cork screw maneuver**
- The physician places 2 fingers on the anterior aspect of the fetal posterior shoulder, applying gentle upward pressure away from the fetal chest.
- The Rubin and Woods Cork screw maneuver may be combined to increase torque forces by using two fingers behind the fetal anterior shoulder and 2 fingers in front of the posterior shoulder.
- Downward traction should be continued during these rotational maneuvers, simulating the rotation of the screw being removed.

M-Manual removal of the posterior arm
- Removal of the posterior arm involves placing the physician's hand in the vagina and locating the fetal arm which, sometimes, is displaced behind the fetus and must be nudged anteriorly.

- The physician's hand, wrist and forearm may need to enter the vagina necessitating an episiotomy or extension.
- The fetal elbow is then flexed, and the forearm is delivered in a sweeping motion over the anterior chest wall of the fetus.
- Grasping and pulling directly on the fetal arm may fracture the humerus.

E-Episiotomy

- Episiotomy should be considered when a shoulder dystocia is encountered, although because the primary problem is a bony impaction, episiotomy by itself will not release the impaction.
- Episiotomy does provide additional room for the physician's hand when internal rotation maneuvers are required.
- Given the success of the McRobert's maneuvers and suprapubic pressure in relieving a large percentage of cases of shoulder dystocia, performing an episiotomy can wait until later in the sequence.

R-Roll-over-**All-fours or Gaskin maneuver**

- Rolling the patient onto her hands and knees known as the all-fours or Gaskin maneuver, is a safe, rapid and effective technique for the reduction of shoulder dystocia.
- Radiographic studies indicate that pelvic diameters increase when laboring women change from the dorsal recumbent position.
- The true obstetric conjugate increases by as nuch as 10 mm, and the sagittal measurement of the pelvic outlet increases by up to 20 mm.
- Once the patient is repositioned, the physician provides gentle downward traction to delivery the posterior shoulder with the aid of gravity.

Zavanelli maneuver: Absolute last resort.

- Head must first be rotated to undo the restitution and flexed to undo the extension and is then replaced in the vagina maintaining a constant firm pressure. Cesarean is performed immediately.

Others

- Cleidotomy
- Symphysiotomy

Obsolete now

Documentation

- Time of birth of the head
- Which arm was impacted against the pubic symphysis-right or left?
- Who (all) were called to help?
- Which maneuvers were performed, their order and the duration of the event?
- Time of birth of the shoulders (baby)
- Condition of the neonate at birth–APGAR, birth trauma and pH.
- Condition of the mother–PPH, tears, etc.

VERSION

EXTERNAL CEPHALIC VERSION

It is manipulation done externally to change breech or transverse lie to cephalic presentation.

Prerequisites

- Informed consent
- Period of gestation >37 weeks
- Singleton pregnancy
- Facility for emergency cesarean section available
- Baby is of average size, no gross anomalies
- Liquor adequate, membranes intact
- Uterus is relaxed
- Pelvis adequate
- No other contraindication for ECV is present.

Contraindications

- Previous uterine scar
- Antepartum hemorrhage
- Intrauterine growth restriction/IUD
- Hypertensive disease complicating pregnancy
- Oligoamnios

Steps

- Should be preferably done under ultrasound guidance.
- Woman in supine position with foot-end elevated.
- Bladder empty
- Check that the fetal heart rate is normal.
- Palpate abdomen/USG to confirm the presentation, position of fetal head, back and hip.
- Grasp the lowest part of the fetus above the pubic bone and gently lift it from pelvic inlet to mobilize the breech. One hand is placed on the head and the other on the breech.

Direction of Version

Forward somersault: The head is moved towards the pelvis and the breech toward the fundus to achieve a transverse lie. This position is maintained, fetal heart is auscultated.

If the heart rate is slow or irregular, the baby is turned back to the original position.

If the heart rate is normal, the version is continued until the head is over the pelvis and the breech is in the fundus.

Following completion of the procedure record an NST.

Version should be performed easily and gently.

Backward somersault: Procedure similar as above but occiput is in the lead in place of face.

There is no role for tocolysis or conduction analgesia for this procedure. But, if the procedure is repeated after a week of failed version then tocolysis to be considered-Inj, Terbutaline 0.25 mg SC the rescue tocolysis. If it fails even with tocolysis the procedure to be abandoned.

- Immunoprophylaxis with anti-D 300 microgram is to be administered in nonimmunized Rh-negative mother.

Complications

- Labor may commence
- PROM
- Antepartum hemorrhage
- Fetal distress
- Fetal death

INTERNAL PODALIC VERSION

In internal podalic version, the fetus is turned by intrauterine manipulation so as to deliver the feet first which enables the obstetrician to effect vaginal delivery by breech extraction.

Indications

- Second baby of twins when lie is transverse or oblique.
- Transverse lie with intrauterine fetal death, baby with congenital anomaly incompatible with life or not salvageable provided the liquor is adequate.

Contraindications

- Obstructed labor with impending rupture
- Reduced liquor

Prerequisites

- Cervix must be fully dilated.
- Liquor must be adequate.
- Baby should be of average size.
- Fetopelvic disproportion ruled out by clinical assessment.

Anesthesia: General anesthesia.

Steps

- Bladder empty, use lithotomy position.
- A hand is introduced into the uterus and membranes are ruptured and both the feet are identified, grasped and gently pulled down towards birth canal. If both the feet are not attainable, then one foot is grasped.
- With other hand applied on abdomen or with the help of an assistant head is simultaneously elevated gently.
- Episiotomy is made or extended if required.
- Legs are drawn till buttocks are visible anteriorly beyond symphysis pubis.
- Breech towel applied and traction maintained till lower third of scapula is visible, keeping back anterior.
- Trunk is slowly rotated to deliver one shoulder and arm, then rotated in reverse direction to deliver other shoulder and arm.

- After coming head may be delivered by simultaneous suprapubic external pressure to flex the head and gentle traction (Burn Marshall) applied or by use of Piper forceps/Low forceps.
- Deliver placenta by CCT/MROP.
- Discontinue uterine relaxants if used, start oxytocin.
- Examine the cervix, vagina, vulva, periurethral region and perineum carefully.

Complications

Maternal

- Tears and lacerations of cervix, vagina, vulva, periurethral region and perineum
- Rupture of uterus
- Abruptio placenta

Fetal

- Asphyxia
- Intracranial hemorrhage
- Other complications of vaginal breech delivery

CHAPTER

21

Episiotomy

DEFINITION

Deliberate incision made into the perineum to increase the outlet area and facilitate delivery.

INDICATIONS

- Not to be performed routinely
- Applied selectively for rigid/scarred perineum, breech, forceps/vacuum delivery, face to pubis delivery and shoulder dystocia.

Timing of episiotomy: At crowning of fetal head, along with a contraction.

PROCEDURE

- Clean the area with antiseptic solution.
  Infiltrate the site of incision on the perineum in a fan-like manner, to include vaginal skin, mucosa and perineal muscles with 10 ml of 0.5–1% xylocaine.
- Perform episiotomy at crowning of fetal head. Place two fingers between baby's head and perineum and cut 3–4 cms of perineum in mediolateral direction from the center of the fourchette (right preferred over left) using a curved/episiotomy scissors, making an angle more than 45° with the midline.
- After delivery of the baby and placenta, examine and identify the apex and look for any extension.
- Examine the cervix, vaginal walls, vulval outlet and paraurethral areas for tears and repair, if any.
- Repair the episiotomy with chromic catgut No. 0/1 or Vicryl rapide 2-0 if available. Close the episiotomy in three layers. The first layer comprised of vaginal mucosa and submucosal tissue, second layer comprised of the perineal muscle and the third layer comprised of subcutaneous tissue and skin.
- Vaginal mucosa is closed with continuous interlocking sutures starting 1 cm above the apex. Perineal muscles are closed with continuous sutures. Skin is closed with mattress or subcuticular sutures. Obliterate all the dead space to prevent hematoma formation.

CARE OF EPISIOTOMY

- Perineal hygiene—clean the area with antiseptic solution after every act of urination and defecation.
- Analgesics for relief of pain
- Sitz bath
- Encourage ambulation and pelvic floor exercises in order to stimulate circulation and speed up healing process.

CHAPTER

22

Active Management of Third Stage of Labor

Third stage of labor: Period from the delivery of the fetus to the complete expulsion of the placenta and membranes.

SIGNS OF PLACENTAL SEPARATION

Abdominal Signs

- Uterus becomes firm and globular
- Suprapubic bulge
- Fundus rises above the umbilicus (Schroeder's sign).

Vaginal Signs

- Fresh bleeding
- Apparent extra vulval lengthening of the cord
- The cord does not recede back when the uterus is raised (Kushner's sign)
- Feeling of placenta per vagina.

STEPS OF ACTIVE MANAGEMENT OF THIRD STAGE OF LABOR

- Do not wait for signs of placental separation.
- Give oxytocin immediately: Within 1 minute of birth of the baby, palpate the abdomen to rule out the presence of an additional baby(s) and give oxytocin 10 units intramuscularly.
- Delayed clamping of the cord if fetus is healthy. After 3 min of delivery of baby/ till cord pulsations stop. Beneficial and causes improved hematocrit, ferritin levels and storage iron in the fetus.
  Clamp cord early if baby asphyxiated, IUGR, thick meconium stained liquor, Rh negative pregnancy, monochorionic twin, infectious diseases of the mother. Quickly dry and wrap the baby and give to mother if appropriate.
- Deliver the placenta by controlled cord traction: Just prior to performing cord traction, clamp the cord close to the perineum using sponge forceps. Hold the clamped cord and the forceps with one hand.
- Keep slight tension on the cord and await a strong uterine contraction (2–3 minutes).
- Place the other hand just above the woman's pubic bone and stabilize the uterus by applying counter-traction during controlled cord traction. This prevents inversion of the uterus.

- When the uterus becomes rounded or the cord lengthens, very gently pull downwards on the cord to deliver the placenta. Do not wait for a gush of blood before applying traction on the cord. Continue to apply counter-traction to the uterus with the other hand.

Name of the drug/ preparation	Dosage and route	Drug action and effectiveness	Cautions and side effects	Storage
Oxytocin	10 units, IM, injection	Acts within 2–3 mins Effect lasts about 15–30 mins	First choice No known contraindications for postpartum use Minimal or no side effects	15–30°C can be stored at room temp for 3 months
Misoprostol (PGE1)	600 mcg	Orally: Acts within 6 mins Peak serum Concentration between 18 and 34 mins	No known contraindications for postpartum use. Common side effects: shivering and fever	Room temperature
Ergometrine	0.2 mg, IM, injection	Acts within 6–7 mins IM Effect lasts for 2–4 hours	Contraindicated in women with preeclampsia, eclampsia, hypertension, heart disease, retained placenta. Causes tonic contractions. Side effects: nausea, vomiting, headaches and hypertension.	2–8°C
Syntometrine	1 ml, IM, injection	Combined rapid action of oxytocin and sustained action of ergometrine	Same caution and side effects as ergometrine	2–8°C

- If the placenta does not descend during 30–40 sec of controlled cord traction (i.e. there are no signs of placental separation), do not continue to pull on the cord.
- Gently hold the cord and wait until the uterus is well-contracted again.
- If necessary, use a sponge forceps to clamp the cord closer to the perineum as it lengthens.
- With the next contraction, repeat controlled cord traction with counter-traction.

Never Pull on the Cord Without Pushing the Uterus up with the Other Hand

- As the placenta delivers, the thin membranes can tear off. Hold the placenta in two hands and gently turn it until the membranes are twisted. Slowly pull to complete the delivery.
- Look carefully at the placenta to be sure none of it is missing. If a portion of the maternal surface is missing or there are torn membranes with vessels, suspect retained placental fragments and manage appropriately.
  [Retained Placenta: If placenta not separated and expelled for 30 minutes or patient is profusely bleeding—Shift to Operation theater and do MROP.]
- Massage the uterus: Immediately massage the fundus of the uterus through the woman's abdomen until the uterus is contracted.

- Repeat the uterine massage every 15 min for the first two hours. Ensure uterus remains hard after you stop uterine massage.

If bleeding continues, check for other causes of PPH (genital lacerations and retained placental fragments) and manage appropriately.

- AMTSL preferred
  - Significantly reduces PPH by 60%.
  - Significantly decreases the need for blood transfusion.
  - Need for therapeutic oxytocics was reduced by 80%.

CHAPTER

23

Nutrition in Labor

- Nutrition in pregnancy plays a crucial role because it influences maternal and perinatal morbidity and mortality.
- **Energy requirements during pregnancy:**
  Energy requirements during pregnancy increase by 12%, because –
  - BMR increases by 10–15%
  - The development of new fetal tissues
  - Maternal physiological changes during pregnancy
  - Building energy reserves for postpartum lactation
- Energy requirement during 1st trimester–No change provided her stores are adequate.
- Energy requirement during 2nd trimester–340 kcal/day more
- Energy requirement during 3rd trimester–352 kcal/day more
- Energy requirement in multiple gestation–150 kcal more than singleton pregnancy
- Energy requirement during lactation–475–500 kcal.

Recommendations for Weight Gain in Singleton Pregnancy

BMI	Weight gain (Kg)
Underweight (<18.5)	12.5–18
Normal (18.5–24.9)	11.5–16
Overweight (25–29.9)	7–11.5
Obese (>30)	5–9.1

Recommendations for Weight Gain in Twin Gestation

BMI	Weight gain (Kg)
Normal (18.5–24.9)	16.8–24.5
Overweight (25–29.9)	14–22.7
Obese (>30)	11.3–19

COMPOSITION OF THE DIET

- Proteins–20% (71 g/day or 1.1 g/kg/day)
- Fats–30%
- Carbohydrates–50%

In diabetics carbohydrates should be of low glycemic index like more of whole grains and soluble fibers like in vegetables which allow slow absorption of glucose and slow rise in blood glucose.

- Food pyramid: 6–11 servings of grains, 3–5 servings of vegetables, 2–4 servings of fruits, 3–4 servings of dairy, 2–3 servings of meat, beans or nuts and 1 serving of sweets.
- Essential fatty acids: 3–6% of total energy intake from fats.
  Ratio of LCPUFA (long chain polyunsaturated fatty acids) omega-6 to omega-3 should be 5:1 to 10:1.
  Docosahexaenoic acid (DHA) is needed for testicular, neural and retinal development of fetus. It is building block for hormones that control immune function, blood clotting, cell growth and it is component of cell membranes. Its deficiency can lead to preterm delivery.
  Recommended dose: 300 mg/day during pregnancy and lactation.
  It is present in fish (salmon, sardines, herring, mackerel, black cod and bluefish). It is advisable to take fish twice weekly. FDA recommends pregnant women not to eat shark, sword fish, king mackerel or Tile fish (high in mercury). Recommended quantity of fish consumption is <6 ounces/week (Albacore tuna) and <12 ounces/week (other fish or shell fish).
- **Dietary sources of essential and long-chain polyunsaturated fatty acids**

	Omega 6	Sources	Omega 3	Sources
Essential fatty acids	Linoleic acid	Corn, soy, safflower and sunflower oils, green leafy vegetables, nuts, seeds	Alpha linolenic acid	Canola, flaxseed, walnut, soybean oil, nuts and seeds
LCPUFA	Arachidonic acid	Egg yolk, meat	Eicosapentaenoic acid	Fish oils, fish
	Gamma linolenic acid	Evening primrose, blackcurrant, oils	Decosahexaenoic acid	Fish oils, fish

- **RDA (Recommended Daily Dietary Allowance) for Adolescent and Adult Pregnant and Lactating Women**

	Pregnant		Lactating	
Age	14–18 years	19–50 years	14–18 years	19–50 years
Fat-soluble vitamins				
Vitamin A	750 μg	770 μg	1200 μg	1300 μg
Vitamin D	5 μg	5 μg	5 μg	5 μg
Vitamin E	15 mg	15 mg	19 mg	19 mg
Vitamin K	75 μg	90 μg	75 μg	90 μg
Water-soluble vitamins				
Vitamin C	80 mg	85 mg	115 mg	120 mg
Thiamine	1.4 mg	1.4 mg	1.4 mg	1.4 mg
Riboflavin	1.4 mg	1.4 mg	1.6 mg	1.6 mg

Contd...

Contd...

Niacin	18 mg	18 mg	17 mg	17 mg
Vitamin B_6	1.9 mg	1.9 mg	2 mg	2 mg
Folate	600 μg	600 μg	500 μg	500 μg
Vitamin B_{12}	2.6 μg	2.6 μg	2.8 μg	2.8 μg
Biotin	30 μg	30 μg	–	–
Pantothenic acid	6 mg	6 mg	–	–
Minerals				
Calcium	1300 mg (2000 mg) in multiple gestation)	1000 mg (1500 mg) in multiple gestation)	1300 mg	1000 mg
Sodium	1.5 g	1.5 g	1.5 g	1.5 g
Potassium	4.7 g	4.7 g	5.1 g	5.1 g
Iron	27 mg	27 mg	10 mg	9 mg
Zinc	12 mg	11 mg	13 mg	12 mg
Iodine	220 μg	220 μg	290 μg	290 μg
Selenium	60 μg	60 μg	70 μg	70 μg
Chromium	29 μg	30 μg	–	–
Copper	1000 μg	1000 μg	–	–
Phosphorus	1250 mg	700 mg		
Others				
Proteins	71 g	71 g	71 g	71 g
Carbohydrates	175 g	175 g	210 g	210 g
Fiber	28 g	28 g	29 g	29 g

- **Sources of vitamins**

Vitamins	Sources
Folic acid	Fortified grains, dried beans, leafy greens, liver, egg, wheat products
Vitamin A	Green leafy vegetables, yellow orange vegetables, carrot, spinach, tomato, papaya, mango
Vitamin B_1	Milk and raw grains
Vitamin B_2	Green vegetables, milk, egg, cheese and fish
Vitamin B_6	Vegetables, grains, legumes, corns
Vitamin B_{12}	Animal proteins, milk, egg, meat
Vitamin C	Fruits, vegetables, amla, orange, sweetlime, lemon
Vitamin D	Fortified milk, fish liver oil, sun light
Vitamin E	Animal proteins and fats, vegetable oils, cereals, meat, eggs, milk, nuts, seeds
Vitamin K	Green leafy vegetables, tomatoes, dairy products, eggs, intestinal flora
Niacin	Poultry, fish and nuts
Iron	Liver, beef, green leafy vegetables, dates
Calcium	Milk, curd, cheese
Zinc	Meat, liver, sea foods

Contd...

Contd...

Iodine	Sea food, iodized salt
Magnesium	Nuts, cocoa, green vegetables
Dietary fiber	Cellulose, hemicelluloses, pectins, lignin and resistant starch
Proteins	Meat, milk, eggs, cheese, poultry, fish

- Iron and calcium require supplementation.
- Well-balanced diet provides RDA of all other vitamins except folic acid. Hence supplementation of only folic acid is recommended during pregnancy.

Unusual requirement of folic acid:
- Hyperemesis gravidarum
- Hemolytic anemia
- Multiple gestation
- Previous history of NTDs.

The Conditions where Supplementation of Other Vitamins and Minerals is Recommended

- **Zinc**
  - Vegetarians
  - Alcoholics
  - Smokers
  - Teenagers
  - Multigravida with impaired intestinal absorption
  - Women receiving diuretics
  - Those with an acute response to infection or trauma
  - Those receiving iron supplementation >60 mg/day
- **Copper** also should be supplemented along with zinc because both zinc and copper compete with iron for intestinal absorption.
- **Iodine**
  - Iodine deficient area
- **Magnesium**
  - Prolonged illness
  - Previous intestinal bypass surgery
- **Vitamin B_{12}**
  - Strict vegetarians
- **Vitamin B_6**
  - Substance abusers
  - Adolescents
  - Multiple gestation
  - Along with antihistaminics as in hyperemesis

A Standard Prenatal Vitamin Formulation

- Iron–30 mg
- Zinc–15 mg
- Calcium–250 mg

- Vitamin B_6–2 mg
- Folate–3 mg
- Vitamin C–50 mg
- Vitamin D–5 μg

MEDICAL CONDITIONS WHERE CONSULTATION WITH REGISTERED DIETICIAN IS ADVISABLE

- Multiple gestation
- Frequent gestation (<3 months interpregnancy interval)
- Tobacco, alcohol of chronic medicinal or illicit drug use
- Severe nausea and vomiting
- Eating disorders
- Inadequate weight gain during pregnancy
- Adolescents
- Restricted eating
- Food allergies/intolerances
- GDM/prior history of GDM
- Prior history of LBW babies/other obstetrical complications
- Social factors that may limit appropriate intake (e.g., religion, poverty)

EFFECT OF NUTRITIONAL PROBLEMS ON PREGNANCY

Maternal–
- Hyperemesis
- Preeclampsia
- Anemia
- GDM

Fetal–
- Low-birth weight
- Preterm birth
- Increased perinatal mortality
- **Barker Hypothesis**
  Some chronic adult diseases originate in utero as a result of fetal adaptation to optimize survival. Low-birth weight has been associated with an increased risk of later development of Type 2 diabetes mellitus, heart disease, hypertension, obstructive lung disease, hypercholesterolemia and renal damage.

NUTRITION DURING LABOR

- Withholding food and drink inappropriately from women in labor may result in dehydration, ketosis, fatigue and can increase levels of stress, which in turn, can affect the neuro-hormonal balance that enables labor to progress unhindered.
- The prophylactic use of antacids or reduction of the volume of stomach contents by restricted oral intake has not been shown to be successful in preventing Mendelson's syndrome.

- For those women for whom a general anesthetic is not anticipated, a light, low residue, low fat diet may be recommended in latent phase. Allow oral fluids to maintain hydration in the active phase.
- For those women for whom a general anesthetic is anticipated, allow only clear liquids.
- The administration of opioids delays stomach emptying. So, allow only liquid diet.

Suggested Drinks for Women in Labor

- Low fat yoghurt drinks
- Fresh fruit juices (avoid apple, pineapple, mango and lemon as they tend to be more acidic)
- Coffee/Tea with skimmed milk
- Soups (cream of tomato or vegetable, etc.)
- Squash drinks–not too concentrated
- Water and ice
- Naturally carbonated mineral water.

Suggested Foods for Women in Labor

- Idli
- Toast with low fat spread, jam/honey
- Cereals with skimmed milk/ganji
- Plain sweet biscuits
- Smooth soup
- Low fat, smooth yoghurt

Parenteral infusions in Labor: Required, if
- Laboring woman declines oral intake
- Repeated vomiting
- Dehydration in case of prolonged labor

Choice of IV Fluids

1. **Normal saline:** Produces sustainable volume expansion with no effect on cell size and function. It causes minimal brain edema and has almost no effect on osmolarity. As it raises, pulmonary capillary wedge pressure by sustained expansion of plasma volume, excess of input, may cause pulmonary edema.
2. **Dextrose 5%:** Dextrose 5% provides a transient volume expansion and if given in large volume, will cause cell edema. This is specially a matter of concern in hypoxic fetus where cerebral edema may aggravate the condition. Given in small quantity, it is a good choice to provide energy in fasting state. Glucose infusions are electrolyte free and an infusion of >3500 ml can cause maternal postpartum cerebral edema, fits and coma.
3. **Dextrose saline:** Combines the effect of both the dextrose as well as saline, but difficult to interpret and predict clinical events. A better option is to give dextrose and saline separately as the condition demands.
4. **Ringer lactate:** An excellent choice for volume expansion as well as an IV drug vehicle. In asphyxia, its use is inappropriate.

5. **Albumin 5%:** Although sparingly used, it produces sustained volume expansion and does not cause any interference in electrolyte balances. When vascular damage is expected, it is best avoided as it will leak into interstitial space and cause a sustained edema there.
6. **Mannitol:** Another excellent choice for volume expansion and being hyperosmolar can help in reducing cellular edema. Has a sustained and relatively long-lasting effect, but may interfere in coagulation mechanism.

RECOMMENDATIONS

- To avoid ketosis as a result of prolonged labor, small amounts of glucose may be given slowly.
- Do not give a large amount of glucose < 6–15 gm/hr
- Intravenous fluids are seldom necessary in first 12 hours of labor and total input is < 3000 ml.
- For expansion of plasma volume, the choice is crystalloid solution like Normal saline.
- Lactated Ringer is also good choice in volume replacements of hemorrhages, but in protracted labors, the lactate may be harmful for the compromised fetus.

SPECIAL SITUATIONS

Preterm labor: The initial therapy for a preterm labor is hydration, in addition to routine oral intake, an infusion of 1500–2000 ml/24 hrs is given. 5% albumin is another good option for a sustained volume expansion.

Preeclampsia and IUGR: A quick volume expansion raises cardiac output and lowers vascular resistance without affecting mean arterial pressure and hence improves hemodynamic stability and increases uterine blood flow.

- The best option is infusion of 500 ml of 0.9% NaCl over 30 mins. 50% of Na deficit should be corrected by giving 3% NaCl. Oxytocin is advantageous due to its antidiuretic properties and resultant volume expansion.
- There is a risk of postpartum pulmonary edema due to sudden volume expansion resulting from sustained uterine contraction and elimination of utero-placental circulation. If dextrose is given, a chance of cerebral edema is likely. These risks are more pronounced in obese and chronically hypertensive patient with very labile hemodynamic system.

Epidural/Spinal analgesia: Before employing either epidural or spinal analgesia, a preload with 500–1000 ml normal saline is greatly beneficial to limit the fall in BP in response to sympathetic block.

Induction and augmentation: Antidiuretic property of oxytocin leads to retention of water and hyponatremia, especially if the delivery solution is glucose. Studies have shown a reduced cord blood Na and higher neonatal jaundice when glucose is used. Saline is the preferred solution for oxytocin infusion, and better to use concentrated infusion.

Fetal distress: After maternal feeding or glucose infusion, due to anaerobic oxidation of glucose, it results in lactate accumulation and cerebral edema.

Glucose and lactated ringer are best avoided and small quantities of saline infusion to expand the blood volume can help by increasing the utero-placental perfusion. Oxygen and lateral position unrestore the cardiac output.

Hypovolemia: To correct hypovolemia of exsanguinations, saline or ringer is the best choice. Blood and/or plasma are reserved only to replace clotting factors, or when there is a marked drop in hemoglobin concentration. Albumin is a good option but has a very short shelf-life. Hemocele having a long shelf-life is an excellent volume expander but interferes with clotting mechanism.

Ketoacidosis: If ketoacidosis is detected, an infusion of N.S 1–2 L in 30 to 60 min given and then maintained at 200–250 ml/hr. Glucose is started only after blood sugar falls below 200 mg%. Insulin is started only after blood sugar falls below 200 mg%. Insulin is started at a rate of 12 U/hr and reduced when blood sugar is <200 mg%. Bicarbonates are given when pH falls <7.1 and potassium is given if serum K^+ is < 3 mEq/L.

Suggested priorities for maternal micronutrient supplementation during lactation:

Priority I	Priority II
Thiamine	Folic acid
Riboflavin	Vitamin D
Vitamin B_6	Calcium
Vitamin B_{12}	Iron
Vitamin A	Copper
Iodine	Zinc
Selenium	

Priority I–The concentration of these nutrients in breast milk and infant status can be readily improved by increasing maternal intake.

Priority II–The concentration of these nutrients in breast milk is unaffected and maternal supplementation benefits the mother than her infant.

EXERCISE IN PREGNANCY

No strenuous exercise during 1st trimester (old concept) –

- Increases core body temperature during embryogenesis
- Shifts oxygenated blood and energy substances to maternal skeletal muscle away from the developing fetus

But now aerobic and strength training exercise during pregnancy are recommended–

- No increase in early pregnancy loss
- No late pregnancy complications
- No abnormal fetal growth
- No adverse neonal outcomes

Benefits of Exercise during Pregnancy

- Strengthens muscles needed for labor and delivery
- Helps reduce backaches, constipation, bloating and swelling
- Improves posture
- Gives energy and improves mood
- Lessens some of the discomforts of pregnancy
- Helps one feel less tired and sleep better
- Increases strength and stamina

Benefits to infants

- Infants have less body fat at birth
- Infants have reduction in the incidence of colic
- Greater neurodevelopmental scores in oral language and motor areas (tested at age 5)

When and How to Start an Exercise Program?

- Second trimester
- Those who are already exercising can continue their exercise throughout pregnancy using guidelines outlined below.

Contraindications for Aerobic Exercise during Pregnancy

Absolute contraindications:

- Hemodynamically significant heart disease
- Restrictive lung disease
- Multiple pregnancy at risk of preterm labor
- Persistent bleeding during 2nd and 3rd trimesters
- Preeclampsia
- Preterm labor (previous/present)
- Cervical insufficiency with or without cerclage
- Placenta previa
- Ruptured membranes

Relative contraindications:

- Heavy smokers (>20 cigarettes/d)
- Orthopedic limitation
- Poorly controlled hypertension
- Extremely sedentary lifestyle
- Chronic bronchitis
- Poorly controlled hyperthyroidism
- Morbid obesity (BMI >40)
- Extreme underweight (BMI <12)
- Poorly controlled diabetes mellitus
- Poorly controlled seizures
- Severe anemia
- Unevaluated maternal cardiac arrhythmia
- IUGR

Warning Signs to Terminate Exercise

- Excessive shortness of breath
- Chest pain or palpitations
- Dizziness
- Painful uterine contractions
- Rupture of membranes
- Vaginal bleeding
- Excessive fatigue
- Backache
- Pelvic girdle pain
- Reduced fetal movements
- Dyspnea
- Headache
- Muscle weakness
- Calf pain or swelling

Which Muscle Groups are Most Important to Exercise?

- Muscles of abdomen, back and pelvis.

Types of Exercise

- Swimming is good as water supports extra pregnancy weight and decreases added strain on joints. It uses all of the major muscle groups in the body.
- Walking is good weight-bearing exercise and increases cardiopulmonary efficiency.

Duration of exercise

- Not more than 30 min (start with 15 min gradually increase by 5 min every 1–2 weeks).

Intensity of Exercise

- Talk test–allowing woman to maintain a conversation during exercise
- Modified heart rate target zones for aerobic exercise in pregnancy

Maternal age (years)	Heart rate (beats/min)
<20	140–155
20–29	135–150
30–39	130–145
>40	125–140

- Borg's rating of perceived exertion: should be 12–14.

Perceived exertion	Level of activity
6	No exerting at all
7	Very very light
8, 9	Somewhat light

Contd...

Contd...

10, 11	Fairly light
12,13	Somewhat
14,15	Hard
16,17	Very hard
18,19	Very very hard
20	Maximal exerting

The Actual Plan

- Warm up–8 min of slow walk
- Aerobic activity–brisk walk/stationary bicycle/swimming/aerobics (20 min)
- Cool down–same activity for 5 min at a slower pace followed by 5–10 min of stretching

Postpartum Exercise: Started

- Immediately after delivery following uncomplicated delivery
- 6 weeks postpartum following cesarean section

Benefits

- Improves cardiovascular fitness
- Facilitates weight loss
- Raises positive mood
- Reduces anxiety and depression
- Gives more energy
- Reduces stress urinary incontinence

CHAPTER

24

Induction of Labor

DEFINITION

Labor induction is stimulation of regular uterine contractions before the spontaneous onset of labor by using mechanical or pharmacological methods after period of fetal viability (28 weeks of gestation) in order to generate progressive cervical dilatation and aims delivery by vaginal route.

Indications

Maternal

- Pregnancy-induced hypertension
- Diabetes mellitus
- Antepartum hemorrhage
- Hydramnios
- Congenital fetal malformations
- Premature ruptures of membranes
- Suspected chorioamnionitis

Fetal

- Placental insufficiency
- IUGR
- Prolonged pregnancy
- Rh isoimmunization
- Previous unexplained stillbirths

Contraindications

- Placenta previa or cord presentation
- Abnormal lie
- Prior classical or inverted "T" incision
- Active genital herpes
- Uterine surgery involving full thickness of myometrium
- Pelvic structural deformities
- Invasive cervical carcinoma
- Contracted pelvis and CPD
- Persistent malpresentation
- Pregnancy with previous cesarean section for recurrent indication
- Elderly primigravida with complicating factors
- High-risk pregnancy with compromised fetus and pelvic tumors.

FACTORS TO BE CONSIDERED BEFORE INDUCTION

Maternal Consideration

- Pre-induction cervical score
- Exclude contraindication of induction of labor
- Receptivity of the uterus to the proposed agent of induction
- Perform clinical pelvimetry to assess pelvic adequacy
- Gestational age
- Maternal condition

Fetal Consideration

- To ensure fetal gestational age
- To estimate fetal weight
- Ensure fetal lung maturity
- Ensure fetal presentation and lie
- Confirm fetal wellbeing

Prerequisites for Induction of Labor

- Valid indication
- Informed written consent (Explain purpose of induction, methods and complications and consequences if not done)
- Known gestational age
- Established fetal lung maturity
- Rule out contraindications for vaginal delivery (Active genital herpes, previous classical cesarean section, major degree placenta previa, cephalo-pelvic disproportion, malpresentation and VVF repair)

Procedure

- Detailed history
- Per-abdominal examination
- Preinduction cervical status assessment, according to Bishop's score
- Pelvic adequacy and elimination of fetopelvic disproportion

  Modified Bishop's score (Calder score)

Score	0	1	2	3
Cervical dilatation in cms	<1	1-2	2-4	>4
Cervical effacement (length) in cms	>4	2-4	1-2	<1
Cervical position	Posterior	Midposition/ Anterior		
Consistency of cervix	Firm	Medium/soft		
Station of presenting part	-3	-2	-1/0	+1, +2

Total score: 11

Calder score <6: Cervical ripening to be done with PGE2/Foley's bulb >6: Induce with PGE1/ oxytocin + amniotomy

COMPLICATIONS OF INDUCTION OF LABOR

Maternal

- Uterine hyperstimulation
- Uterine rupture
- Hyponatremia
- Operative delivery
- Postpartum hemorrhage

Fetal

- Fetal distress
- Umbilical cord prolapse
- Hyperbilirubinemia

CLASSIFICATION OF METHODS OF INDUCTION OF LABOR

1. Non-Pharmacological

A. Natural

- Herbal compounds
- Castor oil
- Hot baths
- Enemas
- Sexual intercourse
- Breast stimulation
- Acupuncture
- Acupressure
- Transcutaneous nerve stimulation

B. Mechanical

- Hygroscopic dilators: Laminaria tents
- Transcervical catheter: Foley's catheter
- Extra-amniotic saline infusion

C. Sweeping of membranes

2. Surgical methods

a. Artifical rupture of membranes

3. Medical or Pharmacological Methods

a. Oxytocin
b. Prostaglandins
c. Nitric oxide
d. Cytokines
e. Relaxin

Mechanical Methods

Not used in modern obstetrics

a. Hygroscopic dilators: Laminaria tents

Types

1. Natural: Originates from stems of laminaria digitalis and laminaria japonicum, stems are cut, peeled, shaped, dried, sterilized and packed according to their size
   a. Small size: 3 to 5 mm in diameter
   b. Medium: 6 to 8 mm
   c. Large: 8 to 10 mm
2. Synthetic: Lamicel and Dilapan S
   a. Lamicel: Slender rod-shaped polyvinyl acetyl sponge impregnated with anhydrous magnesium sulfate (450 mg)
   b. Dilapan-S: Acrylic-based hydrogel rod
   Advantage: These inserts can be used on an outpatient basis without the need of fetal monitoring.

Steps of Insertion

Step 1: Cervix is cleansed with Povidone-Iodine solution and is grasped with a Tenaculum.
Step 2: A Hygroscopic dilator of appropriate size is then inserted using a uterine packing forceps so that the tip rests at the level of internal os.
Step 3: After 4 to 6 hours the Laminaria will swell and dilate the cervix.

- Overnight, laminaria will approximately double in diameter and Dilapan swells more.
- Lamicel increases in diameter 1.5-fold over 2–4 hours.

Complications

- Infection
- Anaphylaxis
- Migration into uterine cavity
- Breakage
- Dumb-bell shaped swelling of the laminaria tent (if inserted beyond the internal os)–difficulty in removal

b. Transcervical Catheter

- A fluid filled balloon is inserted inside the cervix.
- The balloon provides mechanical pressure directly on the cervix which responds by ripening and dilation.
- A Foley's catheter inflated with 20–30 ml fluid is used.

Technique of balloon placement:
Step 1: After sterilization and draping, the catheter No. 12F is introduced into the endocervix either by direct visualization or blindly by sliding it over fingers through the endocervix into the potential space between the amniotic membrane and the lower uterine segment.

Step 2: The balloon is inflated with 30 to 50 mL of normal saline and is retracted so that it rests on the internal os.
Step 3: An intermittent pressure may also be exerted on the catheter end at 2–4 times per hour.
Step 4: Catheter is removed at the time of rupture of membranes or may be expelled spontaneously which indicates a cervical dilatation of 3–4 centimeter or removed at the end of 12 hrs whichever is later.

c. Extra-amniotic Saline Infusion Procedure

Step 1: Done by 16 F Foley's catheter placed through cervix.
Step 2: 30 ml balloon is inflated with saline and pulled snugly against the internal os and catheter taped to thigh.
Step 3: At room temperature normal saline is infused through the catheter port of Foley at 30 or 40 ml/hr by infusion pumps.
Recommendation on mechanical methods: Mechanical procedures (balloon catheters and laminaria tents) should not be used routinely for induction of labor.

d. Sweeping of Membranes: One of the old methods of induction.

The index finger is introduced into cervical os and sweeped in a circular motion stripping the lower pole of membranes off the uterine segment.
Mechanism of action: It releases phospholipase A2 and increases the production of PGF2α besides mechanical dilation of cervix.

- Sweeping the membranes increased the likelihood:
  - Spontaneous labor within 48 hours
  - Birth within one week.

According to NICE guidelines 2013, all pregnant women who do not go into spontaneous labor by 40 completed weeks, sweeping to be done and reassessed after 1 week for sweeping and formal induction.

- Membrane sweeping reduced the frequency of using other methods to induce labor (formal induction of labor)
- The risk of operative delivery is not changed by the intervention.
- No major maternal adverse effects were reported in the trials.
- There was no increase in neonatal infection.
- If begun at 38 completed weeks, stripping should be done once a week. If begun at 40 weeks, stripping to be done once in 72 hours.

2. Surgical Methods

Artificial Rupture of Membranes: Also called as amniotomy, simple method of augmentation of labor.

Under aseptic precautions, a long curved Kocher's forceps or alternatively a disposable plastic amnihook is passed along side the finger into cervix and tweaked. Controlled ARM using needle in case of polyhydramnios/ mobile head.

3. Pharmacological Agents

A. **Oxytocin:** Oxytocin alone cannot be used for induction of labor
- Bishop score <6: Cervical ripening with prostaglandin followed by amniotomy and oxytocin.

- Bishop score >6: Oxytocin administered followed by amniotomy when favorable (fully effaced).

Amniotomy with oxytocin is used primarily only when prostaglandins are contraindicated

B. Misoprostol:

25 µg vaginally 4 hourly max of 6 doses

Or

50 µg orally 4 hourly max of 6 doses

Or

20 µg of oral solution 2 hourly for max. 12 hrs 0 [A single misoprostol tablet is dissolved in drinking water so that 1 ml contains 1 µg (e.g.: 200 µg in 200 ml water). If there is no response after 2 doses in nulliparous woman, the dose can be doubled. The solution is stable for up to 24 hours at room temperature but then should be discarded].

Sublingual versus vaginal misoprostol:

- Sublingual route of administration is as effective as the vaginal route.
- The safety, adverse effects, optimal dose and perinatal outcome remain to be established.

Contraindications

- Previous LSCS

Pre-requisites

1. Normal CTG
2. Para <4
3. No malposition
4. Not a big baby/ No CPD

Monitoring

- After each dose, monitor vitals of mother
- Take CTG trace
- If contractions >3/10 min—no further doses, continue with oxytocin augmentation
- Oxytocin 2 hrs after last oral dose and 4 hrs after last vaginal dose.
- If Cx remains unfavorable after 24 hrs—switch over to other method or repeat course of misoprostol

Complications

1. Uterine hyperstimulation
2. Uterine rupture
3. Meconium-stained liquor

C. Prostaglandin E2: Used for cervical ripening.

The recommended regimens are:

- One cycle of intracervical PGE2 gel: one dose, followed by two doses 6 hours apart (up to a maximum of three doses)
- One cycle of vaginal PGE2 tablets: one dose, followed by a second dose after 6 hours if labor is not established (up to a maximum of two doses)

- One cycle of vaginal PGE2 controlled release pessary: one dose over 24 hours.
  - The gel form is available in a 2.5 ml preloaded syringe for intracervical application. It contains 0.5 mg of dinoprostone.
  - Application: The gel is then instilled into the cervix. The patient is kept in a reclining position for the next 30 minutes. The dose may be repeated every 6 hours, maximum of 3 doses. Perform a pelvic examination and assess the state of the cervix before the next dose is instilled.
  - Oxytocin should be started after 6–12 hours after the last dose of dinoprostone to prevent hyperstimulation (ACOG 2009).

Comparison of intracervical PGE2 versus intravaginal PGE2:

- Intracervical gel is less effective than intravaginal prostaglandins. The risk of not achieving vaginal delivery within 24 hours was increased with intracervical PGE2 when compared to intravaginal PGE2. There was no change in the risk of cesarean section, risks of hyperstimulation, with or without FHR changes between the two groups.

Comparing induction of labor using either oxytocin (alone or in combination with amniotomy) or PGE2 (vaginal or intracervical), overall induction with PGE2 was associated with –

- An increase in successful vaginal delivery within 24 hours
- A reduction in cesarean section
- A reduction in the risk of the cervix remaining unfavorable/unchanged at 24–48 hours
- A reduction in the use of epidural analgesia
- An increase in the number of women satisified with the method of induction.

Failed induction–When uterus does not respond to stimulation at all or when uterus contracts abnormally and cervix does not dilate.

INDUCTION OF LABOR IN SPECIAL CASES

Induction in IUFD

13–17 weeks

- 200 μg vaginally 6th hourly max of 4 doses
- If no effective contractions with 1st dose—double to 400 μg
- Maximum daily dosing not to exceed 1600 μg
- Halve the dose in previous LSCS and monitor closely.

18–26 weeks

- 100 μg vaginally 6th hourly max of 4 doses
- If no effective contractions with 1st dose—double to 200 μg
- Maximum daily dosing not to exceed 800 μg
- Halve the dose in previous LSCS and monitor closely

>26 weeks

- 25–50 μg vaginally 4th hourly max of 6 doses
- If no effective contractions with 1st dose—double to 50–100 μg
- Maximum daily dosing not to exceed 600 μg
- Halve the dose in previous LSCS

- If contractions >2/10 min—dose not to be repeated. Start oxytocin after 4 hrs of last dose
- If no expulsion within 24 hrs, repeat 2nd time
- Not to be used in previous LSCS
- Success—75% within 24 hrs. The reminder will expel in next 24 hrs
- Placenta not to be handled, wait for 2 hrs, if not expelled within 2 hrs 10 U oxytocin in 500 ml saline at 20–30 drops/min. If still not expelled, manual removal of placenta.

Induction in Previous LSCS

- Induction of labor with vaginal PGE2/ Foley's bulb at 40 weeks of gestation. Misoprostol is contraindicated.

Women should be informed of the following risks with induction of labor:
- Increased risk of need for emergency cesarean section during induced labor
- Increased risk of uterine rupture.

Induction in Diabetic Pregnancies

- GDM with diet management with excellent gestational dating in a well-controlled patient, wait spontaneous labor upto 40 weeks
- GDM with insulin treatment at 38 completed weeks
- Overt diabetic well-controlled with no other complications—at 38 completed weeks
- Uncontrolled diabetes—whenever indicated
- Method of induction used depends on Bishop score
- Labor induction when fetus is not excessively large and cervix is considered favorable.

Induction of Labor in Hypertensive Disorders of Pregnancy

- Gestational hypertension: 40 weeks
- Mild preeclampsia: 38 weeks
- Severe preeclampsia: 34 weeks
- Maternal /Fetal complications: Immediate delivery
- Method of induction used depends on Bishop score

Induction of Labor to Prevent Prolonged Pregnancy

- Women with uncomplicated pregnancies — induction of labor between 41 and 42 weeks
- Method of induction used depends on Bishop score
- From 40 weeks, at least twice-weekly cardiotocography and ultrasound estimation of maximum amniotic pool depth.

Induction in Preterm Prelabor Rupture of Membranes

- Induction of labor should not be carried out before 34 weeks unless there are additional obstetric indications (for example, infection or fetal compromise)

- After 34 weeks, discuss the following factors with her before a decision is made to induce labor.
- Risks to the woman (for example, sepsis, possible need for cesarean section)
- Risks to the baby (for example, sepsis, problems relating to preterm birth)
- Local availability of neonatal intensive care facilities.

The recommended regimens are:
- Misoprostol is the drug of choice (See regimens under misoprostol)
- One cycle of vaginal PGE2 tablets : one dose, followed by a second dose after 6 hours if labor is not established (up to a maximum of two doses)
- One cycle of vaginal PGE2 controlled-release pessary: one dose over 24 hours
- Induction of labor is appropriate approximately 6 hours after prelabor rupture of the membranes at term.

Induction of Labor in CHD

- Induction of labor done only for obstetric indications or at 40 weeks of gestation.
- Can use prostaglandin E1 and E2 [Method of induction used depends on Bishop score]
- Caution:
  - Minimum dose to be used
  - Prolonged treatment must be avoided

Induction in Breech Presentation

- Induction of labor is not generally recommended if a woman's baby is in the breech presentation.
- If external cephalic version is unsuccessful, declined or contraindicated, and the woman chooses not to have an elective cesarean section, induction of labor should be offered, if delivery is indicated, after discussing the associated risks with the woman.
- Method of induction used depends on Bishop score.

Induction in Fetal Growth Restriction

- The time of delivery is the most crucial decision as there is risk of intra-uterine demise because of chronic oxygen deprivation and the risk of preterm labor
- Consider delivery, if

Oligoamnios [AFI< 5]
  - At 38 weeks or more
  - If <38 weeks, AFI should be combined with other indicators of fetal status such as umbilical artery Doppler
- Method of induction used depends on Bishop score. Foley's bulb is preferred over misoprostol.

Induction in Multiple Gestation

- Induce at 38 weeks of gestation if uncomplicated, earlier in presence of complications
- Method of induction used depends on Bishop score

Induction in Rh Negative Pregnancy

- Induce at 40 weeks in nonimmunized pregnancies and after fetal lung maturity in isoimmunized pregnancies
- Method of induction used depends on Bishop score

Maternal Request for Induction of Labor

- Induction of labor should not routinely be offered on maternal request alone However, under exceptional circumstances (for example, if the woman's partner is soon to be posted abroad with the armed forces), induction may be considered at or after 40 weeks.
- Method of induction used depends on Bishop score.

FORMAT OF CONSENT FOR INDUCTION

Patient's name: .... Date: ....
I.P. No: ....
Unit: ....

I have been explained in my vernacular language regarding the need for induction in view of ...., the risks (in the form of non-reassuring fetal status, rupture uterus, intrauterine death) and benefits associated with it. I may be considered for emergency LSCS for maternal or fetal indication at any time during the process of induction (fetal distress/non-progress of labor/failed induction). I understand that the above procedure is being undertaken in the good interest of mine (including my fetus) and give my valid consent for the induction after completely reading and understanding. I will not hold the doctor or the hospital authorities responsible for any untoward consequences arising as a result of the process of induction.

Witness | Signature

CHAPTER

25

Labor Analgesia

INTRODUCTION

Although the use of anesthesia or analgesia during labor and delivery must be individualized to each patient, the common goal is to maximize outcomes for both the mother and the neonate. Some laboring patients may not want or need anesthesia; however, others may desire a higher level of pain control or the mode of delivery may necessitate anesthetic intervention.

DEFINITIONS

Analgesia is defined as relief of pain without the loss of consciousness or motor function. Anesthesia is defined as the loss of feeling or sensation and can include the loss of consciousness, motor power, and autonomic reflex activity.

Types of Analgesia or Anesthesia

The spectrum of anesthetic techniques useful in obstetrics includes the following: systemic, local infiltration, peripheral nerve block, major regional analgesia and anesthesia (spinal and epidural blocks), and general anesthesia. Each technique entails varying levels of pain control, alterations to the progression of labor, and effects on the parturient and fetus.

Analgesia for labor: The goal is to achieve adequate pain control without depressing the parturient or fetus or affecting the progress of labor.

1. **Analgesia and anesthesia for vaginal delivery:** For an anticipated vaginal birth, the caregiver must consider various factors when selecting an analgesic or anesthetic, including effectiveness of analgesia, maternal safety, fetal safety, alterations to maternal pushing efforts, and alterations to the musculature of the birthing canal. Major regional anesthesia (epidural or spinal block) is the technique of choice; local infiltration of the perineum and paracervical and pudendal blocks are used less frequently. Rarely, general anesthesia can be used for emergency forceps delivery, shoulder dystocia, or difficult vaginal breech delivery.
2. **Analgesia and anesthesia for cesarean section:** The anticipated length of surgery, medical conditions of the mother, maternal and fetal safety, and urgency of the delivery should dictate the type of anesthesia administered. Major regional anesthesia and, less often, general anesthesia are used. Rarely, local infiltration can be used in cases of emergency cesarean section in which rapid general anesthesia is not possible.

3. **Analgesia for postoperative pain:** Systemic and regional pain control methods have been found to be quite effective. In particular, patient-controlled intravenous (IV) and epidural anesthesia are often used until the patient can tolerate oral analgesics.

I. **Nonpharmacologic techniques:** Some patients may prefer to use nonpharmacologic methods to help prepare for and manage the pains of labor and vaginal delivery. The goal is to minimize the amount of pharmacologic intervention, as tolerated.

- Inexpensive, easy-to-use and devoid of side effects.
- Quality of pain control is poor and lacks scientific validity.
  - Continuous labor support: Emotional support by husband/friends/mother
  - Touch and massage: Include effleurage, counter pressure to alleviate back discomfort, reassuring patting or light stroking.
  - Vertical maternal position: Allow women to adapt position she is most comfortable. No specific recommendations from any studies.
  - Transcutaneous electrical nerve stimulation–transmission of low voltage current to skin via wide surface area over lumbosacral region: No consistent evidence to prove impact on interventions and outcomes in labor.
- Acupuncture: No standardization of points for relief of labor pain.
- Hypnosis.

II. **Systemic analgesia:**

A. Indications. Systemic medications can be given in the latent or active phase of labor for effective pain relief. They can also be used for postoperative pain control.

1. Narcotics are the most effective systemic medication for pain control.

a. Pethidine:
  - Most frequently used opioid, no effect on labor.
  - Intramuscular route
  - Onset of action within 45 minutes after IM administration.
  - Dose: 1–2 mg per kg body weight repeated every 4–6 hrly
  - Side effect–Nausea
    Respiratory depression in neonates born 2–3 hrs after administration
    Neurobehavioral changes in neonate
  - Contraindication
    Mother with liver disease on antidepressants.

b. Morphine:
  - Historically used
  - Currently not used due to excess sedation, maternal and neonatal respiratory depression

c. Fentanyl:
  - Rapid onset of action: 2–3 minutes
  - Intravenous administration
  - Dose—25–50 μm every hour or as continuous infusion 0.25 μm per kg per hour
  - In doses of 1 μm/kg body weight, has no effect on Apgar scores or neurobehavioral scores
  - Suitable for patient controlled intravenous analgesia.

d. Tramadol:
   - Onset of action 10 minutes after IM, lasts for 2–3 hours.
   - Intramuscular route
   - Dose-1–2 mg per kg body weight, no significant respiratory depression.
   - Low incidence of maternal side effects

e. Butorphanol:
   - Intramuscular administration
   - Dose: 1–2 mg IM
   - Side effect—excess maternal sedation, respiratory depression at doses of 2 mg.

f. Remifentanil:
   - Intravenous administration, rapid onset of action.
   - T1/2: 6 minutes, used for patient controlled analgesia.
   - Infusion of 0.025 μm per kg per minute was increased in step-wise manner to maximum dose of 0.15 μm per kg per minute.
   - Minimal maternal and no fatal/neonatal side effects.

Appropriate time for delivery of the baby–Between 1 and 4 hrs of drug administration during which time respiratory depression is least 1st hour-drug effect After 4 hrs-accumulation of metabolites.

Naloxone

- Opioid antagonist of choice for reversing the neonatal effects of maternal opioid administration.
- No benefit with maternal administration of naloxone during labor/ delivery.
- Administered to newborn if any respiratory depression. Dose = 0.1 ml/kg, IV.
- If intravenous route is not accessible, IM route can be used. Endotracheal administration not recommended.
- Can precipitate withdrawl in newborn of opioid dependent mother.
- For reversing maternal respiratory depression, dose is 0.4 mg IV.

1. At 4 cm dilatation with established labor–Inj. Diazepam 2 mg + Inj Pentazocine 6 mg diluted in 10 ml of Normal Saline IV slowly, every hour
2. If no pain relief with above regime: Inj. Tramadol 50 mg for 60 kg wt {If wt > 60 kg, add 1 ml/kg}; Antispasmodics IV{Inj. Buscopan/Epidosin/Anafortan/ Drotin}

   Better to deliver baby between 1–4 hrs of Inj Tramadol
3. In second stage of labor

Inj. Ketamine 0.5 mg/kg every ½ hourly{after counseling the patient}

III. Inhalational methods:
   - Used in mother remaining awake and intact laryngeal reflex
   - Entonox–50% oxygen and 50% nitrous oxide: commonly used.
     - Administered through a mouth piece/face mask
     - Does not interfere with uterine contractions/neonatal Apgar scores

IV. Regional analgesia in labor

Classification:

1. Neuroaxial techniques: most effective
   - Epidural analgesia
   - Combined spinal epidural analgesia [CSEA]

- Spinal analgesia
- Continuous spinal analgesia

2. Alternate regional analgesia
    - Pudendal block
    - Paracervical block
    - Lumbar sympathetic block
    - Perineal infiltration

Indication for Neuraxial Techniques

- Maternal request
- Hypertensive disorders
- Co-morbid medical diseases
- Multifetal gestation
- Trail of labor
- Prolonged labor
- Mother with anticipated difficult airway
- IUFD/presumed fetal compromise
- Obesity and/or anticipated shoulder dystocia

Contraindications for Neuraxial Analgesia

- Maternal refusal
- Coagulopathy and thrombocytopenia
- Local infection

Pre-requisites

- Informed consent
- Pre-anesthetic assessment
- Resuscitation equipment and emergency drugs
- Maternal and fetal monitoring:
- BP every 5 minutes for first 20–30 minutes after every dose
- Continuous CTG monitoring
- Adequate hydration: Avoid dextrose containing fluids.

Drugs Used

Epidural: Bupivacaine: 0.0625–0.1%, both for activation and maintenance, combined with fentanyl or sufentanil. Total dose: 15–20 ml
CSEA: Fentanyl 20–25 mcg or sufentanil 5–10 mcg.

Epidural Analgesia

Indications

An epidural block can be used for establishing analgesia during labor, analgesia and anesthesia for nonoperative, operative vaginal delivery, and anesthesia for cesarean section. After a cesarean section, postoperative pain can be managed with epidural patient-controlled anesthesia quite successfully.

Application: A 19- or 20-gauge plastic indwelling catheter is placed into the epidural space at the level of L2–L5. Verification of placement into the epidural space includes the inability to aspirate blood or cerebrospinal fluid and the administration of a test dose that does not indicate IV or subarachnoid placement. Repeated epidural injections, patient-controlled pumps, and continuous infusion of a mixture of local anesthetic plus narcotic analgesic (e.g., bupivacaine and fentanyl) has allowed lower concentration of medications to be used for effective pain control with minimal risk to patient and fetus.

Advantages

- There is often less fetal depression and respiratory compromise to the mother than with general anesthesia or systemic narcotics.
- The epidural anesthetic can be titrated to fulfil the pain control needs of the parturient, maintain her full consciousness, and allow her to push in a vaginal delivery.
- It is the only mode of anesthesia that can be used throughout all stages of labor and vaginal delivery as well as be dosed for preanesthesia for a cesarean section.

Limitations

- An epidermal block takes longer to initiate than spinal or general anesthesia. Therefore, it is not indicated for expected imminent vaginal delivery or an emergent cesarean section.

Timing of Epidural Analgesia

- In the absence of medical contraindication, maternal request is a sufficient medical indication for pain relief during labor. [Opinion of ACOG and reaffirmed by American Society of Anesthesiologist in 2006].
- Epidural given early in labor does not increase the incidence of cervical dystocia or the cesarean section rate, and it should not be delayed to achieve an arbitrary cervical dilation of 5 cms.
- Epidural per se does not increase incidence of cesarean section.

Effect on Fetal Heart Rate

- Epidural can decrease baseline variability, cause transient bradycardia, but has no effect on Apgar scores.

Effect on Duration of Labor and Instrumental Delivery

- Epidural is associated with lower rates of spontaneous vaginal delivery, prolonged second stage of labor, a higher rate of instrumental vaginal delivery, but does not affect the neonatal outcome.
- Insufficient evidence to support the hypothesis that discontinuing epidural analgesia during late labor reduces the rate of instrumental delivery, may cause inadequate pain relief in labor.

Complications and Side Effects of Regional Analgesia

a. Maternal hypotension: This can cause uteroplacental insufficiency and can lead to fetal distress. Prophylactic intravascular volume expansion with 500–1000 ml of lactated Ringer's solution is usually administered before placing an epidural catheter. If hypotension still occurs, additional IV fluids, ephedrine (10.0 mg IV), or both may be needed. Left uterine displacement (placement of the patient in left lateral tilt position) can be helpful.
b. Accidental dural puncture ("wet tap") and post-dural puncture headache: Complications after a wet tap include spinal headache. Headache occurs 24–48 hrs after epidural and is severe in 65–70% of the cases: is postural, i.e. subsides on lying down and aggravates in upright position. Treatment includes administration of abdominal binders, administration of caffeine, and increased fluid intake. Severe cases may require injection of autologous blood in the epidural space near the dural puncture (i.e., "blood patch").
c. Accidental intravascular injection: CNS toxicity from intravascular injection of an anesthetic includes dizziness, slurred speech, metallic taste, tinnitus, convulsions, and in rare cases, cardiac arrest. Treatment is supportive and may involve establishing an airway to provide assisted ventilation and administering short-acting benzodiazepines or barbiturates for seizure control.
d. Accidental subarachnoid injection: If accidental subarachnoid placement of the catheter is not detected by a test dose, a usual epidural dose may result in high or total spinal anesthesia, leading to apnea and hypotension that must be rapidly treated with supportive care.
e. Backache: Epidural per se does not result in persistent postpartum backache. Short-term local tenderness (3–7 days) may be seen in about 30% of the cases. Proper positioning and an experienced anesthetist can minimize this side effect.
f. Bladder dysfunction: Mothers receiving epidural narcotic and local anesthetic can have difficulty in voiding urine. Checking for bladder distension and encouraging women in labor to void urine best prevents this problem. Offer bed pan or urinary catheter if duration of labor >6 hrs.
g. Maternal pyrexia: Incidence of intrapartum fever with epidural = 10–15%, rise in temperature <1°C. Rule out and treat any underlying cause if temperature >1°C. Treat intrapartum pyrexia aggressively with hydration, antipyretics and other appropriate measures.
h. Miscellaneous: Other side effects are shivering, pruritus and delayed gastric emptying.

Spinal Anesthesia and Analgesia

Indications

Spinal analgesia may be administered for labor and vaginal delivery. Spinal anesthesia can be used for cesarean sections.

Application

For cesarean section, a local anesthetic (tetracaine hydrochloride, bupivacaine, or lidocaine) is injected into the subarachnoid space through a needle placed at the level of L2–L5. A sensory level of T5 is preferable for adequate anesthesia for a cesarean section. For labor and vaginal delivery, small amounts of narcotic (fentanyl, sufentanil citrate, or morphine sulfate) or local anesthetic or both can be used for analgesia. T10–L1 block is needed to minimize the pain of uterine contractions and S2–S4 block is needed for perineal analgesia.

Combined Spinal-Epidural Anesthesia (CSE)

Indications

This type of anesthesia is useful for providing analgesia or anesthesia or both for labor, vaginal deliveries, or cesarean sections.

Application

The most frequently used technique is the needle-through-needle method. The epidural space is identified, a spinal needle is then passed through the epidural needle and advanced beyond its tip to puncture the dura, and spinal anesthesia is administered. The spinal needle is then removed, and an epidural catheter is placed through the remaining needle.

Advantages

The CSE combines the rapidity, density, and reliability of the spinal block with the facility to modify or prolong the anesthesia with the use of the epidural catheter.

Risks

In addition to the risks of spinal and epidural anaesthesia, there may be difficulty interpreting the epidural test dose after a spinal block has been administered.

Major Regional Anesthesia and Analgesia

This is the most commonly used form of anesthesia today. It involves the injection of anesthetic/analgesic agents into the epidural or subarachnoid (spinal) space to achieve adequate analgesia for vaginal delivery or anesthesia for cesarean section.

Peripheral Nerve Block

This form of analgesia involve injection of a local anesthetic agent in the vicinity of discrete peripheral nerves in the pelvis (paracervical or pudendal areas) to achieve pain control.

Paracervical Block

Indications

The paracervical block is a rarely used method of analgesia that can provide relief from uterine contractions. This block involves the transvaginal injection of a total of 10–20 ml of 1% lidocaine (or 2% chloroprocaine) just lateral to the cervix bilaterally at the 4 and 8 o'clock positions).

This technique blocks the sensory nerves from uterus, cervix, and upper vagina.

Limitations

The sensory fibers from the perineum are not affected. Therefore, the paracervical block has no benefit outside of the first stage of labor. In addition, it is difficult to administer late in the first stage.

Risks

Although it is easy to perform and does not cause maternal hypotension, paracervical anesthesia can cause local vasoconstriction, increased uterine tone, and decreased perfusion to the uterus. There is an increased risk for fetal depression and transient fetal bradycardia.

Pudendal Block

Indications

This method is used to achieve perineal analgesia and help the patient tolerate the pain of the second stage of labor and any post-delivery repairs. It is administered by transvaginally injecting a total of 10–20 ml of 1% lidocaine (or 2% chloroprocaine) just posterior to the ischial spines bilaterally. This method blocks the pudendal nerve, which provides afferent fibers to the genitalia and perineum.

Limitations

Complete analgesia may require infiltration of the perineum with a local anesthetic. In addition, if a complicated vaginal delivery or possible cesarean section is predicted, major regional anesthesia should be recommended.

Risks

The pudendal block carries little risk to the fetus. Its rare complications to the mother include accidental sciatic nerve block, formation of a hematoma, or puncture of the rectum.

V. General Anesthesia

This form of anesthesia is used far less than regional anesthesia. It requires endotracheal intubation to protect the parturient's airway and minimize the risk of aspiration.

Indications

Because of its rapid induction, general anesthesia is usually used for extremely emergent cesarean sections and less often for emergent vaginal deliveries (forceps delivery, severe shoulder dystocia, difficult breech delivery). It may also be used when a patient is hypovolemic or has a contraindication to use of regional anesthesia.

Application

The most popular regimen is to use sodium thiopental (3–4 mg/kg) or ketamine hydrochloride (1–2 mg/kg) as the induction agent, followed by succinylcholine chloride (1 mg/kg) for muscle relaxation to facilitate intubation. Pre-oxygenation with 100% oxygen increases the oxygen stores in the maternal lungs. Additional inhalation agents (halothane, isoflurane, nitrous oxide) are commonly used.

Advantages

General anesthesia has the advantages of providing rapid induction and producing less hypotension.

Limitations

Because of its increased risks to the mother and fetus, general anesthesia is usually reserved for situations when all other forms of anesthesia are contraindicated or inadequate.

Risks

Data suggest that the rate of maternal death contributable to general anesthesia may be at least double the rate due to regional anesthesia. The primary cause of death associated with general anesthesia is difficulty with airway management.

1. Failed intubation or aspiration.
2. Increased uterine bleeding.
3. Fetal depression

CHAPTER

26

Prolonged Labor

PROLONGED LABOR

When labor (first and second stage together) duration lasts for more than 24 hours, labor is said to be prolonged.

Classification

- Prolonged latent phase
- Prolonged active phase
- Disorders of dilatation
- Disorders of descent

Causes

1. Power:
    - Hypotonic uterine contractions – intrinsic, excessive sedation, regional analgesia
    - Inadequate maternal bearing down, epidural analgesia
2. Passenger:
    - Macrosomia
    - Malpresentation
    - Malposition
    - Deflexed attitude
    - Fetal anomalies
3. Passage:
    - Cephalopelvic disproportion
    - Pelvic tumors

Criteria Used for Diagnosis of Labor

1. Presence of painful uterine contractions 1–2 C/≥20 sec/10 minutes
2. Dilatation of cervix 1–3 cms, along with effacement

Prolonged Latent Phase

- Prolonged Latent Phase is defined differently in primigravida and multigravida
    - Nullipara: >20 hr (normal about 12 hr)
    - Multipara: >14 hr (normal about 8 hr)

Differentiate it from False Labor Pains

	False labor pain	Prolonged latent phase
1. Observe the patient for 4–6 hr	Irregular contraction which gradually decreases in frequency and intensity. No associated cervical dilatation.	Persistent regular uterine contractions that increase in intensity, frequency and duration. Cervical changes may or may not be present.
2. Therapeutic rest–give injection pethidine 50 mg and injection phenergan 25 mg intramuscular	Sleep for a few hours and awake with no contractions.	Contractions continue and cervical changes start.

Management

No active intervention is required.

Prolonged Active Phase

Disorders of dilatation and descent cannot always be separated and usually overlap.

Disorders of Dilatation

Diagnosis

Protracted dilatation: Slow cervical dilatation in active phase:
- Primi: <1.2 cm/hr
- Multi: <1.5 cm/hr

Secondary arrest of dilatation: No cervical dilatation for 2 hr or more in active phase.

Disorders of Descent

Usually occurs in late first stage of labor.

Diagnosis

- **Prot racted descent:** Maximum slope of descent
  - Primi ≤ 1 cm/hr
  - Multi ≤ 2.0 cm/hr
- **Arrest of descent:** No progress in movement of fetus through the birth canal in the second stage of labor for 1 hour.

Management

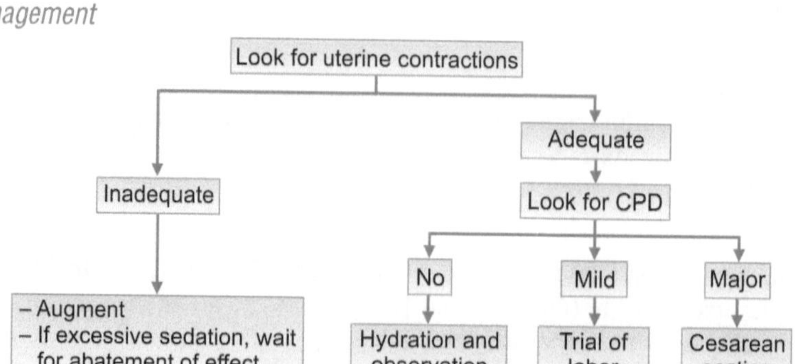

Labor Pattern	Nulliparas	Multiparas	Preferred Treatment	Exceptional Treatment
Prolongation Disorder - prolonged latent phase	>20hr	>14hr	Bed rest	Oxytocin or cesarean delivery for urgent problems
Protraction Disorders			Expectant and support	Ceserean delivery for CPD
- protracted active-phase dilatation	<1.2cm/hr	<1.5cm/hr		
- protracted descent	<1cm/hr	<2cm/hr		
Arrest Disorders			Evaluate for CPD: CPD: cesarean delivery No CPD:oxytocin	Rest if exhausted Cesarean delivery
- Prolonged deceleration phase	>3hr	>1hr		
- Secondary arrest of dilatation	>2hr	>2hr		
- Arrest of descent	>1hr	>1hr		
Failure of descent	No descent in deceleration phase or second stage	No descent in deceleration phase or second stage		

CPD = cephalopelvic disproportion.

Prolonged Second Stage of Labor

- Duration of second stage
  - >2 hr in primigravida (>3 hrs with analgesia)
  - >1 hr in multipara (>2 hrs with analgesia)

  (Absolute duration of second stage is not relevant if mother and baby are stable. Management should be based on the condition of the mother and the fetus rather than the duration of labor).
- Women should be discouraged from lying supine or semi-supine in the second stage of labor and should be encouraged to adopt any other position that they find most comfortable.
- Women should be informed that in the second stage they should be guided by their own urge to push.
- If full dilatation of the cervix has been diagnosed in a woman without epidural analgesia, but she does not get an urge to push, further assessment should take place after 1 h.
- Augment the uterine contractions with the use of oxytocin, this should not be contemplated where uterine activity is already effective and if disproportion or obstructed labor is suspected.
- A routine episiotomy should not be carried out during spontaneous vaginal birth.
- An episiotomy should be performed if there is a clinical need, such as instrumental birth or suspected fetal compromise.

- Where an episiotomy is performed, the recommended technique is a mediolateral episiotomy originating at the vaginal fourchette and usually directed to the right side. The angle to the vertical axis should be between 45 and 60 degrees at the time of the episiotomy.

Operative Vaginal Delivery in Second Stage of Labor

The following prerequisites must be fulfilled when assessing a woman before attempting an operative vaginal delivery.

- Not more than one-fifth of the head should be palpable on abdominal palpation.
- Cervix fully dilated and membranes ruptured.
- Station at level of ischial spines or below.
- Exact position of fetal head should be determined.
- Excessive caput or moulding should not be present.
- There should be noticeable descent of head with uterine contraction and bearing down efforts.
- **Vacuum v/s Forceps:** Choice of instrument should depend on the expertise of the obstetrician, vacuum and forceps having their own advantages and disadvantages. There are no recommendations regarding the preference of the instrument.

Instrumental delivery v/s C-section: Cesarean section at full dilatation with anhydramnios and an engaged fetal head is a difficult procedure. This is reflected in high rates of major obstetric hemorrhage, extension of the uterine incision and prolonged hospital admission. These risks must be balanced with the potential for pelvic floor trauma and neonatal injury following operative vaginal delivery.

Serious Complications of Second Stage Section

Maternal
• Lateral extension of the uterine incision during disimpaction of the fetal head in deep transverse arrest/deflexed occipitoposterior position. • Uterine artery laceration, resulting in significant hemorrhage. This requires significant skill and technique to tamponade. In cases of extreme hemorrhage, hysterectomy may be indicated. • Ureteric injury due to inadvertent suturing to stop hemorrhage. • Broad ligament hematoma. • Bladder injury due to an overstretched lower uterine segment. • Postpartum hemorrhage secondary to atonic uterus, a result of prolonged second stage and augmentation. This may be exacerbated by uterine incision. • Accidental suturing of the lower uterine incision with the posterior wall of the cervix, resulting in occlusion.
Fetal
• Craniofacial/intracranial injury • Cephalohematoma and subgaleal hemorrhage • Intracranial hemorrhage • Skull fracture • Seizures • Jaundice

CHAPTER

27

Obstructed Labor

DEFINITION

Condition where the progress of labor is at a standstill, with the fetal presenting part arrested due to mechanical factors and further progress in the delivery is impossible without professional assistance.

ETIOLOGY

- Maternal causes:
  - Bony obstruction, e.g.
    - Contracted pelvis
    - Tumors of pelvic bones
  - Soft tissue obstruction:

  i. Uterus:
    - Impacted subserous pedunculated fibroid.
    - Constriction ring opposite the neck of the fetus.

  ii. Cervix: Cervical dystocia, prolapsed edematous cervix, cicatrized cervix following Manchester operation, cervical encirclage.

  iii. Vagina: Septa, Stenosis, Tumors.

  iv. Ovaries: Impacted ovarian tumors.
- Fetal causes:
  1. Malpresentations and malpositions, e.g.
     –Persistent occipito-posterior and deep transverse arrest,
     –Persistent mento-posterior and transverse arrest of the face presentation.
     –Impacted frank breech.
  2. Large sized fetus (macrosomia).
  3. Congenital anomalies: e.g.
     –Hydrocephalus.
     –Fetal ascitis.
     –Fetal tumors.
  4. Locked and conjoined twins.

COMPLICATIONS

Maternal

- Maternal distress
- Sepsis

- Atonic PPH
- Rupture uterus
- Remote complications like VVF, RVF
- Dehiscence of symphysis pubis, shock and death

Fetal

- Birth asphyxia
- Intracranial hemorrhage
- Sepsis
- Hypoxic encephalopathy
- Remote: Cerebral palsy

CLINICAL FEATURES

General Examination

- Maternal exhaustion
- Tachycardia
- Dehydration
- Acidotic breath
- May be febrile

P/A Examination

- Tonic uterine contraction, uterus tender, LUS stretched
- Bladder distended, gut distension
- Rising retraction ring
- FHS regular or irregular or absent
- Fetal poles may be palpable P/A

P/V Examination

- Vulval edema
- Hot dry vagina
- Purulent discharge may be present
- Cervix may or may not be fully dilated
- Offensive meconium-stained discharge
- Large caput
- Moulding+++

Look for malpresentation, malposition, deflexed attitude of head, meconium and cause of obstruction.

On catheterization, blood stained urine is seen.

Investigation

- CBC
- Blood group and type
- Urine-ketones, sugar, albumin
- HIV, HbsAg, VDRL

Management

Prevention

- Early recognition, Early referal
- Partogram

TREATMENT

General Measures

- Vaginal swab for culture and sensitivity
- Exclude rupture uterus
- No wait and watch
- No oxytocics
- Hydrate the patient—IV fluids—NS/RL. No dextrose containing fluids
- Arrange blood
- I/V antibiotics
- Foley's catheter to be inserted

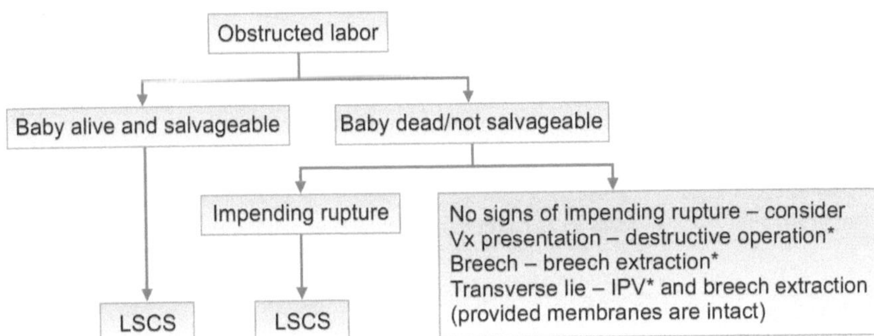

Figure 27.1: Management of obstructed labor

[* To be considered and done only by senior experienced obstetrician]

Anticipated Problems in LSCS for Obstructed Labor

- Advanced edematous bladder may get injured while opening abdomen
- Presenting part deep in pelvis, may be difficult to deliver—can be pushed from below or baby delivered by (Patwardhan) in case of cephalic presentation.
- **Patwardhan's**—back anterior—upper limb followed by opposite upper limb→fetal back followed by lower limbs and head is last to be delivered.
- **Modified Patwardhan**—used when back is posterior—lower limb is delivered such that back becomes anterior—then other lower limb is delivered followed by remaining fetus as in breech presentation.
    - Extension of incision
    - Atonic PPH more common
    - Postoperatively Foley's catheter has to be retained for 5 days if ischemia of bladder wall is suspected.

Third stage: In all cases of prolonged labor, manage third stage actively as there are increased chances of PPH.

CHAPTER

28

Instrumental Delivery

Operative or assisted vaginal delivery aims at use of an instrument either to help by traction or by reducing the diameter of the head to achieve vaginal delivery without causing significant damage to mother of fetus.

Operative vaginal deliveries include:

- Forceps
- Vacuum extraction

FORCEPS DELIVERY

Classification (American College of Obstetrics and Gynecology)

Two important factors are taken into consideration:
Station and Rotation of the head

Procedure	Criteria
Outlet forceps	• Scalp is visible at the introitus without separating the labia • Fetal skull has reached pelvic floor • Sagittal suture is in anteroposterior diameter, right, or left occiput anterior or posterior position • Fetal head is at or on perineum • Rotation does not exceed 45 degrees
Low forceps	Leading point of fetal skull is at station >= +2, and not on the pelvic floor. • Rotation is 45 degrees or less (left or right occiput anterior to occiput anterior, or left or right occiput posterior to occiput posterior) • Rotation is greater than 45 degrees.*
Midforceps High	• Station above +2 but*head is engaged. • Not included in classification.
*To be decided and done only by consultant.	

Anesthesia

- Pudendal block
- Local infiltration for episiotomy
- Regional anesthesia
- General anesthesia

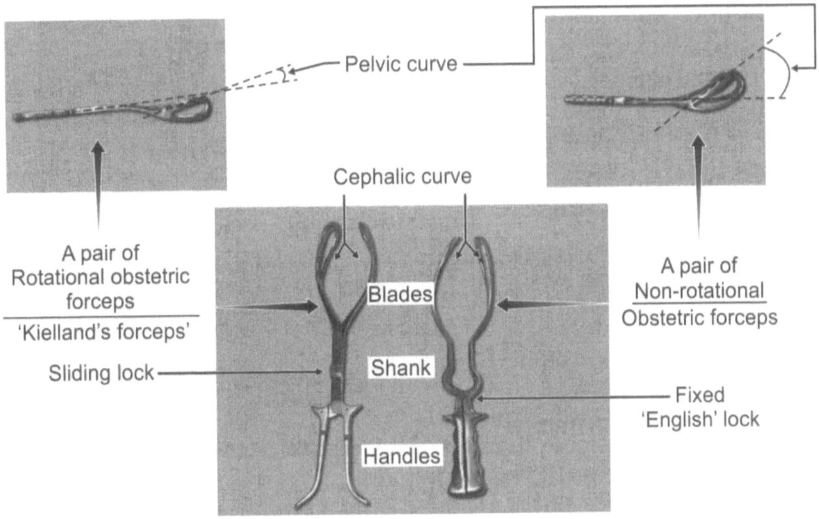

Figure 28.1: Parts of forceps

Clinical Classification

- **Indicative Forceps**
  Definite indications present
- **Elective**
  Always outlet, hence safe delivery, decided in advance to prevent certain complications.
  - Used in maternal disease
  - Controversial benefits in small for date or premature babies.
- **Trial of Forceps**
  When it is likely but not certain that forceps delivery will be successful.
  - To be done in OT with full preparation for CS.

Failure of Trial

- Failure may be defined as the inability to apply the intended instrument or the inability to deliver the baby, hence necessitating the use of a different instrument or, perhaps, cesarean section.
- If there is no progress following three traction attempts, cesarean section should be considered.
- The success of instrumental delivery is dependent on skill, adequate training and clear understanding of the position and station of the fetal head.
  The following are factors that may contribute to failure:
  - Failure to select the correct cup type
  - Inappropriate use of the silastic cup especially in the presence of deflexion of the fetal head, excess caput, or a macrosomic infant
  - Failure of the equipment to provide adequate traction as a consequence of a leakage of the vacuum
  - Inadequate initial case assessment of high head, misdiagnosis of the position and attitude of the head

- Incorrect cup placement too anterior or lateral or inclusion of maternal soft tissue within the cup
- Traction along the wrong plane
- Poor maternal effort with inadequate use of syntocinon to aid expulsive efforts in the second stage
- Choice of the wrong instrument
- Cephalopelvic disproportion.

INDICATIONS FOR ASSISTED VAGINAL DELIVERY

Fetal

- Malpositions of the fetal head (occipito-lateral and occipito-posterior). Such positions occur more frequently with regional anesthesia—a consequence of an alteration in the tone of the pelvic floor that impedes spontaneous rotation to the optional occipito-anterior position.
- Fetal 'distress' is a commonly cited indication for instrumental intervention, however, presumed fetal compromise is a more comprehensive term.
- Elective instrument intervention for infants of reduced weight. In infants weighing <1.5 kg, delivery with forceps does not confer advantage over spontaneous delivery and may increase the incidence of intracranial hemorrhage. Ventouse carries the same risks, but in addition should be avoided in infants if <35 completed weeks of gestation.
- Vaginal breech delivery. Forceps can be applied to the aftercoming head to control the delivery of the vertex, a situation where the ventouse is contraindicated.

Maternal

- The commonest maternal indications are those of maternal distress, exhaustion, or prolongation of the second stage of labor (>2 h in a primigravida (3 h if an epidural is *in situ*), or >1 h in a multipara (2 h if an epidural is *in situ*)).
- Medically significant conditions such as: aortic valve disease with significant outflow obstruction; myasthenia gravis; significant APH due to placental abruption or vasa previa; severe hypertensive disease; and previous cesarean section (to minimize the risk of scar rupture) are less common.

CONTRAINDICATION TO AN INSTRUMENTAL VAGINAL DELIVERY

Absolute

- The vertex is ≥1/5th palpable abdominally.
- The position (occipito-anterior/posterior or lateral) of the fetal head is unknown.
- Before full dilatation of the cervix (although a possible exception occurs with the vacuum delivery of a second twin).
- When the operator is inexperienced in instrumental vaginal delivery.

The Ventouse should not be Used–

- In gestations of less than 35 completed weeks because of the increased risk of intracranial hemorrhage in the fetus.

- With the fetus presenting by the face.
- If there is a significant degree of caput that may either preclude correct placement of the cup or, more sinisterly, indicate a substantial degree of cephalopelvic disproportion.

Relative Contraindications (for Forceps or Ventouse)

- Fetal bleeding disorders (e.g. alloimmune thrombocytopenia) or a predisposition to fractures (e.g. osteogenesis imperfecta) are relative contraindications, however, the comparative risks of a difficult second stage cesarean section must also be considered.
- There is minimal risk of fetal hemorrhage if the vacuum extractor is employed following fetal blood sampling or application of a scalp electrode.

PREREQUISITES

- Informed consent should be obtained and documented
- Engaged fetal vertex: the head should be ≤1/5 palpable in the abdomen
- Ruptured membranes
- Fully dilated cervix
- Position precisely known
- Assessment of maternal pelvis (should be adequate)
- Adequate maternal analgesia
- Empty bladder
- Experienced operator
- Willingness to abandon the procedure if necessary
- Episiotomy should be performed where perineal laceration is anticipated
- Necessary support personnel and equipment must be present.

SUMMARY

F—Full dilatation
O—Occipitoanterior
R—Rupture of membranes
C—Contractions–uterine, good, catheterization
E—Engagement: Empty bowel
P—Position: Pelvis adequate
S—Station of presenting part

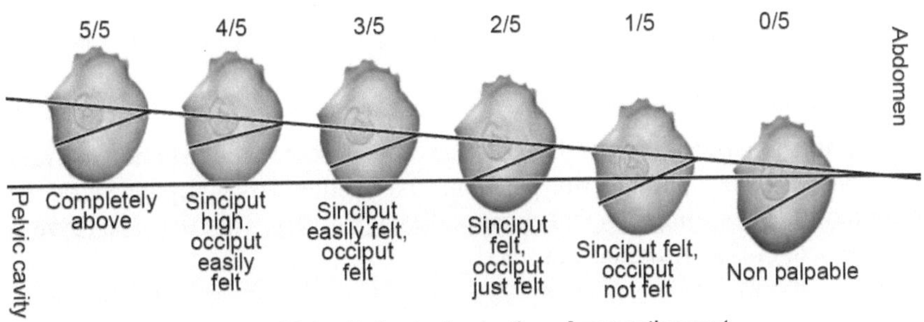

Figure 28.2: Abdominal palpation of presenting part

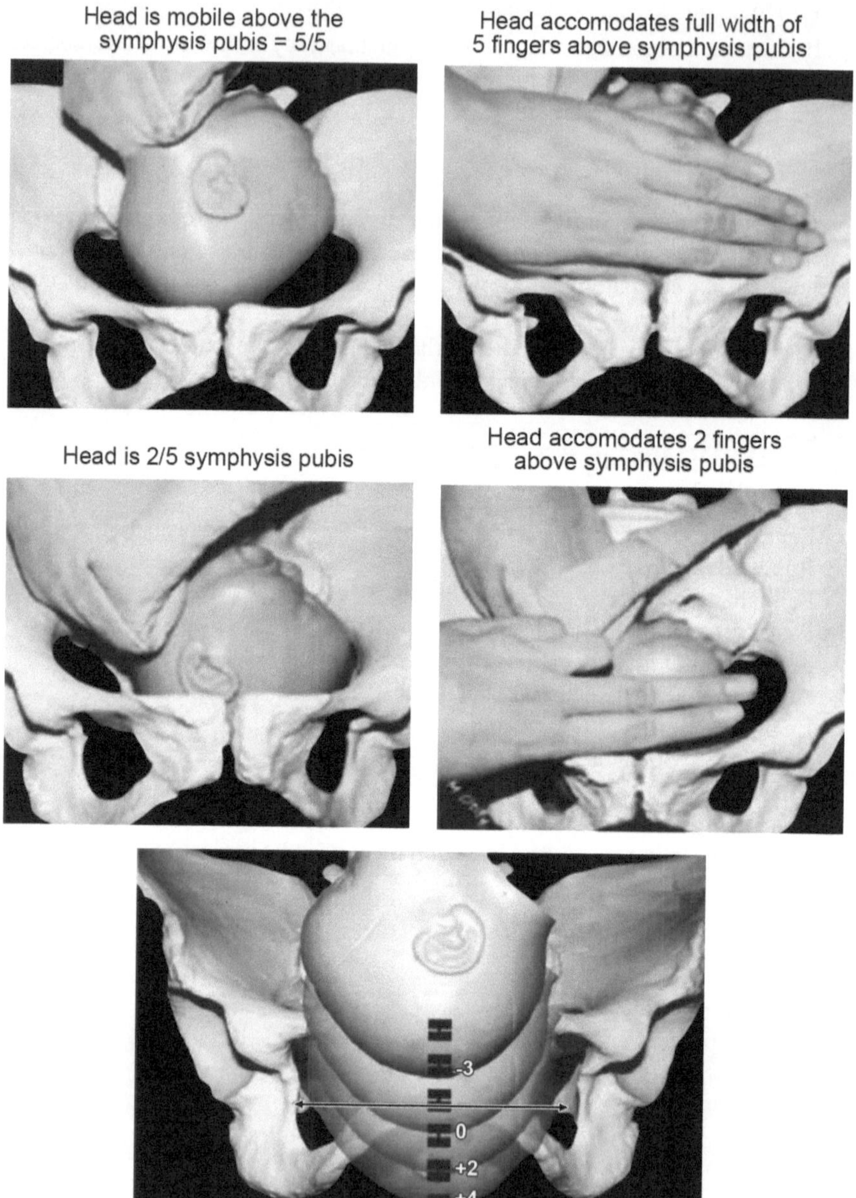

Figure 28.3: Abdominal palpation of presenting part

APPLICATION

Axis of traction. Illustration of the direction of the forces required during delivery of a fetus in an occipito-anterior position. The traction axis is dependent on the station of the presenting part and changes during delivery. This 'J' shape curve is independent of the instrument chosen.

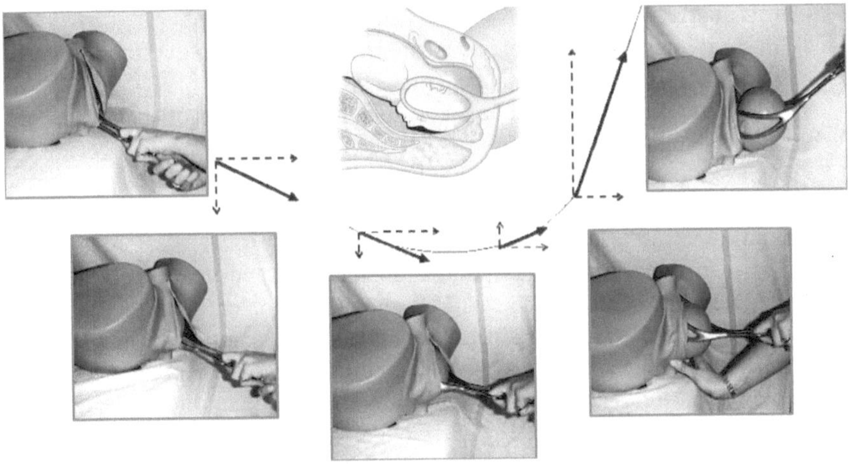

Figure 28.4: Correct application of forceps

Application should be cephalic in which long axis of the blades corresponding to the occipitomental plane of fetal head (biparietal application).

- Confirm position and station of head
- Identification of blades–"Ghosting" or "Phantom" application: The instrument should be placed in front of the pelvis with the tip pointing upwards and pelvic curve forwards.
- Blades are identified.
- First the left blade should be applied guided by the right hand and then the right blade with the left hand.
- Application of left blade–Hold the handle of left blade by pen grip vertically near right groin of the mother. Pelvic curve is directed downward and cephalic curve inward toward the vulva with plane of shank perpendicular to the floor. Fingers of right hand are placed in the vagina between fetal head and left vaginal wall. Left blade is inserted at 5 o'clock positon between head and fingers. The handle is lowered slowly to the horizontal and moved up by the vaginal finger giving an occipitomental position. Middle and index finger of the right hand guide the toe of blade along the side of head. Right thumb is placed on heel of blade and provides the necessary force for guiding into vagina and not the left hand at handle which merely guides the handle over an arc from right thigh towards midline. Fingers are removed and handle is supported by an assistant.
- Right blade held in right hand and applied similarly except that toe is guided more anteriorly to avoid the brow which, if caught, would displace the head and make it LOT thus good application of first blade is lost making it brow mastoid application. When right is in place, handles are locked.
- The left is not moved as it is more correct position and right is guided to fit the left. After handles are locked satisfactorily, the application is checked after correction of rotation.
- Locking should be easy.
- Preextraction examination: FHS auscultation, Vaginal examination to rule out cord, membrane or cervical entrapment and check the application.

- **Check points:**
  - Posterior fontanellae should be located midway between the sides of blades and one finger breadth above the plane of shanks
  - The sagittal suture should be perpendicular to the plane of shanks through out its length
  - Fenestrations of blade felt should be equal and not more than finger tip on either side
- Readjustment:
  - When first check is wrong—handles are unlocked and elevated one at a time and relocked at a desired level. This avoids traction on deflexed head axis
  - When second check is defective oblique sagittal suture—signifies 'Brow mastoid' application, correction is done by unlocking and adjusting each blade at a time—moving them towards midline along the curve of head. Sometimes blades have to be taken out and reapplied.
  - If third check is at fault — one-half inch of fenestration is felt — signifies "short application" in this case, toe of blade is not well-anchored on bimalar eminence, thus may slip during traction. Correction done by unlocking and pushing the blades higher up one at a time.
- Episiotomy is given before traction
- Traction applied preferably during uterine contraction
  - Force of traction should be in line with birth canal. First outwards and posteriorly until the occiput comes under the symphysis pubis and neck pivots in the subpubic angle, then the direction is changed to outward and anteriorly to promote extension of the head. Traction must be intermittent, every 1–2 minutes for 30–40 seconds. Forceps need not be unlocked iin between contractions.
- Traction should not be more than force exerted at wrist joint.
- Not more than 3 attempts.
- Have a clear endpoint and exit strategy.
- Birth of the head: Traction is continued with extension of the head, forehead, face and chin are born.
- Removal of forceps:After the birth of head forceps is removed in reverse process as application.
- After delivery, examine cervix or vagina for any injury.

Face to Pubis Delivery by Forceps

- Head in occipitosacral position
- Rule out pelvic contraction
- Head is engaged
- Long forceps are used
- Make large episiotomy
- Traction force should be horizontal until base of nose is under symphysis, then handles are elevated till occiput emerges followed by downward motion at handles, with delivery of nose, face and chin successively.

Forceps in the After-coming Head of Breech

- Provides controlled and guarded delivery

- Piper forceps or any mid cavity forceps can be used
- Head should be completely rotated and engaged
- Body of the fetus is lifted up by assistant and blades are applied from below
- Left blade applied first followed by right blade
- Rest of the procedure same

Amount of Traction

- In biomechanical studies, a safe limit of 45 lb in primigravidae and 30 lb in multigravidae has been suggested when using forceps and up to 550–600 mmHg (11.6 psi) when using a vacuum cup.
- The aim should be to apply the minimum amount of effective traction necessary to accomplish safe delivery.
- A recent invention uses wireless technology. A strain gauge in the handle grip measures the traction force between the grip assembly and the forceps shank. This may help to avoid excessive traction force, minimizing injury to the fetus and the mother.

Recording of Forceps Operations

- The indications for the forceps operation, including the position and station of the vertex at the time of application of forceps, should be specified in a detailed operative description in the patient's medical record.
- Indication, discussion with parents, relatives, the progress chart, informed consent—all these are protection. Also document the pre- and post-delivery status, procedure in detail, degree of difficulty. Also use lab for—scalp, cord PH, HPE of placenta.

Complications

Maternal

- Lacerations of vulva, vagina, cervix and extension of episiotomy
- Rupture of uterus
- Postpartum hemorrhage due to trauma or atony
- Injury to bladder or rectum
- Infection of genital tract
- Fracture coccyx
- Sepsis [febrile episodes (16%)]
- Urinary and rectal incontinence

Fetal

- Brain damage and intracranial hemorrhage, falx and tentorial tears
- General depression and asphyxia
- Late neurological sequellae, CP
- MR and behavioral problems too
- Bruising, brachial palsy
- Cord compression

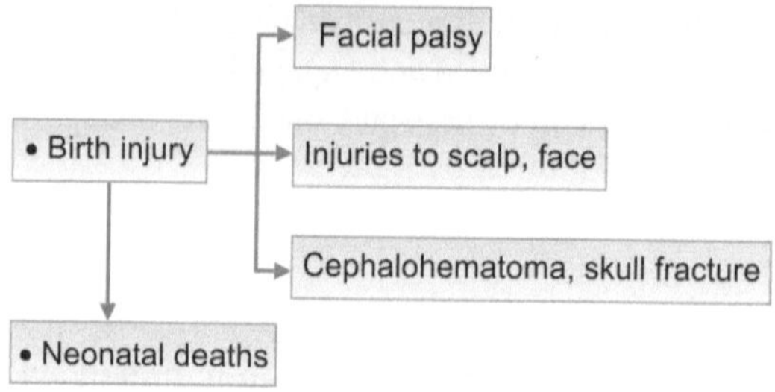

Postoperative Care

- Prophylactic antibiotics
- The patient to be kept in labor room or postoperative ward for minimum of 4–6 hr
- Pulse – ½ hrly, BP record – 2 hrly
- Watch for bleeding PV
- Analgesia and laxative are given as per requirement
- Urine output in initial 6–8 hr
- Care of episiotomy

Kielland forceps: These are usually utilized for rotational deliveries. Specific techniques are required and only properly trained personnel should use them. The design is unique, with a minimal pelvic curve to allow rotation around a fixed axis, and a sliding lock to enable correction of asynclitism.

Procedure: The method of application of the Kielland's blades for occipito-transverse positions is described as the 'wandering method'. As with the standard technique, the forceps are assembled and held in position to enable visualization of their final position prior to application. The anterior blade is chosen, introduced in the standard manner, but subsequently maneuvered over the fetal face until it comes to lie over the anterior parietal bone below the maternal symphysis pubis. The internal hand is used for guidance and protection of the maternal soft tissues from trauma during manipulation of the blade into the correct position. The posterior blade, which occupies the sacral hollow, can be directly inserted in most instances, but if this proves difficult, application in the manner of the anterior blade should be performed, but in reverse. Rotation should be carried out between contractions and may be accomplished by pushing the head 'up' to the level of the pelvic mid-cavity, or by gentle traction at the level at which the head has reached. The axis of traction is more in the vertical plane in the first instance than described with the standard forceps, but extra care must be taken towards the end of the delivery as the lack of the forceps pelvic curve makes perineal damage more likely. Rotational forceps deliveries have been abandoned in favor of manual rotation, rotational ventouse or cesarean section in many institutions because they have been associated with spiral tears of the vagina and other soft tissue injuries, and in some cases uterine rupture. However, they still have a role with the experienced clinician, as the ventouse is associated with a higher incidence of failure of delivery in occipito-posterior and occipito-transverse positions, and second stage deliveries by cesarean section are fraught with difficulties.

Use of Kielland forceps for rotation and delivery of the head can minimize the risk of second-stage cesarean section and its complications. This instrument has been abandoned as it has a reputation for being dangerous; however, it is a safe instrument in experienced hands.

VENTOUSE OR VACUUM EXTRACTION

Principle

Traction on a metal or soft cup, so designed that the suction creates an artificial caput or chignon within the cup and holds it firmly and allows adequate traction on scalp.

Kiwi OmniCup Recent developments have removed the need for cumbersome external suction generators and have incorporated the vacuum mechanism into 'hand held' pumps. Such devices are safe and may be useful for rotational deliveries because they are low profile and are easily maneuvered into the correct position. However, they have a significantly higher failure rate than the conventional ventouse, with cup detachments occurring more frequently.

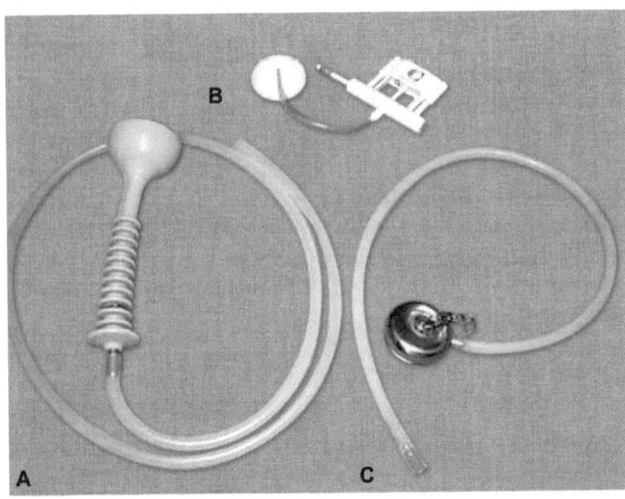

Figure 28.5: Three different types of ventouse: (A) A silastic cup ventouse and (B) A hand-held ventouse (pump incorporated in the handle, (C) A metal cap ventouse — for posterior application 'The Bird cup'. Both of these require external vacuum generators.

Indications

- Same as that of forceps
- Can be used in unrotated head also
- Special indications
    - Occipito-posterior position–POP and DTA
    - In second twin when head is presenting
    - Cord prolapse with incomplete dilatation of cervix
    - LSCS
    - Non-obstetrical indication–Ovarian cyst removal

Contraindications

- Non-vertex presentation
- Fetal coagulopathies
- Known macrosomia
- Following recent scalp blood sampling
- Prematurity <34 weeks
- Fetus with bone demineralization condition

Components

- Suction machine (foot operated/automatic)
- Tubing with locking shoulder
- Cup (rigid or soft)

Prerequisites

- Informed consent
- Experienced person should be present (Senior Resident or Consultant)
- Vertex presentation, station 0 or lower [P/A: Head < 1/5th palpable]
- Term fetus
- Rule out CPD, presence of good uterine contractions
- Cervix should be fully dilated [Application in < fully dilated cervix and midpelvic or higher application previously suggested are not recommended now (except second baby of twin)]
- Membranes should be ruptured
- Bladder should be empty
    - Operator certain about position of head

Application

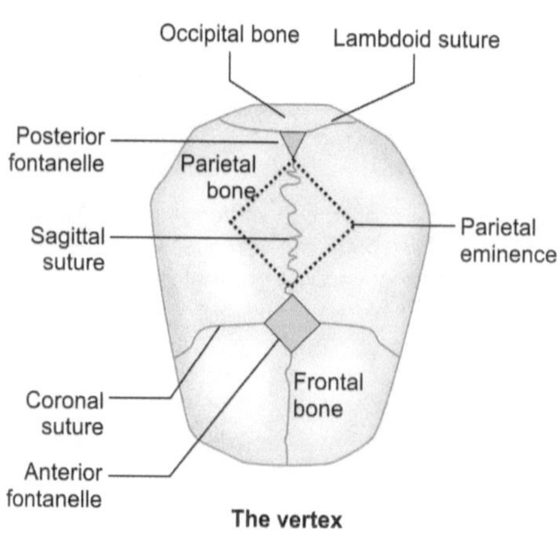

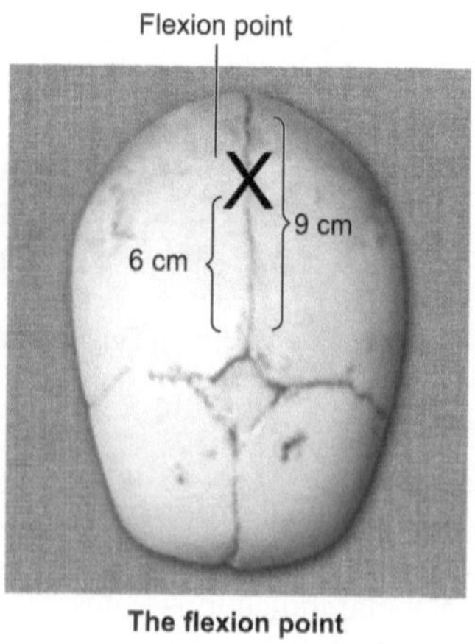

Figure 28.6: Application of ventouse

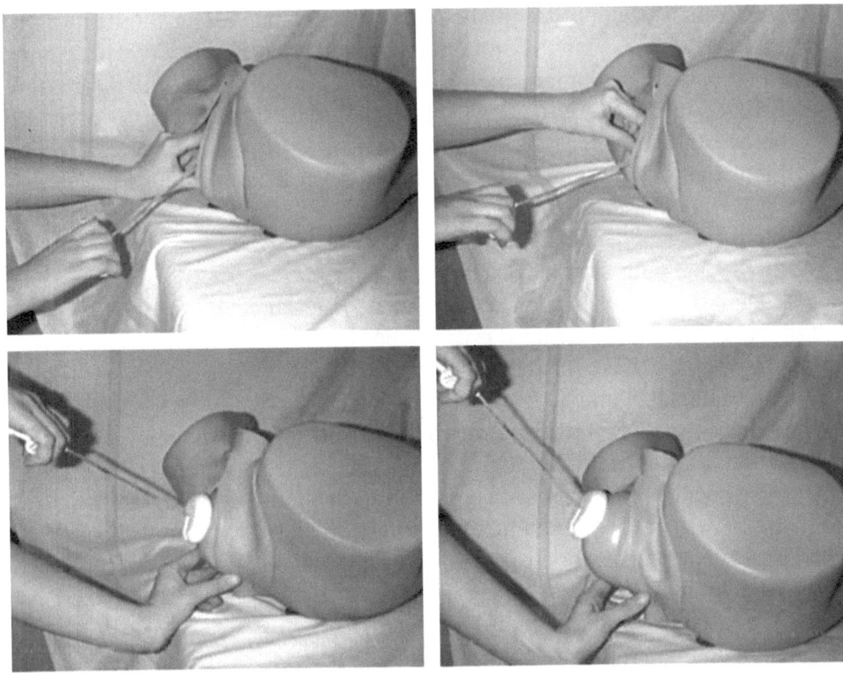

Figure 28.7: An assisted vertex delivery employing a hand-held ventouse (kiwi OmniCup^{TM}). The cup should be positioned over the flexion point to ensure optimal delivery technique.

- Dorsal position. Adequate regional analgesia
- The largest possible size of the cup should be used
- Episiotomy is optional
- Proper placement is most important:
  - Center of the cup should be on flexion point and 3 cm in front of the posterior fontanelle in an average term infant, along the sagittal suture (and thus 6 cm posterior to the anterior fontanelle). In midline, so that the cup is more on occiput. If small caput is present, go more posterior (The ventouse cup should be placed at the leading point of the fetal head: the flexion point is located 3 cm below the posterior fontanelle on the sagittal suture for the occipito-anterior position or 3 cm above the posterior fontanelle for the occipitoposterior position).
  - Anterior placement will enhance extension of head during traction.
  - Asymmetrical placement on one side of sagittal suture may worsen asynclitism.
- The operating vacuum pressure for nearly all ventouse is between 0.6 and 0.8 kg/cm^2 (60 – 80 kPa/500 – 800 cm H_2O). No evidence exists that step-wise incremental increases in pressure improve the rate of successful delivery when compared with a linear increase. Using the latter technique with a silastic cup, a caput secundum is formed instantly, and with the metal cup or OmniCup, an adequate chignon is produced in <2 min. It is important to note that a cup of 5 cm is suitable for nearly all deliveries. Check for proper application and see that no maternal tissues included.

- Traction must occur in the plane of least resistance along the axis of the pelvis: the traction plane. Gentle traction is applied in concert with uterine contractions and voluntary expulsive efforts, minimizing undue pressure and risk of trauma to the fetus. Traction should be intermittent. Two-handed technique—three-finger grip, should be synchronous with uterine contraction and maternal bearing down efforts. Should be in the direction of pelvic axis and perpendicular to cup.
- Episiotomy when the head is bulging the perineum
- Normally 2–3 pulls are required
- Procedure should be abandoned after 2–3 cup detachments
- Release vacuum once the head is delivered
- Inspect vagina and cervix after delivery for any lacerations or tear
- Average time is 15 min
- If no descent with first pull or 2 cup detachments re-evaluate clinical situation
- Abandon the procedure, if:
  - No evidence of progressive descent with each pull
  - When delivery is not imminent following 3 pulls of experienced operator
  - 3 cup detachments (pop-off)
  - Time limit of 30 min
- Rigid cup–better result but more fetal trauma
- Soft cup–more failure rate [Cochrane database]

Complications

Fetal

Direct Injuries

- Scalp abrasions, lacerations
- Cephalohematoma
- Intracranial hemorrhage
- Subperiosteal hemorrhage
- Extradural hemorrhage
- Subdural hemorrhage
- Linear or depressed skull #
- Spinal cord injury
- Facial nerve palsy
- Retinal hemorrhage

Indirect Injuries

- Anemia
- Hemorrhagic shock
- Vascular collapse
- Infection/septicemia
- Jaundice

Maternal

Direct Injuries

- Birth canal lacerations

- Episiotomy extensions
- Bladder/paraurethral/urethral injuries
- Vaginal/vulvar/perirectal hematomas

Indirect Injuries

- Perineal scarring, dyspareunia
- Rectal sphincter dysfunction
- Bladder atony
- Uterine atony
- Fistula formation
- Anemia, hemorrhagic shock
- Endometritis

VACUUM EXTRACTION AS COMPARED TO FORCEPS

Advantages of Ventouse over Forceps

- Can be used on unrotated and OP position
- Can be applied even in undilated cervix
- It is not space occupying
- Lesser traction force (10 kg) is required
- Can be used safely on heads at high level as in 2nd twin
- Minimal risk to mother and fetus
- Requires less technical skill and anesthesia
- Less changes in intracranial pressure during traction

Disadvantages

- More failure than forceps
- Increased risk of cephalhematoma
- Increased risk of retinal hemorrhage
- No difference in long-term fetal morbidity as compared to forceps and spontaneous delivery.

Advantages of Forceps over Ventouse

- In suspected pelvic contraction, where moderate traction is required
- Forceps can quickly expedite delivery in case of fetal distress where ventouse takes longer time
- Safer in premature baby-protective
- Can be applied on face, after coming head
- Simplicity of instrument less costly, handy

Disadvantage

More maternal trauma

Sequential Use of Instruments

- Use of VE to gain pelvic station which may convert a difficult mid-forceps procedure into a presumably safer low or outlet forceps operation.

- Most common reason for abandonment of a VE is repeated cup detachment and for forceps it is as a result of poor application.
- Restricted to selected cases conducted only by highly experienced surgeon.
- Associated with an increased risk of trauma to the infant-intracranial hemorrhage.
- The operator must balance the risks of a C/S following failed vacuum extraction with the risks of forceps delivery following failed vacuum extraction.
- Viable alternative to C/S in certain circumstances in trained hands.
- But chances of ICH and retinal hemorrhage are comparatively more.

Comprehensive documentation is a critical part of carrying out any operative delivery and should include, as a basic minimum–

- A statement of the indication for the procedure
- The anesthesia used
- The personnel involved and an outline of the procedure performed
- The difficulty of the extraction
- The performance of rotation
- Fetal injuries
- Trauma to soft tissue of the mother and its repair
- An estimate of the blood loss.

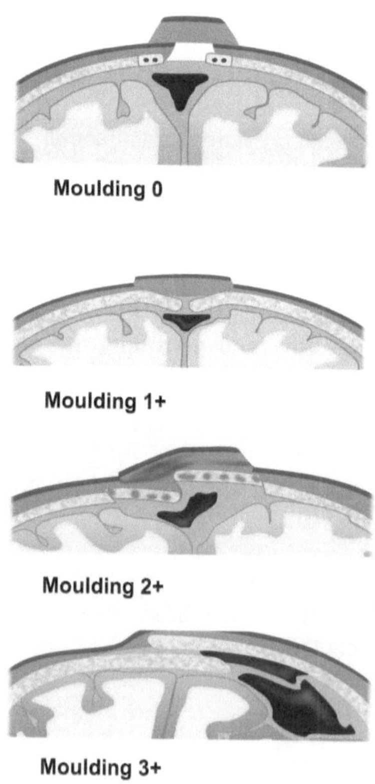

Figure 28.8: Grades of moulding

CHAPTER

29

Cesarean Delivery

WHO recommends cesarean delivery rate not more than 15%.

Pregnant women should be given evidence-based information on cesarean including indications, the procedure involved, risks and benefits of cesarean and implications for future pregnancies.

INDICATIONS

Absolute

0. Major degree CPD
1. Major degree placenta previa
2. Previous history of classical cesarean
3. Advanced carcinoma cervix
4. Vaginal stenosis/atresia
5. Transverse lie uncorrected by ECV
6. Brow presentation in labor
7. Pelvic mass causing obstruction

Relative

- Previous lower segment uterine scar not fit for VBAC
- Nonreassuring fetal status
- Cord accidents
- Abruptio-placenta with poor Bishop score
- Obstructed labor
- Failed induction
- Eclampsia with poor Bishop score
- Genital HPV/HIV/HSV infections
- Fetal macrosomia (>4 kg)
- Fetal congenital anomalies amenable to correction
- Maternal demand
- Malpresentation—breech, shoulder, brow.
- Previous history of repair of fistula (VVF, RVF)

Cesarean Section

Pregnant women should be given evidence-based information on cesarean section (CS), as 1 in 5 will have indications, what the procedure involves, risks and benefits of CS and implications for future pregnancies.

Offer planned CS to women with:
- A term singleton breech (if external cephalic version is contraindicated or has failed)
- A twin pregnancy with first twin breech
- HIV
- Both HIV and hepatitis C
- Primary genital herpes in the third trimester
- Grade 3 and 4 placenta previa

Do not routinely offer planned CS to women with:
- Twin pregnancy (first twin is cephalic at term)
- Preterm birth
- A 'small for gestational age' baby
- Hepatitis B virus
- Hepatitis C virus
- Recurrent genital herpes at term

Maternal request for CS:
- Is not on its own an indication for CS
- Explore and discuss specific reasons
- Discuss benefits and risks of CS
- Offer counselling if fear of childbirth
- The clinician can decline a request for CS, but should offer referral for a second opinion

Planning place of birth

Inform healthy pregnant women with anticipated uncomplicated pregnancies that:
- Home birth reduces CS
- Birth in a 'midwifery-led unit' does not affect CS

Reducing CS rates
- Offer external cephalic version if breech at 36 weeks
- Facilitate continuous support during labor
- Offer induction of labor beyond 41 weeks
- Use a partogram with a 4-hour action line in labor
- Involve consultant obstetricians in CS decision
- Do fetal blood sampling before CS for abnormal cardiotocograph in labor
- Support women who choose vaginal birth after cesarean section (VBAC)

No influence on likelihood of CS
- Walking in labor
- Non-supine position during the second stage of labor
- Immersion in water during labor
- Epidural analgesia during labor
- Active management of labor or early amniotomy to augment the progress of labor
- Raspberry leaves during labor

These may affect other outcomes that are outside the scope of this guideline.

Summary of the effects of CS compared with vaginal birth for women and their babies

Increased with CS	No difference after CS	Reduced with CS
• Abdominal pain • Bladder injury • Ureteric injury • Need for further surgery • Hysterectomy • ITU/HDU admission • Thromboembolic disease • Length of hospital stay • Readmission to hospital • Placenta previa • Uterine rupture • Maternal death • Antepartum stillbirth in future pregnancies • Not having more children • Neonatal respiratory morbidity	• Hemorrhage • Infection • Genital tract injury • Fecal incontinence • Back pain • Dyspareunia • Postnatal depression • Neonatal mortality (excluding breech) • Intracranial hemorrhage • Brachial plexus injuries • Cerebral palsy	• Perineal pain • Urinary incontinence • Uterovaginal prolapse
	This table shows the direction of the effects of CS on risks and benefits but not the size of the effects. The risks do not apply to all women in all circumstances. Details of the absolute and relative risks and benefits are available in the full guideline.	

Pregnancy and childbirth following CS

The decision about mode of birth should consider maternal preferences and priorities, general discussion of the overall risks and benefits of CS (specific risks and benefits uncertain), risk of uterine rupture and perinatal mortality and morbidity.

Women who want VBAC should be supported and:
- be informed that uterine rupture is very rare but is increased with VBAC (about 1 per 10,000 repeat CS and 50 per 10,000 VBAC)
- be informed intrapartum infant death is rare (about 10 per 10,000 the same as the risk for women in their first pregnancy), but increased compared with planned repeat CS (about 1 per 10,000)
- be offered electronic fetal monitoring during labor
- should labor in a unit where there is immediate access to CS and on-site blood transfusion
- if having induction of labor should be aware of the increased risk of uterine rupture (80 per 10,000 if non-prostaglandins are used, 240 per 10,000 if prostaglandins are used)
- be informed that women with both previous CS and a previous vaginal birth are more likely to give birth vaginally

CS is the end-point of a number of care pathways This algorithm includes the common reasons for CS, but this list is not exhaustive. CS may be required for complex or rare conditions that are outside the scope of this guideline

INDICATIONS FOR CLASSICAL CESAREAN DELIVERY

- Inaccessibility of the lower uterine segment as in fibroids, dense adhesions or placenta percreta
- Advanced cervical cancer
- Postmortem cesarean delivery
- Repair of high VVF

Making the decision for CS

- Communication and information should be provided in a form that is accessible
- Consent for CS should be requested after providing pregnant women with evidence-based information
- A competent pregnant woman is entitled to refuse the offer of treatment such as CS, even when the treatment would clearly benefit her or her baby's health

Timing of planned CS: CS should be carried out after 39 weeks of gestation to decrease the risk of respiratory morbidity. **Emergency CS:** In cases of suspected or confirmed acute fetal compromise, delivery should be accomplished as soon as possible. The accepted standard is within 30 minutes.	Document the urgency of CS using: 1. Immediate threat to the life of a woman or fetus 2. Maternal or fetal compromise which is not immediately life-threatening 3. No maternal or fetal compromise but needs early delivery 4. Delivery timed to suit woman or staff

Procedural aspects of CS

Preoperative assessment • Check hemoglobin • Prescribe antibiotics (one dose of first-generation cephalosporin or ampicillin) • Assess risk for thromboembolic disease (offer graduated stockings, hydration, earty mobilization and low molecular weight heparin) • Site an indwelling bladder catheter For healthy women with an uncomplicated pregnancy, don't offer: • Grouping and saving of serum • Cross-matching of blood • Clotting screen • Preoperative ultrasound to localize the placenta	**Anesthetic care** • Discuss post-CS analgesia options • Offer antacids and H_2 receptor analogues • Offer antiemetics • Offer regional anesthesia • Reduce risk of hypotension using: – intravenous ephedrine or phenylephrine infusion – volume pre-loading with crystalloid or colloid – lateral tilt of 15 degrees • General anesthesia for emergency CS should include preoxygenation and rapid sequence induction to reduce the risk of aspiration *Maternity units should have a drill for failed intubation*

Surgical techniques

(For pregnancies at term, where there is a lower uterine segment. These may need modification in situations such as repeat CS, placenta praevia)

Do	Don't
• Wear double gloves for CS for women who are HIV-positive • Use a transverse lower abdominal incision (Joel Cohen incision) • Use blunt extension of the uterine incision • Give oxytocin (5IU) by slow intravenous injection • Use controlled cord traction for removal of the placenta • Close the uterine incision with two suture layers • Check umbilical artery pH if CS performed for fetal compromise • Consider women's preferences for birth (such as music playing in theatre) • Facilitate early skin-to-skin contact for mother and baby	• Close subcutaneous space (unless >2 cm fat) • Use superficial wound drains • Use separate surgical knives for skin and deeper tissues • Use routinely used forceps to deliver babies head • Suture either the visceral or the parietal peritoneum • Exteriorise the uterus • Manually remove the placenta The effects of different suture material or methods of skin closure are uncertain.

A practitioner skilled in the resuscitation of the newborn should be present at CS with a general anesthetic or with presumed fetal compromise

Postoperative monitoring

- Recovery area — one-to-one observations until the woman has airway control, cardiorespiratory stability and can communicate
- In the ward — half-hourly observations (respiratory rate, heart rate, blood pressure, pain and sedation) for 2 hours then hourly if stable
- Intrathecal opioids — hourly observation of respiratory rate, sedation and pain scores for 12 hours for diamorphine and 24 hours for morphine
- For epidural opioids and patient-controlled analgesia with opioids — hourly monitoring during the CS, plus 2 hours after discontinuation

Care of the woman and her baby after CS
- Provide additional support to help women to start breastfeeding as soon as possible
- Offer diamorphine (0.3–0.4 mg intrathecally or epidural diamorphine (2.5–5 mg) to reduce the need for supplemental analgesia
- Offer non-steroidal anti-inflammatory analgesics to reduce the need for opioid analgesics
- Women who are feeling well and have no complications can eat or drink when they feel hungry or thirsty
- After regional anesthesia remove catheter when woman is mobile (>12 hours after top-up)
- Remove wound dressing after 24 hours, keep wound clean and dry
- Discuss the reasons for the CS and implications before discharge from hospital
- Offer earlier discharge (after 24 hours) to women who are recovering, apyrexial and have no complications

Recovery following CS
- Offer postnatal care, plus specific post-CS care, and management of pregnancy complications
- Prescribe regular analgesia
- Monitor wound healing
- Inform women they can resume activities (such as driving, exercise) when pain not distracting or restricting

Consider CS complications:
- Endometritis if excessive vaginal bleeding
- Thromboembolism if cough or swollen calf
- Urinary tract infection if urinary symptoms
- Urinary tract trauma (fistula) if leaking urine

This algorithm should, where necessary, be interpreted with reference to the full guideline

ANESTHESIA FOR CESAREAN DELIVERY

The following techniques are used in relation to the degree of urgency:

1. 15–30 minutes are available from the time of decision to operate is made until the time of delivery—General anesthesia
2. 30–40 minutes—Subarachnoid block (spinal anesthesia)
3. 45–60 minutes—Extension of an existing epidural/Spinal anesthesia
4. 60–90 minutes—New epidural block can be contemplated

Anesthetic Care

- Discuss post-cesarean delivery analgesia options
- Offer antacids and H_2-receptor analogues
- Offer antiemetics
- Reduce risk of hypotension using:
  - Intravenous ephedrine or phenylephrine infusion
  - Volume pre-loading with crystalloid or colloid
  - Lateral tilt of 15 degrees
- General anesthesia for emergency cesarean delivery should include preoxygenation and rapid sequence induction to reduce the risk of aspiration
- Timing of delivery of the baby:
  - Induction delivery interval: 10–20 minutes
  - Skin incision delivery interval: 7 minutes
  - Uterine incision delivery interval: 90 seconds

Timing of Cesarean Delivery

- Elective cesarean delivery–38 completed weeks of gestation to decrease the risk of respiratory morbidity
- Emergency cesarean delivery
- Document the urgency of cesarean delivery using:
  - Immediate threat to the life of the woman or fetus (cesarean delivery within 30 min)

- ◆ Maternal or fetal compromise which is not immediately life-threatening
- ◆ No maternal or fetal compromise but needs early delivery
- ◆ Delivery timed to suit woman or staff

Pre-operative Assesment

- Check hemoglobin
- Prescribe antibiotics (one dose of first-generation cephalosporin or ampicillin)
- Assess risk for thromboembolic disease (offer graduated stockings, hydration, early mobilization and low molecular weight heparin)
- Site an indwelling bladder catheter for 6–12 hrs

For healthy women with an uncomplicated pregnancy, don't offer:
- Cross-matching of blood
- Clotting screen
- Pre-operative ultrasound to localize the placenta

Cesarean Delivery Procedure

- Hair removal with depilatory cream or with clipping results fewer surgical infections than shaving.
- Vaginal preparation with povidonc-iodinc docs not rcducc post-ccsarcan infectious modality.
- There is no evidence that adhesive drapes confer benefits over conventional linen drapes.

Skin Incision

- Transverse incisions are associated with lower maternal morbidity, including dehiscence, than vertical incisions
- Pfannenstiel incisions result in faster operations than Maylard incision
- Joel-Cohen incision is faster than Pfannenstiel incision but cosmetically less acceptable. There is no other difference.
  a. **Low midline vertical incision:** It permits fast access to LUS, better exposure, less blood loss and easier access to upper abdomen.
  b. **Pfannenstiel incision:** It is a curvilinear transverse incision placed 3–4 cm above the symphysis pubis at upper border of pubic hair. It is cosmetically appealing and carries less risk of incisional herniation and wound dehiscence. It involves separation of rectus muscle from its anterior sheath and hence takes slightly more time than vertical incision and may be associated with more blood loss.
  c. **Joel-Cohen incision:** It is tranverse abdominal incision positioned higher than Pfannenstiel incision, about 3 cm below an imaginary line drawn between anterior superior iliac spines, it is straight rather than arched, the tendon plate is not freed longitudinally. The fascia is not separated from the muscles and there is minimal handling of subcutaneous tissues. This incision is associated with decreased duration of surgery and less postoperative febrile morbidity.
     - ◆ Size of the skin incision should be at least 15 cm (about the length of Allis clamp)

Misgav Ladach Technique

1. Joel Cohen's incision. Not recommended in previous CS and obesity.
2. Minimal use of instruments – Using the index and third fingers, abdominal wall layer is stretched in a caudal cranial direction thereby enabling separation of layers. Parietal peritoneum is also opened in the same way transversely to avoid damage to the bladder.
3. Manual lateral stretching of the uterine incision.
4. The placenta is removed manually.
5. The uterus is exteriorized.
6. Single layer uterine closure.
7. Non-closure of the visceral and parietal peritoneal layers.
8. Closure of the abdomen in two layers – Skin and rectus fascia.
9. The skin is closed with two or three mattress sutures. Between these sutures, the skin edges are approximated with Allis forceps, which are left in place for about five minutes while the drapes are being removed.

Modified Misgav Ladach Technique

1. Pfannenstiel skin incision
2. Lateral extension of the subcutaneous tissue, rectus sheath incision, and separation of the two rectus muscles are performed digitally.
3. Opening of the parietal peritoneum at the upper level of the intermuscular space is performed digitally.
4. A transverse 2–3 cm lower uterine segment incision in the midline, using a scalpel and blunt dissection of the remaining uterine fibers and opening of the fetal membranes.
5. Lateral digital extension of the uterine incision, the fetus is extracted
6. Placenta is removed by transabdominal uterine massage combined with light cord traction.
7. Exteriorization is optional.
8. Single layer uterine closure
9. The visceral and parietal peritoneum is left unsutured.
10. The rectus sheath is closed using a continuous suture.
11. The subcutaneous tissue is sutured if its depth exceeds 2 cm.
12. The skin is closed with mattress stitches, continuous subcuticular suture, or clips, according to the surgeon's choice.

Dextro-rotation of uterus should be corrected.

Uterine Incisions

- Transverse lower uterine incision is associated with less maternal morbidity.
- Absorbable staples for uterine wound cannot be recommended at present for routine practice.
- There is no evidence of benefit of blunt versus sharp dissection/extension of uterine incision.

a. **Transverse incision in LUS (Kerr technique):** It is the most common uterine incision used in CS. The myometrial incision is positioned entirely in the thin

LUS. There is less peroperative blood loss compared to other incisions and risk of uterine rupture is <1% at attempted vaginal birth in subsequent pregnancy.

b. **Low vertical uterine incision (Kronig's/Delee's technique):** The myometrial incision is positioned in the LUS. May be used in cases of malpresentation (oblique, transverse, breech). It is occasionally used when LUS is thickened.
c. **Classical uterine incision:** A midline incision is made in the upper uterine segment.
d. **Variations:**

J-shaped incision: Incision is extended upwards from only one uterine angle.

U-shaped incision (trap door incision): Incision is extended upwards from both the uterine angles.

Inverted T incision: Extension of incision is done from the center of upper edge of the incision.

DELIVERY OF THE FETUS

a. **Uncomplicated cephalic presentation:** Hand is introduced into the uterine cavity to elevate the fetal head, while maintaining flexion of fetal head is brought out through the incision. After the delivery of the fetal head, the nose and oropharynx are suctioned and rest of the delivery accomplished.

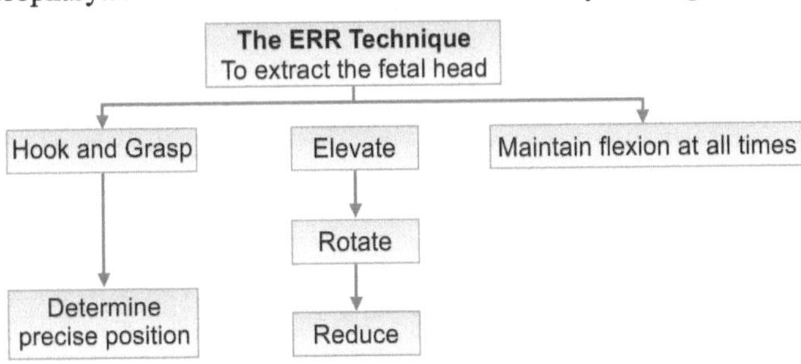

b. **Floating head:** After membranes are ruptured, the amniotic fluid is suctioned out and the fetal head is allowed to descend till it reaches the incision made in LUS. Then fetal head is delivered as described above.
   (or)
   - Forceps-short forceps: Wrigley's or Simpson's
     Single-blade forceps: Vectis or Vacuum: Silastic cups

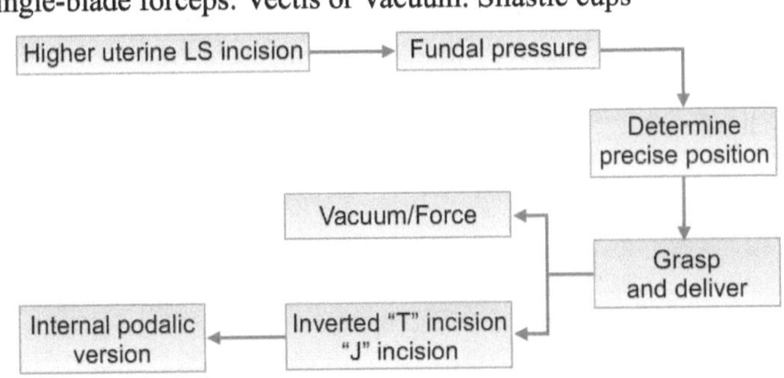

c. **Deeply engaged head:**

Abdomino-vaginal method: In this technique, an extra assistant is kept ready, and after making the uterine incision, pushes the fetal head upwards per vaginam. This enables the operating surgeon to reach beyond the leading edge of the fetal presenting part, which is then elevated and brought out of uterine incision.

Patwardhan's maneuver: In this technique one of the fetal upper limbs is delivered and brought out of the incision. If the back is is not already anterior, then the arm which is out of the incision is gently pulled so that the fetal back rotates anteriorly and the fetal arm is now closer to the midline. The other arm is delivered. The operating surgeon, with both the hands, now holds the fetal trunk and applies gentle traction so that successive parts of the fetal trunk, buttocks and the lower limbs are delivered. Fetal trunk should be held firmly yet no compression of the fetal abdomen should be caused. The fetal trunk should be held so that the thumbs of both hands of the operating surgeon are parallel to the fetal spine and gentle traction should be applied downwards which invariably results in delivery of successive fetal parts. After the fetal trunk and lower limbs have been delivered, the head is then pulled out, and suction of nose and oropharynx is done.

Modified Patwardhan's method: This is done when back is posterior, one lower limb delivered followed by back is made anterior then other lower limb is delivered followed by trunk, upper limbs and at last head is delivered.

Delivery of deeply engaged head

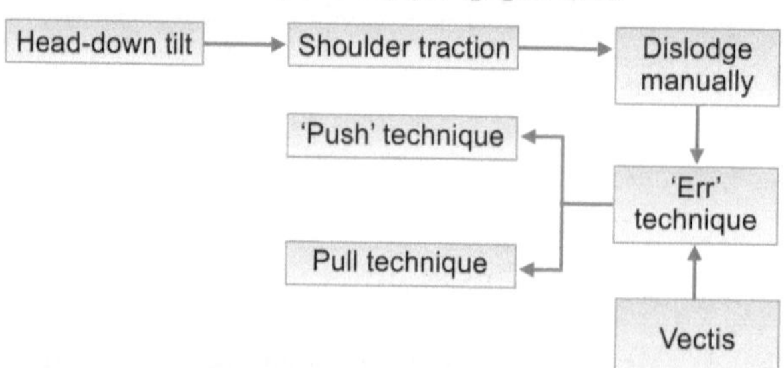

d. **Breech presentation:** Flexed breech-one or both feet are grasped and gently pulled out of the incision. In case of an extended breech, gentle groin traction can achieve the same. Fetal back should be anterior delivery of the shoulders should be conducted one followed by the other, as in vaginal delivery. Then assistant should maintain fundal pressure and operating surgeon can use one of the two methods: Mauriceau-Smellie-Veit or Burns-Marshall. Alternatively, Piper's or a long Simpson's forceps can also be used for delivery of the after-coming head.

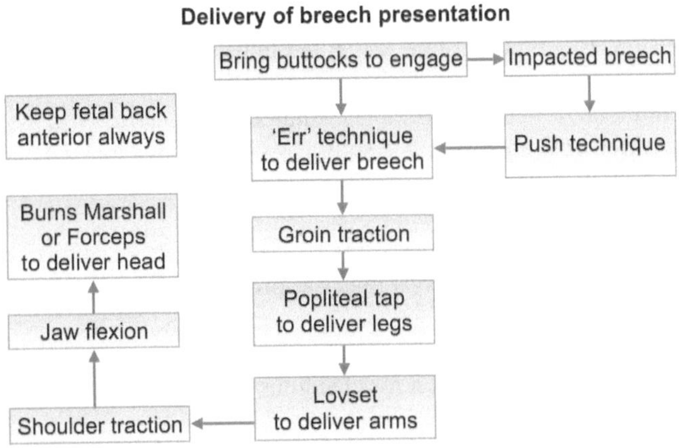

e. **Transverse lie:** A hand is introduced in the uterine cavity and the lower limb is grasped and delivered out of the incision and rest of the delivery is accomplished as a breech. If by error the upper rather than the lower limb is brought out inadvertently, it should be reposited and the lower limb subsequently delivered. In desperate situations, the uterine incision should be extended as a J-shaped incision, the hand brought out, followed by the lower limb of the same side. This should be followed by a gentle pull on the lower limb already delivered and then delivery of second lower limb and rest of the delivery can be conducted as in breech **(Modified Patwardhan technique).**

Placental Delivery

Spontaneous placental delivery should be preferred to manual removal of placenta as the former causes less blood loss and is associated with a decreased incidence of post-op infection.

Exteriorization of Uterus Versus in-situ Repair

Uterine exteriorization at CS allows for ease of suturing, manual uterine massage, observation of uterine tone and allows for routine examination of the adnexa.

In-situ repair without exteriorization can also be done. In this post-operative pain will be less.

There is no evidence of increased morbidity associated with exteriorization of the uterus of repair.

Uterine Closure

As an initial step, the angles of the uterine incision are identified and held with Allis's forceps and the lower edge of the incision with Green Armytage clamps.

Application of this clamp controls bleeding and identifies the lateral limit of uterine incision. Beginning at one angle, the upper margin is followed upto the other angle and in the same way, the lower margin of the incision is followed from one to the other angle. The uterus can be sutured in a double layer, the first layer should be sutured with an absorbable suture in a continuous locking and a second continuous layer (Lambert or Cushing) is used to invert the first layer; the inverting stitch may be horizontal or vertical.

If uterus is closed in single layer (during concurrent sterilization), it should be sutured with an absorbable (vicryl) material preferably in a continuous locking fashion.

A single layer closure is not associated with increased maternal morbidity; but trials are small and no justification for changing practice exists.

Abdominal Closure

- Peritoneal closure usually not recommended.
    - Closure is not necessary in routine practice.
- Rectus muscle may or may not be approximated.
- Rectus sheath
    - If the incision is vertical closure in a mono-layer fashion with non-absorbable suture.
    - In transverse incision, use of non-absorbable suture provides the strong fascial support, however, delayed absorbable sutures may be used.
    - In patients undergoing repeat CS with transverse incision non-absorbable sutures should be used.
    - The stitches are 1 cm from the edge and 1 cm from each other.

Fascial closure: The angles of incision should be identified and should be secured individually. The knot should be tied beyond the angles and should be surgical knot.

- It could be interrupted fashion or
- Continuous interlocking or
- Continous running stitch if used every third stitch should be reinforced with a cobbler knot.

Subcutaneous tissue: It should be closed if depth is ≥2 cm. Closure is associated with less superficial wound dehiscence, especially in obese.

Subrectus Suction Drainage

This reduces the rate of wound infection in high-risk cases.

Skin Closure

Closure of the skin–Sub-cuticular using delayed absorbable suture material.
Mattress suture—non-absorbable sutures
Skin staples–associated with less pain
The effects of different suture material or methods of skin closure are uncertain.
Skin staples may be superior to subcuticular sutures.

Surgical Technique

Do's

- Wear double gloves for CS for women who are HIV-positive
- Use a transverse lower abdominal incision (Joel Cohen incision)
- Use blunt extension of the uterine incision
- Give oxytocin (5 IU) by slow intravenous injection
- Use controlled cord traction for removal of the placenta
- Close the uterine incision with two suture layers
- Check umbilical artery pH if CS performed for fetal compromise
- Consider women's preferences for birth (such as music playing in Theater)
- Facilitate early skin-to-skin contact for mother and baby

Don'ts

- Close subcutaneous space (unless >2 cm fat)
- Use superficial wound drains
- Use separate surgical knives for skin and deeper tissues
- Use routinely forceps to deliver baby's head
- Suture either the visceral or the parietal peritoneum
- Exteriorize the uterus
- Manually remove the placenta

Perioperative Measures

- Prophylactic antibiotics are associated with reduced incidence of endometritis in elective cesarean delivery.
  Antibiotic regimens: Ampicillin and first generation cephalosporins are equally effective.
- Oral intake: There is no justification for withholding early oral intake.

Post-operative Monitoring

- Recovery area–one-to-one observations until the woman has airway control, cardiorespiratory stability and can communicate.
- In the ward—half-hourly observations (respiratory rate, heart rate, blood pressure, pain and sedation) for 2 hours, hourly if stable for 4 hours, and then 2nd hourly for 24 hrs.
- Intrathecal opioids—hourly observation of respiratory rate, sedation and pain scores for 12 hours for diamorphine and 24 hours for morphine.
- For epidural opioids and patient-controlled analgesia with opioids—hourly monitoring during the CS, plus 2 hours after discontinuation.

Care of the Baby and the Woman after CS

- Women should start breastfeeding as soon as possible.
- Offer diamorphine (0.3–0.4 mg intrathecally) or epidural diamorphine (2.5–5 mg) to reduce the need for supplemental analgesia.

- Offer non-steroidal anti-inflammatory analgesics to reduce the need for opioid analgesics.
- Women who are feeling well and have no complications can eat or drink when they feel hungry or thirsty.
- After regional anesthesia remove catheter when woman is mobile (>12 hours after top-up).
- Remove wound dressing after 48 hours, keep wound clean and dry.
- Discuss the reasons for the CS and implications before discharge from hospital
- Offer earlier discharge (after 24 hours) to women who are recovering, apyrexial and have no complications.

THROMBOPROPHYLAXIS GUIDELINES FOLLOWING CS

High Risk

- **Three or more moderate risk factors**
- Extended major pelvic or abdominal surgery (Ex.cesarean hysterectomy)
- Personal history of DVT or pulmonary embolism
- Thrombophilia
- Family history of DVT, pulmonary embolism, thrombophilia
- Paralysis of lower limbs
- Antiphospholipid antibody syndrome

Prophylaxis

- Knee high compression stockings
- Calf stimulation by a calf stimulation device during surgery
- Subcutaneous low molecular weight heparin (minimum 5 days)
- Early mobilization
- Adequate hydration

Moderate Risk

- Age >35 years
- Weight >80 kg at booking visit
- Severe varicose veins
- Current infections
- Preeclampsia
- Immobility prior to surgery (≥5 days)
- Major current illness (ex: heart or lung disease, cancer)
- Emergency cesarean delivery in labor

Prophylaxis

- Knee high compression stockings
- Calf stimulation by a calf stimulation device during surgery
- Subcutaneous low molecular weight heparin
- Early mobilization
- Adequate hydration
- Consider subcutaneous low molecular weight heparin

Low Risk

- Includes women having an elective cesarean delivery and who have had an uncomplicated pregnancy with no other risk factors

Prophylaxis

- Knee high compression stockings
- Calf stimulation by a calf stimulation device during surgery
- Subcutaneous low molecular weight heparin
- Early mobilization, adequate hydration

Classification of Urgency

The NCEPOD classification system recommended the categorization of operations into four grades of urgency.

- A clear classification of the perceived degree of urgency of the CS can facilitate communication and reduce misunderstanding between health care professionals.
- The categorization also independently predicted baby outcome
  The categories are:
  1. Immediate threat to the life of the woman or fetus
  2. Maternal or fetal compromise which was not immediately life-threatening
  3. No maternal or fetal compromise but needs early delivery
  4. Delivery timed to suit woman or staff
     - Grade 1 (immediate threat to the life of the woman or fetus) includes CS for acute severe bradycardia, cord prolapse, uterine rupture, fetal blood sampling, pH less than 7.2.
     - Grade 2 (maternal or fetal compromise which was not immediately life-threatening), there is 'urgency' to deliver the baby in order to prevent further deterioration of either the mother or baby's condition (e.g. antepartum hemorrhage, 'failure to progress' in labor with maternal or fetal compromise).
     - Grade 3 (no maternal or fetal compromise but needs early delivery) includes CS carried out where there is nomaternal or fetal compromise but early delivery is necessary (e.g. a woman booked for elective CS who is admitted with pre-labor SROM or 'failure to progress' with no maternal or fetal compromise).
     - Grade 4 (delivery timed to suit woman or staff) includes all CS carried out 'electively' at a planned time to suit the mother and clinicians.

SECTION 3

POSTPARTUM

- Postpartum Hemorrhage
- Shock in Obstetrics
- Blood Transfusion
- Maternal Collapse
- Venous Thromboembolism
- Cortical Vein Thrombosis
- Postpartum Contraception

CHAPTER

30

Postpartum Hemorrhage

DEFINITION

Loss of 500 ml or more of blood from the genital tract within 24 hours of the birth of a baby following vaginal delivery, 1000 ml or more following cesarean delivery.

Or

Any amount of blood loss causing hemodynamic instability

- Primary PPH involving an estimated blood loss of 500–1000 ml (and in the absence of clinical signs of shock) should prompt basic measures (close monitoring, intravenous access, full blood count, group and screen) to facilitate resuscitation should it become necessary.
- If a woman with primary PPH is continuing to bleed after an estimated blood loss of 1000 ml (or has clinical signs of shock or tachycardia associated with a smaller estimated loss), this should prompt a full protocol of measures to achieve resuscitation and hemostasis.

Incidence 2–11% of all deliveries

Obstetric hemorrhage is the second most common cause of direct maternal mortality.

Prophylactic oxytocics should be offered routinely in the management of the third stage of labor in all women as they reduce the risk of PPH by about 60%.

Table 30.1: Risk factors for PPH

• Presenting antenatally and associated with a substantial increase in the incidence of PPH; women with these factors should be advised to deliver in a consultant-led maternity unit		
Risk factor	**Four T's**	**Approximate odds ratio for PPH (99% CI)**
Suspected or proven placental abruption	Thrombin	13 (7.61–12.9)
Known placenta previa	Tone	12 (7.17–23)
Multiple pregnancy	Tone	5 (3.0–6.6)
Pre-eclampsia/gestational hypertension	Thrombin	4
• Presenting antenatally and associated with a significant (thought smaller) increase in the incidence of PPH; these factors should be taken into account when discussing setting for delivery		

Contd...

Contd...

Risk factor	Four T's	Approximate odds ratio for PPH (99% CI)
Previous PPH	Tone	3
Asian ethnicity	Tone	2 (1.48–2.12)
Obesity (BMI >35)	Tone	2 (1.24–2.17)
Anemia (<9 g/dl)	–	2 (1.63–3.15)
• Becoming apparent during labor and delivery; these factors should prompt extra vigilance among clinical staff		
Risk factor	**Four T's**	**Approximate odds ratio for PPH (99% CI)**
Delivery by emergency cesarean section	Trauma	4 (3.28–3.95)
Delivery by elective cesarean section	Trauma	2 (2.18–2.80)
Induction of labor	–	2 (1.67–2.96)
Retained placenta	Tissue	5 (3.36–7.87)
Mediolateral episiotomy	Trauma	5
Operative vaginal delivery	Trauma	2 (1.56–2.07)
Prolonged labor (>12 hours)	Tone	2
Big baby (>4 kg)	Tone/Trauma	2 (1.38–2.60)
Pyrexia in labor	Thrombin	2
Age (> 40 years, not multiparous)	Tone	1.4 (1.16–1.74)

ATONIC PPH

Responsible for 80% of primary PPH
Once PPH has been identified, management involves four components, all of which must be undertaken simultaneously: communication, resuscitation, monitoring and investigation, arresting the bleeding.

Basic measures for MINOR PPH (blood loss 500–1000 ml, no clinical shock):
- Intravenous access (14-gauge cannula x1).
- Commence crystalloid infusion.

Full protocol for major PPH (blood loss > 1000 ml and continuing to bleed OR clinical shock):
- Assess airway.
- Assess breathing.
- Oxygen by mask at 10–15 liters/minute.
- Intravenous access (14-gauge cannula x 2, orange cannulae).
- Position flat.
- Keep the woman warm using appropriate available measures.
- Transfuse blood as soon as possible.
- Until blood is available, infuse up to 3.5 liters of warmed crystalloid Hartmann's solution (2 liters) and/or colloid (1–2 liters) as rapidly as required.

- The best equipment available should be used to achieve RAPID WARMED infusion of fluids.
- Special blood filters should NOT be used, as they slow infusions.
- Recombinant factor VIIa therapy should be based on the results of coagulation.

Fluid therapy and blood product transfusion
Crystalloid—Up to 2 liters Hartmann's solution
Colloid—Up to 1–2 liters colloid until blood arrives
Blood—Cross-matched, if cross-matched blood is still unavailable, give uncrossmatched group-specific OR give 'O RhD negative' blood
Fresh frozen plasma—4 units for every 6 units of red cells or prothrombin time/ activated partial thromboplastin time >1.5 × normal (12–15 ml/kg or total 1 liters)
Platelets concentrates—If PLT count < 50 × 10^9
Cryoprecipitate—If fibrinogen < 1 g/l

The main therapeutic goals of management of massive blood loss are to maintain:
- Hemoglobin >8 g/dl
- Platelet count >75 × 10^9/l
- Prothrombin <1.5 × mean control
- Activated prothrombin times <1.5 × mean control
- Fibrinogen >1.0 g/l.

Determine the Amount of Blood Loss

- Visual assessment is inaccurate: more when blood loss is less and less when blood loss is more.
  Measurement: Standard with sponges, pads with weight, BRASS –V drape
- Should blood loss be routinely quantified during management of the third stage of labor for the purpose of diagnosing PPH?
- After childbirth, blood loss and other clinical parameters should be closely monitored. At present, there is insufficient evidence to recommend quantification of blood loss over clinical estimation.

Classify According to the Stage of Shock

Classification	Class 1	Class 2	Class 3	Class 4
Blood loss (% Volume Lost)	10–15%	15–30%	30–40%	>40%
Conscious state	Alert, Mild Thirst	Anxious and Restless	Agitated or Confused	Drowsy, Confused Unconscious
Respiratory	Normal	Mildly elevated	Raised	Raised
Rate				
Complexion	Normal	Pale	Pale	Markedly pale
Extremities	Normal	Cold	Cold	Cold
Capillary refill	Normal	Slow >2 sec	Slow >2 sec	Minimal or Absent
PR	Normal	Normal	Elevated	Fast but Thread
Systolic BP	Normal	Normal	Normal/Low	Hypotensive
Urine output	Normal	Normal	Reduced	Oligoanuric

Determine the Etiology of Hemorrhage

Remember 4 T's:

- Tone—Uterine atony (commonest)
- Trauma—Lacerations, Rupture, Inversion
- Tissue—Retained Placenta/clots
- Thrombin—Coagulopathy

For practical management, we propose a 'rule of 30' or a change in the 'shock index' to be valuable in monitoring women with hemorrhage. If the systolic blood pressure falls by 30 mmHg, pulse rate rises by 30 beats/min, respiratory rate increases to 4 X 30 breaths/min and hemoglobin (Hb) or hematocrit drop by 30%, then the patient is most likely to have lost at least 30% of her blood volume and is in moderate shock leading to severe shock. Shock index (SI) refers to pulse rate divided by the systolic blood pressure. The normal value is 0.5–0.7, but with significant hemorrhage the SI increases to 0.9–11.1.

Monitoring and Investigation

Basic measures for minor PPH (blood loss 500–1000 ml, no clinical shock and bleeding ceasing):

- Consider venepuncture (20 ml) for:
  - Group and screen
  - Full blood count
  - Coagulation screen including fibrinogen
  - Pulse and blood pressure recording every 15 minutes.

Full protocol for major PPH (blood loss greater than 1000 ml and continuing to blood OR clinical shock).

- Consider venepuncture (20 ml) for:
  - Cross-match (4 units minimum)
  - Full blood count
  - Coagulation screen including fibrinogen
  - Renal and liver function for baseline.
- Monitor temperature every 15 minutes.
- Continuous pulse, blood pressure recording and respiratory rate (using oximeter, electrocardiogram and automated blood pressure recording).
- Foley catheter to monitor urine output.
- Two peripheral cannulae, 14- or 16-gauge.
- Consider arterial line monitoring (once appropriately experienced staff available for insertion).
- Consider transfer to intensive therapy unit once the bleeding is controlled or monitoring at high dependency unit on delivery suite, if appropriate.
- Recording of parameters on a flow chart such as the modified obstetric early warning system charts.
- Documentation of fluid balance, blood, blood products and procedures.

Lab Reports and their Correction

Investigations	Indications	Blood/Blood Products	Quantity	Effect (Per unit)
Hb	< 8 g%	Packed red cell (150 ml)	4 units*	Increase in PCV by 3%, Hb by 1 g%
PT	>1.5 times	FFP (150–200 ml/unit)	4 units	Increase fibrinogen by 10 mg/dl and coagulation factors by 3–5%
APTT	>1.5 times			
INR	>2			
S.fibrinogen	<100 mg%	Cryoprecipitate (15–20 ml/unit)	4 units	Increase fibrinogen by 10 mg/dl
Platelets	<50,000	RDP (100 ml/unit)	4 units	Increase in platelet count by 5000–10000/mm^3 per unit
		SDP (350 ml/unit)	1 unit	Increase in platelet count by 40000–50000/mm^3 per unit

*4 units of FFP for every 6 units of PCV & 1 amp of inj. Calcium gluconate for every 4 units of PCV

Gauge	Color code	External diameter (mm)	Catheter length (mm)	Flow rate (ml/min)
14G	Orange	2.1	45	300
16G	Grey	1.7	45	200
17G	White	1.5	45	140
18G	Green	1.3	45	95
20G	Pink	1.1	45	62
22G	Blue	0.9	45	33
24G	Yellow	0.7	45	20

Diagnosing the Etiology of PPH

Immediate PPH Uterus soft not contracted	Shock	Atonic PPH
Immediate PPH	Contracted uterus Placenta complete	Tears of vagina, cervix or perineum
Placenta not delivered within 30 min	Immediate PPH Contracted uterus	Retained placenta
Portion of maternal surface of placenta missing	Immediate PPH Contracted uterus	Retained placental fragments
Uterus not palpable per abdomen Slight pain	Immediate PPH Inverted uterus obvious at vulva	Inverted uterus
Bleeding not controlled for >24 hrs of delivery Uterus soft and size more than the elapsed time since delivery	Bleeding continuous irregular, heavy, foul smelling Anemia	Delayed PPH
Immediate PPH (intra-abdominal and/or vaginal) Abdominal pain may decrease after rupture	Shock Rapid pulse Tender abdomen	Ruptured uterus

The most common cause of primary PPH is uterine atony. However, clinical examination must be undertaken to exclude other or additional causes:

- Retained products (placenta, membranes, clots)
- Vaginal/cervical lacerations or hematoma
- Ruptured uterus
- Broad ligament hematoma
- Extragenital bleeding (for example, subcapsular liver rupture)
- Uterine inversion.

Algorithm for the Management of Postpartum Hemorrhage (Hemostasis)

H—Call for **H**elp

A—**A**ssess (haemodynamic status and blood loss) and resuscitate

E—**E**stablish **E**tiology, **E**cbolics (syntocinon/syntometrine/ergometrine bolus), Ensure availability of blood

M—**M**assage the uterus

O—**O**xytocics (syntocinon infusion/prostaglandins, IM, per rectum, intra-myometrial)

S—**S**hift to theater, EUA, exclude trauma/retained products, bimanual compression

T—**T**amponade (balloon or uterine packing)

A—**A**pply compression sutures (B·lynch/modified)

S—**S**ystemic pelvic devascularization

I—**I**nterventional radiology (uterine artery embolization)

S—**S**ubtotal or total abdominal hysterectomy

Management of Atonic PPH

When uterine atony is perceived to be a cause of the bleeding the following mechanical and pharmacological measures should be instituted, in turn, until the bleeding stops:

- Bimanual uterine compression (rubbing up the fundus) to stimulate contractions
- Ensure bladder is empty (Foley catheter, leave in place).
- Syntocinon 5 units by slow intravenous injection (may have repeat dose).
- Ergometrine 0.5 mg by slow intravenous or intramuscular injection (contraindicated in women with hypertension).
- Syntocinon infusion (40 units in 500 ml Hartmann's solution at 125 ml/hour) unless fluid restriction is necessary.
- Carboprost 0.25 mg by intramuscular injection repeated at intervals of not less than 15 minutes to a maximum of 8 doses (contraindicated in women with asthma).
- Direct intramyometrial injection of carboprost 0.5 mg (contraindicated in women with asthma), with responsibility of the administering clinician as it is not recommended for intramyometrial use.
- Misoprostol 1000 micrograms rectally.

If pharmacological measures fail to control the hemorrhage, initiate surgical hemostasis sooner rather than later. Intrauterine balloon tamponade is an appropriate first line 'surgical' intervention for most women where uterine atony is the only or main cause of hemorrhage. If this fails to stop the bleeding, the following conservative surgical interventions may be attempted, depending on clinical circumstances and available expertise:

- Balloon tamponade
- Hemostatic brace suturing (such as using procedures described by B-lynch or modified compression sutures)
- Bilateral ligation of uterine arteries
- Bilateral ligation of internal iliac (hypogastric) arteries
- Selective arterial embolization.

  Resort to hysterectomy sooner rather than later (especially in cases of placenta accreta or uterine rupture).

  A second consultant clinician should be involved in the decision for hysterectomy.

Note

- For management of PPH, oxytocin should be preferred over ergometrine alone, a fixed dose combination of ergometrine and oxytocin, carbetocin, and prostaglandins.
- If oxytocin is not available, or if the bleeding does not respond to oxytocin, ergometrine or oxytocin-ergometrine fixed-dose combination should be offered as second-line treatment.
- If the above second-line treatments are not available, or if the bleeding does not respond to the second-line treatment, a prostaglandin should be offered as a third line of treatment.
- There is no added benefit of offering misoprostol as adjunct treatment for PPH in women who have received oxytocin during the third stage of labor. Where oxytocin is available, and is used in the management of the third stage of labor, oxytocin alone should be used in preference to adjunct misoprostol for the management of PPH.
- In women who have not received oxytocin as a prophylactic during the third stage of labor, oxytocin alone should be offered as the drug of choice for the treatment of PPH.
- Tranexamic acid may be offered as a treatment for PPH if: (i) administration of oxytocin, followed by second-line treatment options and prostaglandins, has failed to stop the bleeding; or (ii) it is thought that the bleeding may be partly due to trauma.
- Recombinant factor VIIa for the treatment of PPH should be limited to women with specific hematological indications.
- Uterine massage should be started once PPH has been diagnosed.
- Bimanual uterine compression may be offered as a temporizing measure in the treatment of PPH due to uterine atony after vaginal delivery.
- Uterine packing is not recommended for the treatment of PPH due to uterine atony after vaginal delivery.

- In women who have not responded to treatment with uterotonics, or if uterotonics are not available, intrauterine balloon or condom tamponade may be offered in the treatment of PPH due to uterine atony.
- External aortic compression for the treatment of PPH due to uterine atony after vaginal delivery may be offered as a temporizing measure until appropriate care is available.
- The research is ongoing on nonpneumatic antishock garments to evaluate the potential benefits and harms of this intervention.
- If other measures have failed and resources are available, uterine artery embolization may be offered as a treatment for PPH due to uterine atony.
- If bleeding does not stop in spite of treatment with uterotonics, other conservative interventions (e.g. uterine massage), and external or internal pressure on the uterus, surgical interventions should be initiated. Conservative approaches should be tried first, followed – if these do not work – by more invasive procedures. Compression sutures may be attempted first and, if that intervention fails, uterine, utero-ovarian and hypogastric vessel ligation may be tried. If life-threatening bleeding continues even after ligation, subtotal (also called supracervical or total hysterectomy) should be performed.

Oxytocics	Dose and route	Maintenance dose	Max dose	Fre-quency	Side effects	Contra-indica-tions
Oxytocin	IV infusion 10–40U in 500 ml crystalloid @ 60 drops/min	IV Infusion 10 U/500 ml @ 40 drops per min	Not more than 3 liters		Hypoten-sion, Water intoxication	None
Ergome-trine/ Methergin	0.2 mg IM/ Slow IV	0.2 mg after 15 min	5 doses	4th hourly	Nausea, vomiting, hypertension	Hyperten-sion, Heart disease, Severe anemia Rh –ve pregnancy
15 Methyl PGF 2α	250 µg	250 µg after 15 min	8 doses	15–90 min	Nausea, vomiting, diarrhea, pyrexia, broncho-constriction	Asthma, heart disease
Misoprostol	600–1000 µg oral/ rectal		2400 µg		Shivering, fever, tachycardia,	None

Never give prostagladins intravenously, it might be fatal.

Onset of Action

Route	Ergometrine	Methergin	Syntometrine	Oxytocin
IV	45–60 sec	1 1/2 min	Not to be used	30 sec
IM	6–7 min	7 min	2 1/2 min	2 1/2 min
Oral	10 min	10 min	–	–
		Duration of action		
	3 hours	3 hours	3 hours	8 min

- **Uncontrolled bleeding** (even after 30 min of oxytocics — oxytocin, methergin, PGF2α and misoprostol) — maintain intravenous oxytocin infusion and consider:

External compression for 30 min

- Uterine massage
  - Massage the fundus of the uterus through the woman's abdomen until the uterus is contracted.

Bimanual Uterine Compression

- It is indicated when uterine massage is not successful in arresting bleeding.
- Wearing sterile gloves, insert a hand into the vagina and remove any blood clots from the lower part of the uterus or cervix.
- Form a fist, place the fist into the anterior fornix and apply pressure against the anterior wall of the uterus.
- With the other hand, press deeply into the abdomen behind the uterus, applying pressure against the posterior wall of the uterus.
- Maintain compression until bleeding is controlled and the uterus contracts.

Compression of Aorta

- Apply downward pressure with a closed fist over the abdominal aorta directly through the abdominal wall.
- The point of compression is just above the umbilicus and slightly to the left.
- Aortic pulsations can be felt easily through the anterior abdominal wall in the immediate postpartum period.
- With the other hand, palpate the femoral pulse to check the adequacy of compression.
- If the pulse is palpable during compression, the pressure exerted by the fist is inadequate.
- If the femoral pulse is not palpable, the pressure exerted is adequate.
- Maintain compression until bleeding is controlled.

If the External Compression is not Effective, then –

Internal compression/surgical method whichever is appropriate depending on the general condition of the patient:

Internal compression: If the patient is stable, can be used for 12–24 hours until the bleeding stops.

Surgical methods: If the patient is not stable.

Condom Tamponade

- Insert Foley's catheter in the bladder prior to the procedure.
- Clean the vagina and cervix with antiseptic solution.
- Under aseptic precautions a size 16 sterile rubber catheter is inserted in the condom and tied near the mouth of the condom by a silk thread, inner end of the catheter remaining within the condom.
- Cervical lips held with sponge holder.
- Condom tied over the catheter is introduced into the uterine cavity. The outer end of the catheter is connected with a saline set and saline is kept 60–70 cms above the level of abdomen and the condom is inflated.
- Pack the vagina with gauze.
- Inflate the condom with 250–500 ml of Normal saline.

Foley's catheter: With a balloon of 30 ml capacity (which may be inflated up to 100 ml) is effective in controlling PPH. But the shape of the balloon may not correspond to the elongated uterine cavity.

Additional Foley catheters can be inserted if necessary to control postpartum hemorrhage resulting from atony, may be useful in cases where cervical lacerations have been repaired but bleeding is still present and placental bed bleeding.

Note: Use Sengstaken-Blakemore tube (after cutting the tube distal to the stomach balloon to facilitate insertion), Rusch urological balloon or Bakri balloon if available.

Care after Tamponade

- Keep woman nil by mouth.
- Monitor pulse, blood pressure, uterine fundal height and signs of vaginal bleeding or bleeding via the lumen of the catheter.
- Record temperature 2nd hourly and urine output hourly.
- Oxytocin infusion is continued.
- Give broad spectrum antibiotics.
- Catheter is kept inflated for 6–24 hours.
- During removal, first deflate the balloon, observe for bleeding for 30 minutes. If no bleeding, stop oxytocin infusion for 30 minutes; and if still no bleeding, the catheter is to be removed. If the woman starts bleeding, reinflate the balloon.

Conservative surgical methods: Reduce the need for hysterectomy.

Surgical methods: If the patient is not stable.

1. **Uterine compression sutures (B-Lynch surgery):**
   Bimanual compression of uterus stops bleeding—compression sutures will help.
   This is called compression test.

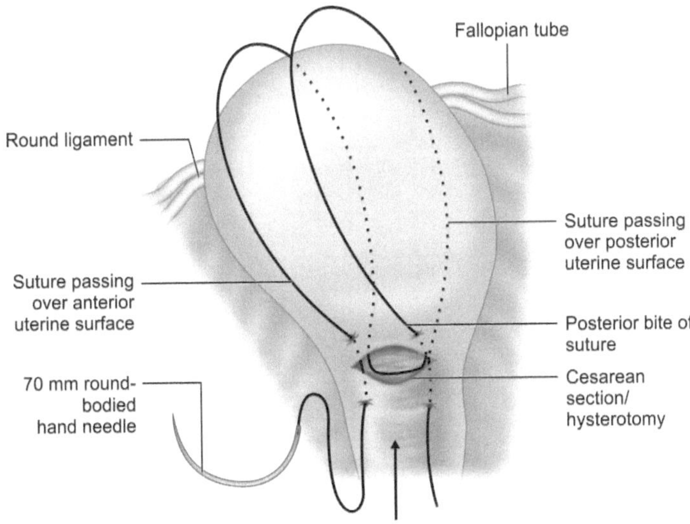

- Patient in lithotomy position with an assistant to observe the degree of vaginal bleeding.
- Apply pressure to the exteriorized uterus below the inferiorly displaced bladder.
- If bleeding stops, patient is a good candidate for the B-lynch suture.
- Uterine cavity checked, explored and evacuated.
- Monocryl/Catgut No. 1 or any other rapidly absorbable suture material with a long needle to be used.
- First suture is placed 3 cm below the transverse hysterotomy incision on the right, passed through the uterine cavity to a point above the incision and about 4 cm from the lateral border of the uterus, at which point it is passed through the anterior uterine wall.
- The suture is then carried vertically over the fundus of the uterus, with the assistant maintaining compression of the uterus. The suture is then passed through the posterior uterine wall at the level of the hysterotomy incision and the uterosacral ligament.
- The suture is carried horizontally to the corresponding position on the left side of the uterus and passed back through the posterior uterine wall on the left, over the fundus and down the side of the uterus anteriorly, again approximately 4 cm from the lateral side of the uterus.
- The suture is then passed through the uterine wall into the cavity at a point symmetrical to that previously done on the opposite side.
- The suture is passed through the wall below the transverse hysterotomy incision at a point corresponding to the initial entry point on the opposite side.
- After closure of the hysterotomy incision, the two ends of the suture are tied.
- The compression on the uterus is maintained throughout so that suture placement results in the greatest degree of compression possible.
- Slippage of the uterine brace suture is best avoided by fixing the sutures at the uterine fundus.

- Transverse compression sutures are applied to the lower segment for abnormal placentation to control bleeding.

Hayman's Uterine Compression

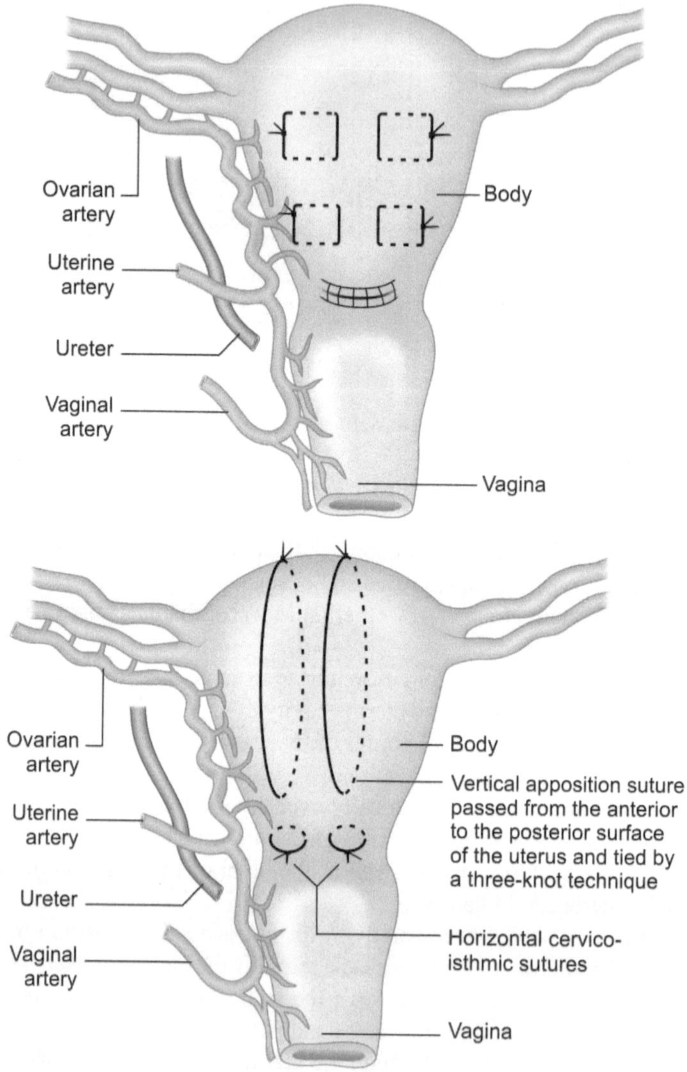

- Modification of the B-lynch suture that can be placed without a hysterotomy incision, useful in patients who deliver vaginally.
- Involves placement of 4 sutures, 2 on each side at the approximate location at which the B-lynch sutures are placed.
- The placement is started with the suture passed anterior to posterior through the entire thickness of the uterus at a point where a transverse uterine incision would be made.

- Compression is maintained on the uterus when sutures are tied down over the fundus.

Advantages

- Safe to perform because no important structures nearby
- Needs less expertise
- Requires less time

Cho Square Stitch

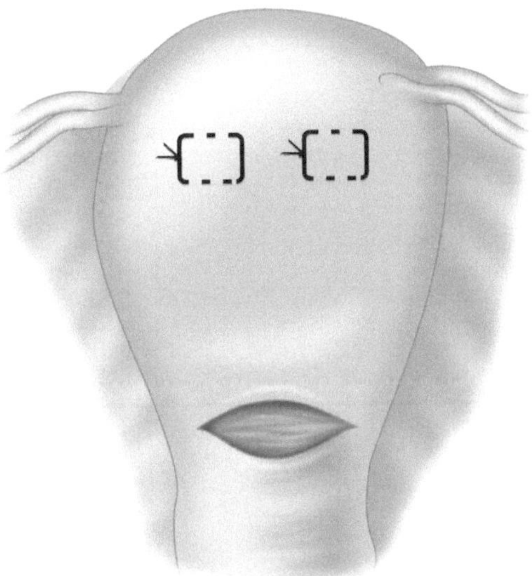

Procedure

- Interrupted circular stitch for placenta accreta using chromic catgut.
- Multiple square sutures along the horizontal axis of uterus taking the full thickness of uterine musculature 2 cm long and the interval between the sutures 2 cm, sutures placed in several tiers depending upon surface of bleeding; may be useful for placenta previa (make sure to leave a drainage portal).
- Sub-endomyometrial injections of 1–2 ml of dilute vasopressin (5 units in 20 ml saline) may reduce local bleeding in the lower uterine segment.
- Check that compression sutures have worked by observing blood loss per vaginum before closing the abdomen (Lithotomy position).

Gunasheela Global Cerclage

Serial encircling stitches taken on a superficial plane at a depth about 2–3 mm in the myometrium, taken at an interval of 2 cm along the horizontal axis from fundus to 1 cm from the lower uterine segment of the uterus and tying in the midline anteriorly (four parallel sutures may be required at an interval of 1 inch) + modified B Lynch vertical sutures (above the LUS near midline and taken through the myometrium – this will still allow a window for inspection to assess the success of the operation). Success rate 75 – 80.

Ligation of artery

Perform uterine and utero-ovarian artery ligation. (Procedure given below)

a. Step-wise devascularization: (Salah Abrabdo) – Success rate 100%
   1. Unilateral uterine artery ligation
   2. Bilateral uterine artery ligation (at upper part of lower uterine segment)
   3. Low uterine artery ligation (after mobilization of bladder)
   4. Unilateral ovarian vessel ligation
   5. Bilateral ovarian vessel ligation

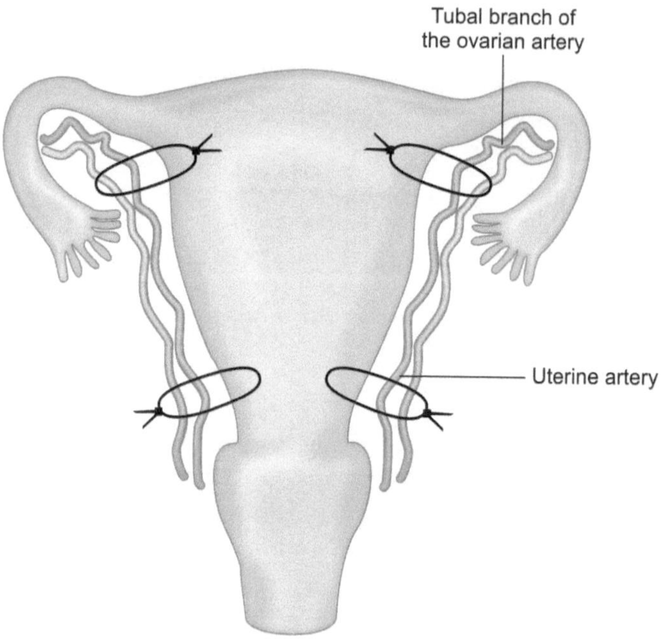

- For direct ligation of the uterine artery, the uterus is elevated by an assistant and deviated laterally.
- An area close to the uterine isthmus is exposed, and a No. 1 absorbable suture (chromic or polyglycolic acid) is then passed through 1 cm of the myometrium, at approximately the level of the endocervix.
- The suture is next passed through an avascular segment of the broad ligament, with the appropriate site chosen by transillumination.
- This suture is then firmly tied either anteriorly or posteriorly, with attention to not inadvertently incorporating neither the bowel nor the omentum.
- *Advantage:* When the body of the uterus is the source of hemorrhage, uterine artery ligations (O'Leary) are much easier and safer to perform and more likely to be effective than ligating the hypogastric arteries, as no retroperitoneal dissection is required and the course of the ureter is not of concern and surgical access is difficult at best.
- To ligate the cervical branch, stitches are placed 2–3 cms below the initial stitches after mobilizing the bladder.
- If despite bilateral uterine artery ligation, bleeding remains uncontrolled, ligation of utero-ovarian anastomosis is done just below the ovarian ligament.

Internal Iliac artery ligation

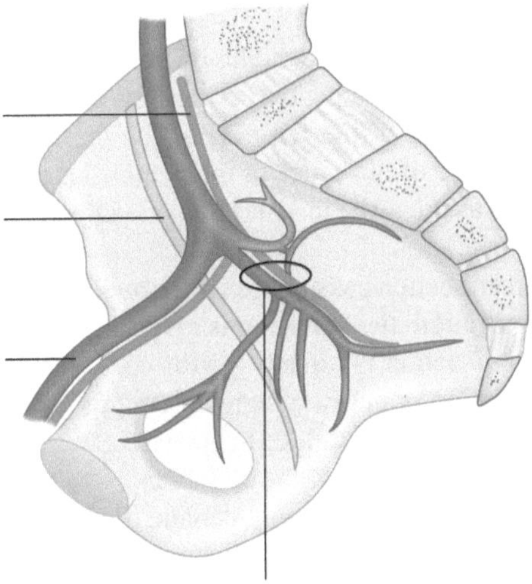

- Causes 85% reduction in pulse pressure in the arteries distal to the point of ligation.
- Highly effective in controlling PPH due to uterine atony, ruptured uterus and placenta accreta. Success rate is 40–75%.
- The peritoneum over the common iliac vessels is opened and dissected for about 5 cm from the point of origin. A blunt tipped right-angled clamp (mixter forceps) is gently placed under the artery from lateral to medial side (to prevent injury to the underlying vein), 5 cm distal to the common iliac artery bifurcation (should be distal to the origin of the posterior division of internal iliac artery).
- Identify the common, external and internal iliac arteries. The ureter passes over the bifurcation of the common iliac artery and reflected medially.
- Doubly ligate the internal iliac artery with non-absorbable material (Silk No 1-0 or Chromic catgut no 2) distal to the bifurcation by at least 3 cm (to avoid the posterior division) at two sites 1 cm apart. Secure the vessel, do not cut the vessel.
- Ligate the contralateral vessel similarly.
- Following the ligation, palpate the dorsalis pedis and femoral vessels to ensure that the external/common iliac arteries have not been inadvertently ligated.

  Complications:
  - Long-term buttock pain
  - Ischemic damage to pelvis
  - Accidental ligature of adjacent structures.

Hysterectomy

- Peripartum hysterectomy proceeds in the same fashion as a routine non-pregnant hysterectomy with some additional changes.
- Due to the increasing size of pedicles secondary to peripartum tissue edema and hypertrophy, pedicles may have to be taken in 2 portions in what otherwise might suffice as a single pedicle.

- Additionally, pedicles should be doubly clamped and doubly ligated and/or suture ligated taking care that hemostasis is certain before moving onto the next pedicle.
- It may be appropriate depending on circumstances to consider a supracervical
- hysterectomy in emergency peripartum procedures. This allows for a more rapid completion of the removal of the major portion of the uterus and to a certain remedy of the cause of the hemorrhage unless the vesico-cervical area is involved as it may be in a placenta previa/percreta where a total hysterectomy is to be done.
- If a cesarean section has not been performed prior to the hysterectomy, a vertical midline infraumbilical incision is given and abdomen is opened in layers.
- If cesarean section is already performed, with continued bleeding, close the uterine incision or apply sponge holding or green armytage forceps at margin of uterine incision to achieve hemostasis.
- Uterus is delivered out of the abdomen.
- Round ligaments are clamped, cut and doubly ligated.
- From the cut edge of the round ligament, the anterior leaf of the broad ligament is opened and incised up to the bladder peritoneum is reflected onto the lower uterine surface in the midline. The posterior leaf of the broad ligament is similiarly reflected down.
- A hole is made in the broad ligament and clamp is applied to include the fallopian tube and ovarian ligament, cut and ligated on both sides.
- Dissect the bladder downwards off the lower uterine segment.
- The uterine vessels on each side are clamped at right angles on each side of the cervix, cut and ligated.

To perform subtotal hysterectomy, it is necessary only to amputate the body of the uterus immediately below the level of uterine artery ligation. The cervical stump is closed with interrupted 2-0 or 3-0 chromic catgut or polyglycolic sutures.

To perform total hysterectomy, uterosacral and cardinal ligaments are clamped and cut.

Indication: Bleeding from lower uterine segment as it happens in placenta previa

- Extensively mobilize the bladder (to prevent injury to the ureters and laceration or suturing of the bladder during cervical excision and vaginal cuff closure).
- If the cervix is effaced and dilated appreciably, the cervicovaginal junction after delivery may be identified through a vertical uterine incision made anteriorly in the midline, either through the open hysterotomy incision or through an incision created at the level of the ligated uterine vessels. A finger is directed inferiorly through the incision to identify the free margin of the dilated, effaced cervix and the anterior vaginal fornix. The contaminated glove is replaced. Circumscribe the vagina close to the cervix. Close the vaginal cuff, before closing the abdomen, ensure hemostasis. Close abdomen in layers.

Role of Factor VII

Recommendations on the management of PPH with this agent are the following:

- Consider the use of rFVIIa only after the failure of medical (treatment of hemodynamic instability, hypothermia, and metabolic abnormalities; uterine

massage/compression; and uterotonic agents), blood component (transfusion of RBC, platelet, and fresh-frozen plasma to correct anemia, thrombocytopenia, and coagulopathy), and conservative surgical/invasive (B-lynch suture, internal iliac or uterine artery ligation, internal uterine tamponade, and uterine artery radiologic embolization) therapies.
- Administer rFVIIa 90 mg/kg as an intravenous bolus over 3 to 5 minutes.
- Before the rFVIIa injection, check that all abnormal parameters influencing rFVIIa efficacy (i.e., acidosis, thrombocytopenia (<20,000), hypofibrinogenemia (<1 gm/L) hypothermia, and hypocalcemia) have been corrected.
- If 20 minutes after the first dose of rFVIIa, there is no response, administer a second dose of rFVIIa (90 mg/kg), ensuring before that temperature, acidemia, serum calcium, platelets, and fibrinogen have been optimized.
- If bleeding persists after 2 doses of rFVIIa, consider hysterectomy.

SECONDARY PPH

Secondary PPH is often associated with endometritis. When antibiotics are clinically indicated, a combination of ampicillin (clindamycin if penicillin allergic) and metronidazole is appropriate. In cases of endomyometritis (tender uterus) or overt sepsis, then the addition of gentamicin is recommended.

Surgical measures should be undertaken if there is excessive or continuing bleeding, irrespective of ultrasound findings.

A senior obstetrician should be involved in decisions and performance of any evacuation of retained products of conception as these women are carrying a high risk for uterine perforation.

Causes of Secondary PPH

- Abnormalities of placentation
    - Idiopathic subinvolution of uteroplacental vessels
    - Retained placental tissue
    - Placenta accreta
- Infection
    - Endometritis, myometritis, parametritis
    - Infection/dehiscence of cesarean scar
- Preexisting uterine disease
    - Leiomyomata
    - Cervical neoplasm
- Trauma: Rupture of vulvar or vaginal hematoma
- Coagulopathy

Management Options

- Clinical features important in making diagnosis.
- Ultrasonography of uterine contents does not distinguish blood clot from placenta; echogenic masses are found in asymptomatic women. Empty uterus on scan may allow a conservative approach.
- IV fluids and blood for hemodynamic stabilization may be necessary in some patients; correct coagulation defects.

- Antibiotics for 12–24 h prior to surgical evacuation.
- Uterotonics and antibiotics may reduce need for curettage.
- Surgical/suction evacuation of uterus.
- Embolization may be tried in persistent bleeding after evacuation before resorting to hysterectomy.
- Send surgical products for histologic examination.

TRAUMATIC PPH

- Tears of the birth canal are the second most frequent cause of PPH. Tears may coexist with atonic uterus.
- Postpartum bleeding with a contracted uterus is usually due to a cervical or vaginal tear.
- Examine the woman carefully and repair tears of the cervix or vagina and perineum, with good exposure using adequate light, assistance and instruments.

Classification of Perineal Tears

- First degree: Involves the vaginal mucosa only
- Second degree: Involves the vaginal mucosa and perineal muscles sparing the sphincters
- Third degree: Involves the anal sphincter
  3A—Less than 50% of external anal sphincter is torn
  3B—More than 50% of external anal sphincter is torn
  3C—Internal anal sphincter is involved
- Fourth degree:involves the anal sphincter complex and rectal mucosa
- Rectal mucosal tear (buttonhole) without involvement of the anal sphincter is rare and not included in the above classification.

Repair of First and Second Degree Perineal Tears/Episiotomy-Principle

Action	Rationale
Check maternal baseline observations, assess uterus is well contracted	To ensure stable condition prior to commencing procedure
Explain procedure to mother and her partner	To psychologically prepare mother and obtain informal verbal consent
Assess extent of perineal trauma and classify degree of laceration	To acknowledge personal limitations and ensue repair is undertaken by most appropriate person
Rectal examination	To check if anal sphincter and mucosa is intact unless only minor trauma
Prepare trolley and equipment – check and record with nursing staff, the number of tampons, swabs, sutures, needles and the expiry date, concentration and amount of local anesthetic	To ensure the equipment is correct prior to the commencement and that count is correct at the end of the procedure
Position of the mother to enable accurate vision and access while endeavoring to maintain dignity	Ensure whole extent of laceration is visible and accessible

Contd...

Contd...

Use aseptic technique	To minimize the risk of infection/wound breakdown
Identify anatomical landmarks: • Infiltrate local anesthetic into exposed edges of traumatised tissue ensuring equal distribution	• To ensure anatomical approximation • To facilitate pain free perineal repair
A tampon may be inserted into the vagina	To ensure area to be sutured is not obscured by blood loss
Identify apex of trauma and insert 1 stitch 1 cm above this point	To ensure hemostasis of small vessels that may have retracted beyond the apex
Suture posterior vaginal trauma using a continuous interlocking or nonlocking suture down to fourchette	To achieve apposition without shortening of the vagina
Do not penetrate rectal mucosa	Risk of rectovaginal mucosa
Identify hymenal remnants at fourchette	Misalignment of introitus may cause dyspareunia
Repair perineal muscles in one or two layers, either use interrupted or continuous suture	Realign perineal muscles
Do not pull sutures too tight	Loose sutures allow for normal reactionary edema
Perineal skin: Subcuticular suturing or interrupted sutures 1 cm apart starting at the fourchette and finishing at the anal end of the trauma	To complete repair
Following completion of the repair	
Remove tampon and inspect repair	Ensure correct suturing, hemostasis, check uterine blood loss
Insert 2 fingers into vagina	Check introitus and vagina, if sutured too tightly
Perform rectal examination	Check no sutures have penetrated rectal mucosa
Clean and dry perineal area	Minimize infection rate
Check and record all swabs, needles and instruments are correct after the procedure	To confirm all equipment and materials used are accounted for
Make the mother comfortable, give advice regarding perineal discomfort, personal hygiene, pain relief, pelvic floor exercises, avoidance of constipation and dyspareunia	Health education
Complete documentation	Provide accurate record of procedure

Preparation

- All repairs must be conducted in the operating theater. If there is any doubt about the diagnosis, it is safer to examine the woman in theater and perform a full assessment.
- Written consent must be obtained and serious risks of the procedure should include bleeding, infection, anal incontinence and fistula formation.

- Effective epidural or spinal anesthetic is necessary.
- Emotional support of the mother is paramount.

Repair Procedure

1. **First degree perineal tear/Vaginal lacerations:**
   - If the laceration is not bleeding, can be left unsutured.
   - If bleeding, identify the apex of the laceration. If the upper edge is not visible, place a suture as high as possible and apply traction to bring the apex of the laceration into view.
   - A continuous locking suture with chromic catgut No 1-0 is done.
   - In case of extensive lacerations, the vagina can be packed tightly following suture for hemostasis to avoid hematoma formation. If vagina is packed, the bladder should be catheterized with Foley's catheter (to avoid retention of urine) and maintain a chart for the fundal height (because the vaginal pack can cause outflow obstruction and lead to pooling of blood in the uterus leading to atonic PPH).

   The vaginal pack and catheter can be removed after 12–24 hours. Broad spectrum antibiotics are prescribed.
2. **Second degree perineal tear:**
   - Repair of second degree repair resembles repair of an episiotomy.
   - Repair with chromic catgut No. 0/1 or Vicryl rapide 2-0 if available. Close in three layers. The first layer comprising vaginal mucosa and submucosal tissue, second layer comprising the perineal muscle and the third layer comprising subcutaneous tissue and skin.
   - Vaginal mucosa is closed with continuous interlocking sutures starting 1 cm above the apex. Perineal muscles are closed with continuous sutures. Skin is closed with mattress or subcuticular sutures. Obliterate all the dead space to prevent hematoma formation.

Repair of Third and Fourth Degree Perineal Tears

Procedure

1. The full extent of the injury should be evaluated by a careful vaginal and rectal examination in lithotomy and the tear should be classified as above.
2. The torn anal epithelium must be repaired with a continuous vicryl 3-0 sutures via the vagina with the knots tightly secured. Interrupted sutures can also be used. Ensure that the apex of the tear has been identified and there are no additional mucosal tears. The sutures are placed through the submucosa of the anorectum starting above the apex of the tear and extending down until the anal verge, with knots placed inside the lumen.
3. An internal anal sphincter tear must be repaired separately by end to end approximation with interrupted 3/0 PDS sutures. These sutures are monofilamentous, and therefore, less likely to precipitate infection compared to a braided suture. The internal anal sphincter is identified as the thickening of the circular smooth muscle layer at the distal 2-3 cm of the anal canal. It appears as the glistening white fibrous structure lying between the anal canal

submucosa and the fibres of external anal sphincter. The internal anal sphincter tends to retract laterally, they need to be identified and sutured.

4. If less than 50% of the external anal sphincter (EAS) thickness is torn (3a tear) an end-to end repair should always be performed with mattress sutures to approximate the muscle ends. When more than 50% of the EAS thickness is torn (3b) then you can chose to perform an overlap repair only if the EAS is completely torn and you are confident in performing an overlap repair. Otherwise you should still perform an end-to-end repair with mattress sutures to approximate the muscle ends. A proper overlap repair is not possible unless the EAS is completely torn in length and thickness. The torn ends of the EAS must be identified and grasped with Allis tissue forceps. The muscle is then mobilized and pulled across to overlap in a 'double-breast' fashion with 3/0 PDS sutures.
    - There are two techniques for repair of the torn external anal sphincter muscle:

    A. End-to-end technique:
    - The torn edges of the external anal sphincter are identified and held with allies forceps and approximated with 4–6 interrupted sutures, placed through the edges of the external anal sphincter and its connective tissue capsule at 3, 6, 9 and 12 o' clock positions. The sutures are first placed through the inferior and posterior portions of the sphincter, these are tied in last in order to facilitate the repair.

    B. Overlapping technique:
    - The overlap method involves taking two sets of sutures. The first row of sutures is taken 1.5 cm from the edge on one side and 0.5 cm on the other side in such a way that when the sutures are tied, the free ends overlap one another. The free end is then sutured to the rest of the sphincter.
    - The remainder of the tear is closed using the same principles and suture material as for repair of episiotomy.
5. Great care must be exercised in reconstructing the perineal muscles to provide support to the sphincter repair. Remember that the anal sphincter would be more likely to be traumatized during a subsequent vaginal delivery in the presence of a short deficient perineum. Also ensure that the knots and suture ends of PDS sutures are completely buried with overlying tissue to avoid suture migration.
6. Prophylactic antibiotics should be given intraoperatively:
   Inj. Taxim 1 gm + Inj. Metronidazole 500 mg IV followed by oral for 3–5 days
    - As the consequences of anal sphincter disruption can result in litigation, document the extent of injury (per vaginal and per rectal examination findings), technique of repair (type of repair, material used and method used), time procedure commenced and completed, analgesia used, instruments/swabs and tampoon counts, blood loss during the procedure and the name/designation of the person completing the repair.
    - A diagram demonstrating the extent of the injury and technique of repair will serve to substantiate that a careful examination has been performed.
    - We may even take pictures to be taken of the trauma and of the muscles grasped for repair.

Care after Repair of Third/Fourth Degree Tears

- Immediately following surgery, advise liquid diet for a day and convert to low residue diet over 2–3 days.
- Prescribe stool softeners for about 10 days (Lactulose 15 ml bd or enough to keep stools soft) from 3rd day. Avoid use of enemas/purgatives.
- To maintain perineal hygiene.
- Clean the area with antiseptic solution after every act of urination and defecation.
- Analgesics are prescribed for relief of pain.
- Sitz bath to be given.
- Encourage ambulation and offer physiotherapy pelvic floor exercises for 6–12 weeks in order to stimulate circulation and speed up healing process.
- Vaginal/rectal examination and sexual intercourse must be avoided for at least 6 weeks following the repair.
- All women who have had obstetric anal sphincter repair should be reviewed 6–12 weeks postpartum.
- If there is disruption, we have to wait for 3 weeks till tissue becomes healthy and edema subsides.

Subsequent Delivery Following Repair

Group I: Third or fourth degree tear with no symptoms
Group II: Third or fourth degree tear with symptoms
Group III: History of second degree anal sphincter repair
Group IV: Asymptomatic but with demonstrable anal sphincter defect or abnormal manometry

Group I

i. Risk of further anal sphincter damage 4% in subsequent vaginal delivery
ii. In patients who are transiently incontinent after first delivery 17 to 24% may develop worsening of symptoms after subsequent delivery

Group II

i. Risk of worsening of symptoms
ii. Avoid operative vaginal delivery and lengthening of second stage

Groups III and IV: Delivery by cesarean section.

- The risk of recurrence of a 3rd/4th degree tear is 5%.
- All women will have anal ultrasound and manometry.
- In general, continent women who have no evidence of significant anal sphincter compromise would be allowed to have a normal vaginal delivery by a senior obstetrician.
- Women with mild anal incontinence with evidence of anal sphincter compromise would be counseled and offered cesarean section.
- Women with significant fecal incontinence need to be counseled about a secondary sphincter repair.
- There is no evidence that prohylactic episiotomy prevents a recurrence of sphincter rupture, and therefore, an episiotomy should only be performed if

there are predisposing factors such as big baby, OP position, shoulder dystocia, fibrotic band or inelastic perineu.

Periurethral and Periclitoral Tears

- If there is light bleeding, pressure for 1–2 minutes will usually arrest the bleeding.
- If there is significant bleeding, these lacerations should be repaired by continuous suture with a chromic catgut No 2-0/3-0. Place a urethral catheter to avoid urethral injury and to guide placement of sutures.

Cervical Lacerations

- The cervix is inspected by using three-ring/sponge forceps. The anterior lip of the cervix is grasped with one forceps at 12 o'clock position, the second forceps is placed at 2 o'clock position and the third forceps is placed at 4 o' clock position. The position of the second and third forceps is progressively changed keeping the first one static, i.e. second one is placed at 4 o' clock position and third one at 6 o'clock position. In this manner, the entire cervix is closely inspected (walking around the cervix).
- Lacerations usually occur laterally and if they are less than 2 cm and not bleeding, do not require suture.
- Identify the angle/apex of the tear and place the first suture proximal to the angle. Suture with chromic catgut No 1-0 by either interrupted or running sutures. Overzealous suturing in an attempt to restore the normal cervical appearance, may lead to subsequent stenosis during uterine involution.
- If the upper edge is not visible, place a suture as high as possible and apply traction to bring the angle of the laceration into view and suture from above downwards.
- If the cervical tear extends partially or completely into the vault of the vagina, the condition is known as colporrhexis. Rarely extend up to the lower uterine segment and uterine artery or its branches and sometimes even through the peritoneum. This may result in extensive external hemorrhage requiring laparotomy.

Note: If bleeding continues, assess clotting status using a coagulation profile.

Retained Placenta

- There is no fixed definition for retained placenta. If placenta is not delivered within 30 min of delivery of baby is usually taken as retained placenta (96% placentae are delivered by 30 minutes).

Types

A. Trapped/Incarcerated: Placenta has separated from the uterine wall but is retained in the uterus because of atony, or more commonly by a constriction ring between the upper and lower uterine segments or in one uterine cornua.

B. Simple adherent placenta/Placenta adherens: It is due to failure of the normal separation through the decidua spongiosa layer. Until separation occurs, either partially or completely, these cases do not bleed excessively.

C. Pathological adherent placenta/Morbidly adherent placenta: Can be partial or complete. May be of three degrees:
   1. Placenta accreta: Invasion of the decidua basalis and adherence to the myometrium
   2. Placenta increta: Invading the myometrium
   3. Placenta percreta: Invasion through the myometrium to the serosal layer

Predisposing factors:
- Multiparity
- Prior missed abortion
- Severe postpartum endometritis
- Retained placenta in previous pregnancy
- Preterm labor
- Uterine fibroids
- Uterine anomaly: such as Bicornuate uterus
- Uterine scar: Previous cesarean section, curettage, myomectomy, hysteroscopic surgery.

Management of retained placenta:
- If the placenta is not expelled spontaneously, clinicians may offer 10 IU of oxytocin in combination with controlled cord traction.
- Ergometrine is not recommended, as it may cause tetanic uterine contractions, which may delay expulsion of the placenta.
- The use of prostaglandin E2 (dinoprostone or sulprostone) is not recommended.
- Intraumbilical vein injection of oxytocin with saline may be offered for the management of retained placenta.
- If, in spite of controlled cord traction, administration of uterotonics and intraumbilical vein injection of oxytocin + saline, the placenta is not delivered, manual extraction of the placenta should be offered as the definitive treatment.
- A single dose of antibiotics (ampicillin or first-generation cephalosporin) should be offered after manual removal of the placenta.

Trapped placenta:
- Clinically fundus feels small, contracted placental edge is felt through the tight cervical os.

USG: Myometrium thickened around the uterus and clear demarcation seen (in placenta accreta myometrium invisible or thin at the placental site).
- The urinary bladder should be catheterized.
- Controlled cord traction must be repeated to deliver the placenta.
- For a simple cervical closure or for a constriction ring that could have entrapped the placenta, administer 150 μg to 350 μg of nitroglycerin IV or 250 μg of terbutaline SC to assist removal. If terbutaline is chosen, uterine relaxation usually occurs within 2 to 3 minutes of the administration of the drug. When the placenta is detached but entrapped, myometrial relaxation normally permits an easy manual removal.

Simple adherent placenta/Placenta adherens
- Pipingas technique: Nasogastric tube No.10 is inserted in umbilical vein and inject 30 units of oxytocin in 30 ml of normal saline or 20 mg PGF 2α in 50 ml normal saline or 800 μg of misoprostol in 30 ml NS.

Manual removal of placenta (MROP):

- Resuscitate the woman in shock and simultaneously prepare to shift to operation theater.
- Informed and written consent to be taken.
- Adequate anesthesia (usually general anesthesia).
- Aseptic surgical technique, in lithotomy position.
- Grasp the fundus through the abdominal wall with the left hand.
- Introduce the right hand into the vagina in the shape of a cone (to prevent rupture of thinned out lower uterine segment accidentally) and pass into the uterus along the umbilical cord.
- Locate the margin of placenta and insinuate ulnar border of hand between the placenta and the uterine wall gently separating placenta from the uterine wall, using the sideways slicing movement of the hand.
- Grasp separated placenta with entire hand, withdraw gradually with membranes.
- Use sponge holder to strip off membranes if necessary.
- Uterus is re-explored to ensure that there are no placental fragments remaining and that the uterine wall is intact. If small pieces are encountered, remove piecemeal as best as possible.
- Massage uterus bimanually and start oxytocin infusion. Explore cervix, vagina for any injury.
- Observe vitals and for PV bleeding for at least 6 hours.
- Continue oxytocin infusion for 1 hour and administer broad spectrum antibiotics for 12–24 hours.

Morbidly adherent placenta:

- If a distinct cleavage plane between the placenta and the uterine wall cannot be located and if the tissue plane between the uterine wall and placenta cannot be developed through blunt dissection with the edge of the gloved hand, a diagnosis of invasive placenta should be considered.
- The retained placenta interferes with uterine contractions that is necessary to control bleeding after delivery, resulting in PPH.

Total placenta accreta:

Conservative management:

- In case of densely adherent placenta, the clinician must not try to remove any nonadherent portions of the placenta.
- Cut the cord as high as possible and leave the placenta.
- Patient's vital signs and amount of bleeding should be closely observed.
- Patient should be given antibiotics and methotrexate, 50 mg IM single dose in hope of autolysis.
- β hcG levels used for monitoring (monitored till undetectable).
- MRO/Curettage is done after 1–2 weeks.

Surgical management:

If bleeding continues despite conservative management, the following options are used:

- Bilateral uterine artery ligation (both upper and lower)
- Ligation of internal iliac artery vessels
- Uterine artery embolization

Retained placental fragments:

- If on examination of placenta, a cotyledon or a succenturiate lobe is found missing, anesthetize the woman and explore the uterine cavity.
- Avoid sharp curettage.
- If further hemorrhage: gentle curettage to remove any retainted fragments of placenta.
- If bleeding not controlled even after that resort to surgical methods as explained under the management of atonic PPH.

Management of placenta accreta diagnosed in antenatal period:

- Can be managed conservatively if fertility is to be preserved.
- Increase in the rates of placenta accreta is because of the increasing rate of cesarean deliveries.
- Risk of placenta accreta with placenta previa by number of prior cesarean deliveries.
  With
  - One prior section 11%
  - Two prior sections 40%
  - Three 61%
  - Four 67%

Diagnosis:

- **Ultrasound features of placenta accreta**
  - Loss of the echolucent area between the uterus and placenta
  - Multiple placental lacunae (Swiss-cheese appearance)
  - Loss of echolucent line between uterus and bladder
  - Focal exophytic masses extending into bladder
- **Color Doppler**
  - Retroplacental vessels invade the myometrium and obscure the bladder-serosal interface.
  - Abnormal intraplacental venous lakes are commonly seen in this setting.
- **MRI:** is costly, usually used in cases where placenta cannot be adequately assessed by sonography and there is increased risk of abnormal placentation.
  - Uterine bulging
  - Heterogeneous signal intensity within the placenta
  - Presence of dark intraplacental bands on T-2 imaging
  - A multidisciplinary approach is needed involving the obstetrician, urologist/ surgeon anesthethist, interventional radiologist, neonatologist, senior nursing staff and with facilities for high volume blood transfusion. Ensure adequate availability of blood products.
  - The 2 most important decisions that need to be made early in the planning process are timing of delivery, and conservative versus radical management
  - Favor delivery at 34 weeks after fetal lung maturity; earlier delivery may be indicated in women with repetitive antepartum bleeding (after administering betamethasone for fetal lung maturity).
  - Do a cesarean hysterectomy for all patients with placenta accreta and placenta previa, reserving attempts at conservative management for those without placenta previa and with suspected areas of focal accreta remote from the lower uterine segment.

- Abdomen is opened by a midline infraumbilical incision (which can be extended if needed) under GA, keep prophylactic catheters ready for embolization prior to surgery.
- Uterus is opened by a vertical incision away from the placental site, baby extracted. No attempt is made to deliver the placenta.
- Uterus is closed and a subtotal/total hysterectomy is done.

- **Conservative management**: Preservation of uterus is individualized to few cases. Same procedure is done as above and after delivery of the baby, if the woman is hemodynamically stable with no active bleeding; the cord is cut close to the placenta and placenta left in-situ. Monitor serum β-hCG.
  - Can be combined with uterine artery or internal iliac artery ligation or methotrexate therapy may be attempted. (Adjunctive uterine artery embolization can be done if facilities are available).

Vulval Hematoma

Incidence: 1 in 500 to 2000 deliveries

Risk facors for pelvic hematoma:
- Nulliparity
- Episiotomy
- Forceps delivery
- Vulval varicosities
- Eccessive ironing of the perineum
- Pudendal nerve block
- Coagulation defects: rare

Types: Depending on the anatomical location, whether above or below the levator ani is divided as –
1. Infralevator—common
2. Supralevator—rare

(The other classification: Puerperal hematomas may be classified as vulvar, vulvovaginal, paravaginal, or retroperitoneal.)

Infralevator hematoma:
- Cervical laceration extending into the vaginal vault or a small rupture of the lower segment are the possible causative factors.
- It involves vulva, perineum, paravaginal space and ischiorectal fossa.
- Causes severe persistent severe pain in perineal region. Can be associated with rectal tenesmus and urinary retention.
- Local examination reveals a tense swelling at the vulva which becomes dusky in color and tender to touch. May be associated with shock.

Treatment:
- General management: Fluid replacement, blood transfusion, analgesics and antibiotics
- Small hematomas (<5 cms) treat conservatively with cold compresses

Larger hematomas: For hematomas that are expanding or more than 5 cm in size, surgical intervention is recommended.
- Resuscitate if in shock and explore under general anesthesia.

- Where possible, the surgical incision should be made via the vagina to minimize visible scarring. Distinct bleeding points should be under-run with figure-of-eight absorable sutures. Closure of hematoma cavity by tyre mattress to obliterate the dead space.The presence of any residual bleeding or a hematoma in cavity is an indication for insertion of a Minivac or corrugated rubber drain, it should be left in place for at least 24 hours. If no distinct bleeding point can be seen (paravaginal venous plexus), cavity should be tightly packed and the pack should be left in place for 48 hours.
- Continuous drainage of bladder for 3–5 days
- Chymotrypsin TID for 5–7 days

Supralevator hematoma:

- Hematoma surfaced inside the vaginal wall presents with copious serosanguinous discharge.
- Can present with unexplained shock following delivery. May be associated with extensions into broad ligament during cesarean section/ extension of cervical or vaginal tear/with rupture of uterus.
- Abdominal examination reveals a swelling above the inguinal ligament pushing the uterus to the opposite side.
- Vaginal examination reveals occlusion of the vaginal canal by a bulge or a boggy swelling which can be felt through the fornix. Rectal examination confirms the findings.
- Ultrasonography CT/MRI helps to localize the hematoma.

Treatment: Resuscitative measures are taken to treat shock.

- Conservative treatment—for hematoma which is not increasing in size. The state of hematoma to be judged both clinically and sonologically. Adequate blood transfusion to be given.
- Emergency laparotomy is done for increasing hematoma and anterior leaf of broad ligament is incised and blood clot is scooped out. Bleeding points are identified and secured. Random blind sutures are to be avoided to prevent injury to ureter. If bleeding is not controlled, internal iliac artery ligation is done. If there is continuous bleeding from the upper vagina, then the anterior division of the internal iliac artery should be ligated. A vaginal pack should be inserted.
- **Selective arterial embolization**: When there is continuous expansion of a supralevator hematoma without extension into the cervix or uterus, selective arterial embolization is seen as the treatment of choice over internal iliac artery ligation, which in itself, has an uncertain chance of success and involves imposing a laparotomy on an already unstable patient.
- Total abdominal hysterectomy is indicated where there is any possibility that a supralevator/broad ligament hematoma is due to a rupture uterus or where a cervical tear appears to have extended up into the uterus.

Inversion of Uterus

Uterine fundus not felt abdominally or visible in vagina.

Types

- Acute: inversion within 24 hrs of delivery
- Subacute: inversion within 24 hrs to 4 weeks of delivery

- Chronic: inversion after 4 weeks of delivery or in non-pregnant state

OR

- Incomplete inversion—fundus of the uterus turned inside out, but the inverted fundus has not descended through the cervix.
- Complete inversion—inverted fundus has passed completely through the cervix to lie within the vagina or, less often, outside the introitus.

Degrees of Inversion

- 1st degree—incomplete inversion
- 2nd degree—complete inversion in the vagina
- 3rd degree—complete inversion outside the introitus

Causes

- Mismanagement of third stage of labor involving fundal pressure and/or cord traction before placental separation and while the uterus is still relaxed.
- Abnormally short umbilical cord, or functionally shortened by wrapped around the fetal body.
- Sudden rise in intra-abdominal pressure due to maternal cough once or vomiting.
- Morbid adherence of a fundally implanted placenta.
- Manual removal of placenta.
- Connective tissue disorders like Marfan's syndrome.

Clinical Features

- Large boggy mass appearing at introitus, with or without placenta attached.
- Severe sustained hypogastric pain in the third stage of labor
- Shock.
- In complete inversion the uterus is not palpable per abdomen.
- In incomplete uterine inversion, the fundus may appear to be normal.

Management

- If acute uterine inversion (occurs when myometrium and cervix is relaxed) is diagnosed immediately after it occurs, same degree of relaxation may allow immediate manual replacement.
- However within 1–2 min, the cervix and lower uterine segment clamp down and, along with increasing congestion, edema, contraction of the inverted uterine fundus, this makes manual replacement difficult, painful and usually impossible without anesthesia.
- If one attempt of immediate manual replacement of uterus fails, move to the following sequence –
    - Summon assistance (anesthesia, nursing, obstetrician)
    - Although the initial shock in these cases is usually of neurogenic type, it is wise to be prepared for the hemorrhage and the hypovolemia that will follow in many cases.
    - If pain is a dominant symptom, then small doses of IV morphine may be given.

To facilitate manual replacement:

Use general anesthesia or wait for effect of any uterotonic to wear off).

Use tocolysis:

1. Nitroglycerin IV: 150–200 µg, can repeat 100–150 µg (Max:500 µg)

- ◆ Can cause hypotension
- ◆ Contraindicated in women with low vascular volumes

- Manual replacement of uterus should be undertaken once anesthesia and tocolysis have been established. If placenta is still attached to fundus do not remove it, if placenta is partially attached to the fundus, it should be peeled off.

Manual Replacement of the Uterus

- The uterine fundus, with or without the attached placenta, is cupped in the palm of the hand, the fingers and thumb of which are extended to feel the uterocervical junction.
- The whole uterus is lifted up towards and beyond the umbilicus.
- Additional pressure is exerted with the finger tips to systematically and sequentially push and squeeze the uterine wall back through the cervix. This pressure may have to be sustained for 3–5 min to achieve complete replacement.
- Once the fundus has been replaced, keep the hand in the uterus while a rapid infusion of oxytocin is given to contract the uterus. When the uterus is felt to contract the hand is slowly withdrawn.
- The sooner manual replacement is undertaken the more likely, it is to succeed with relative ease. With suitable anesthesia and tocolysis within 2 hrs of diagnosis, it is usually successful.

In Case of Delay and/or Manual Replacement Unsuccessful

1. O'Sullivain's hydrostatic replacement technique

- Before using this procedure, it is important to make sure that the uterus and vagina have no lacerations, and if these are found they should be sutured.
- The principle of this technique is to instill a large volume of warm fluid (3–5 L) into the upper vagina, thus distending the fornices which serves to pull open the cervical ring, allowing replacement of the uterine fundus.
- The intravenous tubing is guided into the posterior fornix by one hand which also cups the fundus.
- The other hand seals the introitus around the wrist so that there is no egress of fluid.
- Alternatively, the tubing can be attached to a silastic vacuum extractor cup which is placed inside the introitus and may help provide a better seal.

In case of failure of manual replacement and hydrostatic technique, proceed with surgical management: The operations done are either abdominal or vaginal route:

1. Abdominal route:

Huntington's procedure:

- Allis or similar forceps are used to grasp the myometrium just inside the dimple of the inverted fundus.
- Before using the Allis forceps the cervical ring may be stretched, either with the fingers or by opening the blades of a large forceps.
- Systematically and sequentially, using forceps on both sides, the inverted fundus is then withdrawn from crater to fully correct the inversion.

Haultain's operation:

- Done when Huntington's technique is unsuccessful.
- This involves incision of the posterior cervical ring followed by withdrawl of the fundus using Allis forceps as described in Huntington's procedure.

- The fundus is replaced and the incision is sutured.

2. Vaginal route:

Spinelli procedure:

- Bladder is dissected upwards and pushed out of way.
- The ring and lower part of the inverted uterus i.e. near the cervix is divided anteriorly.
- Inversion is replaced and incision is closed with interrupted sutures.

Kustner procedure:

- Similar to Spinelli but ring is divided posteriorly.
- Whatever method of uterine replacement is used, it should be followed by an oxytocic to keep the uterus well-contracted for 8–12 hours followed by longer acting prostaglandins like 15-mthyl PGF 2α or misoprostol.
- Broad spectrum antibiotic should be given and for 24–48 hrs because of manipulation and large uterine area traumatized and exposed to vaginal bacterial flora.

If treatment not successful – Laparotomy to correct inversion

If laparotomy correction not successful – Hysterectomy

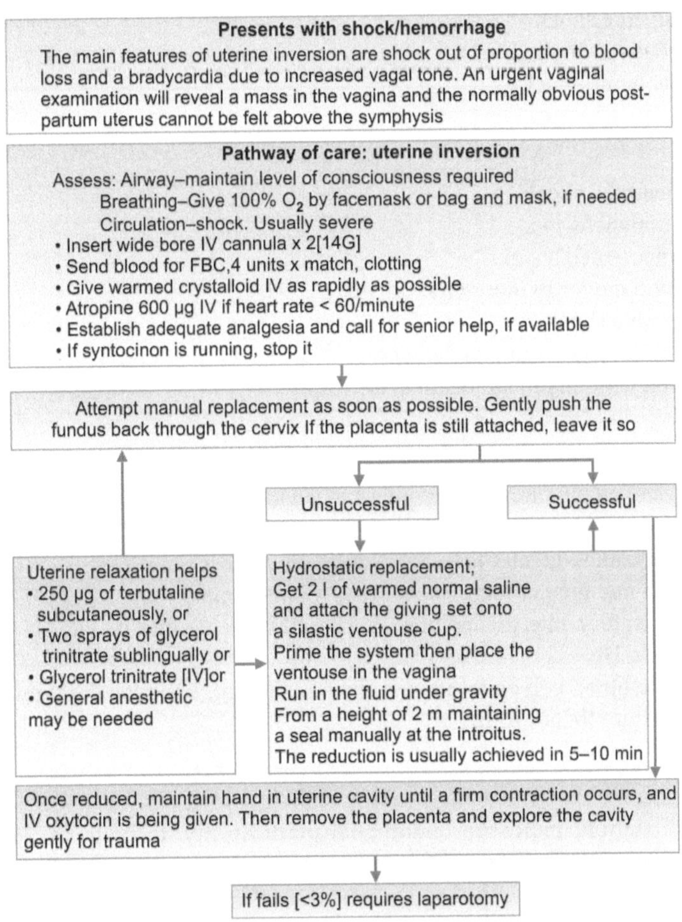

CHAPTER

31

Shock in Obstetrics

Shock is characterized by failure of the circulatory system to maintain adequate perfusion of the vital organs.

CLASSIFICATION

- Hypovolemic shock
- Septic shock
- Cardiogenic shock
- Distributive shock
- Hypovolemic shock

Stages of the Shock

- Compensated shock
  - Autotransfusion
- Decompensated shock
  - Blood moves to more vital organs
- Irreversible shock
  - Multiple system/organ damage
  - Even with treatment, death is the result

SIRS (Systemic Inflammatory Response Syndrome)

- The systemic inflammatory response to a wide variety of severe clinical insults manifested by two or more of the following features:
  - Temperature greater than 38°C or less than 36°C
  - Heart rate greater than 90 beats per minute (bpm)
  - Respiratory rate greater than 20 breaths per minute or $PaCO_2$ less than 32 mm Hg
  - White blood cell count greater than 12,000/ml, less than 4000/ml, or 10% immature (band) forms

Pathophysiology

- Vasodilatation, increased endothelial permeability, thrombosis, leukocyte migration and activation

- Altered cytokines level, abnormal NO synthesis, abnormal arachidonic acid metabolism, neutrophil activation, free radical production, altered complement activation, failure to have localization of inflammation

Multiple Organ Dysfunction Syndrome (MODS)

- This is the presence of altered organ function in a patient who is acutely ill and in whom homeostasis cannot be maintained without intervention.

HYPOVOLEMIC SHOCK

Antepartum	Intrapartum	Postpartum
Ectopic pregnancy Incomplete abortion Molar pregnancy Hyperemesis gravidarum Gastroenteritis, intractable diarrhea Abruptio placenta, placenta previa Diabetic ketoacidosis Burns Peritonitis	Rupture of uterus	Uterine atony Lacerations of genital tract Chorio amnionitis Large placental site Acute uterine inversion Uterine leiomyoma Puerperal sepsis

Determining and Managing the Cause of Shock

Determine the cause of shock after the woman is stabilized, manage accordingly.

Reassess the woman's condition for signs of improvement

- Reassess the woman's response to fluids within 30 minutes to determine if her condition is improving.

Signs of improvement include:

- Stabilizing pulse (rate of 90 per minute or less)
- Increasing blood pressure (systolic 100 mm Hg or more)
- Improving mental status (less confusion or anxiety)
- Increasing urine output (30 ml per hour or more)
- Consider vasoconstrictor agents (in consultation with the intensivist) if hypotension not corrected with IV fluid replacement
- Transfuse blood/blood components as required.

If the woman's condition improves:

- Adjust the rate of infusion of IV fluids to 1 L in six hours.
- Continue management for the underlying cause of shock.

If the woman's condition fails to improve or stabilize, provide further management

- Continue to infuse IV fluids, adjusting the rate of infusion to 1 L in six hours and maintain oxygen at 6–8 L per minute.
- Closely monitor the woman's condition.
- Perform laboratory tests including repeat hemoglobin determination, serum electrolytes, serum creatinine and blood gas analysis.

SEPTIC SHOCK

- A subset of individuals with severe sepsis who develop hypotension despite adequate fluid resuscitation.
- Features of sepsis are present. Inotropic/vasopressor support required for combating hypotension.
- Patients receiving inotropic or vasopressor agents may not be hypotensive by the time that they manifest hypoperfusion abnormalities or organ dysfunction.

Risk Factors for Maternal Sepsis

- Obesity
- Impaired glucose tolerance/diabetes
- Impaired immunity/immunosuppressant medication
- Anemia
- Vaginal discharge
- History of pelvic infection
- Amniocentesis and other invasive procedures
- Cervical cerclage
- Prolonged spontaneous rupture of membranes
- Vaginal trauma, cesarean section, wound hematoma
- Retained products of conception
- GAS infection in close contacts/family members
- Black or minority ethnic group origin

Etiology

- Puerperal sepsis
- Septic abortion
- Chorioamnionitis
- Pyelonephritis
- Necrotizing fasciitis
- Prolonged rupture of membranes
- Post-cesarean endometritis
- UTI
- Toxic shock syndrome

The major pathogens causing sepsis in the puerperium are:

- GAS, also known as *Streptococcus pyogenes*
- *Escherichia coli*
- *Staphylococcus aureus*
- *Streptococcus pneumoniae*
- Meticillin-resistant *S. aureus* (MRSA), *Clostridium septicum* and *Morganella morganii.*

Clinical Features Suggestive of Sepsis

- Fever or rigors
- Diarrhea or vomiting—may indicate exotoxin production (early toxic shock)

- Rash (generalized streptococcal maculopapular rash or purpura fulminans)
- Abdominal/pelvic pain and tenderness
- Offensive vaginal discharge (smelly suggests anaerobes; serosanguinous suggests streptococcal infection)
- Productive cough
- Urinary symptoms

Clinical signs suggestive of sepsis include one or more of the following: pyrexia, hypothermia, tachycardia, tachypnea, hypoxia, hypotension, oliguria, impaired consciousness and failure to respond to treatment. These signs, including pyrexia, may not always be present and are not necessarily related to the severity of sepsis.

Mastitis must never be overlooked.

Common symptoms of sepsis during puerperium:

- Fever, rigors (persistent spiking temperature suggests abscess). Beware: normal temperature may be attributable to antipyretics or NSAIDs
- *Diarrhea or vomiting:* May indicate exotoxin production (early toxic shock)
- Breast engorgement/redness
- Rash (generalized maculopapular rash)
- Abdominal/pelvic pain and tenderness
- Wound infection–spreading cellulitis or discharge
- Offensive vaginal discharge (smelly: suggestive of anaerobes; serosanguinous: suggestive of streptococcal infection)
- Productive cough
- Urinary symptoms
- Delay in uterine involution, heavy lochia
- General–non-specific signs such as lethargy, reduced appetite.

'Red flag' signs and symptoms (see below) should prompt urgent referral for hospital assessment and, if the woman appears seriously unwell, by ememgency ambulance:

- Pyrexia more than 38°C
- Sustained tachycardia more than 90 beats/minute
- Breathlessness (respiratory rate more than 20 breaths/minute; a serious symptoms)
- Abdominal or chest pain
- Diarrhea and/or vomiting
- Uterine or renal angle pain and tenderness
- Woman is generally unwell or seems unduly anxious or distressed.

Early presentation of sepsis (less than 12 hours post-birth) is more likely to be caused by streptococcal infection, particularly GAS, and severe continuous pain suggests necrotizing fasciitis.

Investigations

Blood cultures are the key investigation and should be obtained prior to antibiotic administration; however, antibiotic treatment should be started without waiting for microbiology results.

Serum lactate should be measured within 6 hours of the suspicion of severe sepsis to guide management. Serum lactate ≥4 mmol/l is indicative of tissue hypoperfusion.

Any relevant imaging studies should be performed promptly in an attempt to confirm the source of infection. This could include a chest X-ray, pelvic ultrasound scan or computed tomography scan if pelvic abscess is suspected.

Other samples taken should be guided by the clinical suspicion of focus of infection as appropriate.

Routine blood tests should include full blood count, urea, electrolytes and C-reactive protein (CRP).

Any woman with symptoms of tonsillitis/pharyngitis should have a throat swab sent for culture.

If the MRSA status of the woman is unknown, a premoistened nose swab may be sent for rapid MRSA screening where such testing is available.

- Give the woman a combination of antibiotics to cover aerobic and anaerobic infections and continue until she is fever-free for 48 hours.
- Penicillin G 2 million units OR ampicillin 2 g IV every six hours OR Cefotaxim/ Ceftriaxone 1 gm IV every 12th hourly.
  (If allergic to give Vancomycin or Ofloxacin)
  - PLUS Gentamicin 1.5 mg/kg body weight IV every 24 hours
  - PLUS Metronidazole 500 mg IV every eight hours.
- A combination of either piperacillin/tazobactam or a carbapenem plus clindamycin provides one of the broadest ranges of treatment for severe sepsis.
- MRSA may be resistant to clindamycin, hence if the woman is or is highly likely to be MRSA-positive, a glycopeptide such as vancomycin or teicoplanin may be added until sensitivity is known.

Antimicrobial choices and limitations of antimicrobials

Antimicrobial	Limitations
Co-amoxiclav	Does not cover MRSA, Pseudomonas or ESBL-producing organisms
Metronidazole	Only covers anaerobes
Clindamycin	Covers most streptococci and staphylococci, including many MRSA, and switches off exotoxin production with significantly decreased mortality Not renally excreted or nephrotoxic
Piperacillin/tazobactam and carbapenems	Covers most organisms except MRSA and are renal sparing (in contrast to aminoglycosides) Piperacillin/tazobactam does not cover ESBL producers
Gentamicin (as single dose of 3–5 mg/kg)	Poses no problem in normal renal function but if doses are to be given regularly, serum levels must be monitored

Abdominal pain, fever (greater than 38°C) and tachycardia (greater than 90 beats/ minute in the puerperium) are indications for intravenous antibiotics and senior clinical review.

Non-steroidal anti-inflammatory drugs (NSAIDs) should be avoided for pain relief in cases of sepsis as they impede the ability of polymorphs to fight GAS infection.

Tasks to be performed within the first 6 hours of the identification of severe sepsis:

- Obtain blood cultures prior to antibiotic administration.
- Administer broad-spectrum antibiotic within 1 hour of recognition of severe sepsis
- Measure serum lactate.
- In the event of hypotension and/or a serum lactate greater than 4 mmol/l:
  - Deliver an initial minimum 20 ml/kg of crystalloid or an equivalent.
  - Apply vasopressors for hypotension not responding to initial fluid resuscitation to maintain mean arterial pressure above 65 mmHg.
- In the event of persistent hypotension despite fluid resuscitation (septic shock) and/or serum lactate greater than 4 mmol/l:
  - Achieve a central venous pressure of ≥8 mmHg
  - Achieve a central venous oxygen saturation ≥70% or mixed venous oxygen saturation ≥65%.
- Treat hypotension if present, as mentioned above.
- Oxygen should be administered to all patients.
- If there is evidence of respiratory distress and arterial blood gases, acid base balance is deranged, endotracheal intubation is undertaken to maintain adequate oxygenation.
- Invasive monitoring is helpful in patients with refractory shock or underlying complex cardiac lesions. The goal of therapy is to maintain the vital parameters as follows.
  - Mean arterial pressure >60 mm Hg
  - Systolic BP >90 mm Hg
  - CVP 8–12 cm
  - PCWP 14–18 cm H_2O
  - Urine output >30 ml/hr (at least 0.5 ml/kg/hr)
  - Hematocrit >30%, Hb 8–10 g/dl
- Blood transfusion is required in cases associated with hemorrhage or when hematocrit <30%.
- If the patient does not respond to IV fluids, hypotension persists, inotropic and vasoconstrictor agents are required. Dopamine is most commonly used agent (use after adequate fluid replacement, or else can cause profound hypotension), started at the rate of 5 μg/kg/min and increased gradually by 5–10 μg/kg/min increments upto a rate of 20–50 μg/kg/min. Once blood pressure is stabilized, reduce to 2–5 μg/kg/min.
- If the response to dopamine is unsatisfactory, start norepinephrine at a dose of 0.5–1 μg/kg/min and titrated to maintain a systolic blood pressure of 90 mm Hg.
- Correction of acidosis/electrolyte imbalance/myocarditis to be treated in consultation with intensivist.

Vasopressor/Inotropic Support

- Aim: To improve tissue perfusion without causing hypoxia
  If MAP <65 mm of Hg
- Noradrenaline: 0.2–1 ugm/kg/min

- Dobutamine: 2.5–20 μgm/kg/min
- Dopamine: 5–20 ugm / kg/min
- Vasopressin: 0.01–0.04 U/min
- Cardiac index: >4.0 L/min/m^2

Stress Dose Glucocorticoids

- Beneficial results of stress-dose administration of corticosteroids demonstrated in patients with severe and refractory septic shock.
- Low-dose hydrocortisone 50 mg every 8 hrs recommended if vasopressor support required for >48 hrs.
- No support exists in the medical literature for the routine use of high doses of corticosteroids in patients with sepsis or septic shock.

Maintenance of Euglycemia

- Plasma glucose should be maintained in the reference range (80 – 110 mg%), with insulin infusion if necessary.
- Aggressive glycemic control improves outcome in severe sepsis and septic shock.

Nutritional Support

- The enteral route is preferred, unless the patient has an ileus or other intestinal abnormality
- The benefits of enteral nutrition are:
  - Protection of gut mucosa
  - Avoiding translocation of organisms from the GI tract
- Enteral nutrition with immunomodulatory substances like glutamine and omega-3 fatty acid containing formulas is recommended for gut protection

Indications for Admission of the Woman to the ICU

Sytem	Limitations
Cardiovascular	Hypotension or raised serum lactate persisting despite fluid resuscitation suggesting the need for inotropic support
Respiratory	Pulmonary edema Mechanical ventilation Airway protection
Renal	Renal dialysis
Neurological	Significantly decreased conscious level
Miscellaneous	Multiorgan failure Uncorrected acidosis Hypothermia

Role of Surgery

Remove the foci of infection, after 24 hours of antibiotic coverage.

IVIG

- It is recommended for severe invasive streptococcal or staphylococcal infection if other therapies have failed.
- IVIG has an immunodulatory effect and in staphylococcal and streptococcal sepsis also neutralizes the super-antigen effect of exotoxins and inhibits production of tumor necrosis factor and interleukins.
- High-dose IVIG has been used in pregnant and postpartum women and is effective in exotoxic shock (i.e. toxic shock attributable to streptococci and staphylococci), but there is little evidence of benefit in Gram-negative (endotoxin-related) sepsis.
- The main contraindication to IVIG use is a congenital deficiency of immunoglobulin A.

Recombinant Human Activated Protein C

- Administration of recombinant activated protein C modulates coagulation and inflammation
  - Inhibits thrombosis
  - Inhibits neutrophil recruitment
  - Promotes fibrinolysis
  - Inhibits platelet activation
- Inhibits mast cell degranulation

Response Evaluation While Managing Shock

- Cardiovascular/Hemodynamic parameters
  - Systolic BP >90 mm of Hg, MAP >60 mm of Hg
  - Hb >8 gm%; >10 gm% in patients with cardiac compromise
  - Oxygen saturation > 92% (Pulse oximetry)
  - Central venous oxy Hb saturation >70%
  - Pulmonary capillary wedge pressure 14–18 mm of Hg
  - Central venous pressure 12–15 cm of water
- Metabolic parameters
  - pH >7.35
  - PaO_2 : 80–100 mm Hg
  - $PaCO_2$: 30–35 mm Hg
- Renal parameters
  - Maintain urine output 20–30 ml/hr (0.5 ml/kg/hr)

Infection Control Issues

The woman should be isolated in a single room with en-suite facilities to reduce the risk of transmission of infection.

Healthcare workers (defined as doctors, midwives, nurses, anesthetists and members of the wound care team) should wear personal protective equipment including disposable gloves and aprons when in contact with the woman, equipment and their immediate surroundings.

Breaks in the skin of the woman or carer must be covered with a waterproof dressing.

Fluid-repellent surgical masks with visitors must be used at operative debridement/change of dressings of GAS necrotizing fasciitis and for other procedures where droplet spread is possible.

Visitors should be offered suitable information and relevant personal protective equipment while the woman is isolated.

Monitoring of the Fetus and Delivery of the Baby

In a critically-ill pregnant woman, birth of the baby may be considered if it would be beneficial to the mother or the baby or to both. A decision on the timing and mode of birth should be made by a senior obstetrician following discussion with the woman if her condition allows.

If preterm delivery is anticipated, cautious consideration should be given to the use of antenatal corticosteroids for fetal lung maturity in the woman with sepsis.

During the intrapartum period, continuous electronic fetal monitoring is recommended. Changes in cardiotocography (CTG), such as changes in baseline variability or new onset decelerations, must prompt reassessment of maternal mean arterial pressure, hypoxia and acidemia.

Epidural/spinal anesthesia should be avoided in women with sepsis and a general anesthetic will usually be required for cesarean section.

Neonatal Issues if Sepsis Develops in the Puerperium

The baby is especially at risk of streptococcal and staphylococcal infection during birth and during breastfeeding. The umbilical area should be examined and a pediatrician consulted in the event of sepsis in the puerperium.

If either the mother or the baby is infected with invasive GAS in the postpartum period, both should be treated with antibiotics.

The Indications for Prophylaxis to Family/Staff

Close household contacts should be warned about the symptoms of GAS infection and told to seek medical attention should symptoms develop. Asymptomatic contacts may warrant prophylaxis.

DISTRIBUTIVE SHOCK

Neurogenic Shock and Anaphylaxis

- Treatment same as for hypovolemic shock.
- In addition, correct and eliminate the cause of neurogenic shock, (e.g. inversion of uterus, myocardial infarction and pulmonary embolism).

CHAPTER

32

Blood Transfusion

- A blood transfusion is a procedure in which blood is given to a patient through an intravenous (IV) line in one of the blood vessels. Blood transfusions are done to replace blood lost during the surgery or a serious injury.
- Conditions that may require blood transfusion include:
    - Postpartum hemorrhage leading to shock;
    - Loss of a large volume of blood at operative delivery;
    - Severe anemia, especially in later pregnancy or if accompanied by cardiac failure.

Note: For anemia in early pregnancy, treat the cause of anemia and provide hematinics.

THE PURPOSE AND SCOPE OF BLOOD TRANSFUSION

- Maternal mortality due to obstetric hemorrhage is 25–30% and anemia is 15%, both these conditions require blood transfusion.
- Studies show that there is inappropriate transfusion in 15–45%, either transfusion done in not indicated cases or too late or too little done in indicated cases.
- Rising cost and nonavailability of blood, risk of transfusion reaction and transmission of infections have made us to limit transfusion only in indicated cases.

Anemia in the Antenatal Period

- **Pregnancy <36 weeks:**
    - Hb - 5 gm% or below
    - Hb - 5–7 gm% in presence of established or incipient cardiac failure or clinical evidence of hypoxia, pneumonia or any other serious bacterial infection and malaria.
- **Pregnancy >36 weeks:**
    - Hb <7 gm%
    - Hb - 7–9 gm% or below in presence of clinical evidence of hypoxia, pneumonia or any other serious bacterial infection and malaria.

Anemia in the Intranatal/Postnatal Period

- If the Hb is less than 7 gm%

- Patient needing major surgery and Hb less than 8 gm%
- Ongoing bleeding or risk of further bleeding with Hb less than 8 gm%
- If BP <70 mm Hg and symptoms/signs of hypovolemic shock
- BP persistently <90 mm Hg (systolic) within ½ hour of admission even when 2 liters of crystalloids have been infused.
- Anemia tolerated well even at a hematocrit of 18–25%, myocardial lactate flux not affected with Hb 6 g/dl.
- Heart failure occurs only when hematocrit is <10%. Chronic anemia is better tolerated.
- There is increase in 2,3-diphosphoglycerate in RBCs which facilitates oxygen delivery.
- There is no change in cardiac output until Hb <7g/dl. Obstetric women tolerate well with no adverse affect on mother and fetus.
- Thus blood transfusion is indicated in antenatal period if Hb is <6g/dl four weeks prior to delivery where there is no time to give iron.
- This improves anemic status and oxygen carrying capacity to withstand the strains of labor and blood loss during labor.
- When Hb is <7 g/dl in labor or immediate postpartum period, blood transfusion depends on the medical history, age and symptoms. Fit and healthy women require no blood transfusion even with Hb of <7 g/dl.
- Exchange transfusion rarely done, only in desperate cases of cardiac failure with anemia, severe anemia requiring surgery, severe anemia with hematocrit of 13% near term.
- In sickle cell anemia repeated transfusion indicated thus partial exchange transfusion done. In patients who refuse blood transfusion or Jehovah's witnesses optimize Hb before delivery.
- Antenatal planning required to keep Hb above 10.5 g/dl. Blood sparing techniques are acceptable in these patients.

GENERAL PRINCIPLES OF BLOOD TRANSFUSION

- All women should have their blood group and antibodies status checked at booking and at 28 weeks of gestation.
- If any blood component therapy is contemplated, a sample for group-and-save must be sent to the blood bank.
- Patient blood samples used for crossmatching should be no more than 7 days old.
- In pregnancy, pre-autologous deposit is not recommended.
- Cell salvage is recommended for women in whom an intraoperative blood loss of more than 1500 ml is anticipated. Cell salvage should only be used by healthcare teams who use it regularly and have the necessary expertise and experience. Consent should be obtained and its use in obstetric patients should be subject to audit and monitoring.

Compatibility Testing

Compatibility testing is done in three steps:

1. ABO-Rh typing

2. Cross-match
3. Antibody screening

ABO-Rh Typing

- Determination of patient's correct blood type is exceedingly important and is done by testing red blood cells for A and B antigens and the serum for A and B antibodies.Rh typing is also carried out.

Cross-matching

- Cross-match is essentially a trial transfusion in which donor cells are mixed with recipient serum to detect potential for serious transfusion reactions. It takes about 45–60 minutes for cross-matching.

Screening for Infectious Agents

- Every unit of donated blood should be screened for transfusion-transmissible infections using the most appropriate and effective tests, in accordance with both national policies and the prevalence of infectious agents in the potential blood donor population.
- All donated blood should be screened for the following:
  - HIV-1 and HIV-2
  - Hepatitis B surface antigen (HBsAg)
  - *Treponema pallidum* antibody (syphilis)
  - Hepatitis C
  - Malaria
- No blood or blood product should be released for transfusion until all nationally required tests are shown to be negative.
- Perform compatibility tests on all blood components transfused even if in life-threatening emergencies, the tests are performed before the blood products are issued.

WHO Prescribes a Checklist Before Prescribing Blood

1. What improvement in the patient's condition am I to achieve following the blood transfusion?
2. Can I minimize the blood loss to reduce the transfusion?
3. Are there any other treatment like IV replacement fluid and oxygen?
4. What are the specific clinical and lab indications for transfusion?
5. What are the risks of transmitting infectious agent?
6. Do the benefits of transfusion reaction outweigh the risks?
7. What other options are there if no blood is available in time?
8. Will the trained person monitor and respond immediately if any acute transfusion reactions occur?
9. Have I recorded my decision and reasons for transfusion on patient's chart and the blood request form?

RCOG Recommends Reduction of Blood Transfusion By–

1. Treatment of anemia a must.
2. Hb% of 10.5 g/dl indicates hematinic deficiency, excludes hemoglobinopathies.
3. Oral iron preferred in the treatment of anemia. Parenteral iron only in intolerance to oral, absorption defects, doubtful compliance of patient.
4. Recombinant human erythropoietin (rHuEPO) used only in end-stage renal disease.
5. Hemoglobinopathies and bone marrow failure syndrome treated by blood transfusion in close conjunction with hematologist.
6. Active management of 3rd stage of labor proved to decrease incidence of blood transfusion.
7. High risk of hemorrhage patients advised hospital delivery only.
8. Optimal management of women on anticoagulants.

General Principles of Blood Transfusion are (RCOG):

- Blood grouping and antibodies should be done at booking and at 28 weeks.
- Patient's blood sample for cross-matching should be ideally fresh, group and save sample in case of high risk patients (placenta previa, accreta), sample should not be more than 7 days old.
- Only Kell negative blood should be used in women of child-bearing age.
- CMV seronegative red cells and platelets for seronegative women. Minimize the use of banked blood by
  - Pre-autologus deposit of blood. In pregnancy, this is not advised.
  - Acute normovolemic hemodilution: Removal of predetermined volume of blood prior to surgery, replaced by crystalloids and subsequent reinfusion of the removed blood.
  - Intraoperative blood salvage: If blood loss of >1500 ml expected. In pregnancy, there is a risk of amniotic fluid embolism and contamination with fetal cells.
  - Autologus blood transfusion in ruptured ectopic and reactionary hemorrhage in postoperative cases.
- Normal blood volume is 7% of ideal body weight and it increases to 8–9% in pregnancy. Massive blood loss is loss of 1 blood volume in 24 hours or 50% of blood volume loss in 3 hours or loss at a rate of 150 ml/minute.

1. Whole blood

Indications

- Red cell replacement in acute blood loss with hypovolemia
- Exchange transfusion
- Patients needing red cell transfusions where red cell concentrates or suspensions are not available

Contraindications

Risk of volume overload in patients with:

- Chronic anemia
- Incipient cardiac failure

Description	Preparation	Storage	Transfusion	Obstetric indication
Quantity: 350 ml	For human donors by venesection	Between 2°C–6°C in approved blood bank	One unit of whole blood increases Hb by 0.75 to 1 g/dl and hematocrit by 3 to 5%	Postpartum hemorrhage
No functional platelets	Collected into a sterile, disposable, plastic pack containing anticoagulant CPDA (40 ml) 14.2%	If stored <2°C freezing injury to RBC	Administer without warming	Ectopic pregnancy
No labile coagulation factors (V and VIII)		>8°C growth of bacteria	Transfusion should be started within 30 minutes of issue	Antepartum hemorrhage
Tested for HBsAg, HIV, VDRL, malarial parasite and hepatitis C virus		Shelf life: 35 days	Complete transfusion idoally within 2 hours not more than 4 hours	DIC
Components prepared from whole blood used commonly in obstetrics Packed red blood cells Platelet concentrates Fresh frozen plasma Cryoprecipitate				

In an extreme situation and when the blood group is unknown, O RhD negative red cells should be given (although these may be incompatible for patients with irregular antibodies). The decision to perform blood transfusion should be made on both clinical and hematological grounds.

Blood Components

- Packed red cells,
- Platelet concentrate,
- Fresh frozen plasma,
- Cryoprecipitate,
- Human plasma proteins such as albumin, coagulation factor concentrates, immunoglobulins.
- Specialized products: CMV negative or leuko-reduced blood and type specific or HLA-matched platelets.

Red cell concentrates

Description	Preparation	Storage	Transfusion	Obstetric indication
Quantity: 150–200 ml	Prepared from single blood donor collected in plastic bags	Between 2°C–6°C in approved blood bank	Single unit of PRBC raises the Hb% by 1g and hematocrit by 3% in a non-bleeding patient	For Hb <6g/dl–severe anemia
Hemoglobin approximately 20 g/100 ml	Plasma is separated from RBCs by either centrifugation or undisturbed sedimentation	Shelf life: 35 days	Transfusion should be started within 30 minutes of issue	In acute blood loss
Hematocrit 55%–70%	Preparation time: 20 minutes		Give 1 ampoule of calcium after each 5 units of PRBC	

FFPs/Cryoprecipitate

- It is essential that regular full blood counts (CBCs) and coagulation screens are performed during the bleeding episode. FFP, cryoprecipitate and platelets should not be given on clinical suspicion alone unless there is delay in obtaining blood results.
- FFP contains stable clotting factors, albumin, immunoglobulin and no platelet.
- Full blood count (CBC) and coagulation screening advised before advising FFP.
- FFP takes 30 minutes to thaw, once thawed, used in 6 hours.
- In the bleeding woman with disseminated intravascular coagulation (DIC), a combination of FFP, platelets and cryoprecipitate is indicated.
- The FFP and cryoprecipitate should ideally be of the same group as the recipient. If unavailable, FFP of a different ABO group is acceptable, provided that it does not have a high titer anti-A or anti-B activity.
- No anti-D prophylaxis is required if an Rh D negative woman receives Rh D positive FFP or cryoprecipitate.
- Fibrinogen levels should be maintained above 1.0 g/l by the use of FFP or two pools of cryoprecipitate.
- There is insufficient evidence to suggest that FFP is useful in major blood loss in the absence of DIC. Its use should be guided by the use of coagulation tests.

RCOG Recommends

- Infusion of FFP ideally before 1 blood volume is lost.
- In DIC, a combination of FFP, platelets and cryoprecipitate indicated.
- FFP indicated when fibrinogen is <100 mg/dl and maintain fibrinogen >1 g/dl.
- FFP and cryoprecipitate ideally should be of same group of the recipient. No need of anti-D prophylaxis in Rh-ve.
- FFP administered as 12–15 ml/kg, to keep the activated partial thromboplastin time (aPTT) and PT time ratio <1:5.
- Contraindicated for augmentation of plasma volume or albumin concentration.

Fresh Frozen Plasma

Description	Preparation	Storage	Transfusion	Obstetric indication
Quantity: 100 ml	Plasma separated from one whole blood donation within 6 hours of collection	At 25°C or colder	1 unit raises the fibrinogen level by 5–10 mg%	DIC TTP
Contains all the coagulation factors specially fibrinogen Factor VIII level at least 70% of normal fresh plasma level No platelets	Plasma placed at -65°C to -75°C for 30 min to 1 hr and frozen sold	Shelf-life: 12 months	Thawing takes 20 minutes Issued in thawed form for immediate transfusion Complete transfusion within 20 min	Liver diseases INR >2x normal Activated partial thromboplastin time >1.5x normal Following massive blood transfusion (1 FFP for every 4 to 5 units of whole blood/ packed cells)

Cryoprecipitate

- It is cold precipitable protein fraction derived from thawed FFP at 1–6°C. Contains factor VIII, fibrinogen, fibrinonectin, vW factor and factor XIII.
- 1 unit/kg body weight raises plasma fibrinogen by approximately 50 mg/dl in the absence of consumption or massive bleeding.

Cryoprecipitate Indicated in ACOG

- In von Willebrand's, unresponsive to desmopressin and congenital fibrinogen deficiency in perioperative or peripartum period
- Bleeding with fibrinogen of 80–100 mg/dl.

Description	Preparation	Storage	Transfusion	Obstetric indication
Quantity: 15 ml	From FFP by collecting the precipitate during controlled thawing at 2°C to 6°C and resuspending it in 10 ml to 20 ml of plasma	Frozen within 1hr after precipitation at -1°C or colder	Each unit increases fibrinogen by 5 to 10 units	DIC (as a source of fibrinogen) Administer when fibrinogen is <100 mg/dl

Contd...

Contd...

As much fibrinogen as in FFP but in a volume of only 15 ml		Shelf-life: 12 months	A large amount of fibrinogen can be administered through small volume of cryoprecipitate	Clinical hemorrhage and fibrinogen <150 ml/dl von Willebrand factor deficiency
Factor VIII, XIII & von Willebrand factor			To infuse within 6 hrs of thawing Transfusion time: within 20 min	Factor XIII deficiency

Platelets:

- The platelet count should not be allowed to fall below 50 x 10^9/l in the acutely bleeding patient.
- A platelet transfusion trigger of 75 x 10^9/l is recommended to provide a margin of safety. Platelets may not be on-site in many units, so their need should be anticipated and good communication with the transfusion laboratory maintained.
- Rh D-negative women should receive Rh D-negative platelets. The platelets should ideally also be group compatible.
- 50 x 10^9/l anticipated when 2 volume replaced by fluids or 5–10 units of red cell component transfusion.
- Platelet transfusion not effective when thrombocytopenia is due to platelet destruction as in ITP, TTP, untreated DIC.

Contraindications

Not generally indicated for prophylaxis of bleeding in surgical patients, unless known to have significant pre-operative platelet deficiency.

Dosage

1 unit of platelet concentrate/10 kg body weight: In a 60 or 70 kg adult, 4–6 single donor units containing at least 240 x 10^9 platelets should raise the platelet count by 20–40 x 10^9/L.

Increment will be less, if there is:

- Splenomegaly
- Disseminated intravascular coagulation
- Septicemia

Administration

After pooling, platelet concentrates should be infused as soon as possible, generally within 4 hours, because of the risk of bacterial proliferation.

- Must not be refrigerated before infusion as this reduces platelet function

Description	Preparation	Storage	Transfusion	Obstetric indication
Random donor platelets (RDP)	Separated from single blood donor unit, suspended in 50 ml of plasma	20°C to 24°C	Should be infused in 1–2 ml/min	With/without active bleed if platelet count <20,000/mm^3
Quantity: 50–100 ml	Preparation time: 1 hour	Do not store at 2°–6°C reduces platelet function		Active bleed and platelet count less than 50,000
One unit increases the platelet count by 6,000–8,000 cells	Readily available from blood bank	Continuous gentle agitation is maintained throughout the storage period to prevent platelet aggregation		Platelet function defects DIC Gestational thrombocytopenia
Single donor platelets (SDP)	Only platelets are obtained from a donor by apheresis		4–6 units of platelet concentrates infused over a period of 30 minutes	Severe preeclampsia HELLP syndrome
Quantity: 300–350 ml	Preparation time: 24–48 hrs	Short shelf-life: 72 hrs		ITP
One unit increases the platelet count by 30,000–60,000 cells				SLE

Single donor platelets offer several advantages over random donor platelets. They are:

- Fewer donor exposures, fewer follow ups and investigations post-transfusion
- Risk of bacterial contamination reduced by 10-fold, risk of septic transfusion reaction reduced by 5-fold
- When multiple transfusions are indicated, SDPs are preferred
- Disadvantage: They have a higher processing fee than RDPs

Advantage of RDP: They are readily available for infusion

Complications

Febrile non-hemolytic and allergic urticarial reactions are not uncommon, especially in patients receiving multiple transfusions.

Factor VII Concentrates

Use of Recombinant Factor VII in Obstetrics

Indication	Dose	Mechanism of action	Response time	Potential complications	Notes
Treatment of coagulopathy associated with massive hemorrhage	50-100 mcg/kg IV	Binds tissue factor at site of injury	Usually within 20-30 min	Thrombosis including CVA, MI, DVT/PE	Requires circulating clotting factors as substrates
Originally developed to treat bleeding in hemophilia patients with factor inhibitors	May be repeated once	Activates factors X-Xa IX-IXa	If no response, consider repeating dose	Rare in obstetric population	Works best in the presence of normothermia

ADMINISTERING BLOOD PRODUCTS

- Check unit of blood details against transfusion slip.
- Check patient details against blood unit.
- Attach unit of blood to transfusion set and run through blood correctly and remove the air column.
- Aseptically attach blood transfusion set to cannula.
- Ensure blood is flowing and set at correct rate.

Disposable equipment for blood administration

- Cannulae for infusing blood products: Must be sterile and must never be reused.
- Use flexible plastic cannulae, if possible, as they are safer and preserve the veins.
- A doubling of the diameter of the cannula increases the flow rate of most fluids by a factor of 16.

Time Limits for Transfusion

Component	Start infusion	Complete infusion
Whole blood and packed red blood cells	Within 30 min of removing pack from refrigerator	Ideally within 2 hrs, not more than 4 hrs
Platelet concentrates	Immediately	Within 20 min
FFP and cryoprecipitate	As soon as possible	Within 20 min

Warming Blood

There is no evidence that warming blood is beneficial to the patient when infusion is slow. Cold blood can cause spasm in the vein used for infusion. Dry warm towels applied locally may help, but take care not to burn the skin. Case reports suggest that, at infusion rates greater than 100 ml/minute, cold blood could be a contributing factor in cardiac arrest. However, keeping the patient warm is probably more important than warming the infused blood.Warmed blood is most commonly required in:

Large volume rapid transfusions:
- Adults: greater than 50 ml/kg/hour
- Children: greater than 15 ml/kg/hour

Exchange transfusion in infants
Patients with clinically significant cold agglutinins.

Blood should only be warmed in a blood warmer. Blood warmers should have a visible thermometer and an audible warning alarm and should be properly maintained. Older types of blood warmer may slow the infusion rate of fluids. Blood should never be warmed in a bowl of hot water as this could lead to the hemolysis of the red cells and liberation of K^+ which could be life-threatening.

Procedure

- Start transfusion at the rate of 6 drops per min
- Increase the rate half an hrly up to 20 d/min
- Complete the transfusion process in 4–5 hrs
- Observe the patient for 2 hrs after transfusion
- No recommendations for routine use of diuretics before/ after transfusion.

Time limits for infusion

	Start infusion	**Complete Infusion**
Whole blood/red cells	Within 30 minutes of removing pack from refrigerator	Within 4 hours (or less in high ambient temperature)
Platelet concentrates	Immediately	Within 20 minutes
Fresh frozen plasma	Within 30 minutes	Within 20 minutes

MONITORING THE TRANSFUSED WOMAN

For each unit of blood transfused, monitor the woman at the following stages:
- Before starting the transfusion
- At the onset of the transfusion
- 15 minutes after starting the transfusion;
- At least every hour during the transfusion
- At four-hour intervals after completing the transfusion.
- Closely monitor the woman during the first 15 minutes of the transfusion and regularly thereafter to detect early symptoms and signs of adverse effects.
- At each of these stages, record the following information on the woman's chart:
  - General appearance
  - Temperature
  - Pulse
  - Blood pressure
  - Respiration
  - Fluid balance (oral and IV fluid intake, urinary output).
- In addition, record:
  - The time the transfusion is started
  - The time the transfusion is completed
  - The volume and type of all products transfused

- The unique donation numbers of all products transfused
- Any adverse effects.

Does Hypocalcemia Occur with Administration of Blood?

With 4–5 units of transfusion, calcium binds with citrate preservatives. This is self-resolving with metabolism of citrate by liver and kidney. Hypocalcemia will not impede blood coagulation. Hypocalcemia with hypothermia and acidosis is dangerous and will decrease cardiac output cause bradycardia and dysrhythmia thus calcium gluconate indicated here (WHO).

Responding to a Transfusion Reaction

Transfusion reactions may range from a minor skin rash to anaphylactic shock. Stop the transfusion and keep the IV line open with IV fluids (normal saline or Ringer's lactate) while making an initial assessment of the acute transfusion reaction and seeking advice. If the reaction is minor, give promethazine 10 mg by mouth and observe.

Managing Anaphylactic Shock from Mismatched Blood Transfusion

- Manage as for shock and give:
  - Adrenaline 1:1000 solution (0.1 ml in 10 ml normal saline or Ringer's lactate) IV slowly;
  - Promethazine 10 mg IV;
  - Hydrocortisone 1 g IV every two hours as needed.
- If bronchospasm occurs, give aminophylline 250 mg in 10 ml normal saline or Ringer's lactate IV slowly.
- Combine resuscitation measures above until stabilized.
- Monitor renal, pulmonary and cardiovascular functions.

Documenting A Transfusion Reaction

- Immediately after the reaction occurs, take the following samples and send with a request form to the blood bank for laboratory investigations.
  - Immediate post-transfusion blood samples
  - One clotted
  - One anticoagulated (EDTA/sequestrene) taken from the vein opposite the infusion site
  - The blood unit, giving set containing red cell and plasma residues from the transfused donor blood
  - The first specimen of the woman's urine following the reaction.
- If septic shock is suspected due to a contaminated blood unit, take a blood culture in a special blood culture bottle.
- Complete a transfusion reaction report form.
- Immediately report all acute transfusion reactions, with the exception of mild skin rashes, to a medical officer and to the blood bank that supplied the blood.

Record the following information on the woman's chart:
- Type of transfusion reaction
- Length of time after the start of transfusion that the reaction occurred
- Volume and type of blood products transfused
- Unique donation numbers of all products transfused.

TRANSFUSION REACTIONS

Acute Complications of Transfusion

Acute transfusion reactions occur during or shortly after (within 24 hours) the transfusion. They can be broadly classified in the following three categories according to their severity and the appropriate clinical response.

Category 1: Mild Reactions

- Mild hypersensitivity: Allergic, urticarial reactions

Category 2: Moderately Severe Reactions

- Moderate–severe hypersensitivity (severe urticarial reactions)
- Febrile non-hemolytic reactions:
  - Antibodies to white cells, platelets
  - Antibodies to proteins, including IgA
- Possible bacterial contamination (early signs)
- Pyrogens

Category 3: Life-threatening Reactions

- Acute intravascular hemolysis
- Bacterial contamination and septic shock
- Fluid overload
- Anaphylactic reactions
- Transfusion-associated lung injury

Delayed Complications of Transfusion

Delayed complications of transfusion essentially fall into two categories.

Transfusion-transmitted Infections

- HIV-1 and HIV-2
- HTLV-I and II
- Viral hepatitis B and C
- Syphilis
- Chagas disease
- Malaria
- Cytomegalovirus
- Other rare infections, e.g. human parvovirus B19 and hepatitis A

Other Delayed Complications of Transfusion

Other delayed complications of transfusion which occur days, months or even years after the transfusion has been completed, include:

- Delayed hemolytic reaction
- Post-transfusion purpura
- Graft-vs-host disease
- Iron overload (in patients who receive repeated transfusions)

Massive Transfusion Protocol

The Massive Transfusion Protocol is used to identify and manage patients at risk of bleeding by standardizing blood orders for component replacement during the bleeding episode.

Morbidity and mortality tend to be high among such patients, not because of the large volumes infused but, in many cases, because of the initial trauma and the tissue and organ damage secondary to hemorrhage and hypovolemia.

Criteria for Activation of Massive Transfusion Protocol

- Actual or anticipated 4 units of RBC in <4 hrs + hemodynamically stable, +/- ongoing blood loss.
- In children ≥30 ml/kg of red cells in <4 hours with ongoing uncontrolled bleeding.
- Major obstetric, surgical, gastrointestinal bleeding.

Investigations

- CBC
- Coagulation profile (PT, aPTT, INR, fibrinogen)
- Ionized calcium
- Arterial blood gas

Aim

- Temperature >35°C
- pH >7.2
- Base excess < -6
- Lactate <4 mmol
- Calcium – >1.1 mmol/l
- Platelets >50,000
- PT/aPTT <1.5 x normal
- INR ≤1.5
- Fibrinogen >1 g/l

Protocol

RBC: FFP: Platelets = 1:1:1

- Tranexamic acid - loading dose 1 gm over 10 min, then infusion of 1 gm over 8 hrs

- Cryoprecipitate if fibrinogen <1 gm/L
- Monitor CBC, coagulation profile, ionized calcium, arterial blood gas every ½ hr

Complications of Massive or Large Volume Transfusion

- Acidosis
- Hyperkalemia
- Citrate toxicity and hypocalcemia
- Depletion of fibrinogen and coagulation factors
- Depletion of platelets
- Disseminated intravascular coagulation (DIC)
- Hypothermia
- Reduced 2,3 diphosphoglycerate (2,3 DPG)
- Microaggregate

Acidosis

During blood storage, red cell metabolism generates acids which result in a small but significant reduction in its pH. If acidosis is present in a patient receiving a large volume transfusion, it is much more likely to be the result of inadequate treatment of hypovolemia than due to the effects of transfusion.

Management

Under normal circumstances, the body can easily neutralize this acid load from transfusion and the routine use of bicarbonate or other alkalizing agents, based on the number of units transfused, is unnecessary.

Hyperkalemia

The storage of blood will result in a small increase in extracellular potassium concentration, which will increase the longer it is stored. This rise is rarely of clinical significance, other than in neonatal exchange transfusions.

Management

Give Inj. Calcium gluconate 10%, 10 ml (1 amp) over 10 minutes slow IV.

- Salbutamol nebulization 15 mg every 30–45 min for first 2 hrs, then 4 hrly
- 25% Dextrose 100 ml + 10 units of rapid acting insulin given over half an hour
- Potassium binder
- Dialysis is last resort

Prevention

Use the freshest blood available in the blood bank and which is less than 7 days old.

Citrate Toxicity

Citrate toxicity is a rare problem, but it is most likely to occur during the course of a large volume transfusion of whole blood. Citrate binds calcium which reduces the body's ionized calcium level. Hypocalcemia, particularly, in combination with hypothermia and acidosis, can cause a reduction in cardiac output, bradycardia, and other dysrhythmias.

Management

Following transfusion, the anticoagulant citrate is usually rapidly metabolized to bicarbonate. It is, therefore, unnecessary to attempt to neutralize the acid load of transfusion. There is very little citrate in red cell concentrates and red cell suspension. The routine prophylactic use of calcium salts, such as calcium chloride, is not recommended. However, their use should be considered if there is clinical or biochemical evidence of a reduced ionized calcium.

Depletion of Fibrinogen and Coagulation Factors

Plasma undergoes progressive loss of coagulation factors during storage, particularly factors V and VIII, unless stored at –25°C or colder. Red cell concentrates and plasma-reduced units lack coagulation factors which are found in the plasma component. In addition, dilution of clotting factors and platelets will occur following administration of large volumes of replacement fluids. Massive or large volume transfusions can, therefore, result in disorders of coagulation.

Management

In order to avoid the indiscriminate use of fresh frozen plasma and cryoprecipitate, use these products only when there is clinical or laboratory evidence that they are needed. If there is prolongation of the prothrombin time (PT or INR), give ABO-compatible fresh frozen plasma in a dose of 15 ml/kg. If the APTT is also prolonged, heat-treated Factor VIII/fibrinogen is recommended in addition to the fresh frozen plasma. If none is available, give 10–15 units of ABO-compatible cryoprecipitate, which contains Factor VIII and fibrinogen.

Depletion of Platelets

Platelet function is rapidly lost during storage of blood and there is virtually no platelet function after 48 hours.

Management

Platelet concentrates should only be given when: Patient shows clinical signs of microvascular bleeding, i.e. bleeding and oozing from mucous membranes, wounds, raw surfaces and catheter sites and patient's platelet count falls below 20×10^9/L.

Give sufficient platelet concentrates to stop the microvascular bleeding and to maintain an adequate platelet count.

Platelet transfusion should be considered in cases where the platelet count falls below 20×10^9/L, even if there is no clinical evidence of bleeding, because there is a danger of hidden bleeding, such as into the brain tissue.

Prevention

The prophylactic use of platelet concentrates in patients receiving large volume blood transfusions is not recommended.

Disseminated Intravascular Coagulation (DIC)

Disseminated intravascular coagulation (DIC) is the abnormal activation of the coagulation and fibrinolytic systems, resulting in the consumption of coagulation factors and platelets. DIC may develop during the course of a massive blood transfusion, although its cause is most likely to be related to the underlying reason for transfusion, such as hypovolemic shock, trauma or obstetric complications, rather than the transfusion itself.

Management

Treatment should be directed at correcting the underlying cause and at correction of the coagulation problems as they arise.

Hypothermia

The rapid administration of blood or replacement fluids directly from the holding refrigerator can result in a significant reduction in body temperature. Hypothermia can result in various unwanted effects.

Management

If there is evidence of hypothermia, every effort should be made to warm blood and intravenous fluids during large volume transfusions.

Reduced 2, 3 Diphosphoglycerate (2, 3 DPG)

The presence of 2,3 DPG in blood facilitates the release of oxygen from the hemoglobin molecule to the tissue. Levels of 2,3 DPG in stored blood are usually well-maintained with modern anticoagulant additive solutions.

Microaggregates

White cells and platelets can aggregate together in stored whole blood, forming microaggregates. During transfusion, particularly a massive transfusion, these microaggregates embolize to the lung, their presence has been implicated in the development of adult respiratory distress syndrome (ARDS). However, ARDS following transfusion is most likely to be primarily caused by tissue damage from hypovolemic shock.

Management

Filters are available to remove microaggregates, but there is little evidence that their use prevents this syndrome. The use of buffy coat-depleted packed red cells will decrease the likelihood of ARDS.

Recombinant Factor VII a Transfusion

Can be considered in life-threatening PPH but this should not delay life-saving procedure for PPH. Whether it reduces blood loss during cesarean section is doubtful. It has a pivotal role in initiating coagulation but efficacy and safety still to be established. One can consider keeping a stock in the blood bank.

Routine use not recommended due to its lack of effect of mortality (Grade B), and variable effect on morbidity (Grade C).

- Uncontrolled hemorrhage in salvageable patient
- Failed surgical or radiological measures to control bleeding
- Adequate blood component replacement
- pH >7.2, temperature >34°C

FUTURE TRENDS

Increasing demand and nonavailability of blood has brought blood analogues still in research process, like –

- Cell-free purified hemoglobin solution
- Perfluorocarbon emulsions an inert liquid with high oxygen solubility, oxygen delivered by simple diffusion.
- Liposome-encapsulated hemoglobin.

CHAPTER

33

Maternal Collapse

Maternal collapse is defined as an acute event involving the cardiorespiratory systems and/or brain, resulting in a reduced or absent conscious level (and potentially death), at any stage in delivery and up to six weeks after delivery.

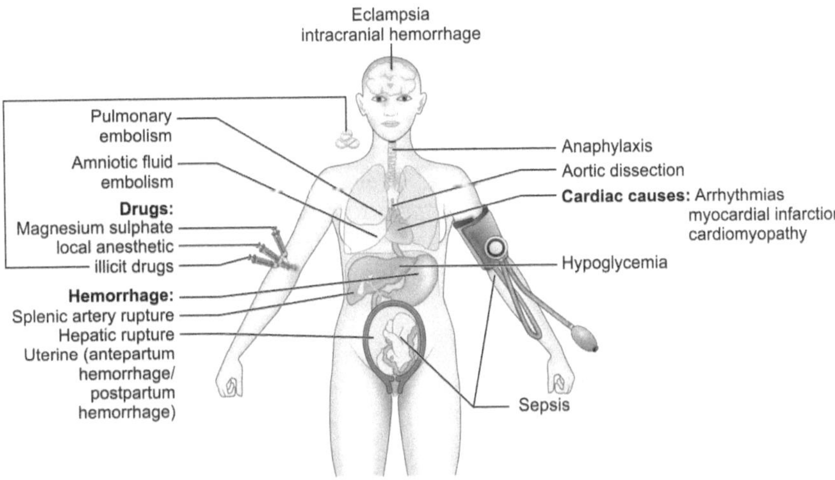

Reversible cause		Cause in pregnancy
4 H's	Hypovolemia	Bleeding (may be concealed) (obstetric/other) or relative hypovolemia of dense spinal block; septic or neurogenic shock
	Hypoxia	Pregnant patients can become hypoxic more quickly
		Cardiac events: Peripartum cardiomyopathy, myocardial infarction, aortic dissection, large-vessel aneurysms
	Hypo/hyperkalemia and other electrolyte disturbances	No more likely
	Hypothermia	No more likely
4 T's	Thromboembolism	Amniotic fluid embolus, pulmonary embolus, air embolus, myocardial infarction
	Toxicity	Local anesthetic, magnesium, other
	Tension pneumothorax	Following trauma/suicide attempt
	Tamponade (cardiac)	Following trauma/suicide attempt
Eclampsia and pre-eclampsia		Includes intracranial hemorrhage

Causes of obstetric collapse			
	Antepartum	Intrapartum	Postpartum
Obstetric hemorrhage	Antepartum hemorrhage (abruptio, placenta previa, uterine rupture)	Intrapartum hemorrhage, uterine rupture	Postpartum hemorrhage
Other hemorrhage	Aortic dissection	Aortic dissection	Aortic dissection
	Splenic artery aneurysm rupture	Splenic artery aneurysm rupture	
	Hepatic rupture	Hepatic rupture	
Other obstetric	Eclampsia	Eclampsia	Eclampsia
	Vasovagal episodes	Vasovagal episodes	Uterine inversion
Intra-cerebral events	Epilepsy, brain tumor, sub-arachnoid hemorrhage intracranial hemorrhage or thrombosis, cerebral vein, sinus thrombosis	Epilepsy, sub-arachnoid hemorrhage intracranial hemorrhage or hemorrhage or thrombosis, cerebral vein sinus thrombosis	Epilepsy, brain tumor, sub-arachnoid hemorrhage intracranial hemorrhage or thrombosis, cerebral vein sinus thrombosis
Cardiac events	Myocardial infarction (MI), pre-existing cardiac disease	MI, cardiomyopathy, pre-existing cardiac disease	MI, cardiomyopathy, bacterial endocarditis
Pulmonary events	Pulmonary embolism (PE)	PE	PE
	Anaphylaxis	Anaphylaxis	Anaphylaxis
		Amniotic fluid embolism	

AMNIOTIC FLUID EMBOLISM

Also known as **anaphylactoid syndrome of pregnancy.**

It is a form of embolism which is brought about by strong uterine contractions forcing the liquor with its contained particles of meconium, lanugo and vernix caseosa into a patent uterine sinus from where it is carried in the lungs.

- 1 in 8,000 to 1 in 80,000 pregnancies.
- 10% of maternal deaths in USA and 16% in UK.

Risk Factors

- Advanced maternal age
- Multiparity
- Meconium
- Cervical laceration
- Intrauterine fetal death
- Very strong frequent or uterine tetanic contractions
- Sudden fetal expulsion (short labor)

- Placenta accreta
- Polyhydramnios
- Uterine rupture
- Maternal history of allergy or atopy
- Chorioamnionitis
- Macrosomia
- Male fetal sex
- Oxytocin (controversial)

Timing

- Labor–Late in first stage or during second stage at the time of delivery. If the fetus is alive at the time of the event, nearly 70% will survive the delivery but 50% of the survived neonates will incur neurologic damage.
- Cesarean delivery

Clinical Manifestation

- Cough
- Headache
- Chest pain
- Dyspnea
- Hypotension
- Cyanosis
- Seizure
- Uterine atony
- Bronchospasm
- Transient hypertension
- Altered mental status
- Disseminated intravascular coagulation
- Adult respiratory distress syndrome
- Cardiopulmonary arrest

- Rapid deterioration and death occurs in most patients in the first one hour of the onset of symptoms. Amniotic fluid embolism is a diagnosis of exclusion.
- Postmortem finding of amniotic fluid contents in the pulmonary vessels is the best proof for diagnosis.

Investigations

Non-specific

- Complete blood count
- Coagulation parameters including FDP, fibrinogen
- Arterial blood gases
- Chest X-ray
- Electrocardiogram
- Echocardiogram

Specific

- Serum tryptase
- Serum sialyl Tn antigen
- Zinc coproporphyrin

Management

It is supportive rather than specific as there is no proven effective therapy.

Goals of Management

- Restoration of cardiovascular and pulmonary equilibrium
  - Maintain systolic blood pressure >90 mm Hg.
  - Urine output >25 ml/hr
  - Arterial pO_2 >60 mm Hg.
- Re-establishing uterine tone
- Correct coagulation abnormalities
- As intubation and CPR may be required, it is necessary to have easy access to the patient, experienced help, and a resuscitation tray with intubation equipment, DC shock, and emergency medications.

Immediate Measures

- Set up IV infusion, O_2 administration.
- Airway control→endotracheal intubation (ET tube 6–6.5)→maximal ventilation and oxygenation.
- Medication for sedation is thiopental 3–5 mg/kg IV and succinyl choline 1–1.5 mg/kg upto 150 mg IV.
- Treat hypotension, increase the circulating volume and cardiac output with crystalloids.
- After correction of hypotension, restrict fluid therapy to maintenance levels since ARDS follows in up to 40 to 70% of cases.
- Steroids may be indicated (recommended but no evidence as to their value)
- Dopamine infusion if patient remains hypotensive (myocardial support) -2–5 mcg/kg/min IV; titrate to BP and cardiac output
- Vasopressor therapy such as noradrenaline may be used (reduced systemic vascular resistance) noradrenaline – 2–4 mcg/hr infusion

Management in ICU

- Continuous monitoring of ECG, pO_2, CO_2, and urine output.
- Early placement of arterial, central venous, and pulmonary artery catheters to provide critical information and guide specific therapy.
- Central venous pressure monitoring is important to diagnose right ventricular overload and guide fluid infusion and vasopressor therapy. Blood can also be sampled from the right heart for diagnostic purposes.
- Pulmonary artery and capillary wedge pressures and echocardiography are useful to guide therapy and evaluate left ventricular function and compliance.
- An arterial line is useful for repeated blood sampling and blood gases to evaluate the efficacy of resuscitation.

Management of Coagulopathy

- DIC results in the depletion of fibrinogen, platelets, and coagulation factors, especially factors V, VIII, and XIII. The fibrinolytic system is activated as well.
- Most patients will have hypofibrinogenemia, abnormal PT and aPTT and low platelet counts.
- Treat coagulopathy with FFP for a prolonged aPTT, cryoprecipitate for a fibrinogen level less than 100 mg/dL, and transfuse platelets for platelet counts less than 20,000/mm^3.

Restoration of Uterine Tone

- Uterine atony is best treated with massage, uterine packing, and oxytocin or prostaglandin analogues.
- Improvement in cardiac output and uterine perfusion helps restore uterine tone.
- Extreme care should be exercised when using prostaglandin analogues in hypoxic patients, as bronchospasm may worsen the situation.

DRUG OVERDOSE/TOXICITY

Magnesium Sulphate

The antidote to magnesium toxicity is 10 ml 10% calcium gluconate given by slow intravenous injection.

Local Anesthetic Agents

If local anesthetic toxicity is suspected, stop injecting immediately.

Lipid rescue should be used in cases of collapse secondary to local anesthetic toxicity.

Intralipid 20% should be available in all maternity units.

Manage arrhythmias as usual, recognizing that they may be very refractory to treatment.

Intracranial Hemorrhage

Expert neuroradiology is required to establish an accurate diagnosis. Management is the same as in the nonpregnant state, although delivery may be necessary to facilitate this. The appropriate experts should be involved at the earliest opportunity.

Anaphylaxis

In cases of anaphylaxis, all potential causative agents should be removed, and the A, B, C, D, E approach followed.

If the anaphylactic reaction occurs in the community, the woman should receive basic life support and be transferred to a hospital setting as quickly as possible, unless a suitably trained healthcare professional is present with appropriate equipment/drugs, in which case definitive resuscitation and treatment should be commenced.

The definitive treatment for anaphylaxis is 500 micrograms (0.5 ml) of 1:1000 adrenaline intramuscularly. **Please note this dose is for intramuscular use only.**

CHAPTER

34 Venous Thromboembolism

RISK FACTORS

Obstetrical

- Cesarean delivery
- Diabetes
- Hemorrhage and anemia
- Hyperemesis
- Immobility–prolonged bed rest
- Multiparity
- Multifetal gestation
- Preeclampsia
- Puerperal infection

General

- Age 35 years or older
- Cancer
- Connective tissue disease
- Dehydration
- Immobility–long distance travel
- Infection and inflammatory disease
- Myeloproliferative disease
- Nephrotic syndrome
- Obesity
- Oral contraceptive use
- Orthopedic surgery
- Paraplegia
- Prior thromboembolism
- Sickle cell disease
- Smoking
- Thrombophilia

DIAGNOSIS

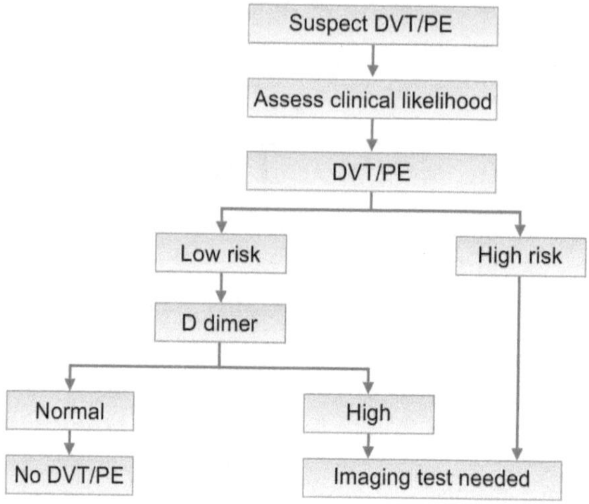

DEEP VEIN THROMBOSIS

Symptoms

Unilateral swelling and discomfort of one leg

Signs

Homans' sign (no predictive value)
1. Homans' sign: Relaxed foot abnormally plantar flexed
2. Pseudo-Homans': Pain on passive dorsiflexion of foot

Other Unreliable Signs

- Tenderness
- Distal extremity edema
- Lower leg circumference >2 cm difference is significant
- Superficial phlebitis may occur
- Left leg affected in up to 90% of cases
- Mosse's sign–pain on pressing the calf–should not be done–risk of dislodgement of the clot–pulmonary embolism

Clinical Likelihood of DVT

Scoring for DVT–Clinical decision rules	
Clinical variable	**Score**
Active cancer	1
Paralysis, paresis, or recent cast	1
Bedridden for >3 days; major surgery <12 weeks	1
Tenderness along distribution of deep veins	1
Entire leg swelling	1

Contd...

Contd...

Unilateral calf swelling >3 cm	1
Pitting edema	1
Collateral superficial nonvaricose veins	1
Alternative diagnosis at least as likely as DVT	–2

- Low—Zero or Less
- Moderate—1 to 2
- High—3 or Greater

DVT Evaluation

1. Venography: Investigation of choice, but time consuming and associated with complications, not done.
2. Impedance plethysmography: This is an extremely accurate test to assess thromboses in the lower iliac, femoral, and popliteal veins. It is only 50 percent sensitive for detection of clots in the small calf veins, with increased false-positive results during pregnancy (due to decreased venous return). Given these limitations as well as the wide availability of ultrasonography, it is seldom used today.
3. Compression ultrasonography: This noninvasive technique is currently the most-used first-line test to detect deep-venous thrombosis. The diagnosis is based on the noncompressibility and typical echoarchitecture of a thrombosed vein.

Criteria for establishing the diagnosis of acute DVT
• Lack of vein compressibility (principal criterion) • Vein does not "wink" when gently compressed in cross-section • Failure to appose walls of vein due to passive distention
Direct visualization of thrombus
• Homogeneous • Low echogenicity
Abnormal Doppler flow dynamics
• Normal response: Calf compression augments Doppler flow signal and confirms vein patency proximal and distal to Doppler • Abnormal response: Flow blunted rather than augmented with calf compression

4. Computed tomography: Spiral computed tomography (CT) scanning is widely available and very useful for detecting lower extremity deep venous thrombosis as well as those within the vena cava and iliac and pelvic venous systems.
5. Magnetic resonance (MR) imaging: This imaging technique allows excellent delineation of anatomical detail above the inguinal ligament. MR imaging is immensely useful for diagnosis of iliofemoral and pelvic vein thrombosis.
6. D-dimer assay: The test is limited by factors that may contribute to false-positive testing, including pregnancy, the postpartum and postoperative periods, and superficial thrombophlebitis. In particular, normal pregnancy causes a physiologic increase in D-dimer, with levels exceeding the threshold for normal in 78% and 100% of patients in the second and third trimesters, respectively.

The value of D-dimer testing in pregnancy appears to be its ability to rule out disease because negative predictive value of 100%. The value of D-dimer testing in the late-second and third trimesters is likely to be lower than in the first half of pregnancy because the former patients will likely have levels above the threshold.

Differential Diagnosis

- Ruptured Baker's cyst
- Cellulitis
- Postphlebitic syndrome/venous insufficiency.

Evaluation of Suspected DVT

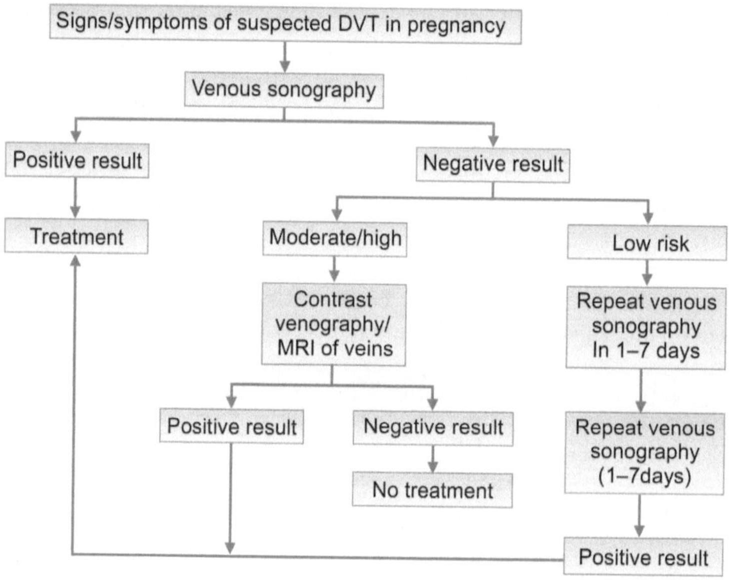

Management

Anticoagulation is initiated with either unfractionated or low-molecular-weight heparin. During pregnancy, heparin therapy is continued, and for postpartum women, anticoagulation is begun simultaneously with warfarin. Recall that pulmonary embolism develops in about 25 percent of patients with untreated venous thrombosis, and anticoagulation decreases this risk to less than 5 percent.

Before anticoagulant therapy is commenced, blood should be taken for a full blood count, coagulation screen, urea and electrolytes and liver function tests.

Performing a thrombophilia screen prior to therapy is not routinely recommended. When undertaken, thrombophilia screens should be interpreted by clinicians (usually hematologists) with specific expertise in the area.

After symptoms have abated, graded ambulation should be started. Elastic stockings are fitted and anticoagulation is continued. Recovery to this stage usually takes 7 to 10 days.

Unfractionated Heparin (UFH)

Treatment is with an intravenous heparin bolus followed by continuous infusion titrated to achieve full anticoagulation.

Antenatal Management

- Initial bolus of intravenous unfractionated heparin at a dose of 80 units/kg, followed by a continuous intravenous infusion of 18 units/kg/hour.
- If a woman has received thrombolysis (see below), the loading dose of heparin should be omitted and an infusion started at 18 units/kg/hour.
- It is mandatory to measure activated partial thromboplastin time (APTT) 4–6 hours after the loading dose, 6 hours after any dose change and then at least daily when in the therapeutic range. The therapeutic target APTT ratio is usually 1.5–2.5 times the average laboratory control value.
- Women receiving therapeutic-dose unfractionated heparin should have their platelet count monitored at least every other day until day 14 or until the unfractionated heparin is stopped, whichever occurs first.
- Pregnant women who develop heparin-induced thrombocytopenia or have heparin allergy and require continuing anticoagulant therapy should be managed with the heparinoid, danaparoid sodium or fondaparinux, under specialist advice.
- Because of their adverse effects on the fetus, oral anticoagulants should not be used for antenatal VTE treatment.

Using this weight-adjusted regimen, the infusion rate should be adjusted according to the APTT

Infusion rates according to activated partial thromboplastin time (APTT)			
APTT ratio	**Dose change (units/kg/hour)**	**Additional action**	**Next APTT (hours)**
<1.2	+ 4	Re-bolus 80 units/kg	6
1.2–1.5	+ 2	Re-bolus 40 units/kg	6
1.5–2.5	No change		24
2.5–3.0	- 2		6
> 3.0	- 3	Stop infusion 1 hour	6

Low Molecular Weight Heparin (LMWH)

Enoxaparin 1 mg/kg SC every 12 h or Enoxaparin 1.5 mg/kg SC every 24 hrs
Dalteparin 200 U/kg SC every 24 hr or 100 U/kg SC every 12 hrly
Tinzaparin 175 U/kg SC every 24 hours

Calculation of initial doses of drugs by early pregnancy weight				
Initial dose	**<50**	**50–69**	**70–89**	**>90**
Enoxaparin	40 mg bd	60 mg bd	80 mg bd	100 mg bd
Dalteparin	5000 IU bd	6000 IU bd	8000 IU bd	10,000 IU bd
Tinzaparin		175 units/kg once daily (all weights)		
bd = twice daily				

- Routine measurement of peak anti-Xa activity for patients on LMWH for treatment of acute VTE in pregnancy or postpartum is not recommended except in women at extremes of body weight (less than 50 kg and 90 kg or more) or with other complicating factors (for example with renal impairment or recurrent VTE) putting them at high risk.
- Routine platelet count monitoring should not be carried out (unless unfractionated heparin has been given).

Note:

1. Low Molecular Weight Heparin (1 mg/kg SC every 12 hours) – Preferred option over unfractionated heparin
2. Avoid warfarin until postpartum (contraindicated in pregnancy)
3. Duration: First Venous Thromboembolism: 6 months (including at least 6 weeks postpartum)–Recurrent Venous Thromboembolism or Thrombophilia: Long-term anticoagulation
4. Peripartum anticoagulation management
    1. Spontaneous labor: Stop anticoagulation at onset of labor.
    2. Elective induction, planned cesarean delivery: Stop anticoagulation 24 hours before delivery for LMWH.
    3. A common approach is to transition from LMWH to UFH at 36–38 weeks gestation. If the patient goes into spontaneous labor and is receiving UFH subcutaneously, she should be able to receive regional analgesia if the aPTT is normal. If significantly prolonged, protamine sulfate may be administered at 1 mg/100 U of UFH. If the patient is at very high risk for VTE, IV UFH can be started and then discontinued 4–6 hrs before expected delivery.
    4. Regional anesthesia (Epidural and intrathecal anesthesia)
        - Avoid regional anesthesia within 24 hours of last LMWH when twice daily dosing or within 12 hours of last LMWH when daily dosing (prophylaxis).
        - Restart within 4–6 hours of normal delivery and 12 hours after cesarean section.
        - Withhold LMWH for 2–4 hrs after removal of epidural catheter.
5. In women receiving therapeutic doses of LMWH, wound drains (abdominal and rectus sheath) should be considered at cesarean section and the skin incision should be closed with staples or interrupted sutures to allow drainage of any hematoma.

Thromboprophylaxis

Unfractionated Heparin

- Low dose prophylaxis
    1. First trimester: 5000 to 7000 Units q12 hours
    2. Second trimester: 7500 to 10,000 Units q12 hours
    3. Third trimester: 10,000 Units q12 hours
- Adjusted dose prophylaxis to aPTT of 1.5 to 2.5 times normal

Low-Molecular Weight Heparin

Suggested thromboprophylactic doses for antenatal and postnatal LMWH

Postpartum

- Therapeutic anticoagulant therapy should be continued for the duration of the pregnancy and for at least 6 weeks postnatally and until at least 3 months of treatment has been given in total.
- Women should be offered a choice of LMWH or oral anticoagulant for postnatal therapy after discussion about the need for regular blood tests for monitoring of warfarin, particularly, during the first 10 days of treatment.
- Women should be advised that neither heparin (unfractionated or LMWH) nor warfarin is contraindicated in breastfeeding.
- Postpartum warfarin should be avoided until at least the third day and for longer in women at increased risk of postpartum hemorrhage.
- Warfarin with target INR of 2–3 with initial UFH or LMWH overlap until INR ≥2 for 2 days.

COMPLICATIONS WITH ANTICOAGULANT TREATMENT

Unfractioned Heparin

- Bleeding
- Osteopenia
- Thrombocytopenia

Advantages of LMWH over Unfractionated Heparin

- Fewer bleeding complications
- Lower risk of heparin induced thrombocytopenia (HITT) and osteoporosis
- Longer plasma half-life
- Predictable dose response relationship
- Patient compliance–SC injections

Prevention of Post-Thrombotic Leg Syndrome

Graduated elastic compression stockings should be worn on the affected leg for 2 years after the acute event, if swelling persists, to reduce the risk of post-thrombotic syndrome.

Antenatal Assessment and Management (to be Assessed at Booking & Repeated if Admitted)

- Single previous venous thromboembolism (VTE) +
  - Thrombophilia or family history
  - Unprovoked/estrogen-related
- Previous recurrent VTE(>1)

→ **High risk**
- Requires antenatal prophylaxis with LMWH
- Refer to trust nominated thrombosis in pregnancy expert/team

- Single previous VTE with no family history or thrombophilia
- Thrombophilia + no VTE
- Medical comorbidities, e.g: heart/lung disease, SLE, cancer, inflammatory conditions, nephritic syndrome, sickle cell disease, intravenous drug user
- Surgical procedure (e.g: appendicectomy)

→ **Intermediate risk**
- Consider antenatal prophylaxis with LMWH
- Seek trust nominated thrombosis in pregnancy expert/team advice

- Age >35 yrs
- Obesity (BMI >30 kg/m^2)
- Parity ≥3
- Smoker
- Gross varicose veins
- Current systemic infection
- Immobility, e.g:paraplegia, symphysis pubis dysfunction (SPD), long distance travel
- Preeclampsia
- Dehydration/hyperemesis/ OHSS (Ovarian hyperstimulation syndrome)
- Multiple pregnancy
- ART (Assisted Reproductive Therapy)

→ • 3 or more risk factors • 2 or more if admitted → **Intermediate risk**

→ < 3 risk factors → **Lower risk**
Mobilization and avoidance of dehydration

Postnatal Assessment & Management (to be Assessed on Delivery Suite)

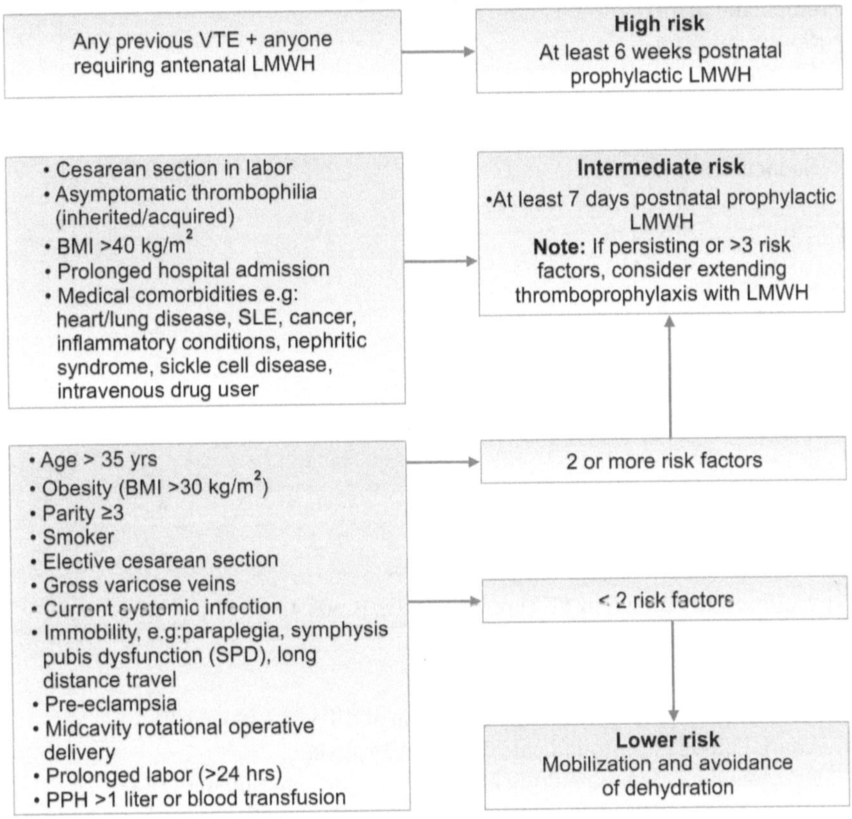

PULMONARY THROMBOEMBOLISM

Pulmonary embolism occurs due to thrombus blocking the pulmonary artery. Women are at higher risk in pregnancy more so in puerperium compared to non-pregnant women.

Symptoms

Small to moderate embolus (Normal right ventricular function and normal arterial pressure)

- Dyspnea
- Pleuritic chest pain–acute or sub-acute
- Hemoptysis
- Low-grade fever

Larger embolus (Right ventricular hypokinesia with normal systemic arterial pressure)

- Sudden onset of dyspnea
- Arterial oxygen desaturation
- Increased jugular venous pressure

Massive embolism (systemic arterial hypotension and anatomically widespread thromboembolism)
- Severe dyspnea
- Cyanosis
- No chest pain or central chest pain
- Collapse
- Sudden death

Clinical Likelihood of PE

Clinical variable	Score
Signs and symptoms of DVT	3.0
Alternative diagnosis less likely than PE	3.0
Heart rate >100/min	1.5
Immobilization >3 days; surgery within 4 weeks	1.5
Prior PE or DVT	1.5
Hemoptysis	1.0
Cancer	1.0

High clinical likelihood of PE if point score exceeds 4.

Investigations

- ECG–S wave in lead 1, Q wave inversion and T wave in lead 3.
- Arterial blood gas—to indicate degree of hypoxia.
- Ultrasound examination of the lower extremities—to rule out DVT.
- Chest X ray with lead apron to shield fetus—mostly normal, sometimes decreased bronchovascular markings. Not diagnostic but helps to rule out other causes like pneumothorax and pneumonia. Well-established abnormalities include focal oligemia (Westermark's sign), a peripheral wedged-shaped density above the diaphragm (Hampton's hump), and an enlarged right descending pulmonary artery (Palla's sign).
- Ventilation perfusion scan—first do perfusion scan only if that is abnormal a ventilation scan is needed. But this method lacks specificity.
- CT scan, CT angiography—embolus, decreased bronchovascular markings. Greatest sensitivity. Radiation scatter to abdomen low so safe in pregnancy. RV enlargement on chest CT indicates an increased likelihood of death within the next 30 days compared with PE patients who have normal RV size on chest CT.
- MRI
- D dimer assay—sensitive but not specific

Differential Diagnosis

- Pneumonia, asthma, chronic obstructive pulmonary disease
- Congestive heart failure
- Pericarditis
- Pleurisy: "Viral syndrome," costochondritis, musculoskeletal discomfort

- Rib fracture, pneumothorax
- Acute coronary syndrome
- Anxiety

Evaluation: Suspected Pulmonary Embolism

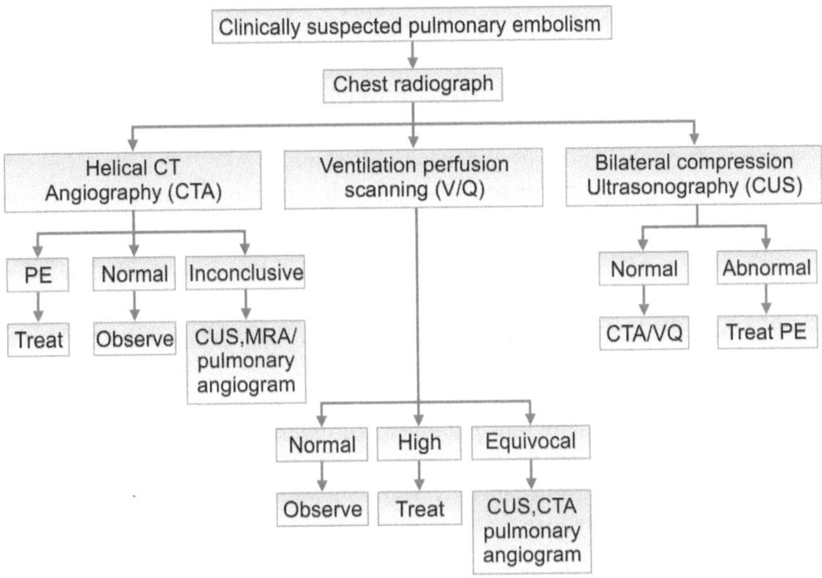

Management

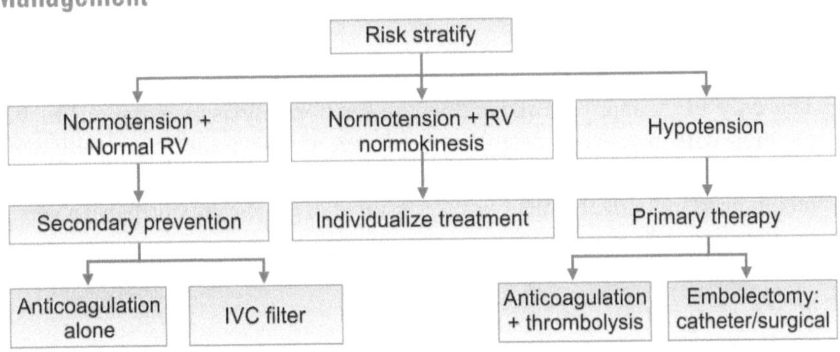

Primary therapy–Consists of clot dissolution with thrombolysis or removal of PE by embolectomy.

Secondary prevention–Anticoagulation with heparin and warfarin or placement of an inferior vena caval filter.

Thromboprophylaxis is recommended based on the risk scoring. As mentioned above intravenous unfractionated heparin is the preferred treatment in massive PTE with cardiovascular compromise.

The on-call medical team should be contacted immediately. An urgent portable echocardiogram or CTPA within 1 hour of presentation should be arranged. If massive PTE is confirmed or, in extreme circumstances prior to confirmation, immediate thrombolysis should be considered.

Venacaval Filters

Indications

- The woman who has very recently suffered a pulmonary embolism and who must undergo cesarean delivery, reversal of anticoagulation may be followed by another embolus, and surgery while fully anticoagulated frequently results in life-threatening hemorrhage or troublesome hematomas. In these, placement of a vena caval filter should be considered before surgery.
- In the very infrequent circumstances in which heparin therapy fails to prevent recurrent pulmonary embolism from the pelvis or legs, or when embolism develops from these sites despite heparin treatment.
- Filters can also be used with massive emboli in patients who are not candidates for thrombolysis.

Fibrinolysis

- Successful fibrinolytic therapy rapidly reverses right heart failure and may result in a lower rate of death and recurrent PE by (1) dissolving much of the anatomically obstructing pulmonary arterial thrombus, (2) preventing the continued release of serotonin and other neurohumoral factors that exacerbate pulmonary hypertension, and (3) lysing much of the source of the thrombus in the pelvic or deep leg veins, thereby decreasing the likelihood of recurrent PE.
- The preferred fibrinolytic regimen is 100 mg of recombinant tissue plasminogen activator (tPA) administered as a continuous peripheral intravenous infusion over 2 hours. Patients appear to respond to fibrinolysis for up to 14 days after the PE has occurred.
- Contraindications to fibrinolysis — intracranial disease, recent surgery, and trauma. The overall major bleeding rate is about 10%, including a 1–3% risk of intracranial hemorrhage.
- The only FDA-approved indication for PE fibrinolysis is massive PE. For patients with preserved systolic blood pressure and submassive PE with moderate or severe RV dysfunction, ACCP guidelines for fibrinolysis recommend individual patient risk assessment of the thrombotic burden versus the bleeding risk.

Embolectomy

- Surgical embolectomy is uncommonly indicated with the use of thrombolysis and filters. Published experience with emergency embolectomy during pregnancy is limited.

RADIATION EXPOSURE IN PREGNANCY

Fetal Exposure

The diagnosis of DVT and PE in pregnant patients poses unique challenges because of concerns about fetal radiation exposure. The ACOG advises that exposure to less than 5 cGy has not been associated with increases in pregnancy loss or fetal anomalies. Exposure to ionizing radiation doses above 1 cGy, however, may create a marginally increased risk for childhood leukemia (from 1/3000 base-line to 1/2000). Judicious use and selection of tests is advised.

Radiologic modality	Fetal radiation exposure (cGy)
Chest radiograph	<0.01
Venography	
Limited, shielded	<0.05
Full (unilateral), unshielded	0.31
Pulmonary angiography	
Brachial vein	0.05
Femoral vein	0.22–0.37
V/Q scan	0.007–0.031
Ventilation scan	0.001–0.019
Perfusion scan	0.006–0.012
CTPA (spiral CT)	0.013

Maternal Exposure

Radiation exposure to the maternal breast is also an important consideration when choosing tests because the increased glandularity and proliferative state of the pregnant breast presumably make it more radiosensitive. This is an important concern with respect to cumulative radiation exposure and cancer risk. V/Q scanning results in substantially lower maternal breast radiation exposure. CTPA is estimated to expose maternal breast tissue to 150 times more ionizing radiation than V/Q scanning, with doses estimated at 2 to 6 cGy. This dose can be reduced about 50 to 60% with breast shielding, without significant reduction in image quality.

CHAPTER

35

Cortical Vein Thrombosis

- Cerebral vein and dural sinus thrombosis (CVT) is less common than most other types of stroke but can be more challenging to diagnose.
- CVT is more common in women than men with a female to male ratio of 3:1 due to the increased risk of CVT associated with pregnancy and puerperium and with oral contraceptives.

ETIOLOGY

- Prothrombotic conditions, either genetic or acquired
- Oral contraceptives
- Pregnancy and the puerperium
- Malignancy
- Infection
- Head injury and mechanical precipitants

Clinical Aspects

Cerebral vein and dural sinus thrombosis (CVT) has a highly variable clinical presentation. The onset can be acute, subacute, or chronic. Symptoms and signs of CVT can be grouped into three major syndromes:

- Isolated intracranial hypertension syndrome (headache with or without vomiting, papilledema, and visual problems)
- Focal syndrome (focal deficits, seizures, or both)
- Encephalopathy (multifocal signs, mental status changes, stupor, or coma)
- Headache—Headache is the most frequent symptom of CVT. The features of CVT-related headache are quite variable:
  - Headache is more often localized than diffuse. However, the site of the headache has no relationship with the localization of the occluded sinus or the parenchymal lesions.
  - Headache onset is usually gradual, increasing over several days. However, some patients with CVT have sudden explosive onset of severe headache (i.e., thunderclap headache) that mimics subarachnoid hemorrhage.
  - Headache caused by intracranial hypertension from CVT is typically characterized by severe, dull, generalized headache that worsens with valsalva maneuvers and with recumbency. Visual obscurations may occur, coinciding with bouts of increased headache intensity.
- Headache may resemble migraine with aura.

Encephalopathy–Disturbances of consciousness and cognitive dysfunction, such as delirium, apathy, a frontal lobe syndrome, multifocal deficits, or seizures, can be present in severe cases of CVT.

Focal symptoms and signs–Motor weakness with monoparesis or hemiparesis, sometimes bilateral, is the most frequent focal deficit associated with CVT. Aphasia, in particular of the fluent type, may follow sinus thrombosis, especially when the left lateral sinus is affected. Sensory deficits and visual field defects are less common.

Seizures–Focal or generalized seizures, including status epilepticus, are more frequent in CVT than in other stroke types. Variables associated with seizures include supratentorial parenchymal brain lesions, sagittal sinus and cortical vein thrombosis, and motor deficits.

Isolated sinus and vein thrombosis–Isolated thrombosis of the different sinus and veins produces diverse clinical pictures.

- In cavernous sinus thrombosis—ocular signs dominate the clinical picture with orbital pain, chemosis, proptosis, and oculomotor palsies.
- Isolated cortical vein occlusion produces motor/sensory deficits and seizures.
- In sagittal sinus occlusion—motor deficits, bilateral deficits, and seizures are frequent.
- Isolated lateral sinus thrombosis frequently present with isolated headache or isolated intracranial hypertension. Less often, they may also present with focal deficits or seizures. Aphasia often follows if the left transverse sinus is occluded.
- Jugular vein or lateral sinus thrombosis may present as isolated pulsating tinnitus.
- Multiple cranial nerve palsies may occur in thrombosis of the lateral sinus jugular, or posterior fossa veins thrombosis.
- When the deep cerebral venous system (i.e., the straight sinus and its branches) is occluded, the signs and symptoms of CVT are generally severe, with coma, mental problems, and motor deficits, often bilateral.

DIAGNOSIS

- Brain MRI in combination with MR venography is the most sensitive technique for demonstrating the thrombus and the occluded dural sinus or vein.
- The combination of an abnormal signal in a venous sinus on brain MRI and the corresponding absence of flow on MR venography confirms the diagnosis of CVT.
- CT scan of brain is normal in up to 30 percent of CVT cases, and most of the findings with CVT are nonspecific. In about one-third of patients, CT demonstrates direct signs of CVT as follows:
    - The dense triangle sign, seen on noncontrast head CT as a hyperdensity with a triangular or round shape in the posterior part of the superior sagittal sinus caused by the venous thrombus.
    - The empty delta sign (also called the empty triangle or negative delta

sign), seen on CT brain with contrast as a triangular pattern of contrast enhancement surrounding a central region lacking contrast enhancement in the posterior part of the superior sagittal sinus.
- The cord sign, usually seen on head CT with contrast as a curvilinear or linear hyperdensity over the cerebral cortex caused by a thrombosed cortical vein.
- CT venography is a useful alternative to MR venography or intra-arterial angiography for the diagnosis of CVT, demonstrating filling defects, sinus wall enhancement, and increased collateral venous drainage. Accuracy of CT brain combined with CT venography is 90 to 100 percent, depending on the occlusion site.

LABORATORY TESTS

Aside from neuroimaging, there is no simple confirmatory laboratory test that can confidently rule out CVT in the acute phase of the disease. Current guidelines from the AHA/ASA recommend obtaining routine blood studies consisting of a complete blood count, chemistry panel, prothrombin time, and activated partial thromboplastin time for patients with suspected CVT. The findings from these tests may suggest the presence of conditions that contribute to the development of CVT such as an underlying hypercoagulable state, infection, or inflammatory process.

PROGNOSIS

Cerebral venous thrombosis (CVT) can result in death or permanent disability, but usually has a favorable prognosis.

Early deterioration and death – Approximately 5 percent of patients die in the acute phase of the disorder. The main cause of acute death with CVT is transtentorial herniation secondary to a large hemorrhagic lesion. Other causes of early death include herniation due to multiple lesions or to diffuse brain edema, status epilepticus, medical complications, and pulmonary embolism.

Predictors of Mortality at 30 Days

- Depressed consciousness
- Altered mental status
- Thrombosis of the deep venous system
- Right hemisphere hemorrhage
- Posterior fossa lesions

Predictors of Poor Long-term Prognosis

- Central nervous system infection
- Any malignancy
- Thrombosis of the deep venous system
- Hemorrhage on CT or MRI brain
- Glasgow coma scale score <9 on admission

- Altered mental status
- Age >37 years
- Male gender

Recurrence – The risk of recurrent CVT appears to be low, ranging from approximately 2 to 7 percent.

TREATMENT

Starts as soon as the diagnosis is confirmed, consists of reversing the underlying cause when known, control of seizures and intracranial hypertension, and antithrombotic therapy. Anticoagulation is the mainstay of acute and subacute treatment for CVT.

Acute Antithrombotic Treatment

Immediate goals of antithrombotic treatment: To recanalize the occluded sinus/vein to prevent the propagation of the thrombus, namely to the bridging cerebral veins; to treat the underlying prothrombotic state, in order to prevent venous thrombosis in other parts of the body, particularly, pulmonary embolism; and to prevent the recurrence of CVT.

Anticoagulation

- Unfractionated heparin or LMW heparin is appropriate treatment for acute CVT in full anticoagulant doses is reasonable, followed by vitamin K antagonists, regardless of the presence of ICH. [Dosage as same as for DVT].
- Antiplatelet drugs may be used as alternatives when anticoagulants are contraindicated, but there is no evidence, even from uncontrolled series, regarding their effectiveness and safety in CVT.
- Endovascular thrombolysis is typically restricted to patients with a poor prognosis who have not responded to anticoagulation with heparin or LMW heparin. Direct thrombolysis aims to dissolve the venous clot by delivering a thrombolytic substance (urokinase or rt-PA) within the occluded sinus through an intravenous catheter.
- For secondary prevention in patients with provoked CVT (associated with a transient risk factor), vitamin K antagonists may be continued for three to six months. For patients with unprovoked CVT, vitamin K antagonists may be continued for six to 12 months. For patients with recurrent CVT, venous thromboembolism after CVT, or a first CVT with severe thrombophilia indefinite anticoagulation may be considered.

Acute Symptomatic Treatment

Elevated Intracranial Pressure

- General recommendations – Elevating the head end of the bed, intensive care unit admission with sedation, administering mannitol, hyperventilation to a target $PaCO_2$ of 30 to 35 mmHg, and ICP monitoring.

- Routine use of glucocorticoids is not recommended, mainly because there is no evidence that they are effective for CVT.
- Patients with impending herniation due to unilateral hemispheric lesion, hemicraniectomy can be life-saving, and limited data suggest that a good functional outcome can be achieved.
- In patients with chronically increased ICP, successful treatment of intracranial hypertension can prevent visual failure and resolve headache. A diagnostic/ therapeutic lumbar puncture will decrease the cerebrospinal fluid (CSF) pressure and offer headache relief.
- Acetazolamide (500 mg twice daily) or furosemide (for patients who cannot tolerate acetazolamide), are therapeutic options for patients with increased ICP.

Repeated lumbar punctures, a lumboperitoneal shunt, or fenestration of the optic nerve sheet should be considered if severe headaches persist, or if visual acuity is decreasing.

Seizures

- Antiepileptic drug prophylaxis was associated with a reduced risk of early seizures in patients with CVT.
- When AED prophylaxis is used, valproate is preferable to phenytoin because it has fewer pharmacologic interaction.

Management After the Acute Phase

- Anticoagulation with warfarin for three to 12 months duration in adults, and three to six months in children, aiming at an international normalized ratio (INR) target of 2.5 (acceptable range: 2 to 3).
- Chronic oral anticoagulation is reserved for patients with recurrent CVT, severe thrombophilia or combined prothrombotic conditions. Antiepileptic drug management, headaches, visual loss, and cognitive and psychiatric complications are additional problems that may complicate the subacute phase of CVT.
- For pregnant women with a history of CVT who have a prothrombotic state or have had an additional previous thromboembolism temporary anticoagulation is recommended. A reasonable regimen is subcutaneous LMW heparin beginning in the third trimester and continuing up to eight weeks postpartum.
- For adolescents and women with a history of CVT, oral contraceptives are not recommended.

Subsequent pregnancy – Pregnancy and the puerperium are risk factors for CVT. Nevertheless, the risk of complications during subsequent pregnancy among women who have a history of CVT appears to be low in the absence of a prothrombotic condition or a previous thromboembolism (i.e., a previous CVT or deep venous thrombosis before the index CVT).

- Based upon the available evidence, CVT and pregnancy or puerperium-related CVT are not a contraindication for future pregnancy.
- The role of antithrombotic prophylaxis during subsequent pregnancies is unproven in women with a history of CVT. There is no worldwide consensus regarding this issue.

CHAPTER

36

Postpartum Contraception

It is the initiation and use of family planning methods during the first year after delivery.

- Post-placental–Within 10 mins after placental delivery.
- Immediate postpartum–Within 48 hours after delivery.
- Early postpartum–48 hrs up to 6 weeks.
- Extended postpartum–6 weeks to up to 1 year after birth.

HEALTHY TIMING AND SPACING OF PREGNANCIES [HTSP]

- Time interval from one child birth to next conception is 2 years and from one child birth to next child birth is 3 years.
- Time interval after miscarriage to conception is 6 months.

Method of postpartum contraception

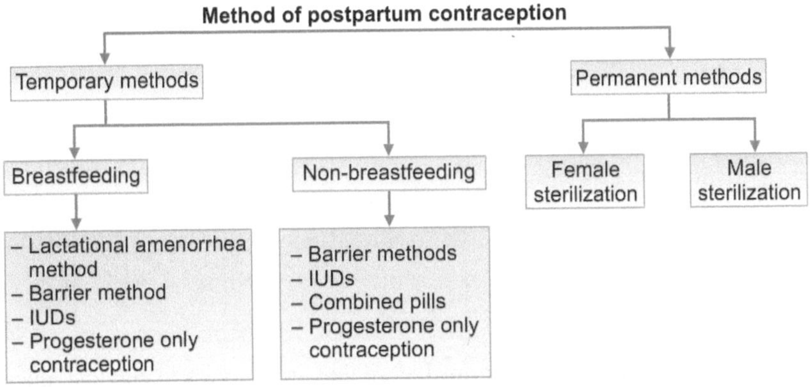

LACTATIONAL AMENORRHEA METHOD (LAM)

Criteria for LAM

- Exclusive or nearly exclusive breastfeeding—on demand around the clock (every 2–3 hours and no supplemental feeding)
- Menstruation has not returned
- Less than 6 months postpartum.

If any of the three factors change, further protection is needed to prevent pregnancy.

Advantages

- Breastfeeding practices required by LAM have other health benefits for mother and baby like bonding, protects baby from diseases, etc.
- Universally available
- Can be used immediately after child birth
- No supplies or procedures needed
- Bridge to other contraceptive methods
- No hormonal side effects

Disadvantages

- No protection against STIs
- Effectiveness after 6 months is uncertain
- Small chance of MTCT if mother is HIV positive
- Failure rate 0.5 to 1.5%

BARRIER METHODS

Male Condoms

When used consistently and correctly male condoms are highly effective against pregnancy and STIs.

Advantages

- Easily available
- Cheap
- Easy to carry
- Free from side effects
- Protection against STIs

Disadvantages

- Failure rate with consistent and correct use is 3%, average failure rate is 12/100 woman years
- May decrease sensation
- Coitus dependent
- Allergy to latex

Spermicidal agents: Kill the sperms before they gain access to cervical mucus, e.g.; nonoxynol-9, octoxynol, menfegol, etc.
Failure rate is high when used alone – 30 per 100 women years.
Effective if used along with barrier methods
Fertility awareness method: Not reliable in postpartum period

IUDs

Commonly used IUDs in postpartum period are:

- Cu-T 380A [lifespan—10 years]
- Multiload Cu-250 [lifespan—3 years]
- Multiload Cu-375 [lifespan—5 years]

Time of Insertion

- Immediately after delivery of placenta
- During cesarean section
- Within 48 hrs of child birth

If not inserted within 48 hrs, insertion should be delayed for 4 to 6 weeks. Expulsion rates are higher with interval insertion [after 6 weeks].

Advantages

- The device requires one time motivation.
- Coitus independent.
- Its cost when spread over several years is low.
- It has no effect on amount or quality of breast milk.
- No systemic side effects.

Disadvantages

Needs trained personnel for insertion

Complications

- Pain due to abnormal position of IUDs, uterine perforation, expulsion, disparity between IUDs size, and uterine cavity
- Bleeding
- Expulsion
- Infection
- Perforation
- Ectopic pregnancy [0.25 to 1.5 per 1000 women years]

Failure rate: 0.1 to 1%

PROGESTERONE-ONLY CONTRACEPTION

Progesterone-only Pills

POP is started 21days postpartum and soon after miscarriage and precaution taken for first 48 hrs.

The tablet is taken daily without a break and at the same time with a leeway of 3 hrs on either side of fixed time each day.

Failure rate is 2 to 3 per 100 women years.

Contraindications

- Previous ectopic pregnancy
- Breast and genital cancers,
- Abnormal genital bleeding,
- Active liver and arterial disease
- Porphyria

Advantages

- Lactating women
- Age over 35 years and smokers

- Those with focal migraine
- Diabetic, hypertensive, sickle cell anemia

Progesterone-only Injectables

Safe to use immediately postpartum if not breastfeeding
Use after 6 weeks postpartum if breastfeeding.
Preparations: 150 mg DMPA IM every 3 months-failure rate–0.4 per 100 women years
Note: 200 mg IM every 2 months, failure rate–0.6 per 100 women years

Advantages

- Easy to administer
- Compliance is good
- Lactating women
- Does not affect lipid and carbohydrate metabolism

Disadvantages

- Menstrual irregularities
- Does not prevent STIs
- Side effects like weight gain, depression, bloated feeling and mastalgia
- Prolonged DMPA leads to osteopenia
- Contraindicated in breast cancer

Implants

Norplant 1 and 2, Implanon, Jadelle, Capronor
Contraindications: Same as POPs
Failure rate: 0.2 to 1.3 per 100 women years

Advantages

- Long-acting with sustained effects
- Coital independent
- Systemic side effects are less
- Lactating mothers
- Women over 40 years

Disadvantages

- Breakthrough bleeding, irregular cycles and amenorrhea
- Expensive
- Local infection can occur
- Requires insertion and removal

Postcoital Contraception

Postcoital contraceptive agents interfere with postovulatory events leading to pregnancy and are, therefore, known as interceptives.
Also known as emergency contraception.

- **Levonorgestrel**: 0.75 mg LNG one tablet taken within 72 hrs of unprotected intercourse and repeated 12 hrs later. Alternatively single dose of 1.5 mg of levonorgestrel can be taken within 72 hrs (commonly used as i-pill now) with same effectiveness.

Failure rate–1.1 per 100 women years

Advantages

- Has no estrogen side effects
- Can be used in hypertensive, cardiac, and diabetic
- Lactating women
- Single dose therapy is an advantage

Ulipristal: A synthetic progesterone hormone receptor modulator, attaches to progesterone receptor and prevents ovulation, suppresses ovulation and prevents implantation 30 mg tablet to be taken within 5 days 2% pregnancy rate is reported.

Centchroman: Two tablets taken twice in within 24 hrs of intercourse can prevent implantation in 99% cases.

- **Yuzpe regimen**: Consists of the oral administration of 2 doses of 100 μg ethinyl estradiol (EE) and 500 μg levonorgestrel 12 hours apart.

Failure rate: 3.2 per 100 women years

Cu-T: Within 5 days of intercourse prevents implantation of fertilized ovum

PERMANENT METHODS

Female Sterilization

Ideal time: 24–48 hours of normal delivery, provided the mother is healthy, it should be delayed for a week in cardiac disease, uncontrolled hypertensive disease, infections, Hb < 7 g%, unexplained vaginal bleeding.

Preoperative Evaluation

Hb% should be preferably >10 g% or at least >7 g%

Consent of the mother alone is enough.

METHODS OF STERILIZATION

Modified Pomeroy Technique

- Loop of the tube made at isthmus of the tube and 0.5 cm of the tube is excised
- Plain catgut is used
- Tube not to be crushed

Failure rate: 1 in 300–400 operations

Parkland Technique

- Tube is separated from the adjacent mesosalpinx at an avascular site
- Freed tube is ligated at the proximal and distal end with 0 chromic catgut suture and the intervening segment of about 0.5 cm removed or the tube is simply divided between the ligated ends.

Failure rate: 1 in 400 operations

Others not commonly done are:
- Irving method
- Aldridge method
- Cornual resection
- Uchida method
- Fimbriectomy

Routes of sterilization: Laparotomy, Minilaparotomy

Laparoscopy: Contraindicated in immediate and early postpartum, can be performed after 2 weeks.

MALE STERILIZATION

Vasectomy

- Safe, convenient and highly effective simple form of contraception for men
- Not effective immediately, WHO recommends backup methods for 3 months
- Can be timed to coincide with postpartum period when the fertility is low
- Ideal with LAM, if not on LAM, couple should use other methods of contraception for 12 weeks

SECTION 4

MEDICAL DISORDERS IN PREGNANCY

- Anemia
- Hypertensive Disorders in Pregnancy
- Heart Disease
- Diabetes
- Epilepsy
- Bronchial Asthma
- Jaundice
- Thyroid Disorders

CHAPTER

37

Anemia

DEFINITION

Anemia is a condition of low oxygen carrying capacity of blood in which Hb concentration is two standard deviation below the median for healthy population of same age, sex, and stage of pregnancy.

Physiological Anemia

During pregnancy normal Hb level is 10–12 gm/dl as compared to nonpregnant women of 12–14 gm/dl due to the increase in plasma volume more than RBCs volume.

WHO Classification

Mild anemia	9.1–11 g/dl
Moderate anemia	7.1–9 g/dl
Severe anemia	<7 g/dl

ICMR Classification

Category	Anemia	Hb level
1	Mild	10–10.9 g/dl
2	Moderate	7–10 g/dl
3	Severe	<7
4	Very severe (decompensated)	<4

CDC CRITERIA

I and III trimester – 11 gm%
II trimester – 10.5 gm %

Iron Deficiency Anemia

It is the most common type of anemia (95%).

	Normal	Negative iron balance	Iron deficient erythropoiesis	Iron deficiency anemia
Marrow iron stores	1 to 3+	0 to 1+	0	0
Serum ferritin (μg/L)	50–200	<20	<15	<15
TIBC (μg/dL)	300–360	>360	>380	>400
SI (μg/dL)	50–150	Normal	<50	<30
Saturation (%)	30–50		<20	<10
Marrow sideroblasts (%)	40–60		<10	<10
RBC protoporphyrin (μg/dL)			>100	>200
RBC morphology	Normal	Normal	Normal	Microcytic/ hypochromic

	S. ferritin	Hb	Diagnosis
Category I	>12 μg/dl	>11 g/dl	Normal
Category II	<12 μg/dl	>11 g/dl	Storage iron deficiency
Category III	<12 μg/dl	<11 g/dl	IDA
Category IV	>12 μg/dl	<11 g/dl	Other causes

Daily Requirements of Iron

Nonpregnant state 1 mg/day of absorbed iron (10% absorption)

During Pregnancy

Iron requirement depends on body weight of the mother and size and maturity of the fetus.

Total requirement	
Basal iron	280 mg
Expansion of red cell mass	570 mg
Fetus	200–350 mg
Placenta	50–150 mg
Blood loss at delivery	100–250 mg
	1200–1600 mg

Iron conserved by amenorrhea 10 × (24–48) = 240–480 mg

Additional iron requirement during pregnancy 500–600 mg/4–6 mg/day of absorbed iron (absorption 10%, in low bioavailability diets 3–4%)

- <20 weeks 2.5 mg/day
- 20–32 weeks 5.5 mg/day
- >32 weeks 6–8 mg/day

Expected Hb at 40 weeks of gestation can be calculated by the formula:

$$X + (40 - Y) - 3$$

X = current Hb in gm/dl

Y=current gestational age in weeks

Etiology

1. Inadequate intake of iron.
2. Defective absorption of iron, e.g. achlorhydria, drug interaction–calcium, antacids, vitamins, micronutrients, phenytoin, phenobarbitone, food-phytates, oxalates and phosphates.
3. Increased demand, e.g. menstruation and pregnancy.
4. Chronic blood loss, e.g. abnormal uterine bleeding and hemorrhoids, esophageal varices, worm infestation, malaria.

Clinical Picture

A. Symptoms: General symptoms of anemia are:
- Easy fatigability
- Headache
- Dyspnea
- Palpitation

B. Signs: Pallor which can be detected in the palpebral conjunctiva, face, palm of the hand, nail bed and mucus membranes of the mouth.
- Nails are brittle, striated with loss of their luster. Spooning of the nails may occur in chronic cases (koilonychia).

Investigations

- Hemoglobin, RBC, hematocrit (PCV)
- Blood film: Microcytic hypochromic anemia
- Indices MCV (75–95) fl, MCHC (32–35) g/dl, MCH (27–33) pg are reduced, most sensitive being MCHC
- Urine for occult blood, schistosomes and pus cells
- Stool for ova cyst for 3 consecutive days {Helminthiasis}
  Occult blood {Guaiac test}
  Avoid turnip, radish, broccoli, spinach, meat 3 days before.

Type of anemia	Peripheral smear findings
Iron deficiency anemia	Microcytosis, hypochromosis, anisocytosis, poikilocytosis, target cells (central staining of red cells with precipitated Hb)
Megaloblastic anemia	Macrocytosis, hypersegmented neutrophils (at least 3 cells having > 5 nuclear lobes), basophilic stippling, tear drop cells
Dimorphic anemia	Macrocytosis or normocytosis, normochromosis or hypochromosis
Sickle cell anemia	Sickle cells, Howell Jolly bodies (nuclear remnants)
Hereditary spherocytosis and immune hemolytic anemia	Spherocytes
Thalassemia	Microcytosis, hypochromosis, target cells
G6PD deficiency	Heinz bodies (precipitation of denatured globin) and fragmented cells

In Special Circumstances

- Serum iron concentration
- Serum ferritin
- Iron binding capacity
- Transferrin saturation
- Transferrin receptor—to assess cellular iron status
- Tfr + ferritin—complete picture of iron status
- **Megaloblastic anemia**–Serum folate (>5 ng/ml) ↓
  - Red cell folate (160–640 mcg/l) ↓
  - Serum B_{12} levels (200–900 pg/dl) ↓
- **Bone marrow biopsy**–indications
  a. Refractory anemia (no response to therapy in 6 weeks)
  b. Kala azar infection
  c. Aplastic anemia

Adjunctive Tests

- S. proteins–Hypoproteinemia
- RFT–Suspected renal disease
- Fractional test meal analysis
- Osmotic fragility test–Hereditary spherocytosis
- Sputum and chest X-ray for pulmonary TB in suspected cases

Prophylactic Iron Therapy

- National nutritional anemia prophylaxis program recommends 100 tablets of ferrous sulphate 200 mg with 60 mg of elemental iron with folic acid 0.5 mg to all pregnant women in third trimester of pregnancy, lactating women. Presently the recommendation is 100 mg elemental iron per day by giving two tablets daily instead of one.
- WHO recommends universal oral iron supplementation with 60 mg of elemental iron daily for 6 months in pregnancy in areas where the prevalence of iron deficiency is less than 40%. In areas where prevalence is greater than 40%, recommendation is to continue 3 months postpartum.
- Government of India recommendations–100 mg elemental iron + 500 mcg of folic acid in 2nd half of pregnancy for 100 days.

Suggestions for Better Prophylaxis

- Dietary modifications to add iron rich foods: Jaggary, liver, meat, kidney, eggs, dates and green vegetables are rich in iron
- Community-based distribution of tablets
- Fortification of common food stuffs (e.g. wheat and salt)
- Educating adolescent girls about diet, personal hygeine
- Hookworm infestation should be treated–T. Albendazole 400 mg to all anemic patients in 2nd and 3rd trimester. Change in defecation habits and avoid bare-foot walking.
- Chemoprophylaxis for malaria in endemic and high risk areas.

Treatment of Iron Deficiency Anemia

Mild anemia–treat with oral iron irrespective of gestational age

Moderate anemia

- <36 weeks-oral iron
- >36 weeks-parenteral iron

Severe anemia

Local guidelines for blood transfusion in chronic anemia are broadly divided into three groups:

1. Duration of pregnancy <36 weeks gestation
   - Hb ≤5 g%
   - Hb 5–7 g% and in the presence of established or incipient cardiac failure or clinical evidence of hypoxia, pneumonia or any other serious bacterial infection and malaria
2. Duration of pregnancy ≥36 weeks gestation
   - Hb ≤6 g% and in the presence of established or incipient cardiac failure or clinical evidence of hypoxia, pneumonia or any other serious bacterial infection and malaria
3. When elective cesarean section is planned and there is history of antepartum hemorrhage, postpartum hemorrhage, previous cesarean section with Hb 8–10 g%, then 1 unit of blood should be cross-matched and if Hb is <8 g%, then 2 units of blood should be cross-matched.

The specific indication for blood transfusion in pregnancy should be based on national guidelines and can be modified appropriately to the local situation.

PROTOCOL FOR BLOOD TRANSFUSION

- <5 g/dl
- 5–7 g/dl in the presence of established or incipient cardiac failure or clinical evidence of hypoxia, pneumonia or any other serious bacterial infection and malaria–Blood transfusion irrespective of gestational age
- 5–7 g/dl in the absence of established or incipient cardiac failure or clinical evidence of hypoxia, pneumonia or any other serious bacterial infection and malaria

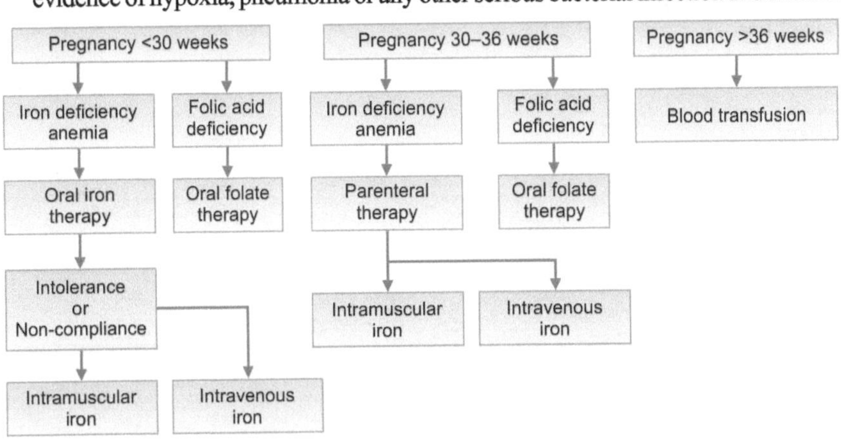

Goal of Iron Therapy

It is to correct Hb deficit and replenish iron stores in tissues.

Choice of therapy depends on three factors:
1. Severity of anemia
2. Gestational age
3. Tolerance of therapy chosen

Oral Iron Therapy

Mild and moderate anemia–ferrous sulphate, ferrous ascorbate, ferrous fumarate, ferrous gluconate

Salt	Dose of salt	Elemental iron
Ferrous sulphate	300	60
Ferrous gluconate	300	35
Ferrous fumarate	200	65
Ferrous ascorbate		100

Advise to patient on iron therapy: To take iron half an hour before meals and avoid drugs and food interfering with iron absorption.

Side effects: Nausea, vomiting and constipation, abdominal cramping and diarrhea.

Disadvantages of Oral Therapy

Intolerance and unpredictable absorption, noncompliance.

Indicators of Response to Therapy

- Feeling of wellbeing
- Improved look
- Better appetite
- Reticulocyte count increases in 5–10 days
- Increase in Hb and hematocrit in 3 weeks.

If no improvement in 3 weeks–Check compliance, absorption and other causes of microcytic hypochromic anemia, like thalassemia, pyridoxine deficiency, lead poisoning.

Therapeutic Trial with Iron and Folate Supplements

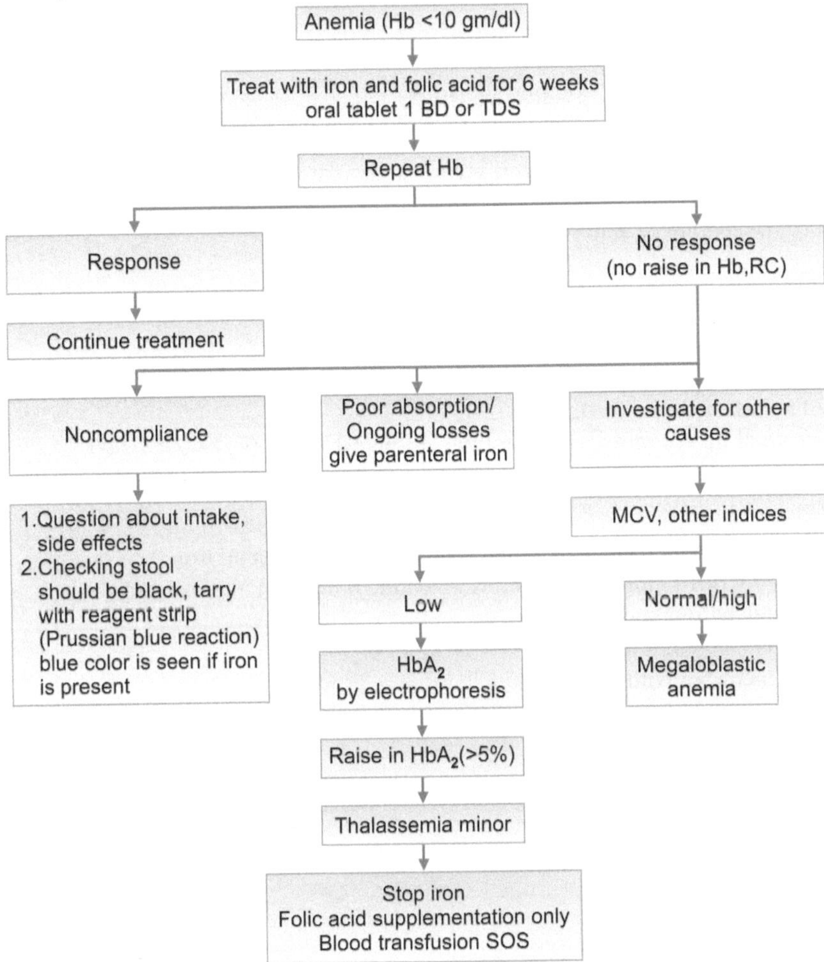

Parenteral Iron Therapy

Indications

a. Intolerance to oral iron
b. Poor compliance to oral iron
c. Malabsorption syndrome
d. Rapid blood loss
e. Inability to maintain iron balance (hemodialysis)

Preparations

Intramuscular

a. Iron-dextran complex (Imferon)
b. Iron-sorbitol-citrate complex (Jectofer)
c. Iron sorbitol citrate + folic acid + Vit B_{12} (Jectofer plus)

Usage: 100 mg of elemental iron given on alternate days after test dose deep IM by Z technique.
Side effects: Fever, muscle pain, discoloration of skin

Intravenous

Newer iron preparations
a. Iron sucrose (Orofer-s)
b. Iron gluconate (Globac)
c. Fractionated iron dextran
Parenteral iron requirement = (normal Hb-pts Hb) × wt (kg) × 2.4 + 500

Iron Sucrose

- Each 5 ml vial contains 20 mg/ml (100 mg) of elemental iron.
- 200 mg in 100 ml NS infusion is given in 20 mins on alternate days
- Excellent tolerance
- Almost no complications
- Hb increases within 3 weeks

Side Effects

SE	Iron dextran	Iron sucrose
Serious life-threatening anaphylaxis	0.6–0.7%	0.002%
Hypersensitivity	0.2–3%	0.005%
Mild adverse reactions	Up to 50%	Up to 35%

Properties of an Ideal Parenteral Iron

Property	Ideal	Iron dextran	Iron sucrose	Ferric carboxy-maltose
Type	I (robust)	I (robust)	II (semi-robust)	I (robust)
Molecular weight	>100 KD	>100 KD	34–60 KD	150 KD
Complex stability	High	High	Moderate	High
Half-life	Long	3–4 days	6 hrs	16 hrs
pH	Neutral	Neutral	High	Isotonic
Osmolality	Isotonic	Isotonic	High	Isotonic
Antigenicity	Low	High	Low	Low
Test dose	No	Yes	No	No
Time for injection	Short	4–6 for 20 mg/kg	15 min for 100 mg	15 min for 1000 mg
Max dose	High	20 mg/kg	600 mg/week	1000 mg/ infusion/week

Ferric Carboxymaltose Injection

- Type I–robust iron
- Not associated with dextran-induced hypersensitivity
- Can be administered in much higher doses than others
- Short infusion time
- A test dose is not required
- Latest parenteral iron–closest to the ideal iron
- Ferric carboxymaltose (FCM) injection contains iron in a stable ferric state as a complex tightly bound within a carbohydrate polymer.
- Due to the stability of the complex, it does not release ionic iron under physiological conditions.
- The iron hydroxide core, with its carbohydrate shell, is taken up by macrophages and enters the lysosomes where Fe^{3+} can be converted into Fe^{2+} as required.
- The Fe^{2+} is released by a divalent metal transporter (DMT1) then by ferroportin and taken up by transferrin after oxidation by ceruloplasmin.
- Iron from FCM is distributed in the liver and spleen and taken up predominantly by the bone marrow from within 60 minutes after administration.
- Within 2–3 weeks of FCM administration, iron utilization rates were 91–99% in the iron-deficient patients, and 61–84% in the patients with functional iron deficiency.

Composition

Each ml contains:

- Ferric carboxymaltose equivalent to elemental iron 50 mg.

Presentation

- Vials of 10 ml [500 mg].

Storage

- Store in the original package
- Do not store above 30°C
- Do not refrigerate or freeze

Dosage

- For IV use only
- Conventionally calculated using Ganzoni formula:

Cumulative iron deficit [mg] = body weight [kg] x (target Hb–actual Hb) [g/dl] x 2.4 + iron storage depot [mg]

- Use simpler regimen as used in FERGIcor study

Hb (g/dl)	Body weight 35 kg to <70 kg	Body weight ≥70 kg
≥10	1000 mg	1500 mg
<10	1500 mg	2000 mg

Note: A cumulative iron dose of 500 mg should not be exceeded for patients with body weight <35 kg.

- Can be injected undiluted @ 100 mg/minute IV

- In case of drip infusion ferric carboxymaltose injection must be diluted only in sterile 0.9% sodium chloride solution as follows:

Iron	Maximum volume of normal saline	Minimum time for administration
200 to <500 mg	100 ml	6 min
500 to 1000 mg	250 ml	15 min

- "FCM's near-neutral pH and physiological osmolarity results in a lower rate of injection-site reactions than observed with other IV iron preparations."
- "Moreover, FCM is stable and does not release large amounts of ionic iron (i.e., non-transferrin-bound iron)."
- "This, together with the low reactivity with other cellular components reduces the likelihood of acute toxicity."
- Further, short infusion time reduces chance of extravasation.

Contraindications

- Known hypersensitivity to ferric carboxymaltose injection or to any of its excipients
- Anemia not attributed to iron deficiency
- Evidence of iron overload or disturbances in utilization of iron
- In pregnancy in the first trimester
- In children below 14 years

Special Population

- Pregnancy
  - Contraindicated–first trimester
  - 2nd/3rd trimesters: careful risk/benefit evaluation
  - Fe from FCM can cross the placental barrier [not FCM per se]
- Lactation: <1% in breast milk
- Children–not studied, contraindicated
- Hepatic dysfunction–caution, iron assessment
- Acute or chronic infection, asthma, eczema or atopic allergies–caution

ERYTHROPOIETIN

Indications

- Anemia of systemic disease
- Anemia of malignancy
- Anemia secondary to chemotherapy
- Anemia of AIDS/HAART
- Anemia of prematurity

Role of Erythropoietin in Iron Deficiency Anemia in Pregnancy

- End stage renal disease
- Antepartum iron deficiency anemia

- Postpartum anemia
- Anemia of pregnant women in chronic hemolytic disorders
- Emerging use of EPO is treatment of moderate to severe iron deficiency anemia during pregnancy as an alternative to patients refusing blood transfusion

Recommended Dose of EPO

50–150 IU/kg SC twice or thrice weekly till the course of parenteral iron is over.

- Darbepoietin alfa, a molecularly modified EPO with additional carbohydrate, has a half-life in the circulation that is three to four times longer than recombinant human EPO, permitting weekly or every other week dosing.

Side Effects

- Polycythemia
- Increased viscosity of blood leads to rise in blood pressure and increases the risk of stroke.

Blood Transfusion

Indications

- Hemorrhage
- Severe anemia >36 weeks without failure
- Severe anemia in failure any period of gestation
- Refractory anemia

Packed Cells

80–100 ml/day not to be repeated in 24 hrs. Packed cells preferred over whole blood because patient will have less volume overload, less reactions one unit will increase hematocrit by 3–4% and Hb by 1 gm% in 3 days.

Exchange Transfusion

- In severe anemia with CCF
- Improvement will be seen in 30 min

Antenatal Care

- More frequent visits
- Be vigilant to detect and manage the complications of anemia such as heart failure, preterm labor, UTI
- Fetal monitoring for growth and wellbeing

Intrapartum Management

First stage: Special precautions that are to be taken during labor–

- The patient should be on bed and should lie in a position comfortable to her.
- Arrangements for oxygen inhalation is to be kept ready to increase the oxygenation of the maternal blood and thus diminish the risk of fetal hypoxia.
- Prophylactic antibiotics to be given.

- Avoid ARM unless indicated.
- Strict asepsis is to be maintained to minimize puerperal infection.

Second stage: Prophylactic outlet forceps or vacuum delivery may be done to shorten the duration of second stage. Methergin is contraindicated in severe anemia.

Third stage: Practice active management of third stage of labor.

Megaloblastic Anemia

It is caused by deficiency of folic acid and/or vitamin B_{12}.

Megaloblastic anemia in pregnancy is nearly always secondary to folate deficiency.

FOLIC ACID DEFICIENCY ANEMIA

Daily Requirement

Nonpregnant women: 50–100 μg/day
Pregnant women: 800 μg/day
Lactation: 600 μg/day

Etiology

1. Inadequate intake
2. Defective absorption
3. Increased demand, e.g. pregnancy
4. Drugs: Phenytoin, primidone, barbiturate, sulphasalazine, nitrofurantoin, tetracycline

Clinical Picture

- General symptoms of anemia (see before)
- GIT manifestations in the form of:
  - Dyspepsia
  - Anorexia
  - Nausea
  - Vomiting
  - Diarrhea
  - Beefy (Red, Glassed) tongue
  - Hepatosplenomegaly

Investigations

1. Blood film
   - Oval macrocytes, anisocytosis, poikilocytosis
   - Hypersegmented neutrophils (>5 lobes)
2. Redcell folate level: It is low measured by radioimmunoassay.
3. Bone marrow: Abnormal red cell precursors (megaloblasts).

For the diagnosis at least 2 of the following features must be present:

- >4% neutrophils must have >5 lobes
- Presence of orthochromic macrocytes (diameter >12 mcg)
- Nucleated RBCs are found.
- Howell Jolly bodies
- Macropolycytes

FOLIC ACID PROPHYLAXIS

- Diet—rich in folic acid like fortified grains, dried beans, green leafy vegetables, liver, egg, wheat products
- All women planning for pregnancy are advised to take 500 μg/day of folate 3 months preconceptionally to prevent neural tube defects. Those who have had a previous fetus with neural tube defects on anticonvulsants or carrying a multiple pregnancy and in malaria endemic areas, are advised to take 5 mg/day of folic acid.
- WHO recommends folic acid intake of 400 μg daily for 6 months during pregnancy and continuing for 3 months postpartum in low risk and 5 mg/day for high risk.
- Vitamin C increases folate absorption by converting it into folinic acid.

Treatment

- If folic acid deficiency is diagnosed, give 5 mg /day orally and continue for 3 months postpartum.

VIT. B_{12} DEFICIENCY ANEMIA (ADDISONIAN PERNICIOUS ANEMIA)

It is rare.

Daily Requirement

Non-pregnant–3 μg/day
Pregnancy, Lactation–4 μg/day

Etiology

1. Inadequate intake (rare)
2. Deficient intrinsic factor as in atrophic gastritis or gastrectomy
3. Malabsorption syndrome
4. Increased demand, e.g. pregnancy

Clinical Features

- General symptoms of anemia
- GIT manifestations: as folic acid deficiency
- Neurological manifestations
- Subacute combined degeneration
- Peripheral neuritis

Investigations

- Decreased serum vit. B_{12}
- MCV >100 fl
- MCHC 30–36 g/dl
- Peripheral smear–Macrocytosis, anisocytosis, poikilocytosis

Treatment

- Oral preparations have unreliable absorption properties and are inadequate for long-term preparation.
- Inj Vit. B_{12} 1000 μg IM is recommended for once a week for 6–8 weeks followed by 1000 μg monthly for maintenance in those who have malabsorption.

(When iron alone is given in iron deficiency anemia folic acid deficiency will get unmasked. When folic acid alone is given in megaloblastic anemia vitamin B_{12} deficiency will become severe and it will increase the neurological manifestations.)

DIMORPHIC ANEMIA

Combined deficiency of iron, folic acid with findings of both anemias but dominance of one.
Blood film may show macrocytic or normocytic, normocytic or hypochromic pictures.
Bone marrow shows megaloblastic changes.
Treatment is correction of all deficiencies.

HEMOLYTIC ANEMIAS

Classification of Hemolytic Anemias

	Intracorpuscular defects	Extracorpuscular factors
Hereditary	Hemoglobinopathies (Thalassemia, sickle cell anemia) Enzymopathies (Pyruvate deficiency, G6PD deficiency) Membrane-cytoskeletal defects (Spherocytosis)	Familial (atypical) Hemolytic uremic syndrome
Aquired	Paroxysmal nocturnal hemoglobinuria (PNH)	Mechanical destruction (microangiopathic) Toxic agents Drugs Infectious Autoimmune

HEMOGLOBINOPATHIES

Inherited disorders of hemoglobin. Abnormalities of quantity of globin chains.

Sickling disorder–qualitative abnormality. Amino acid substitution in an α globin or β globin chain.

Thalassemia–Quantitative disorder. Impaired production and imbalance of globin genes.

Thalassemia

An autosomal inherited disorder results from failure of production of either α chain (α-thalassemia) or β chain (β-thalassemia) of the hemoglobin molecule and their replacement with other polypeptide chains.

α-Thalassemia

a. **α-Thalassemia major (homozygotes):** The fetus with this disorder is affected in utero showing polyhydramnios, erythroblastosis, anemia and hydrops resembling Rh-incompatibility. This fetus does not survive due to inability of oxygen transfer as α-chain is responsible for O_2 carrying capacity.
b. **α-Thalassemia minor (heterozygotes):** Patient develops mild progressive anemia during pregnancy.

1	-α/αα	Silent carier
2	--/ αα	Thalassaemia minor
		Mild hemolytic anemia
3	α–/--	HbH disease moderate to severe hemolytic anemia
4	--/--, γγ/γγ	Thalassemia major or Hb Barts

Effects on Pregnancy

1. Silent carrier state–no effect
2. Thalassemia minor
    - Mild microcytic hypochromic anemia
    - Patient tolerates pregnancy
    - Oral iron and folic acid 5 mg throughout pregnancy
    - Parenteral iron should never be given to prevent iron overload
3. HbH
    - Compatible with extrauterine life
    - Normal life expectancy but chronic hemolytic anemia of moderate to severe degree
    - Anemia worsens during pregnancy and blood transfusion is necessary.
    - Neonate appears well at birth but soon develops hemolytic anemia
    - Severity of hemolytic anemia is similar to thalassemia major.
4. Hb Bart
    - Has increased affinity for oxygen
    - Common cause of stillbirth in south-east Asia
    - Non-immune hydrops
    - USG at 12 weeks is 100% sensitive and specific by measuring cardiothoracic ratio
    - Patient can develop severe preeclampsia if fetus is having hydrops fetalis.

Diagnosis

Low MCV and MCH but normal MCHC.

β-Thalassemia

a. **β-thalassemia major/Cooley's anemia (Homozygotes):** The disorder starts in childhood leading to death of the patient mostly in the 2nd or 3rd decade.
b. **β-thalassemia minor (heterozygotes):** As α thalassemia minor

Incidence

1 in 300–500

Clinical nomenclature	Genotype	Disease
Thalassemia major	Homozygous or compound heterozygous (β0/β0, β0/β+, or β+/β+)	Severe, requires blood transfusions regularly
β-thalassemia trait	β/β+ or β/β0	Asymptomatic, with mild microcytic anemia, or microcytosis without anemia

β-Thalassemia Major (Cooley's Anemia)

A female who thrives to adulthood is usually sterile hence pregnancy is rare due to high maternal mortality. MTP is recommended.

Fetal Effects

- Neonate normal at birth due to HbF but later HbF is replaced HbA_2, hence infant is severely anemic requiring multiple transfusions.
- Iron overload occurring by end of 1st decade—deferoxamine given.
- Thalassemia facies—stunted growth with frontal bossing and maxillary prominence
- Death due to infections
- Contraceptive advice is of paramount importance. In splenectomized women, oral contraceptive should be avoided as they have higher risk of thrombosis.

β-Thalassemia Minor

- Mild microcytic hypochromic anemia which does not respond to iron therapy
- Mild splenomegaly is common
- Folate and oral iron supplements given throughtout pregnancy
- Parenteral iron never to be given
- Decreased MCV and MCH, normal MCHC
- HbA_2 >3.5% conforming β-thalassemia

Diagnosis

- The diagnosis of α or β thalassemia trait may be suspected by finding a low MCV, a low MCH and a normal MCHC (as distinct from iron deficiency when ALL the indices are reduced)
- The diagnosis is confirmed by globin chain synthesis studies, DNA analysis or in the case of β thalassemia, raised concentrations of HbA_2 and HbF
- In the presence of a normal ferritin, α thalassemia is assumed and genetic testing is only performed when both the parents are affected.

Antenatal Management

- Women with α or β thalassemia trait need iron if their ferritin level is low
- Iron therapy may also be indicated if their Hb level falls significantly below booking and the red cell indices fall as this would suggest iron deficiency
- Oral folate should be given throughout pregnancy.
- In cases of severe anemia with proven iron deficiency, parenteral iron may be indicated but these women should be managed jointly with a hematologist.
- Pregnancy in the truly transfusion-dependent girl is very rare.
- See antenatal screening guideline on thalassemia for management if thalassemia is suspected or confirmed in a pregnant woman.

Labor and Thalassemia Trait

In labor for α or β thalassemia trait, no specific management is required apart from a cross-match if anemic (Hb <9 g/dl) in case of the hemorrhage, however, Hb of 6–7 g/dl may be tolerated so long as there is no active bleeding.

β Thalassemia Major and Pregnancy

- Reports of pregnancy in women with homozygous β thalassemia major are rare.
- Several studies have reported a high rate of pregnancy loss, intrauterine growth restriction and prematurity.
- All patients should have been seen by a hematologist specialized in thalassemia prior to embarking on a pregnancy. If iron levels are high, they can be given high intensity chelation regimes to reduce the iron level pre-conceptually.
- A cardiac echo should be preformed if no planning has been possible.
- The mean level of hemoglobin should be maintained above 10 g/dl in an effort to suppress ineffective erythropoiesis (not universally accepted and liaison with the hematologist is paramount)
- The transfusion requirement in pregnancy increases by a mean of two units of washed pack cells every two to three weeks.
- All splenectomized women should continue their penicillin V treatment
- Cross-matching blood can be extremely difficult, and therefore, if at all possible, two or three days' notice of the need for a transfusion should be given to blood bank.
- It is unknown whether deferoxamine is safe during pregnancy. Teratogenic effects such as retardation of bone ossification, vertebral aplasia and bifurcation or fusion of ribs have been observed in animal studies. Only eight women in the world literature have received defercoxamine for several weeks during pregnancy—there were no adverse fetal outcomes. However, termination should be discussed.
- The newer chelating agent L1 deferiprone has been demonstrated to be both teratogenic and embryotoxic in rats and is contraindicated in pregnancy.
- Vitamin C is usually administered to women on desferrioxamine this should be stopped in pregnancy as it increases gastrointestinal absorption of dietary iron and might precipitate cardiac damage.
- Folate supplementation should be given in pregnancy.

- Splenectomy due to hypersplenism is generally performed at a young age. Hypersplenic crises occur more frequently in pregnancy, especially in the last few weeks, so that anemia, leukopenia and thrombocytopenia may occur singly or in combination. Splenectomy should be reserved for those with severe thrombocytopenia.
- There may be a predisposition to venous clotting after splenectomy. Aspirin administration during pregnancy to this group of patients has been suggested but there have been no clinical trials so far.

Fetal Well-being

- Serial growth scans from 28 weeks every two weeks
- Twice weekly biophysical profile and Doppler from 30 weeks

Labor

- Labor with a hemoglobin of less than 10 g/dl can lead to significant morbidity and mortality.
- Thalassemic patients have small stature and CPD is common during labor, thus emergency cesareans are common.
- Therefore elective cesarean at 37–38 weeks is recommended, this also allows blood to be available and optimization of the clinical state prior to delivery.
- Vaginal delivery would be preferable in women with thrombocytopenia in order to avoid bleeding during or after the operation.
- It is probably alright for women to breastfeed on desferrioxamine, as it is poorly absorbed orally but clinical and hematological follow up of the newborn is indicated.
- Breastfeeding is also contraindicated with L1 deferiprone.

Sickle Cell Anemia

- An autosomal recessive inherited disorder in which glutamic acid in position 6 of the β-chain of the hemoglobin molecule is replaced by valine. This leads to production of HbS. HbS on exposure to hypoxia forms insoluble aggregations and RBCs become sickle-shaped and are subsequently fragmented.
- Sickle-shaped cells increase the blood viscosity and occlude blood vessels of various organs.
- The manifestations appear usually in homozygous not in heterozygous state.
- Heterozygous state: sickle cell trait (HbAS)
- Homozygous state: sickle cell disease (HbSS)
- Compound heterozygous hemoglobin variants

Sickle cell anemia is characterized clinically by symptoms of anemia, arthralgia and recurrent painful crises due to occlusion of the microvasculature by sickle cells.

They generally appear to be undernourished and have a short trunk, narrow hips and shoulders and long spindly extremities.

Splenomegaly is frequently noted in children but seldom found in adults.

They may have cardiomegaly and heart murmurs.

A mild to moderate hyperbilirubinemia causes the sclera to be muddy yellow color.

They are often able to tolerate a hemoglobin of 7–8 g/dl.

Sickle cell traits are usually asymptomatic throughout their life.

However, sickling may occur under conditions of severe hypoxia such as at high altitude.

Some studies suggest that they have an increased incidence of asymptomatic bacteriuria and clinical pyelonephritis.

Compound heterozygous – HbS combined with either HbC or beta thalassemia may lead a clinical course resembling that of sickle cell anemia.

- Most common in black people of African origin, also in Saudi Arabians, Asians and people of Mediterranean origin.
- A low hemoglobin in the absence of bleeding in any of these groups may point to a diagnosis of sickle cell disease.
- Crises often precipitated by infection and exacerbated by dehydration, hypoxia, hypotension, hypothermia, acidosis and venous stasis.
- Crises more common in pregnancy because of the hypercoagulable state. The stress of labor may precipitate a sickle cell crisis.

Blood Transfusion

- ALL women with sickle cell disease should have an extended phenotype performed early in their disease because of the likelihood of developing red cell antibodies. If the woman has not had one performed in the past, then it is helpful to do this as soon as possible in the pregnancy. (Send three EDTA tubes down to hematology).
- As a general rule, patients with sickle cell disease should only be transfused because of a particular clinical situation. The final decision on transfusion should be made jointly by the consultant obstetrician and hematologist.
- Possible indications include: Ongoing high transfusion regime, multiple pregnancy, poor fetal growth or a hemoglobin 15% less than steady state level.
- It is important that all blood for patients with sickle cell disease is screened for sickle cell hemoglobin prior to transfusion.
- Many women with sickle cell disease have had multiple transfusions and have red cell antibodies. They should, therefore, be screened before any transfusion and the appropriate blood selected.
- Donor blood is leukocyte depleted and can be classed as CMV safe. CMV negative blood will be supplied to women antenatally who are CMV negative.

For all these reasons, it is very important that:

- The request form for transfusion be clearly marked indicating that the patient has sickle cell disease.
- That the transfusion laboratory be given as much notice as possible that a transfusion is required (often at least three working days) unless the blood is required for a medical emergency.

Antenatal Care

- All women with sickle cell disease have a degree of hemolysis and should routinely be on folic acid 5 mg daily throughout pregnancy.
- Stop hyrdoxy urea 3 months prior to conception.
  Mechanism of action:
  - Increases HbF.
  - Improves red cell hydration.
  - Decreases rate polymerization of HbS.
  - Decreases frequency of crises.
- All women with sickle cell disease are functionally hyposplenic as a result of recurrent splenic infarcts. They should routinely be on hyposplenic prophylaxis with penicillin or equivalent in case of penicillin allergy and this should be continued throughout pregnancy.
- There should be a low threshold for treating infection because of the hyposplenism.
- 1/3 will develop preeclampsia.
- Low-birth weight deliveries are common (>20%) and as such they should have serial growth scans.
- Miscarriage rate is 12% and the stillbirth rate 4%.
- Management should be in liaison with the woman's hematologist.

Intrapartum Care

- Inform the hematologist that the patient is in labor.
- Encourage oral fluids.
- Continuously monitoring the oxygen saturation by pulse oximetry and give oxygen by mask if necessary.
- Continuously monitor the baby.
- If a painful crisis occurs, treat as usual for the patient. Always seek a cause and always send a midstream sample urine for urgent microscopy.
- If strong opiates are needed notify the neonatologist and warn the patient that after delivery the baby may have to go to the special care neonatal unit.

Puerperium

- Crises may occur in the puerperium, therefore, watch infection sites (urine, cesarean section scar, intravenous line sites, perineum and breasts).
- Good hydration should be maintained.

Sickle cell crisis in pregnancy

- Hospital admission to labor ward, ideally the critical care room is recommended for assessment and intervention.

1. Suspect
2. Inform senior obstetrician, anesthetist, hematologist and pediatrician. Close liaison with hematology is crucial.
3. Airway
   - Assess
   - Maintain patency
   - Apply oxygen 15 l/min
   - Attach pulse oximeter
   - Consider arterial blood gas

4. Breathing
    - Assess need for ventilation
    - Protect airway
5. Circulation
    - Assess pulse, BP and whether dehydrated.
    - Put on ECG.
    - Treat per-arrest arrhythmias.
    - Avoid frequent assessment of BP by inflation cuff, if stable; if unstable, consider arterial line.
    - Secure IV access, send blood for FBC, reticulocyte count, U and E, LFT's, cross-match.
6. Rehydrate
    - Ensure adequate hydration with Hartmann's or normal saline.
    - Monitor fluid input and urine output.
    - Avoid CVP line if possible.
7. Consider need for transfusion
    - Advice must be taken from the consultant hematologist. A top-up transfusion is used to maintain the hemoglobin at a reasonable level (> 6 g/dl) or to correct a rapid, significant fall (>2–3 g/dl).

    Indications are as follows:
    - Splenic or hepatic sequestration
    - Aplastic crisis
    - Acute folate deficiency
    - Hemorrhage

    Exchange transfusion is used to reduce maternal hemoglobin to less than 30% to reduce the chance of sickling. Transfuse only to the normal hemoglobin level.

    Indications
    - Acute chest syndrome
    - Eclampsia and pre-eclampsia
    - Central nervous system involvement
8. Monitor FH continuously by cardiotocography if viable and consider timing and method of delivery.
    - Resuscitation of the mother should be carried out before delivery of the baby.
    - Immediate delivery is not necessarily indicated if the CTG is non-reactive or the biophysical profile is unsatisfactory. Fetal parameters tend to improve and return to normal as the crisis improves.
9. Give adequate parenteral analgesia
    - Opiates IV, IM or as patient-controlled analgesia
10. Avoid hypothermia
11. Investigate cause
    - If the temperature is raised take blood for culture and commence antibiotics – augmentin or cefuroxime. A midstream specimen of urine and sputum sample should be taken as necessary. Request CXR as indicated.
12. Treat crisis specifically
    - Painful crisis and acute hepatic or splenic sequestration are more common in the third trimester and postpartum period.

Painful Crisis

- Presenting symptoms are fever, pain in the extremities, back, chest and abdomen.
- Clinical findings are tenderness over the distal bones, lumbar spine, sterum and ribs, generalized abdominal tenderness and dark urine.
- Investigations show evidence of DIC, GGT and total bilirubin will be raised. MRI may show edema and infarction of the bone marrow.

Acute Hepatic or Splenic Sequestration

- Common in HbSC and HbS thalasaemia variants
- Presenting symptoms are fever and abdominal pain and commonly bone pain
- Clinical finding is progressive enlargement of the liver or spleen
- Investigations–serial Hb estimations show a rapid fall to 30% of steady state Hb with a rise in reticulocyte count. Ultrasound will usually show enlargement of the liver and spleen. Gallstones and biliary tree obstruction should be looked for and excluded. Acute cholecystitis should be ruled out.
- Manage as above. If Hb is more than 2 g/dl below steady state give an immediate transfusion. Discuss with hematologist.

Aplastic Crisis

- Presenting symptoms are pallor, fever, weakness, exertional dyspnea.
- May show signs of high output cardiac failure.
- Investigations: Serial Hb estimations show progressive anemia to below 3.5 g/dl with a low reticulocyte count. Bone marrow aspirate shows giant pronormoblasts.
- Management—transfuse to usual level of Hb. Check serum folate level to rule out folate deficiency. Administer folic acid if low. Spontaneous recovery can be expected in around two weeks.
- Check for parvovirus infection.

Acute Chest Syndrome

- Presenting symptoms are fever, chest pain, shortness of breath and a non-productive cough.
- Clinical findings are signs of congestion, basal crepitations and signs of pleural effusions.
- Investigations–CXR shows patchy pulmonary infiltrations mainly in the lower lobes. Blood gases and lung scans show abnormalities.
- Manage as above, exclude pneumonia and PE, commence exchange transfusion, give broad spectrum antibiotics IV if the temperature is persistently above 38°C.

Avascular Necrosis of the Hip

- Presenting symptom is persistent hip; pain made worse by walking and relieved by rest.

- Clinical findings are limited abduction with adduction deformity and apparent shortening of limb.
- Investigate by X-ray or MRI of the hip.
- Management–orthopedic consultation, analgesia and non-weightbearing for 3-6 months

13. Documentation
    - Keep a record of pulse, BP, resp. rate, SaO_2, FH and treatments given
14. Consider differential diagnosis
    - Conditions causing fever pain and anemia, e.g. acute febrile illness such as pneumonia or tonsillitis, obstetric problems such as preeclampsia and abruption and surgical problems such as pyelonephritis, appendicitis, cholecystitis and pancreatitis and DVT.
15. Organize hemoglobinopathy screening for the baby.

Contraception

- OCPs not recommended
- Progesterone–prevent painful sickle crisis
- IUCD contraindicated as it increases risk of infections
- Condoms + foams and diaphragms–safest but high failure rates
- Sterilization with one child due to short lifespan of mother

THROMBOCYTOPENIA IN PREGNANCY

Incidence: 8%

Etiology

Pregnancy specific:

- Gestational thrombocytopenia–70%
- Pre-severe preeclampsia or eclampsia–21%
- HELLP syndrome
- Acute fatty liver of pregnancy

Pregnancy Associated

- Thrombotic thrombocytopenic purpura
- DIC
- Hemolytic uremic syndrome

Non-pregnancy Related

- Immune thrombocytopenic purpura–3%
- Spurious
- Hereditary
- Marrow disorder
- B_{12}/folate deficiency
- Infection
- Drugs
- Malignancy

Evaluation

- Normal platelet count: 150,000–400,000/μL
- Requires assessment when <100,000/μL
- The primary reason for evaluating thrombocytopenia is to assess the risk of bleeding and assess the presence of underlying disorders (TTP, HIT, etc.)

< 20,000 – increased risk of bleeding

20,000–50,000 – rarely have increased risk of spontaneous bleeding but increased risk of bleeding from procedures

50,000–1,00,000 – no increased risk of spontaneous bleeding and can undergo most procedures.

GESTATIONAL THROMBOCYTOPENIA

Five Criteria

1. Mild thrombocytopenia (usually >70,000/μL)
2. Patients are asymptomatic with no history of bleeding
3. There is no preconception history of thrombocytopenia
4. Occurs late in gestation
5. Postpartum resolution–usually by 2–12 weeks and no fetal/neonatal thrombocytopenia

Etiology

Unknown

- Accelerated platelet activation is suspected to occur at placental circulation.
- Accelerated consumption of platelets is due to the reduced lifespan of platelets during pregnancy.

Diagnosis of Gestational Thrombocytopenia is by exclusion.

History

- Current or previous bleeding problems
- Family h/o hemorrhagic disorders
- H/o recent blood transfusion
- H/o viral fever, easy bruising, gingival bleeding and menometrorrhagia-ITP
- H/o hypertension with impending symptoms–severe preeclampsia
- H/o jaundice-AFLP
- H/o of neurologic manifestations, abdominal pain, fever and renal abnormalities-TTP
- H/o drug intake–Quinidine, quinine, sulfa drugs, gold salts, antibiotics (Vancomycin, etc.), Heparin–autoimmune ITP
- H/o skin rashes, oral ulcers, joint pain, seizures-SLE

- H/o recurrent pregnancy loss, deep vein thrombosis, pulmonary embolism, Stroke-APLA syndrome
- H/o onset of thrombocytopenia in pregnancy
    - A mother in the first or early second trimester, who has thrombocytopenia will have immune thrombocytopenic purpura more commonly.
    - Gestational thrombocytopenia—more common in third trimester.

Examination

- Temperature–febrile infections–dengue, malaria
- Petechiae, ecchymosis, gum bleeding, oral ulcers, rashes
- BP-systolic ≥160 mm Hg and diastolic ≥110 mm Hg on two occasions at least six hours apart-Preeclampsia
- Icterus–AFLP, HELLP syndrome.
- Splenomegaly-portal hypertension

Laboratory Evaluation

- Complete blood count and peripheral smear
    - Low platelet counts with otherwise normal smear suggests gestational thrombocytopenia/AITP.
- Peripheral smear is essential to rule out spurious thrombocytopenia
    - Clumping of platelets is common and can artificially lower the total platelet count
- Antiplatelet antibodies—expensive, and has poor standardization
- Urine albumin–proteinuria of 5 grams or greater in a 24-hour urine specimen–suggests preeclampsia
- Fundoscopy–evidence of hypertensive retinopathy
- Elevated LDH–hemolysis seen in preeclampsia, TTP
- Peripheral smear:
    - Schistocytes-suggestive of MAHA
    - Hypersegmented neutrophils and oval macrocytes – Folate deficiency
    - Malarial parasites
- LFT–elevated liver enzymes in HELLP
- RFT–abnormal in severe PE, HELLP syndrome, TTP, HUS
    - S.uric acid—elevated in preeclampsia, HELLP, AFLP
- Blood sugars-hypoglycemia-AFLP
- PT, aPTT, D-dimer deranged–in DIC
- Vit B_{12} levels
- Folic acid levels
- Bone marrow biopsy
- Anticardiolipin antibody, lupus anticoagulant antibody-APLA
  ANA, dsDNA-SLE
- USG abdomen–IUGR, splenomegaly, kidney parameters abnormal
  Doppler–IUGR

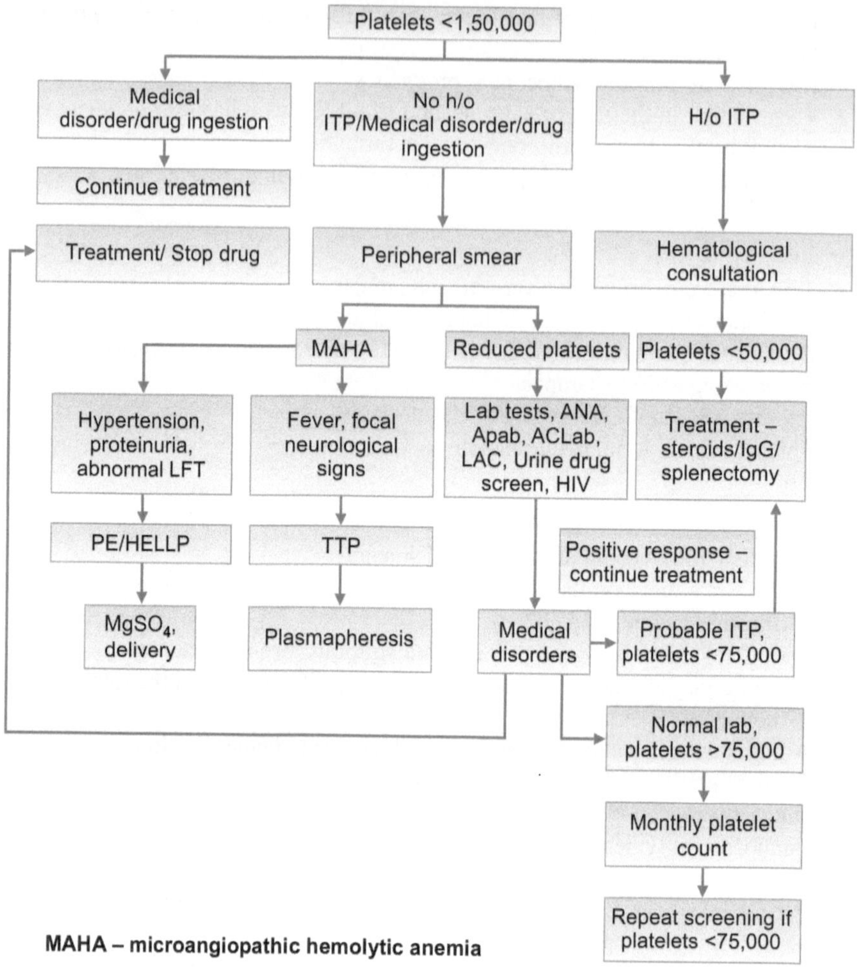

MAHA – microangiopathic hemolytic anemia

Management

Pre-Pregnancy and Prenatal

- Exclude pathological causes
- Monitor platelet counts every 4 weeks antenatally
- No treatment is necessary

Labor and Delivery

- Mode of delivery determined by obstetric considerations.
- Avoid fetal blood sampling and traumatic vaginal delivery
- A safe platelet count for vaginal delivery: >50,000/cu mm
  - Regional anesthesia- >80,000/cu mm
- Cesarean done only for obstetric indications

Postnatal

- Cord blood platelet count. Fetus not affected by the maternal thrombocytopenia.
- Maternal platelet counts followed postnatally
  - Monthly follow up of platelets.
  - Re-evaluate if platelet count falls below 70,000/or falls rapidly.
  - Reassurance.

Note:

- Gestational thrombocytopenia is the commonest cause of thrombocytopenia during pregnancy (70%).
- If no antecedent history of thrombocytopenia is present and platelet counts are >70,000/μL, the condition is more likely to be GT.
- If platelet counts fall to <50,000/μL or if a preexisting history of thrombocytopenia is present, the condition is more likely to be ITP.
- Direct or circulating antiplatelet antibodies have no value in the workup of thrombocytopenia in pregnancy because they usually are nonspecific.
- Invasive procedures to determine fetal platelet counts (scalp sampling, PUBS) are not necessary.
- No risk to mother or fetus.

IDIOPATHIC (IMMUNE) THROMBOCYTOPENIC PURPURA (ITP)

- Acquired disorder
- Thrombocytopenia in the absence of other blood cell abnormalities (normal RBC and WBC, normal peripheral smear)
- No clinically apparent conditions or medications that can account for thrombocytopenia
- Mild cases clinically difficult to differentiate from benign thrombocytopenia of pregnancy
- A previously normal woman can sometimes develop ITP during a pregnancy
- Significant bleeding rare if platelets >10,000/μL
- Spontaneous remission common in children, rare in adults
- 2/3rd have pre-existing disease and 1/3rd are newly diagnosed
- It is a diagnosis of exclusion.

Incidence

- 1 in 1000–10,000 pregnancies
  Childhood form (most <10 yrs old)

Etiology

- Often after **infection** (viral or bacterial)
- Theories:
  - Antibody cross-reactivity
  - *H. pylori*
  - Bacterial lipopolysaccharides

Features

- Peak incidence in winter
- ~50% receive some treatment
- ≥75% in remission within 6 months

Adult Form

Etiology

- ITP plasma induces thrombocytopenia in normal subjects
- Platelet-reactive autoantibodies present in most cases
  - Often specific for a platelet membrane glycoprotein
- Antibody coated platelets cleared by tissue macrophages
  - Most destruction in spleen (extravascular)
- Most subjects have compensatory increase in platelet production
- Impaired production in some patients
  - Intramedullary destruction

Features

- No prodrome
- Chronic, recurrences common
- Spontaneous remission rate about 5%

Pathogenesis

- Increased platelet destruction
- Autoantibodies inhibit platelet production

Diagnosis

- Petechiae, purpura, sometimes mucosal bleeding
- Major internal/intracranial bleeding rare
- Mortality rate <5%
- Absence of constitutional symptoms or splenomegaly
- Other blood counts and coagulation parameters normal
- No schistocytes or platelet clumps on blood smear
- Marrow shows normal or increased megakaryocytes

Rule Out Other Causes

- Lab error/PLT clumping
- Drug/medication interaction
- Infections (HIV, Hepatitis C)
- Thyroid/autoimmune disease
- Destructive/consumptive processes (TTP/HUS)
- Bone marrow disease (leukemias, MDS)

Investigations

Confirmatory testing not necessary in typical cases

- Serum antiplatelet antibody assay (poor sensitivity – not recommended)
- Test for specific anti-platelet glycoprotein antibodies (more specific, negative in 10–30%)

Management of ITP in Pregnancy

- Emergency vs. Chronic treatment

General Principles of Therapy

- Goal–Safe platelet count (30,000–50,000) to prevent major bleed, not normalized count
- Treatment to be initiated only if platelets <20,000–30,000
- Mortality <1%
- Platelet transfusion only if life-threatening bleeding
- Prednisone 1 mg/kg/day to be administered along with blood transfusion
- Most respond within one week (gestational diabetes, fetal toxicity)
- Supplement with calcium and vitamin D if greater than 3 months treatment
- Unresponsive–IV Ig 1 gm/kg/day over 1–2 days
- Unresponsive to medical therapy – splenectomy after 2nd trimester
- Splenectomy–removes primary site of destruction of antibody-coated platelets, and decreases antiplatelet antibody production
- If successful–remission usually within two weeks of surgery
- 65% long-term remission
- Rh AntiD is used to treat if other treatment does not work out. It is still under research.
- Potential for neonatal thrombocytopenia (approx 15% incidence)
  - Consider fetal blood sampling in selected cases
  - Consider Cesarean delivery if fetal platelets <20,000

Complications

- Fetal hemorrhage during delivery as the maternal antibodies cross the placenta.

Chronic Refractory ITP

- Persistent >3 months
- PLT <50,000
- Failure to respond to splenectomy
- Azathioprine, cyclosporine after 2nd trimester
- Rituximab, TPO receptor agonist – still under research

NEONATAL ALLOIMMUNE THROMBOCYTOPENIA (NAIT)

- Mother develops antibodies against fetal platelet antigens
- Maternal IgG crosses placenta and attacks platelet antigen in fetus
- Can occur in first pregnancy
- 1/1000–5000 births
- Mother is asymptomatic–normal platelet count
- 75–90% recurrence rate with increased severity
- 200 cases NAIT
- Anti-HPA-1a—75 percent
- Anti-HPA-5b—16 percent
- Anti-HPA-15b—4 percent

HEMOLYTIC UREMIC SYNDROME

- Microangiopathic hemolytic anemia, thrombocytopenia and uremia.
- Mostly occurs postpartum.

Classic HUS

- Diarrhea-positive (D+) or epidemic HUS-Shiga-like toxins
- Mainly in young children
- Prodrome lasting one or two weeks, during which the children have influenza-like symptoms, or more commonly, diarrhea.
- Then comes an abrupt onset of oliguria or anuria.
- Microangiopathic hemolytic anemia, thrombocytopenia and uremia.

Atypical HUS

- Diarrhea-negative (D–) HUS.
- Occurs mainly in adults
- Triggering factors–Nonenteric bacterial infections, viral infections, chemotherapeutic or immunosuppressive drugs, oral contraceptives, pregnancy, malignancy, autoimmune disorders such as systemic lupus erythematosus, antiphospholipid antibody syndrome
- Severe proteinuria, with microangiopathic anemia and thrombocytopenia

THROMBOTIC THROMBOCYTOPENIC PURPURA

- Fever
- Microangiopathic hemolytic anemia
- Thrombocytopenia
- Neurologic symptoms
- Uremia

Platelet thrombi develop in small arteries and arterioles throughout the body.

Management

- No specific treatment
- Plasma exchange is the treatment of choice
- Termination of pregnancy should be considered
- LMWH only after platelet count becomes normal

THROMBOCYTOPENIA AND INFECTION

- Immune complex-mediated platelet destruction
    - Childhood ITP
    - Bacterial sepsis
    - Hepatitis C, other viral infections

- Activation of coagulation cascade
  - Sepsis with DIC
- Vascular/endothelial cell damage
  - Viral hemorrhagic fevers
  - Rocky Mountain Spotted Fever
- Damage to platelet membrane components by bacterial enzymes (e.g., *S. pneumoniae* sialidase)
- Decreased platelet production
  - Viral infections (EBV, measles)
- Mixed production defect/immune consumption
  - HIV infection

Inherited Thrombocytopenia

- Congenital aplastic anemia/Fanconi's anemia
- Congenital amegakaryocytic thrombocytopenia
- Thrombocytopenia with absent radius syndrome (recessive)
- Bernard-Soulier syndrome (recessive, giant platelets, defective function, GPIb defect)
- May-Hegglin anomaly and related disorders (dominant, leukocyte inclusions, giant platelets, MYH-9 mutation)
- Other autosomal dominant syndromes (platelets may be normal or giant)
- Wiskott-Aldrich syndrome (X-linked, immunodeficiency, eczema)

Pseudothrombocytopenia

- Artifactually low platelet count due to in vitro clumping of platelets
- Usually caused by antibodies that bind platelets only in presence of chelating agent (EDTA)
- Seen in healthy individuals and in a variety of disease states

Diagnosis

- Marked fluctuations in platelet count without apparent cause
- Thrombocytopenia disproportionate to symptoms
- Clumped platelets on blood smear
- "Platelet satellitism"–platelets stuck to WBC
- Abnormal platelet/leukocyte histograms
- Platelet count varies with different anticoagulants

PLATELET TRANSFUSION

Platelet transfusion triggers:
- Without bleeding or any other risk factor - 10,000/mm^3
- Fever, antibiotic therapy, sepsis - 20,000/mm^3
- Major surgeries - 50,000/mm^3
- Neurosurgery and ophthalmic surgery - 1,00,000/mm^3

Contraindications

- Thrombotic thrombocytopenic purpura
- Heparin induced thrombocytopenia

Ineffectiveness of Platelet Transfusions

- In raising the platelet count of patients with ITP or post-transfusion purpura.
- To treat neonatal alloimmune thrombocytopenia unless platelets from specially selected donors, such as the infant's mother, are used.

Harmful Effects of Leukocytes

- Centrifugally separated cellular blood components contain between 10^8 to 10^9 white blood cells (WBC)/unit.
- Sensitize recipients to human leukocyte antigens (HLA) and cause refractoriness to platelet transfusions.
- Cause graft vs. host disease (GvHD) and immune modulation.
- These "passenger" leukocytes may carry such infectious agents as cytomegalovirus (CMV) and HTLV I/II.

CHAPTER

38

Hypertensive Disorders Complicating Pregnancy

CLASSIFICATION

According to National High Blood Pressure Education Program Working Group on High Blood Pressure in Pregnancy:

1. **Gestational Hypertension**
   - Systolic BP ≥140 or diastolic BP ≥90 mm Hg for first time during pregnancy after 20 weeks
   - No proteinuria
   - BP returns to normal before 12 weeks' postpartum
   - Final diagnosis made only postpartum
   - May have other signs or symptoms of preeclampsia, e.g. epigastric discomfort or thrombocytopenia.
2. **Preeclampsia**

   Minimum criteria
   - BP ≥140/90 mm Hg after 20 weeks' gestation on two occasions 4–6 hrs apart in right upper limb in sitting or lateral position
   - Proteinuria ≥300 mg/24 hours or ≥1+ dipstick (≥30 mg/dL)

   Increased certainty of preeclampsia:
   - BP ≥160/110 mm Hg
   - Proteinuria ≥2.0 g/24 hours or ≥2 + dipstick
   - Serum creatinine >1.2 mg/dL unless known to be previously elevated
   - Platelets <100,000/L
   - Microangiopathic hemolysis—increased LDH (>600 U/L)
   - Elevated serum transaminase levels—ALT or AST
   - Persistent headache or other cerebral or visual disturbance
   - Persistent epigastric pain.

Mild Preeclampsia

Preeclampsia which is not severe.

- BP 140/90 to 160/110 mm Hg
- Proteinuria <2+ on dipstick or >300 mg but <5 g in 24 hour urine.

Severe Preeclampsia

- Severe hypertension in association with proteinuria
  - Blood pressure reading, with the patient at rest, of at least 160 mm Hg systolic or 110 mm Hg diastolic pressure on two occasions at least 6 hours

apart. In practice, after a diastolic pressure reading of 110 mm Hg, the clinician should not wait for 6 hours for diagnosis and treatment.

OR

- Hypertension in association with severe proteinuria
    - Proteinuria levels of at least 5 g in 24 hour urine collection or 3+ to 4+ on semiquantitative assay collected at least 4 hours apart.

OR

- If there is multiorgan involvement such as–
  One or more of the following criteria are present:
    - Oliguria, 24 hour urinary output of less than 500 mL
    - Cerebral or visual disturbances, altered consciousness, headache, scotoma, or blurred vision
    - Pulmonary edema
    - Epigastric or right upper quadrant pain caused by stretching of Glisson's capsule. Occasionally pain precedes hepatic rupture.
    - Impaired liver function test of unclear etiology
    - Thrombocytopenia
    - Intrauterine growth restriction.

3. **Eclampsia**
    - Seizures that cannot be attributed to other causes in a woman with preeclampsia.
4. **Superimposed Preeclampsia on Chronic Hypertension**
    - New-onset proteinuria ≥300 mg/24 hours in hypertensive women but no proteinuria before 20 weeks' gestation
    - A sudden increase in proteinuria or blood pressure or platelet count <100,000/L in women with hypertension and proteinuria before 20 weeks' gestation.
5. **Chronic Hypertension**
    - BP ≥140/90 mm Hg before pregnancy or diagnosed before 20 weeks' gestation not attributable to gestational trophoblastic disease, OR
    - Hypertension first diagnosed after 20 weeks' gestation and persistent after 12 weeks' postpartum.

Diagnosis

1. **Blood pressure:** Elevated BP is the traditional hallmark for diagnosis of the disease.
   BP ≥140/90 mm Hg, two readings 4–6 hrs apart.

Blood Pressure Measurement

Equipment

Mercury sphygmomanometer provides the accurate measurement.
The length of the BP cuff bladder should be 3/4th of arm length.
The width should be 2/3rd of the circumference of the upper arm.

Appropriate cuff size—

- Arm circumference 22–26 cm—small adult cuff 12×22 cm
- Arm circumference 27–34 cm—adult cuff 16×30 cm

- Arm circumference 35–44 cm—large adult cuff 16×36 cm
- Arm circumference 45–52 cm—adult thigh cuff 16×42 cm

Technique

- The BP is taken in sitting position with the back supported
- The arm should be supported at the level of the heart
- The mercury sphygmomanometer should be visible but doesn't have to be at the level of the heart
- The BP cuff should be placed with the bladder midline over the brachial artery 2–3 cm above the antecubital fossa
- Check systolic BP by palpatory method, inflate the cuff to a pressure 30 mm Hg greater than systolic BP
- The stethoscope should be placed lightly over the brachial artery
- Deflate the cuff slowly at the rate of 2–3 mmHg per heartbeat
- Systolic BP — Korotkoff phase I, Diastolic BP — Korotkoff phase V.

Errors

- Small cuff–overestimation of systolic BP by 10–50 mmHg in obese patients—pressure generated may not be fully transmitted to the brachial artery. So, pressure in the cuff is higher than the intra-arterial pressure
- Arm below the level of heart–BP will be elevated by 10–12 mm Hg due to the added hydrostatic pressure induced by gravity (1 cm low–0.7 mm Hg elevation)
- Arm above the heart level–BP will be lowered
- Patients' sleeves should not be rolled as this may act as a tourniquet
- Stethoscope is placed almost over the antecubital fossa—minimizes artifactual noise related to stethoscope touching the cuff
- Exerting pressure over brachial artery by stethoscope—turbulence is increased and disappearance of the sound is delayed.

2. **Proteinuria**

   Excretion of 300 mg/24 hour urine protein or if this method is not available, 30 mg/dL (≥1+ on dipstick) or more in at least 2 random urine samples collected at least 4–6 hrs apart in the absence of urinary infection.
   - 1 + 0.3–0.45 g/L
   - 2 + 0.45–1.0 g/L
   - 3 + 1–3 g/L
   - 4 + ≥3 g/L–10 g/L

3. **Excessive Weight Gain and Edema**

   Excessive weight gain (>0.5 kg/week/2 kg/month) and edema are not included in the diagnostic features of preeclampsia, but it should alert the clinician to screen for preeclampsia.

   Edema: After 12 hour of rest in lying down position.

   Grades: I—Ankle
II—Below knee
III—Face, hand, abdominal wall, vulva
IV—Anasarca

4. **Other Signs and Symptoms (Suggestive of Imminent Eclampsia)**
   - **Headache:** Frontal/Occipital, pulsatile/dull, may occur simultaneously with visual symptoms, not relieved by analgesics

Due to abnormal cerebral perfusion pressure usually precedes eclampsia.

- Epigastric/Right upper quadrant pain: May be associated with nausea and vomiting, indicative of imminent eclampsia
  - Due to hepatic ischemia
  - Stretching of hepatic capsule (Glisson's capsule) due to edema and hemorrhage
  - Associated with ↑ SGOT, SGPT and LDH
- Visual disturbances: Scotomas, blurred vision, blindness due to
  - Spasm of retinal vessels
  - Edema
  - Retinal detachment.

Fundoscopy: Keith Wagner Classification

Grade 1—Mild generalized narrowing of arterioles
Broadening of arteriolar light reflex
Vein: Artery = 3:1. In hypertensive retinopathy (normal is 3:2)

Grade 2—Diffuse generalized narrowing of arterioles with focal attenuation and deflection of veins along AV crossings (Salu's signs)

Grade 3—Grade 2 + Bonnet's sign (banking of veins along AV crossings) and Gunn's sign (tapering of veins on either side of AV deflection) + copper wiring

Grade 4—Grade 3 + silver wiring + papilledema

Fundoscopy in Preeclampsia

Grade 0: Normal
Grade 1: Arterial spasm
Grade 2: Arteriovenous crossing
Grade 3: Edema, hemorrhage, exudates
Grade 4: Papilledema

Pre-existing Vascular Disease

Arteriolar sclerosis detected by ↑light reflex, copper wiring and arteriovenous nicking

- **Hyper-reflexia:** Does not correlate with severity of disease.
  - It is due to CNS irritability.
  - Clonus is suggestive of imminent eclampsia.
- **Oliguria:** <500 mL/24 hour

Laboratory Findings

- Thrombocytopenia: <1 lakh/mm^3
  - Incidence 20%
  - Caused by microangiopathy
- Coagulation screening: PT/aPTT prolonged if platelet <10,000/mm^3
- Liver function test
  - SGOT >40 IU/L
  - SGPT >40 IU/L

- LDH >600 U/L

After delivery SGOT and SGPT, decrease by 5 days, LDH by 10 days.

- Renal Function Test (RFT)

Renal Function Test	Normal	Severe preeclampsia
S. creatinine	0.8 mg%	>1.3–1.4 mg%
B. urea	15 mg%	>20–25 mg%
Creatinine clearance	>130 mL/minute	<100 mL/minute
S. uric acid	4–5.5 mg%	>6 mg%

  - ↑ uric acid in preeclampsia in the last trimester is indicative of poor fetal prognosis
  - Hyperuricemia is as a result of ↓ urate clearance by PCT
  - In PE, renal tubular function is affected earlier than glomerular function. ↓ clearance of uric acid precedes changes in GFR
- Hematological abnormalities:
  - ↑ Hb and PCV caused by ↓ plasma volume
  - Fibrinogen usually increases but decreases (<200 mg% in Abruptio placenta
  - D-dimer >0.5 mg%—Severe disease
  - Thrombin time prolonged in 50% of severe preeclampsia [(N) 10 15 seconds].

Diagnostic Difficulties:

1. Multigravida—severe preeclampsia is rare, so look for chronic hypertension; chronic renal disease, APLA
2. Severe hypertension in early gestation
3. Hepatitis, gallstones
4. Epilepsy
5. TTP
6. HUS
7. Acute fatty liver of pregnancy
8. SLE
9. Sepsis
10. Fluctuating BP, episodic headache, sweating and palpitation suspect pheochromocytoma. Estimation of 24 hour urine sample for vanillylmandelic acid (VMA) is important (before this if she is on M dopa, it should be stopped for at least 48 hours, banana, coca foods should be avoided for correct results).

Risk Factors for Preeclampsia

1. Couple-related risk factors:
   - New paternity
   - Limited sperm exposure
   - Pregnancies after donor insemination, oocyte donation, embryo donation
2. Maternal or pregnancy-related risk factors:
   - Extremes of maternal age
   - Multifetal gestation
   - Preeclampsia in previous pregnancy
   - Chronic hypertension and/or renal disease

- Maternal autoimmune conditions (e.g. rheumatological disease, SLE)
- Obesity and insulin resistance (with or without PCOS, the risk is proportionate to BMI)
- Pre-gestational diabetes mellitus
- Preexisting thrombophilias
- Maternal susceptibility genes
- Family history of preeclampsia
- Smoking (reduced risk)
- Hydropic degeneration of the placenta.

Predictive Tests for Preeclampsia Syndrome

Testing related to	Examples
Placental perfusion/ vascular resistance	Roll-over test, isometric hand grip or cold pressor test, angiotensin II infusion test, mid-trimester mean arterial pressure, platelet angiotensin II binding, rennin, 24 hour ambulatory blood pressure monitoring, uterine artery or fetal transcranial Doppler velocimetry
Fetal-placental unit endocrine dysfunction	hCG, AFP, PAPP A, inhibin A, activin A, placental protein 13, CRH
Renal dysfunction	Serum uric acid, microalbuminuria, urinary calcium or Kallikrein, microtrasferrinuria, N-acetyl β-glucosaminidase
Endothelial dysfunction/oxidant stress	Platelet count and activation, fibronectin, endothelial adhesion molecules, prostaglandin, thromboxane, CRP, cytokines, endothelin, neurokinin B, homocysteine, lipids, antiphospholipid antibodies, plasminogen activator inhibitor, leptin, p-selectin, angiogenic factors to include placental growth factor, VEGF, fms-like tyrosine kinase receptor- 1 (sFlt-1), endoglin
Others/miscellaneous	Antithrombin III, atrial natriuretic peptide, β_2 microglobulin, genetic markers, free fetal DNA, serum proteonomic markers

Predictors of Preeclampsia

Test	+ve finding	Sensitivity	Specificity	PPV	NPV
DBP <20 weeks	≥80	32–46%	84–91	20–30	95
	≥85	16–31%	93–97	20–30	95
II trimester MAP (18–26 weeks)	≥90	82%	68	20	98
Hand grip test	SBP ≥15 DBP ≥20	54%	98	79	93
Roll-over test (28–32 weeks)	DBP ≥20	25–88%	92–95	33–93	89–91
Angiotensin sensitivity (28–37 week)	≤80 g/kg/ minute to ↑ DBP	75–76	83–99	45–90	9–95
	≥20 ≤100 g	92	86	50	99
Biochemical screening (serum)					
S.Fe	>100 µg%	83%	87%	–	–

Contd...

Contd...

SAFP	>2 MOM	25% Risk			
Platelet angiotensin II binding	↑	88	87	78	83
Uric acid levels	↑	88	97	–	–
AT-III levels	<70% nonpg control	–	–	80	89
Fibronectin levels	↑ 400 mg/mL	38	97	38	97
Biochemical screening test (urine)					
Ca/Creatinine 24–34 weeks	<0.0.4	70	95	64	96
2, 3 di-6 keto PGF12	<400 pg/mg	–	–	65	82
N acetyl-β-D-glucosaminidase	Creatinine	80	78	21	98
Microalbuminuria	↑↑	83	94	–	–
Kallikrein:Creatinine (16–20 weeks)	≥11 μg/mL	67–70	75–86	–	–
24 hour Ca	≤170 <12 mg%	–	–	85%	91%
Doppler USG					
Uterine and umbilical A. (21–24 weeks)	Abnormal flow RI >0.58	77–93	85–94	7–28	70–90
Arcuate A. (16–18 weeks)	Diastolic notching	68	69	42	87
Arcuate A. (18–20 weeks)	Diastolic notching	64	84	70	80

Prevention of Preeclampsia

	Pregnancy outcome	Recommendations
Diet and exercise	No reduction in preeclampsia	Insufficient evidence to recommend
Protein or salt restriction	No reduction in preeclampsia	Not recommended
Magnesium or zinc supplementation	No reduction in preeclampsia	Not recommended
Fish oil supplementation and other sources of fatty acids	No effect in low risk or high risk populations	Insufficient evidence to recommend
Calcium supplementation 2 g/day	Reduced preeclampsia (30%) in those at high risk and with low baseline dietary supplementation. No effect on perinatal outcome	Recommended for women at high risk of gestational hypertension and in communities with low dietary calcium intake
Low dose aspirin I mg/kg	19% reduction in risk of preeclampsia, 16% reduction in fetal/ neonatal deaths	Consider in high-risk populations
Heparin or low molecular weight heparin 5000–10000 units SC bd	Reduced preeclampsia in women with renal disease and in women with thrombophilia	Lack of randomized trials, not recommended

Contd...

Contd...

Antioxidant vitamins (C,E)	No reduction in preeclampsia	Number of adverse effects including increased risk of stillbirth and of birth weight <2.5 kg. Not recommended
Antihypertensive medications in women with chronic hypertension	Risk of women developing severe hypertension reduced by half, but not risk of preeclampsia	No evidence to recommend

Advise women at high risk of preeclampsia to take 75 mg of aspirin* daily from 12 weeks until the birth of the baby.

Women at high risk are those with any of the following:
- Hypertensive disease during a previous pregnancy
- Chronic kidney disease
- Autoimmune disease such as systemic lupus erythematosis or antiphospholipid syndrome
- Type 1 or type 2 diabetes
- Chronic hypertension.

Advise women with more than one moderate risk factor for preeclampsia to take 75 mg of aspirin* daily from 12 weeks until the birth of the baby.

Factors indicating moderate risk are:
- First pregnancy
- Age 40 years or older
- Pregnancy interval of more than 10 years
- Body mass index (BMI) of 35 kg/m^2 or more at first visit
- Family history of preeclampsia
- Multiple pregnancy.

Tell women who had preeclampsia that their risk of developing —
- Gestational hypertension in a future pregnancy ranges from about 1 in 8 (13%) pregnancies to about 1 in 2 (53%) pregnancies
- Preeclampsia in a future pregnancy is up to about 1 in 6 (16%) pregnancies
- Preeclampsia in a future pregnancy is about 1 in 4 (25%) pregnancies if their preeclampsia was complicated by severe preeclampsia, HELLP syndrome or eclampsia and led to birth before 34 weeks, and about 1 in 2 (55%) pregnancies if it led to birth before 28 weeks.
- Mild hypertension diastolic blood pressure 90–99 mm Hg, systolic blood pressure 140–149 mm Hg
- Moderate hypertension diastolic blood pressure 100–109 mm Hg, systolic blood pressure 150–159 mm Hg
- Severe hypertension diastolic blood pressure 1–10 mm Hg or greater, systolic blood pressure 160 mm Hg or greater.

If an automated reagent-strip reading device is used to detect proteinuria and a result of 1+ or more is obtained, use a spot urinary protein: creatinine ratio or 24-hour urine collection to quantify proteinuria. Diagnose significant proteinuria if the urinary protein:creatinine ratio is greater than 30 mg/mmol or a validated 24-hour urine collection result shows greater than 300 mg protein.

In women with gestational hypertension, take account of the following risk factors that require additional assessment and follow-up:

- Nulliparity
- Age 40 years or older
- Pregnancy interval of more than 10 years
- Family history of preeclampsia
- Multiple pregnancy
- BMI of 35 kg/m^2 or more
- Gestational age at presentation
- Previous history of preeclampsia or gestational hypertension
- Pre-existing vascular disease
- Pre-existing kidney disease.

Management of Gestational Hypertension

- Women with gestational hypertension are at risk for progression to either severe preeclampsia (9.6%), mild preeclampsia (46%) or eclampsia, therefore, require close observation of maternal and fetal conditions.
  Maternal evaluation: Weekly prenatal visits, education about reporting pre-eclamptic symptoms, evaluation of urine albumin. Uncontrolled BP, occurrence of preeclamptic symptoms–Perform CBC, liver function test.
  Fetal evaluation: Ultrasound examination of fluid and estimated fetal weight at the time of diagnosis and repeated every month. NST to be done, from 37 weeks and repeated weekly. Fetal Doppler to be done in cases with IUGR.
- Antihypertensive drugs to be started when BP ≥150/100 mm Hg
- The onset of maternal symptoms or a sudden increase in BP to severe values or development of proteinuria (≥2+ on dipstick) requires prompt hospitalization for close evaluation
- If BP is well-controlled, continue pregnancy until 40 weeks
- Abnormalities in maternal and fetal surveillance is an indication to terminate pregnancy before 40 weeks.

General Principles of Management of Preeclampsia

- The only effective treatment is to deliver the infant and placenta, ciliary therapy is predominantly symptomatic and not directed at underlying cause
- Primary objective must always be the safety of mother
- Decision between immediate delivery and expectant management must be individualized after careful assessment of severity of disease, gestational age, maternal and fetal status at the time of initial evaluation, presence of labor or rupture of membranes.

Management of Mild Preeclampsia

- No salt restriction
- No limitation
- No anti-hypertensives
- No diuretics
- No sedatives
- High-protein diet – 80–100 g/d

	Management of pregnancy with gestational hypertension			Management of pregnancy with preeclampsia		
Degree of hypertension	**Mild hypertension (140/90 to 149/99 mm Hg)**	**Moderate hypertension (150/100 to 159/109 mm Hg)**	**Severe hypertension (160/110 mm Hg or higher)**	**Mild hypertension (140/90 to 149/99 mm Hg)**	**Moderate hypertension (150/100 to 159/109 mm Hg)**	**Severe hypertension (160/110 mm Hg or higher)**
Admit to hospital	No	No	Yes (until blood pressure is 159/109 mm Hg or lower)	Yes	Yes	Yes
Treat	No	With oral labetalol as first-line treatment to keep: • Diastolic blood pressure between 80–100 mm Hg • Systolic blood pressure less than 150 mm Hg	With oral labetalol as first-line treatment to keep: • Diastolic blood pressure between 80–100 mm Hg • Systolic blood pressure less than 150 mm Hg	No	With oral labetalol as first-line treatment to keep: • Diastolic blood pressure between 80–100 mm Hg • Systolic blood pressure less than 150 mm Hg only offer women with gestational hypertension antihypertensive treatment other than labetalol after considering side-effect profiles for the woman, fetus and newborn baby. Alternatives include methyldopa and nifedipine	With oral labetalol as first-line treatment to keep: • Diastolic blood pressure between 80–100 mm Hg • Systolic blood pressure less than 150 mm Hg • Labetalol (oral or intravenous) • Hydralazine (intravenous) (consider using up to 500 mL crystalloid fluid before or at the same time as the first dose of intravenous hydralazine in the antenatal period) • Nifedipine (oral)
Measure blood pressure	Not more than once a week	At least twice a week	At least four times a day	At least four times a day	At least four times a day	More than four times a day, depending on clinical circumstances

Contd...

Contd...

Test for proteinuria	At each visit using automated reagent-strip reading device or urinary protein: creatinine ratio	At each visit using automated reagent-strip reading device or urinary protein: creatinine ratio	Daily using automated reagent-strip reading device or urinary protein: creatinine ratio		Do no repeat quantification of proteinuria	Do not repeat quantification of proteinuria	Do no repeat quantification of proteinuria
Blood tests	Only those for routine antenatal care	Test kidney function, electrolytes, full blood count, transaminases, bilirubin Do not carry out further blood tests if no proteinuria at subsequent visits	Test at presentation and then monitor weekly: Kidney function electrolytes, full blood count, transaminases, bilirubin		Monitor using the following tests twice a week: kidney function, electrolytes, full blood count, transaminases, bilirubin	Monitor using the following tests three times a week: kidney function, electrolytes, full blood count, transaminases, bilirubin	Monitor using the following tests three times a week: kidney function, electrolytes, full blood count, transaminases, bilirubin

Fetal monitoring:

Chronic hypertension

- Ultrasound fetal growth and amniotic fluid volume assessment and umbilical artery doppler velocimetry between 28 and 30 weeks and between 32 and 34 weeks. If results are normal, do not repeat at more than 34 weeks, unless otherwise clinically indicated
- Cardiotocography if fetal activity is abnormal

Mild or moderate gestational hypertension

- Ultrasound fetal growth and amniotic fluid volume assessment and umbilical artery Doppler velocimetry if diagnosis is confirmed at less than 34 weeks. If results are normal, do not repeat at more than 34 weeks, unless otherwise clinically indicated
- Cardiotocography if fetal activity is abnormal

Severe gestational hypertension or pre-eclampsia

- Cardiotocography at diagnosis of severe gestational hypertension or pre-eclampsia
- If conservative management of severe gestational hypertension or preeclampsia is planned, carry out all the following tests at diagnosis:

Contd...

Contd...

- Ultrasound fetal growth and amniotic fluid volume assessment
  - Umbilical artery doppler velocimetry
- If the results of all fetal monitoring are normal do not routinely repeat cardiotocography more than weekly
- Repeat cardiotocography if any of the following occur:
  - The woman reports a change in fetal movement
  - Vaginal bleeding
  - Abdominal pain
  - Deterioration in maternal condition
- Do not routinely repeat ultrasound fetal growth and amniotic fluid volume assessment or umbilical artery doppler velocimetry more than every 2 weeks
- If the results of any fetal monitoring are abnormal, case needs to be individualized

Women at high risk of pre-eclampsia

- Carry out ultrasound fetal growth and amniotic fluid volume assessment and umbilical artery doppler velocimetry starting at between 28 and 30 weeks (or at least 2 weeks before previous gestational age of onset if earlier than 28 weeks) and repeating 4 weeks later in women with previous:
  - Severe pre-eclampsia
  - Pre-eclampsia that needed birth before 34 weeks
  - Pre-eclampsia with a baby whose birth weight was less than the 10th centile
  - Intrauterine death
  - Placental abruption
- Carry out cardiotocography if fetal activity is abnormal

Timing of birth

Severe preeclampsia:

- Manage pregnancy in women with pre-eclampsia conservatively until 34 weeks
- Offer birth to women with pre-eclampsia before 34 weeks, after discussion with neonatal and anesthetic teams and a course of corticosteroids has been given if: severe hypertension develops refractory to treatment maternal or fetal indications develop

Mild or moderate preeclampsia:

At 34 + 0 to 36 + 6 weeks depending on maternal and fetal condition, risk factors and availability of neonatal intensive care

- Recommend birth within 24–48 hours after 37+ 0 weeks

Contd...

Contd...

Gestational hypertension:
- Do not offer birth before 37 weeks to women with gestational hypertension whose blood pressure is lower than 160/110 mm Hg, with or without antihypertensive treatment
- For women with gestational hypertension whose blood pressure is lower than 160/1 10 mm Hg after 37 weeks, with or without antihypertensive treatment, timing of birth, and maternal and fetal indications for birth should be agreed between the woman and the senior obstetrician
- Offer birth to women with refractory severe gestational hypertension after a course of corticosteroids (if required) has been completed

INTRAPARTUM CARE

Blood pressure
- During labor, measure blood pressure: hourly in women with mild or moderate hypertension continually in women with severe hypertension
- Continue use of antenatal antihypertensive treatment during labour
- Hematological and biochemical monitoring
- Determine the need for haematological and biochemical tests during labour in women with mild or moderate hypertension using the same criteria as in the antenatal period even if regional analgesia is being considered
- Care during epidural analgesia
- Do not preload women who have severe pre-eclampsia with intravenous fluids before establishing low-dose epidural analgesia and combined spinal epidural analgesia

Management of the second stage of labor
- Do not routinely limit the duration of the second stage of labor: in women with stable mild or moderate hypertension or if blood pressure is controlled within target ranges in women with severe hypertension
- Recommend operative birth in the second stage of labor for women with severe hypertension whose hypertension has not responded to initial treatment

Anticonvulsants
- Consider giving intravenous magnesium sulphate if birth is planned within 24 hours
- Indications for MGSO4:
  - Severe hypertension and proteinuria
  - Mild or moderate hypertension and proteinuria with one or more of the following:
    - Symptoms of severe headache
    - Problems with vision, such as blurring or flashing before the eyes
    - Severe pain just below the ribs or vomiting
    - Papilloedema

Contd...

Contd...

- Signs of clonus (≥3 beats)
  - Liver tenderness
  - HELLP syndrome
- If considering magnesium sulfate* treatment, use the following as features of severe pre-eclampsia:
  - Platelet count falling to below 100 x 109 per liter
  - Abnormal liver enzymes (ALT or AST rising to above 70 IU/liter).

Regimen for administration of magnesium sulfate:*

- Loading dose of 4 g should be given intravenously over 5 minutes, followed by an infusion of 1 g/hour maintained for 24 hours
- Recurrent seizures should be treated with a further dose of 2–4 g given over 5 minutes
- Do not use diazepam, phenytoin or lytic cocktail as an alternative to magnesium sulphate* in women with eclampsia

Corticosteroids for fetal lung maturation

- If birth is considered likely within 7 days in women with pre-eclampsia: give two doses of betamethasone* 12 mg intramuscularly 24 hours apart in women between 24 and 34 weeks
- Consider giving two doses of betamethasone* 12 mg intramuscularly 24 hours apart in women between 35 and 36 weeks

Postnatal management of women with gestational hypertension	Postnatal management of women with preeclampsia
1. In women with gestational hypertension, who have given birth, measure blood pressure: • Daily for the first 2 days after birth • At least once between day 3 and day 5 after birth • As clinically indicated if antihypertensive treatment is changed after birth • Continue use of antenatal antihypertensive treatment • Consider reducing antihypertensive treatment if their blood pressure falls below 140/90 mm Hg • Reduce antihypertensive treatment if their blood pressure falls below 130/80 mm Hg • If a woman has taken methyldopa to treat gestational hypertension, stop within 2 days of birth • Offer women who have had gestational hypertension and remain on antihypertensive treatment after 2 weeks, a medical review • Offer women who have had gestational hypertension and who still need antihypertensive treatment at the postnatal review (6–8 weeks after the birth) a specialist assessment of their hypertension **2. For women with gestational hypertension, who did not take antihypertensive treatment and have given birth** • Start antihypertensive treatment if their blood pressure is higher than 149/99 mm Hg • Offer women who have had gestational hypertension a medical review at the postnatal review (6–8 weeks after the birth). **Antihypertensives:** • The following antihypertensive drugs have no known adverse effects on babies receiving breast milk: – Labetalol – Nifedipine – Enalapril – Captopril	**1. In women with preeclampsia who did not take antihypertensive treatment and have given birth, measure blood pressure:** • At least four times a day while the woman is an inpatient • At least once between day 3 and day 5 after birth • On alternate days until normal if blood pressure was abnormal on days 3–5 • Start antihypertensive treatment if blood pressure is 150/100 mm Hg or higher • Offer women who have had preeclampsia a medical review at the postnatal review (6–8 weeks after the birth). **2. Ask women with preeclampsia who have given birth about severe headache and epigastric pain each time blood pressure is measured** **3. In women with preeclampsia who took antihypertensive treatment and have given birth, measure blood pressure:** • At least four times a day while the woman is an inpatient • Every 1–2 days for up to 2 weeks until the woman is off treatment and has no hypertension • Continue antenatal antihypertensive treatment (methyldopa should be stopped within 2 days of delivery) • Consider reducing antihypertensive treatment if their blood pressure falls below 140/ 90 mm Hg • Reduce antihypertensive treatment if their blood pressure falls below 130/80 mm Hg • Offer women who have had preeclampsia and remain on antihypertensive treatment after 2 weeks, a medical review • Offer women who have had preeclampsia and who still need antihypertensive treatment at the postnatal review (6–8 weeks after the birth) a specialist assessment of their hypertension

Contd...

Contd...

– Atenolol – Metoprolol • There is insufficient evidence on the safety in babies receiving breast milk of the following antihypertensive drugs: – ARBs – Amlodipine – ACE inhibitors other than enalapril and captopril Avoid diuretic treatment for hypertension if the woman is breastfeeding or expressing milk	**Hematological and biochemical monitoring** • In women who have preeclampsia with mild or moderate hypertension, or after step-down from critical care: measure platelet count, transaminases and serum creatinine 48–72 hours after birth or step-down • Do not repeat platelet count, transaminases or serum creatinine measurements if results are normal at 48–72 hours • If biochemical and hematological indices are improving but stay within the abnormal range in women with preeclampsia who have given birth, repeat platelet count, transaminases and serum creatinine measurements as clinically indicated and at the postnatal review (6–8 weeks after the birth) • If biochemical and hematological indices are not improving relative to pregnancy ranges in women with preeclampsia who have given birth, repeat platelet count, transaminases and serum creatinine measurements as clinically indicated • In women with preeclampsia who have given birth, carry out a urinary reagent—strip test at the postnatal review (6–8 weeks after the birth). • In women with preeclampsia who have given birth and have stepped down from critical care level 2, do not measure fluid balance if creatinine is within the normal range • Offer women who had preeclampsia and still have proteinuria (1+ or more) at the postnatal review (6–8 weeks after the birth) a further review at 3 months after the birth to assess kidney function and consider offering them a referral for specialist kidney assessment

Expectant Management of Severe Preeclampsia

- Preeclampsia remote from term (28–34 weeks) can be managed conservatively with fetal surveillance and monitoring for disease progression
- Average time gained in expectant management is 10–14 days. This reduces perinatal morbidity by 50%.

Principles of Expectant Management

- Reduce BP (main aim is to prevent cerebrovascular accident)
- Prevent convulsions with $MgSO_4$
- Use IV fluids carefully to avoid fluid overload.

Selection of Candidates for Expectant Management

Maternal

- Controlled HTN
- Urinary protein of any amount
- Oliguria <0.5 mL/kg/hour which resolves with routine fluid and food intake
- AST/ALT >2 times normal without epigastric pain or right hypochondrial tenderness.

Fetal

- BPP ≥6
- AFI >2 cm
- USG EFW >5th percentile
- Admission: Administer magnesium sulfate, steroids, antihypertensives
- Determine the eligibility for expectant management in 24 hours.

Indications for Expeditious Delivery (Within 72 Hours)

Maternal

- Uncontrolled severe HTN
- Eclampsia
- Platelet <1 lakh/μl
- AST/ALT >2 times the normal with epigastric pain or RUQ tenderness
- Pulmonary edema
- ↓ Renal function
- Abruptio placenta
- Headache (persistent)
- Visual disturbance.

Fetal

- Repetitive late or severe variable decelerations
- BPP ≤4 on two occasions 4 hour apart AFI ≤2 cm
- USG EFW ≤5th percentile
- Umbilical artery Doppler: Reverse diastolic flow.

Indications for Immediate Delivery

- Fetal distress
- HELLP.

Clinical Monitoring

- Monitor BP 4–6 hourly
- Watch for symptoms of imminent eclampsia
- Headache–paracetamol–persistent after 6 hours–$MgSO_4$–persists–deliver
- Input/Output chart
- Daily weight monitoring
- DFMC
- Fetal heart rate monitoring.

Laboratoy Studies During Expectant Management

- Platelet count
- ALT, AST, LDH, creatinine
- Clotting studies not required in preeclampsia not associated with drop in platelets; D-dimer (not INR and aPTT) useful in detecting early stages of DIC
- 24 hour urine collection for protein and creatinine remains the gold standard.

Fetal Assessment During Expectant Management

- Daily NST
- BPP biweekly
- Fetal Doppler velocimetry biweekly
- Ultrasound documentation of fetal growth at every 2 weeks.

Guidelines for Fetal Surveillance

Hypertension	Modality	Frequency
Chronic hypertension	Early dating ultrasound for fetal growth/AFV/UAD	First trimester as per clinical assessment
Gestational hypertension	Ultrasound for fetal growth/ AFV/UAD	At time of diagnosis and every 3–4 weeks
Preeclampsia	Ultrasound for fetal growth/ AFV/UAD Cardiotocography	At time of diagnosis and every 2–3 weeks Twice weekly
Preeclampsia with IUGR	Cardiotocography AFV/UAD Ultrasound for fetal growth	Twice weekly On admission and twice weekly Every 2 weeks

*AFV, Aminiotic fluid volume; UAD, Umbilical artery Doppler

LABOR AND DELIVERY

Indications for Delivery

Maternal

- Persistent severe HTN

- Persistent cerebral symptoms
- Persistent epigastric pain
- Progressive thrombocytopenia
- Abnormal liver enzymes with hemolysis
- Onset of labor, rupture of membranes/bleeding P/V.

Fetal

- Severe IUGR
- Non-reactive NST with abnormal BPP
- Oligoamnios.

Mode of Delivery

- **Indications for cesarean section:**
  1. Breech <2 kg.
  2. BS <5 and gestational age <30 weeks (should be individualized: Because of ↑ AP, FGR and fetal distress).
  3. Obstetric indications
     - Trial of induction within a limited time frame is warranted >30 weeks
     - Epidural analgesia is not contraindicated unless platelet count <75000 cu/mm^3
     - Close monitoring during labor and delivery
     - Urine output every hours
     - IV fluids <150 mL/hour.

Postpartum Management

- ≤44% of eclampsia occurs postpartum
- Resolution in 24 hours, severe cases take 2–4 days
- Keep the patient in recovery room for 12–24 hours
- Hourly I/O vitals, reflexes monitoring for 24 hours
- Urine albumin daily till it becomes undetectable
- No diuretics (unless there is pulmonary edema) and salt restriction
- Nifedipine is effective in control of BP as well as improving urine output during 24 hours after delivery
- At discharge: If BP is high, prescribe anti-hypertensives
- No need of prophylactic anticonvulsants
- Weekly check up
- After 12 weeks: BP not normal–evaluation of HTN.

Complications of Severe Preeclampsia

Maternal

- Abruptio placenta (1–4%)
- Disseminated coagulopathy/HELLP syndrome (10–20%)
- Pulmonary edema/aspiration (2–5%)
- Acute renal failure (1–5%)
- Eclampsia (<1%)
- Liver failure or hemorrhage (<1%)

- Stroke (rare)
- Death (rare)
- Long-term cardiovascular morbidity.

Fetal

- Preterm delivery (15–67%)
- Fetal growth restriction (10–25%)
- Hypoxia-neurologic injury (<1%)
- Perinatal death (1–2%)
- Long-term morbidity associated with low-birth-weight (fetal origin of adult disease).

Antihypertensives in Pregnancy

Antihypertensives may prevent cerebrovascular accident but do not prevent preeclampsia, alter the natural course of disease in women with mild preeclampsia or improve the perinatal outcome.

Class	Drug	Preparation	Initiating dose	Max dose	Common side effects
Centrally acting	Methyldopa clonidine	250 mg 0.1 mg	250 mg TID 0.1 mg BD	2 g 2.4 mg	Postural hypotension, drowsiness, dryness of mouth, headache, depression, swelling of feet
β-adrenergic blocker	Atenolol Labetolol	25,50 mg 25,100 mg	50 mg OD 100 mg BD	200 mg 2400 mg	Dizziness, drowsiness, insomnia, fatigue, bradycardia, swelling of feet, depression, shortness of breath
Calcium channel blockers	Nifedipine Amlodipine	5,10 mg 5,10 mg	10 mg TID 5 mg OD	120 mg 120 mg	Headache, dizziness, fatigue, flushing, palpitation, heart burn, constipation, nasal congestion, cough, peripheral edema, flushing, headache, vomiting, diarrhea, constipation
Vasodilator	Hydralazine	25 mg	25 mg TID	300 mg	Loss of appetite, eye-tearing, stuffy nose
α-1 blocker	Prazosin	1 mg	1 mg BD	20 mg	Drowsiness, dizziness headache, palpitations, dryness of mouth, unusual tiredness

Drugs in Acute Hypertensive Emergencies

Aim: Bring BP down to 140 systolic and 90 diastolic.

1. **Labetalol:**
   - Start with 20 mg IV as a bolus over 5–10 minutes; if effect is suboptimal after 20 minutes, give 40 mg IV bolus and 80 mg every 10 minutes for additional doses. Use a maximum of 300 mg in 24 hours.
   - For continuous IV administration of 20 mg/hour (200 mg, i.e. 40 mL vial in 160 mL of Ringer lactate). The resulting solution will contain 1 mg/mL. Initial dose is 20 mg/hour, dose can be doubled every 20 minutes up to a maximum of 200 mg/hour.
   - Once the blood pressure is controlled oral labetalol 100–400 mg every 12 hours can be started. If desired BP, levels are not achieved, switch to another drug.

   Contraindication: Bronchial asthma, CCF
2. **Nifedipine:** Start with 10 mg orally and repeat in 30 minutes if necessary. Maximum dose 120 mg. No sublingual nifedipine.
3. **Nitroglycerin**
   - Starting dose: 5 μg/minute
   - Usual dose: 200–300 μg/minute
   - Maximum dose: 400 μg/minute
   - Rate of increase 5 μg every 5 minute
   - Infusion: 200 μg in 500 ml NS in glass bottle via rigid polyethylene tube values in mL/hour microdrops/minute.

Indications for Prophylactic Magnesium Sulfate

- Severe preeclampsia
- Imminent eclampsia.

ECLAMPSIA

Convulsion/coma after 20 weeks of pregnancy, during labor and/or within 7 days of delivery usually associated with signs of preeclampsia.

Until proved otherwise, all pregnant women with convulsions should be considered to have eclampsia.

Types

- Antepartum—50%
- Intercurrent—Patient recovers from the convulsions and pregnancy continues beyond 48 hours (7–10 days) (not seen these days because eclampsia is the indication for termination)
- Intrapartum—30%
- Postpartum—20%, occurs within 4 days, but can occur up to 4 weeks.

Clinical Features

Phases of Eclamptic Seizures

Prodromal phase: There may be aura followed by twitching of the muscles of face, tongue and limbs. This stage lasts for 30 seconds.

Tonic phase: The entire body goes into tonic spasm–trunk opisthotonus, limbs are flexed, hands clenched, respiration ceases and tongue protrudes between the teeth, cyanosis appears, eyeballs become fixed. This stage lasts for 30 seconds.

Clonic phase: Grand mal convulsions occur starting from the facial muscles to involve the entire body. There is frothing at the mouth. This phase lasts for about 1–4 minutes.

Stage of recovery: The convulsions slowly subside, respiration resumes and the patient passes into a stage of coma of variable duration.

Investigations

- CBC with peripheral smear
- Blood group and type
- HIV, HBsAg, VDRL
- PIH profile—urine, albumin, blood urea, serum creatinine, serum uric acid, platelet count
- Liver enzymes—SGOT, SGPT
- If platelet count <1 lakh/cumm, send LDH, PS for hemolysis, DIC profile, fibrinogen
- Fundoscopy
- Neuroimaging studies (CT/MRI) indications are:
  - Neurological deficit
  - Prolonged coma
  - Atypical presentation of eclampsia (convulsion before 20 weeks or more than 48 hours after delivery)
  - Recurrent convulsions.

Prognosis

- Maternal mortality in eclampsia varies from 2–30%, with adequate treatment it should be <2%
- Perinatal mortality varies from 30–50% and is due to prematurity (spontaneous and induced, hypoxia and the effect of drugs used).

The following factors are associated with bad prognosis:

- Antepartum eclampsia
- Long interval between fits and delivery
- Late referrals
- Coma in between convulsions

- Very high blood pressure
- Oliguria
- Abnormal liver function tests and HELLP syndrome.

Management of Eclampsia

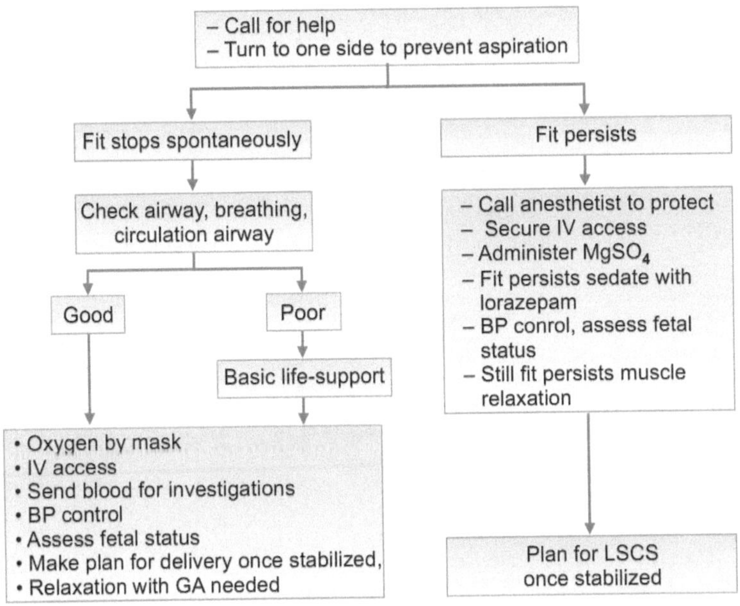

General Management

- Nurse in specialized intensive care units with all necessary equipment
- All external provoking stimuli are reduced to the minimum
- Nursed on railed cots with minimum handling and examinations
- Suction apparatuses, are used to keep the throat clear, and head end may be lowered to facilitate postural drainage. Sometimes a left lateral position may be needed
- Oxygen is always kept at hand. Care is taken to prevent pneumonia
- During a convulsion, soft, firm mouth gag is used to prevent injury to the tongue
- Maintain fluid balance. Fluid replacement should be with Ringer lactate/normal saline at the rate of 75 ml/h up to a maximum of 125 ml/h (Sibai 1999). Any overzealous infusion may precipitate pulmonary/cerebral edema
- Prophylactic antibiotic therapy is given to prevent infection
- Anti-hypertensive management. Same as mentioned for hypertensive crisis.

MEDICAL MANAGEMENT

Anti-convulsant Management

Regimen	Loading dose	Maintenance dose
Pritchard	4 g (20 mL of 20%) over 3–5 mts IV 10 g (20 mL of 50%) IM-5 g in each buttock	5 g 4th hourly IM, after ensuring presence of • Patellar reflex • Respiratory rate >14/minute • Urine output >30 mL/hour continued for 24 hours after the last convulsion or delivery whichever is later
Zuspan	4 g over 5–10 mts IV	1 g/hour IV
Sibai	6 g over 20 mts IV	2 g/hour IV
Suman Sardesai	4 g IV/IM	2 g IM/IV 3 hourly
Dhaka regimen	4 g IV over 10–15 minute + 2.5 g in each buttock	2.5 g IM every 4 hours
Lytic Cocktail Regime (Menon 1950)	25 mg of chlorpromazine + 100 mg pethidine in 20 mL of 5% dextrose IV + 50 mg of chromazine + 25 mg phenergan IM	50 mg of chlorpromazine + 25 mg phenargan IM 4th hourly--24 hours
Diazepam therapy (Lean)	40 mg IV infusion	40 mg in 500 mL 5% D IV
Phenytoin therapy (Reynolds)	10 mg/kg---5 mg/kg 2 hours later	200 mg orally after 12 hours till 48
ICMR low dose regimen (preferred in Indian women with low BMI)	3 gm, 15 ml of 20% $MgSO_4$ solution, IV over 15–20 minutes and 2.5 g of 50% $MgSO_4$ deep IM alternatively in each buttock	Every 4 hours, 2.5 g of 50% $MgSO_4$ deep IM, alternatively in each buttock

Single Dose Regimen

Single dose of 4 g of 20% magnesium sulfate given intravenously over 3 to 5 minutes. (8 mL of 50% $MgSO_4$ diluted in 12 cc of 5% dextrose or distilled water) followed by 4 g of 50% magnesium sulfate IM (undiluted 2 g on each buttock).

Side Effects

Maternal

$MgSO_4$ blood levels		Symptoms and signs
mg/dl	mEq/L	
4–8	4–8	Therapeutic
9–12	10	Nausea, warmth, flushing, somnolence, double vision, slurred speech,weakness, loss of patellar reflex
15–17	12	Muscular paralysis and respiratory difficulty
30–35		Cardiac arrest

Fetal

- No effect on BPP, no neonatal compromise
- Neurological, neuromuscular depression
- Protective effect against cerebral palsy
- Hyporeflexia
- Decreases FHR variability
- Low Apgar score
- Nosocomial infections, neutropenia
- Disturbed fetal calcium hemostasis.

Management of Magnesium Sulfate Toxicity

- Intravenous calcium as 10 mL of 10% calcium gluconate infusion is given slowly over three minutes (Calcium is the antidote for magnesium). If respiratory arrest ensues, prompt endotracheal intubation and ventilation are life saving.

  Serum magnesium levels to be monitored when:
  - IV $MgSO_4$ regimen is given
  - Oliguria and/or serum creatinine >1 mg/dL
  - Recurrent convulsions
  - There are other signs of magnesium toxicity.

If $MgSO_4$ is Contraindicated–

Phenytoin: 10–15 mg/kg body weight, slow IV infusion at 50 mg/minute, followed by 100 mg slow IV bolus every 6–8 hours.

Management of Status Eclampticus

- Convulsion episode persisting for more than 30 minutes or that which occurs in quick success without full recovery of consciousness in between the episodes
- Thiopentone sodium 0.5 g in 20 mL of 5% D IV along with intubation of the patient.

Management of Recurrence of Convulsions

- If convulsions occur half an hour after the loading dose, then it is called recurrence of convulsions
- Maintenance dose of 2 g magnesium sulfate is given IM every 3 hourly till 24 hours after delivery or after last convulsions whichever was later.

Obstetric Management

- Delivery is mandatory irrespective of gestational age
- If cervix is favorable, then induction of labor.

Indication for LSCS

- Unfavorable cervix
- Uncontrolled convulsions
- Deeply unconscious patient
- Uncontrolled blood pressure
- Other obstetrical indications.

HELLP Syndrome

(HELLP = hemolysis, elevated liver enzyme levels and low platelet count)

- 0.2–0.6% of all pregnancies.
- 4–12% of women with preeclampsia/eclampsia
- The syndrome presents antepartum—69% of patients (70%—28–36 weeks, 20% >3 weeks, 10% <28 weeks) postpartum—11–44% of patients.
- Post-partum HELLP: manifestation-few hours to 7 days, majority within–48 hours.

Risk Factors

- Multiparous
- White race
- Maternal age greater than 25 years
- Preeclamptic women—managed conservatively.

Criteria to Establish the Diagnosis of HELLP Syndrome

1. Hemolysis
   - Abnormal peripheral blood smear
   - Increased bilirubin ≥1.2 mg/dL
   - Increased lactic dehydrogenase >twice the upper limit of normal for the laboratory.
2. Elevated liver enzymes
   - Elevated ALT or AST greater than twice the upper limit of normal for the laboratory (≥72 IU/L)
   - Increased lactic dehydrogenase greater than twice the upper limit of normal for the laboratory (600 IU/L).
3. Low platelet count <100,000/mm^3

Clinical Features

- Approximately 90% of patients present with generalized malaise
- Epigastric pain/RUQ: 65% (30–90%)
- Nausea and vomiting: 30%
- Headache: 33–61%
- Visual changes: 17%
- Malaise or a nonspecific viral-like syndrome in the third trimester (evaluated with a CBC and LFT)
- Thrombocytopenia symptoms

- HTN (82–88%), mild HTN: 15–50%, normotensive: 12–18%
- Proteinuria (86–100%)
- No proteinuria 13%
- Hypoglycemia
- Hyponatremia
- Cortical blindness
- Transient nephrogenic diabetes insipidus.

Investigations

- Hemoglobin
- Low platelet count (<1,00,000 cells/mm^3)
- Abnormal peripheral smear (schistocytes, burr cells, echinocytes)
- Low serum haptoglobin levels
- Liver function test
  - Elevated serum bilirubin (indirect form)
  - Liver enzymes (AST/ALT >70 U/L)
  - Elevated lactate dehydrogenase (LDH) levels >600 U/L
- Coagulation profile: PT/aPTT/fibrinogen-normal unless associated with DIC
  - Laboratory abnormalities typically worsen after delivery and peak at 24 to 48 hours postpartum.

Classification

Mississippi Classification

Depending on platelet count, used to predict the rapidity of recovery postpartum, maternal-perinatal outcome, and the need for plasmapheresis.
Class I: Platelet nadir below 50,000/mm^3.
Class II: Platelet nadir between 50,000 and 100,000/mm^3.
Class III: Platelet nadir between 100,000 and 150,000/mm^3.

Tennessee and Memphis Classification

Complete HELLP
1. Platelet <1,00,000/cumm
2. LDH ≥ 600 IU/l
3. AST ≥ 70 IU/l

Partial HELLP
One or two of the above.

Medical and Surgical Disorders Confused with the HELLP Syndrome

- Acute fatty liver of pregnancy
- Appendicitis
- Diabetes mellitus
- Gallbladder disease
- Gastroenteritis
- Glomerulonephritis

- Hemolytic uremic syndrome
- Hepatic encephalopathy
- Hyperemesis gravidarum
- Idiopathic thrombocytopenia
- Kidney stones
- Peptic ulcer
- Pyelonephritis
- Systemic lupus erythematosus
- Thrombotic thrombocytopenic purpura
- Viral hepatitis.

Complications

- Maternal mortality rate—1.1%
- 1–25% of affected women develop DIC, placental abruption hepatorenal failure, pulmonary edema, pleural effusion, ARDS subcapsular hematoma and hepatic rupture
- Severe ascites (>1 lit)-cardiopulmonary complications
- Cerebral edema, retinal detachment
- ARF, sepsis, stroke.

Therapeutic Modalities Used to Treat or Reverse HELLP Syndrome

1. Antihypertensives: Same as for preeclampia.
2. Anticonvulsants: Same as eclampsia, use magnesium sulfate.
3. Bed rest.
4. Plasma volume expansion (crystalloids, albumin 5 to 25 percent).
5. Antithrombotic agents: If associated with DIC
   - Low-dose aspirin (50–150 mg/day)
   - Dipyridamole
   - Heparin
   - Antithrombin III
   - Prostacyclin infusions.
6. Immunosuppressive agents.

Role of Corticosteroids in HELLP

- Insufficient evidence to determine benefit
- Recent Cochrane review revealed no difference in primary outcomes of maternal and perinatal mortality or morbidity between control and study groups
- Few studies reveal that routine use of corticosteroids improve laboratory abnormalities, facilitates maternal transfer to a tertiary care center and also facilitates fetal lung maturity if preterm.

Corticosteroid therapy should be instituted in patients with HELLP platelet count of <100,000/cumm, 1.5 lakhs with eclampsia, epigastric pain, fulminant disease and should be continued until LFTs are resolving and the platelet count >100,000/cumm.

- Steroids given antenatally do not prevent the typical worsening of laboratory abnormalities after delivery. However, laboratory abnormalities resolve more quickly in patients who continue to receive steroids postpartum

- Steroids have to be given for 48 hours before delivery and continued for 24–48 hours postpartum
- Dose in antepartum 5–10 mg IV bd (dexamethasone)
- Miscellaneous
    - Fresh frozen plasma infusions
    - Exchange plasmapheresis
    - Dialysis.

Highlights

- Anticipate the diagnosis
- Evaluate the maternal condition
- Evaluate the fetal condition
- Control the hypertension
- Prophylaxis of convulsions with $MgSO_4$
- Water and electrolyte balance
- Hemotherapy
- Management of labor and delivery
- Optimize perinatal care
- Intensive postpartum treatment of the patient
- Be alert for multiple organ failure
- Advise on future pregnancy.

Obstetric Management

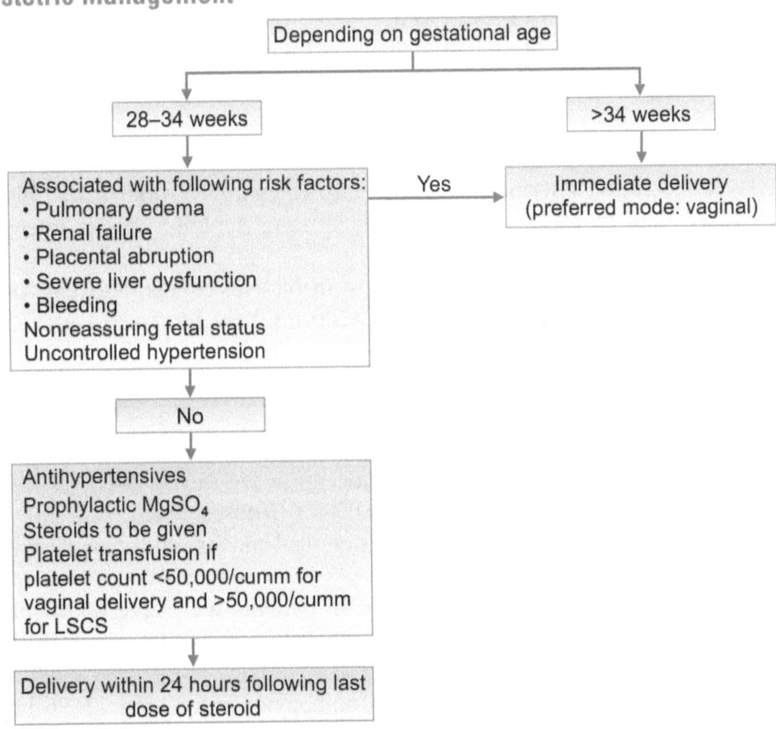

Indications for Cesarean Delivery

- Nonreassuring fetal status
- Abnormal fetal presentation
- <30 weeks and Bishop score <5
- <32 weeks with IUGR or oligohydramnios and Bishop score <5
- Known subcapsular liver hematoma
- Suspected abruptio placentae.

Management During Cesarean Delivery

- General anesthesia for platelet count <75,000/mm^3
- Transfuse 6 units of platelets if count <40,000/mm^3 (in vaginal delivery if <20,000)
- Delee's incision prefer (because scarce development of lower uterine segment)
- Spontaneous expulsion of placenta is preferred
- Do not exteriorize uterus
- Insert subfascial drain
- Secondary skin closure or leave subcutaneous drain
- Observe for bleeding from upper abdomen before closure.

Advise About Future Pregnancies

- The risk of recurrence of preeclampsia 25%-eclampsia is 5–10% and for the HELLP syndrome: 11–25% if <32 weeks
- >32 weeks recurrence of HELLP is 5%
- The risk of recurrence of preterm delivery is high, about 61%.

Postpartum Intensive Care

- Patients with DIC/platelets <20,000/mm^3/severe ascites/renal dysfunction delayed resolution/deterioration, pulmonary edema, ATN (transfusion blood/ products, fluid mobilization, compromised renal function) needs intensive monitoring for several days
- **Goal:** It is to maintain ↓ LDH, increase in platelet counts, adequate urine output, BP <150/100 mm Hg, diuresis >100 mL/hour for 2 consecutive and clinical improvement
- Monitor: Vitals, IP/OP, laboratory values, pulse oximetry–at least for 48 hours
- Maintain adequate hydration
- Administer antihypertensive
- Continue IV $MgSO_4$ 2 g/hour for 24 hours
- Steroids: Dexamethasone 10 mg IV BID for 2 doses, then 5 mg BID for 2 additional doses, suspend when there is clinical and laboratory improvement
- Dialysis: In cases of ARF
- Plasmapheresis: It has been successful in patients with severe laboratory abnormalities, who have required repeat transfusions to maintain their hematocrit at 72 hours postpartum
- The absence of improvement of the thrombocytopenia within 72–96 hours postpartum indicates severe compromise of compensatory mechanisms and possible multiple organ failure.

CHRONIC HYPERTENSION

Pre-pregnancy

- Establish the cause and severity of hypertension
- Detailed history, physical examination and appropriate laboratory and cardiac testing are essential in seeking a possible cause for hypertension and to ascertain end-organ damage, if present
- Evaluate renal function
- In those with mild to moderate hypertension, stop medication or switch to medication with few fetal side effects
- In those with severe or difficult to control hypertension, medication may be needed despite the potential fetal risks
- Encourage early prenatal care in an appropriate setting.

Antenatal

- Provide early and frequent prenatal care
- Discontinue antihypertensive medication unless maternal diastolic pressure >100–110 mm Hg
- Use oral medication in severe hypertension (methyldopa, calcium channel blockers, labetalol) and in those with mild hypertension complicated by risk factors.

Laboratory Studies

All Patients

- Establish baseline level of proteinuria
- Microscopy of centrifuged urinary sediment for white and red blood cells (including red cell morphology) and for casts
- Baseline serum electrolytes, creatinine, uric acid and glucose
- Midstream urine culture
- Complete blood examination.

Selected Patients

- Electrocardiogram
- Renal ultrasound should be considered, particularly, if hypertension is severe
- Fasting free plasma metanephrines or 24 hour urine collection for estimation of catecholamine excretion if there is concern regarding a possible pheochromocytoma. At least two consecutive collections are advised.

Fetal Surveillance with Serial Ultrasound

- Obtain early dating scan
- Start with serial ultrasound for fetal growth, amniotic fluid, and umbilical artery Doppler at 26 weeks in women with severe hypertension or mild hypertension with risk factors
- Maintain vigilance for superimposed preeclampsia.

Labor and Delivery

- Continuous electronic fetal monitoring
- Use antihypertensives to maintain blood pressure <160/110 mm Hg.

Postnatal

- Monitor closely in the first 48 hours to anticipate hypertensive encephalopathy, pulmonary edema, or renal failure
- Most antihypertensive drugs are safe during lactation: avoid thiazide diuretics.

LONG-TERM CONSEQUENCES

Counseling for Future Pregnancies

- Recurrence of pre-eclampsia (25%), more so, if associated with thrombophilia
- Recurrence of HELLP–5 to 25%
- Recurrence of eclampsia–5%.

Long-term of Sequelae

1. Cardiovascular and neurovascular morbidity
   - Ischemic heart disease
   - Stroke
   - Chronic hypertension–3 to 6-fold increased risk
   - Type II DM–3.5-fold increased risk.
2. Renal sequelae
   - Chronic renal disease.
3. Neurological sequelae
   - Persistence of brain white matter lesions.

Pulmonary Edema

- Incidence—3% in patients with severe preeclampsia
- Usually occurs in postpartum period
- Usually resulting from aggressive use of crystalloid solution for intravascular volume expansion.

Causes

1. Cardiogenic pulmonary edema—cardiomyopathy
2. Noncardiogenic pulmonary edema
   a. Acute lung injury
   b. ARDS.

NON-CARDIOGENIC CAUSES OF PULMONARY EDEMA

Unique to Pregnancy

- Preeclampsia/eclampsia/HELLP syndrome
- Tocolytic therapy

- Amniotic fluid embolism
- Sepsis-chorioamnionitis, endometritis, septic abortion.

Clinical Features

- Respiratory distress
- Severe hypoxemia
- Diffuse rales on auscultation.

Indications for Invasive Monitoring in Severe Preeclampsia

Severe preeclampsia with severe cardiac disease, renal disease or both, or in cases of refractive hypertension, oliguria and pulmonary edema (not responding to diuretics).

Investigations

CBC, BUN, creatinine, ALT, AST, LDH, uric acid, urine protein to creatinine ratio, ABG, chest X-ray, ECHO, INR, PT, aPTT.

Treatment

- Intensive care monitoring
- Position—nurse-patient at 45° angle
- Oxygen supplementation to maintain PaO_2 >65 mm Hg and O_2 saturation >95% to avoid hypoxic injuries to fetus, consider intermittent positive pressure ventilation or semi-selective intubation if oxygenation cannot be maintained
- Restriction of IV fluids to avoid fluid overload
- Diuretic: If BP is maintaining, placental perfusion is good; give injection frusemide 10 mg IV and titrate
- Treat the underlying cause of pulmonary edema
- Consider central hemodynamic monitoring line, when
  - Cardiac cause is suspected
  - Patient unresponsive to diuretics
  - Presence of hypotension
- Inotropes and vasoactive agents in selective cases.

RENAL DISEASE

Renal Physiology in Normal Pregnancy

- During normal pregnancy, the maternal cardiovascular system undergoes important changes. Blood volume and red cell mass increase by up to 50%, systemic vascular resistance falls and cardiac output increases by up to 30%. These cardiovascular adaptations have profound effects on renal function:
  - Renal blood flow increases by 50%
  - Glomerular filtration rate (GFR) increases by 30%. Increased GFR, changes in glomerular hemodynamics and possibly alterations in renal tubular function lead to an increase in urine protein excretion in pregnancy from an upper limit of 150 mg/d to 260 mg/d

- Serum creatinine decreases by 20%
- Blood pressure falls in the first two trimesters and gradually returns to baseline as the pregnancy approaches term
- Renal size increases by approximately 1 cm in bipolar length during normal pregnancy
- Smooth muscle relaxation and compression of the ureters by the gravid uterus commonly lead to pelvicalyceal dilatation, more prominently on the right than the left

ACUTE KIDNEY INJURY/ACUTE RENAL FAILURE

New System of Definition and Classification (RIFLE)

Risk	Serum creatinine increases 1.5 times or GFR fall more than 25%	Urine output <0.5 mL/kg/hour for >6 hours
Injury	Serum creatinine increases 2 times or GFR falls more than 50%	Urine output <0.5 mL/kg/hour for >12 hours
Failure	Serum creatinine increases 3 times or GFR falls more than 75% or serum creatinine >4 mg%	Urine output <0.3 mL/kg/hour for >24 hours
Loss	Persistent ARF	
End stage	On dialysis or >3 months	

Causes

- Pre-renal (intravascular volume depletion, renal vasoconstriction)
  - Acute and massive hemorrhage
  - Severe dehydration
  - Septic abortion
- Renal (acute tubular and cortical necrosis)
  - Renal diseases
  - DIC
  - Ischemia, toxins
  - Severe abruption
- Post-renal (obstructive causes)
  - Accidental ligation of ureters during cesarean section.

Acute Tubular Necrosis

- It is the commonest pathology in obstetrics
- Renal medulla is involved
- Epithelium will slowly regenerate and the renal function will usually return to normal in 1–2 weeks if it is taken care of in time.

Acute Cortical Necrosis

- Relatively uncommon
- Seen in abruptio placentae and endotoxin shock following Gram-negative septicemia

- The damage that occurs in the segment of nephron supplied by glomerular afferent vessels are end arteries, and hence irreversible.

Intracranial Bleeding

Leading cause of death in preeclampsia.

Clinical Features

When anuria is reversible, clinical condition can be divided into four phases:

1. **Incipient phase**
   - Short lasting
   - Marked diminution of urine output.
2. **Phase of anuria**
   - Lasts for few hours to 3 weeks
   - Urine output is <400 mL in 24 hours.

   Clinical features:
     - Anorexia, vomiting and diarrhea
     - Raised BP
     - Abdominal distension
     - Drowsiness
     - Cheyne-Stoke respiration
     - Dry furred tongue
     - Muscle twitches
     - Mental confusion and delirium followed by coma
     - Sensory motor deficit, focal neurological deficit such as unilateral papillary dilation.

Investigations

- CBC-leukocytosis present
- Urine
  - Specific gravity is >1,020 in pre-renal causes and ≤1,010 in renal causes
  - Proteins present
  - Casts and red cells present
  - Urine osmolality is increased
  - Plasma creatinine ratio >40 in pre-renal ARF and <20 in renal ARF
- Serum electrolytes-raised
- ABG-decrease bicarbonates
- ECG-peak 'T' wave, absence of 'P' wave, prolonged QRS complex (evidence of raised potassium)
- CT
- MRI

3. **Phase of diuresis**

   a. Early diuresis
      - Tubular reabsorption delayed up to a period of anuria
      - Despite increased urinary excretion there is retention of electrolytes (sodium, potassium).

b. Late diueresis
Causes
- Osmotic diuresis due to high blood urea
- Inadequacy of tubular reabsorption
- Release of surplus fluid and electrolytes.

4. **Phase of recovery**
   - Tubular epithelium regenerate, tubular function and glomerular activity is re-established
   - Electrolytes levels become normal.

Recovey is the exception rather than the rule.

Chronic Renal Disease

- Chronic kidney disease (CKD) is defined as abnormalities in serum biochemistry, urinary constituents (blood and/or protein) or renal structure that are present for 3 months or more
- Incidence—Varies from 2 per 10,000 women to 12 per 10,000 women
- When assessed prepregnancy, women can be arbitrarily considered in three categories:
  - Those with preserved renal function or only mild impairment of renal function (Scr ≤125 pmol/L) and no hypertension
  - Moderate renal insufficiency (Scr 125–250 pmol/L–some use 220 pmol/L as the upper limit)
  - Severe renal insufficiency (serum creatinine ≥250 pmo1/L).
- The outcome of pregnancy in women with chronic renal disease depends on the following factors:
  - The degree of renal impairment
  - The presence of chronic hypertension
  - The presence of proteinuria
  - Underlying renal pathology.
- Renal disease associated with hypertension increases fetal loss by a factor of 10 at comparable serum creatinine levels.

	Degree of renal impairment		
	Mild: Serum creatinine <125 micromol/L (%)	**Moderate: Serum creatinine 125–220 micromol/L (%)**	**Severe: Serum creatinine >220 micromol/L (%)**
Chronic hypertension	20	62	82
Preeclampsia	20	58	64
Anemia	10	73	≤100
Fetal growth restriction	4	35	43
Preterm delivery	5	30	86
Live birth rate	98	88	64
Loss of renal function	5	50	75
Postpartum deterioration	0	50	60
End-stage renal disease	0	23	40

National Kidney Federation K/DOQI Classification of Chronic Kidney Disease		
CKD stage	Estimated GFR	Comment
1	>90 mL/minute	Only classified as CKD if associated
2	60–89 mL/minute	With renal structural or urinary dipstick abnormalities
3	30–59 mL/minute	May be subclassified into: 3a: 45–59 mL/minute 3b: 30–44 mL/minute
4	15–29 mL/minute	
5	<15 mL/minute or on dialysis	
GFR; glomerular filtration rate. Estimated GFR calculations are not valid during pregnancy		

National Kidney Foundation Classification of Chronic Kidney Disease

- This is based on estimated glomerular filtration rate (eGFR). The use of eGFR is not validated in pregnancy. eGFR is calculated from serum creatinine, patient age, gender and ethnicity. Importantly, this calculation is not validated for use during pregnancy and should not be used. Alternatively, renal function during pregnancy can be estimated by creatinine clearance.
- Since the eGFR equation is invalid during pregnancy and creatinine clearance is inconvenient, most centers continue to rely on changes in serum creatinine concentration to identify potential renal dysfunction during pregnancy, mindful that relative changes in creatinine have greater clinical utility than absolute values. Preconception baseline values of eGFR are useful in predicting maternal and fetal outcomes.
- In general nephrological practice and obstetric medicine, the protein creatinine ratio (PCR) or albumin creatinine ratio (ACR) are accepted as surrogates for 24 hour collections. Assuming steady production and excretion of creatinine, this method corrects for variations in urine concentration and correlates closely with complete 24 hour urine collection data, including in pregnant patients with CKD. PCR or ACR can be used for quantitative monitoring of proteinuria during pregnancy.
- **Effects of chronic renal disease on pregnancy**

Renal disease	Effects
Chronic glomerulonephritis and focal glomerular sclerosis	Usually no adverse effects in the absence of hypertension One view is that glomerulonephritis is adversely affected by the coagulation changes of pregnancy Urinary tract infection is more common
IgA nephropathy	Risk of uncontrolled/sudden escalating hypertension and worsening renal function
Pyelonephritis	Bacteriuria in pregnancy can lead to exacerbation Multi-organ failure, including acute respiratory distress syndrome may ensue
Reflux nephropathy	Thought to be at risk of sudden, escalating hypertension; however, the consensus now is that results are satisfactory when preconception function is only mildly affected and hypertension is absent Vigilant screening for urinary tract infection is necessary

Contd...

Contd...

Urolithiasis	Infection may be more frequent Stents can be successfully placed and ureterostomy performed during pregnancy There is limited data on lithotripsy in pregnancy
Polycystic kidney disease	Functional impairment and hypertension are minimal during childbearing years
Diabetic nephropathy	Usually there is no adverse effect on the renal lesion but there is increased risk of infection and preeclampsia
Systemic lupus erythematosus	The prognosis is most favorable if disease is in remission for >6 months preconception Higher doses of steroids may be needed postpartum
Periarteritis nodosa	Fetal prognosis is poor and maternal death often occurs Therapeutic termination should be considered
Scleroderma	If the onset occurs during pregnancy, there can be rapid overall deterioration Reactivation of quiescent disease can occur postpartum
Previous urinary tract surgery	May be associated with other malformations of the urogenital tract Urinary tract infection is common Renal function may undergo reversible decrease Cesarean section may be necessary to maintain continence mechanism if an artificial sphincter is in situ There are no other significant obstructive problems
After nephrectomy, solitary/pelvic kidney	May be associated with other malformations Pregnancy well-tolerated Dystocia rarely occurs with pelvic kidney
Wegener's granulomatosis	Proteinuria and hypertension are common from early pregnancy Immunosuppressive drugs are safe Cytotoxic drugs should be avoided
Renal artery stenosis	May present as chronic hypertension or as recurrent isolated pre-eclampsia if diagnosed, transluminal angioplasty can be performed in pregnancy

Preconception counseling: Ideally, all patients with CKD should be offered counseling prior to conception in order to evaluate the risks of proceeding with pregnancy and the likely outcomes. Medications known to be harmful to the developing fetus can be discontinued or substituted for safer alternatives. Patients with active lupus nephritis or vasculitis, and those with poorly controlled blood pressure should be advised to wait until these are optimized before trying to conceive. Similarly, patients with significant renal dysfunction (serum creatinine >180 mmol/liter) may not accept the risks associated with proceeding with pregnancy and may be better advised to wait until they have received a renal transplant. In the majority of cases, patients need not be discouraged from trying to conceive as long as the potential risks are understood and the pregnancy is closely monitored.

Medication's use in CD and pregnancy		
Antihypertensives		
Commonly used	**Rarely used**	**Contraindicated**
Nifedipine	Beta-blockers	ACE inhibitors
Labetalol	Alpha-blockers	Angiotensin receptor blockers
Methyldopa	Amlodipine	Aliskiren
Hydralazine	Verapamil	Spironolactone
		Moxonidine
		Minoxidil (3rd trimester)
		Thiazide diuretics
		Diltiazem
Immunosuppressants		
Likely to be safe	**Likely to be harmful**	**Contraindicated**
Prednisolone	Anti-thymocyte globulin	Mycophenolate
Azathioprine	Rituximab	Sirolimus
Ciclosporin		Methotrexate
Tacrolimus		
ACE, angiotensin converting enzyme		

Investigations

- Complete blood count
  Maternal anemia in women with renal impairment occurs due to decreased erythropoietin production and shortened red cell survival. This anemia can usually be managed by oral/intravenous iron therapy. Using recombinant erythropoietin when the hematocrit falls below 19%. Erythropoietin can cause hypertension, or aggravate pre-existing hypertension. As such, blood transfusions may be required in rare cases to maintain the hematocrit where erythropoiesis stimulating agents are not felt to be safe to use.
- Urine routine and albumin–24 hours collection or spot test for total urine protein: creatinine ratio
  - **The significance of proteinuria alone:** Proteinuria can be an indicator of renal impairment in pregnancy. There was a preterm delivery rate of 50% and a fetal growth restriction rate of 25%. Importantly, 20% of these women progressed to end-stage renal disease within 5 years.
  - Women with a history of recurrent UTI or structural abnormalities should submit a urine sample for culture every month irrespective of symptoms to identify asymptomatic bacteriuria.
    - Serum urea, creatinine
    - Serum electrolytes
    - Urine culture spot

These tests should be repeated every 4 weeks or more frequently, depending on the clinical situation.

Renal function: Decline in renal function during pregnancy occurs rarely in patients with mild renal impairment at baseline (serum creatinine <125 mmol/liter) and often reflects an episode of obstruction, pyelonephritis or pre-eclampsia. In such cases, return to baseline renal function almost always occurs within 3 months post-partum. In contrast, women with moderate CKD (serum creatinine >125 mmol/liter) have a 25% risk of permanently losing 25% of their kidney function as a result of pregnancy, increasing to a 50% risk in those with baseline creatinine >180 mmol/liter. Furthermore, women with a preconception serum creatinine greater than 180 mmol/liter have a one in three chance of requiring dialysis during pregnancy or within 6 months of delivery.

- A renal ultrasound is required during pregnancy if:
  - There is a sudden decline in renal function
  - There are signs or symptoms suggestive of obstruction or renal stone disease
  - As above, mild pelvicalyceal dilatation is commonly identified during normal pregnancy. Functional ureteric obstruction should only be suspected if there is progressive dilatation on serial renal ultrasound scans, suggestive signs and symptoms or obstruction, or worsening renal function
  - Large kidneys on ultrasound may reflect polycystic kidney disease, diabetic nephropathy or chronic obstruction
  - Focal scarring of kidneys may reflect a congenital abnormality of the kidney and urinary tract (CAKUT) in the mother, most commonly vesicoureteric reflux
  - Small kidneys may be the result of any chronic process and further diagnosis may be difficult.
- Renal biopsy to confirm etiology of intrinsic renal disease should be reserved for:
  - Unexplained decline in kidney function in CKD or acute kidney injury
  - Newly diagnosed nephrotic syndrome
  - Features suggestive of systemic disease or vasculitis.

A renal biopsy is not indicated to investigate stable CKD, nonnephrotic range proteinuria or preeclampsia, and not after 32 weeks' gestation when the pregnancy should be brought to an end prior to renal investigation.

Immunological investigation of suspected intrinsic renal disease	
Test	**Comments**
Anti-nuclear antibodies (ANA)	Associated with connective tissue diseases and SLE. Antibodies against double-stranded DNA (anti-dsDNA) and extractable nuclear antigens (ENA) should be performed if positive
Anti-neutrophil cytoplasmic antibodies (ANCA)	Associated with small vessel vasculitis (Churg Strauss disease, granulomatosis with polyangiitis and microscopic polyangiitis)
Complement components C3 and C4	Decreased levels are found in active SLE, post-infectious glomerulonephritis, mesangiocapilliary glomerulonephritis, subacute bacterial endocarditis, cryoglobulinemia and heavy chain-deposition disease
Other tests	Rheumotoid factor, cryoglobulins and C3 nephritic factor measurement may be indicated

MANAGEMENT

Obstetric Management

- Early dating scan to estimate gestational age accurately
- Need more frequent hospital visits, depending on the clinical situation
- Nuchal and anomaly scans are performed as in all other pregnant women
- Serum screening is not a reliable screening tool in these women
- The anomaly scan must include a detailed scan of the urinary tract to look for evidence of inherited conditions such as obstructive uropathy
- Regular scans are recommended every 4 weeks from 28 weeks of gestation onwards to check growth as well as liquor volume
- Consideration should be given to prophylactic low dose aspirin for the prevention of preeclampsia. Blood pressure monitoring and adequate control are important determinants of outcome.
- There is controversy over 'tight' versus 'non-tight' blood pressure control, based on the fact that every 10 mm fall in mean arterial pressure is associated with a 145 g reduction in mean birthweight. The current consensus is that blood pressure should be maintained at no higher than 140/90 mm Hg. Drugs such as methyldopa, calcium channel blockers, hydralazine and labetalol are safe to use in these women. Preterm labor is common.
- The prompt treatment of bacterial vaginal and urinary tract infections, including asymptomatic bacteriuria, can be helpful in prevention of preterm labor. Women with recurrent urinary tract infections should be given antibiotic prophylaxis throughout pregnancy. The choice of antibiotic is determined by stage of pregnancy, sensitivities of the cultured organisms and local practice. Cephalosporins and penicillins are safe and well-tolerated throughout pregnancy. Gentamicin may be used for severe pyelonephritis with appropriate monitoring. Trimethoprim is a folate antagonist and should be avoided in the first trimester. Nitrofurantoin is associated with neonatal hemolysis if used in the third trimester and should be avoided. Quinolones should not be used throughout pregnancy.
- There is no evidence to suggest safety of the oxytocin receptor antagonist atosiban in women with renal insufficiency
- In the absence of maternal or fetal deterioration, delivery should be planned at or near term
- Early delivery is usually necessary for obstetric indications such as pre-eclampsia and fetal growth restriction or for rapidly deteriorating maternal renal function
- Obstetric considerations should be the main determinant for cesarean section
- Women with nephrotic syndrome should receive prophylactic heparin in pregnancy as well as for 6 weeks postpartum
- Following delivery, women should be seen at a postnatal combined clinic. They should continue their established care with their nephrology team
- Appropriate contraceptive advice must be given at this time.

Dialysis in Pregnancy

Indications for acute dialysis during pregnancy are similar to those in nonpregnant women.

- Severe refractory metabolic acidosis
- Electrolyte imbalance, especially severe refractory hyperkalemia
- Volume overload leading to congestive heart failure
- Pulmonary edema that is unresponsive to diuretics.

- Dialysis may be initiated earlier in pregnancy if there is an acute deterioration in renal function because of the increased risk of fetal demise.

Pregnancy in Women on Chronic Dialysis

- The incidence of pregnancy is lower in women on peritoneal dialysis than on hemodialysis
- Spontaneous miscarriage is common and occurs in 21% of pregnancies reaching the second trimester. Preterm delivery is common. Polyhydramnios is found in 42–79% of pregnancies.
- Maternal complications include hypertension (40–80%), hypertensive crisis, pre-eclampsia, anemia and placental abruption. Approximately half of these women will be delivered by cesarean section.

Recommendations for Management

Nutrition

- Protein intake can be increased to 1.5 g/kg/day in women on hemodialysis and 1.8 g/kg/day in women on peritoneal dialysis. Weight gain of 0.5 kg/week can be expected. Fluid intake should be determined individually, taking into account native urine output and the type/frequency of renal replacement therapy the woman is receiving.
- The calcium requirement in these women is around 1.5 g/day. This can be achieved by using a high calcium dialysate. They also need measurement of 25-hydroxy vitamin D levels in each trimester and supplementation if these are found to be low. Most people on dialysis tend to have high phosphate levels but if the levels are low, oral phosphate supplements can be used. All women will need folate supplementation in the dosage of 5 mg/day.
- In addition, vitamin C, thiamine, riboflavin, niacin and vitamin B_6 need to be supplemented.

Management of hemodialysis: The frequency of dialysis should ideally be increased to at least 20 hours per week. The aim is to maintain a predialysis blood urea of 15–20 mmol/l. Maternal volume depletion and hypotension should be avoided during dialysis and as such, a biocompatible, smaller surface area dialyzer to reduce the ultrafiltration rate per treatment is recommended.

The maternal diastolic blood pressure should be maintained at between 80–90 mm Hg. The amount of bicarbonate and potassium in the dialysate should be adjusted based on serum chemistries to avoid the electrolyte imbalance that can occur as a result of more frequent dialysis.

Peritoneal Dialysis and Pregnancy

Successful pregnancies can proceed in patients using peritoneal dialysis (PD) although there is limited clinical experience worldwide. The continuous nature of the process limits uremia and avoids rapid fluid shifts. As pregnancy progresses, the gravid uterus can reduce peritoneal blood flow and prevent instillation of sufficient fluid to make PD effective. In the absence of residual renal function, patients on PD may be unable to control fluid status adequately during pregnancy, necessitating transfer to hemodialysis (HD). Nevertheless, an elective change from PD to HD is not mandatory for patients who are already established on PD at the time of conception.

Management of peritoneal dialysis: Peritoneal dialysis can be continued safely during pregnancy. It is necessary to increase the number of exchanges during pregnancy and the fill volumes of peritoneal dialysis fluid may need to be reduced to 1–1.5 L. It is more practical to do this by switching to automated peritoneal dialysis. As pregnancy progresses, due to the size of the enlarging uterus, it may become impossible to continue with peritoneal dialysis and there should be a switch to hemodialysis. Although the possibility of peritonitis exists, increased incidence has not been reported during pregnancy. If cesarean section is necessary, it must be performed extraperitoneally. Alternatively, temporary hemodialysis can be instituted postpartum following traditional cesarean section.

Management of anemia: The erythropoietin dose may need to be increased by 50–100% to maintain the hemoglobin between 10–11 g/dL. In addition, intravenous iron supplementation may be required to maintain iron saturation of at least 30%.

Pregnancy in Renal Transplant Recipients

Indications for initiation of renal replacement therapy during pregnancy	
Absolute indications	**Relative indications**
Refractory hyperkalemia	Moderate uremia (urea >25 μmol/liter)
Refractory fluid overload	Resistant hypertension
Refractory metabolic acidosis	
Severe uremia causing encephalopathy or pericarditis	

- Pregnancy is estimated to occur in 12% of transplanted women
- The ectopic pregnancy rate is higher and this is related to adhesions from previous surgery and peritoneal dialysis
- Maternal and fetal outcomes for pregnancies following renal transplantation are far superior to those for mothers on dialysis
- The risks are predominantly related to the level of renal function at conception and blood pressure control

- Transplant rejection and function are not affected by pregnancy assuming the following are met:
  - At least 12 months post-transplant
  - Stable renal function
  - Proteinuria <1 g/d
  - Minimal or well-controlled hypertension
  - No recent or on-going transplant rejection
  - Minimal levels of appropriate immunosuppression
- Hypertension pre-dates pregnancy in about 70% of kidney transplant recipients. Superimposed preeclampsia and urinary tract infection occur in up to 40% of these women. Acute bacterial pyelonephritis is relatively common. There is also a higher risk of developing gestational diabetes. The incidence of preterm delivery, preterm premature rupture of membranes and fetal growth restriction is as high as 60%.
- Opportunistic infections are more common in immunosuppressed, pregnant kidney transplant patients. Of these, rubella, cytomegalovirus, toxoplasmosis, herpes simplex and hepatitis B and C can affect the fetus.

RECOMMENDATIONS FOR MANAGEMENT

Prepregnancy Counseling

- This must include a discussion on the impact of pregnancy on acute rejection and graft loss. The risk of acute rejection correlates with the prepregnancy serum creatinine levels as well as the interval between transplant and pregnancy. Long-term survival of the graft appears similar in those undertaking pregnancy to those who do not become pregnant. Acute rejection in pregnancy occurs in 9–14% of women but the incidence of serious episodes of rejection is 5%, which is similar to the rates observed in nonpregnant transplant patients. Little is known about the impact of pregnancy on chronic rejection.

Management of Immunosuppressive Regimens

- Immunosuppressive agents should be continued at prepregnancy dosages. Prednisolone, azathioprine, ciclosporin and tacrolimus are all safe to use in pregnancy. Mycophenolate mofetil (MMF) has traditionally been considered unsafe in pregnancy. Its use has been associated with an increased risk of malformations and first-trimester pregnancy loss. The most frequent malformations include external ear and other facial malformations such as cleft palate and lip. Current opinion is to avoid using MMF in pregnancy. There is little evidence regarding the safety of rituximab, sirolimus or everolimus and they should be avoided. Breastfeeding while on immunosuppressive drugs is controversial because of concerns for the effects on the baby. However, these recommendations are not absolute. New evidence is emerging regarding low levels of drug excretion into breast milk (for example, on azathioprine).

- Although there is many decades' experience of use of these agents during pregnancy, women should be informed of the recognized patterns of reported side effects:
    - At high doses (>20 mg/d) prednisolone can lead to fetal adrenal insufficiency and risk of maternal infection. Maintenance doses of less than 10 mg/d appear safe and well-tolerated in pregnancy.
    - Cyclosporine and tacrolimus may exacerbate hypertension and limit renal adaptation to pregnancy. Fetal growth restriction may be associated with these agents azathioprine is teratogenic in high doses in animal studies. In humans, it has been used without obvious teratogenicity. It may be associated with fetal growth restriction.
    - Trough serum levels of the calcineurin inhibitors tacrolimus or cyclosporine should be measured at every visit. Altered pharmacodynamics during pregnancy necessitates careful titration of doses of these drugs to maintain adequate levels whilst avoiding toxicity. A dose increase of up to 4-fold may be required and close monitoring in the puerperium is as important as during pregnancy, if not more so.

Antenatal Management

- Women should be tested for cytomegalovirus, HIV, herpes simplex virus and hepatitis B and C. Those found to be cytomegalovirus negative should have their titres rechecked in each trimester. Oral glucose tolerance tests or, in cases where there is strong suspicion, blood sugar monitoring, should be arranged to diagnose gestational diabetes.

Management of Hypertension

- Alpha methyldopa, labetalol and nifedipine are safe to use in these women. Magnesium sulphate prophylaxis can also be used safely in severe pre-eclampsia. The loading dose of magnesium remains the same. The infusion of magnesium must be decreased according to the level of elevated creatinine over the normal pregnancy level. Uric acid is a less helpful marker since it can be raised in transplant patients without preeclampsia.

Labor Management

- In the absence of any obstetric complications, delivery is timed for 38–40 weeks of gestation. Vaginal birth is the preferred route. Prostaglandins and syntocinon are both safe to use for cervical ripening or induction. The allograft, located in the false pelvis, does not obstruct delivery of the fetus. Cesarean section may be necessary for obstetric indications or if there are concerns related to severe pelvic osteodystrophy. If cesarean section is indicated then a lower segment approach may be difficult due to the course of the transplanted ureter. Early liaison with and involvement of the urology surgical team or renal transplant surgeons is advisable when elective cesarean section is planned. Stress dosage steroids should be administered to women who are on immunosuppressive dosages of steroids.

Neonatal Problems

- Neonates can have thymic atrophy, transient leukopenia or thrombocytopenia, adrenocortical insufficiency, septicemia and cytomegalovirus/hepatitis infection.

Lupus Nephritis

It often enters a phase of quiescence during pregnancy as a result of increased endogenous corticosteroid production. Consequently, flares can often occur in the puerperium when increased vigilance is recommended. If lupus flares do occur during pregnancy they can be difficult to distinguish from pre-eclampsia hypertension, proteinuria and decline in renal function, often with thrombocytopenia. The presence of invisible hematuria, depressed serum complement levels, a rise in anti-double-stranded DNA titer and cutaneous manifestations of SLE support a diagnosis of a lupus flare and should be treated promptly. Renal biopsy may be required if renal function declines quickly, or if nephrotic syndrome develops, in order to determine the most appropriate treatment for the renal disease. Patients with SLE and antiphospholipid antibodies are at greatly increased risk of thromboembolic disease and preeclampsia.

Visual Disorders

Cortical Blindness

- Caused by multiple microhemorrhages and micro-infarct in the occipital lobe
- It is equivalent to seizure
- Should be treated as having eclampsia
- Quick recovery is observed after delivery.

Diplopia

- Diplopia may occur as result of functional impairment of 6th cranial nerve
- CT scan to rule out tumor in the brainstem
- This condition improves after delivery.

CHAPTER

39

Heart Disease

HEART DISEASE

Cardiac disorders of varying severity complicate approximately 1 percent of pregnancies and contribute significantly to maternal morbidity and mortality rates. It may be–

- Congenital
- Acquired

Clinical Classification of Heart Disease (NYHA 1979)

Class I. Uncompromised: No limitation of physical activity: These women do not have symptoms of cardiac insufficiency or experience anginal pain.

Class II. Slight limitation of physical activity: These women are comfortable at rest, but if ordinary physical activity is undertaken, discomfort in the form of excessive fatigue, palpitation, dyspnea, or anginal pain results.

Class III. Marked limitation of physical activity: These women are comfortable at rest, but less than ordinary activity causes excessive fatigue, palpitation, dyspnea, or anginal pain.

Class IV. Severely compromised inability to perform any physical activity without discomfort: Symptoms of cardiac insufficiency or angina may develop even at rest. If any physical activity is undertaken, discomfort is increased.

NYHA class should be stepped up with each subsequent pregnancy.

Pre-Pregnancy Counseling

Assessment should be done by both the obstetrician and the cardiologist:

- Confirm the nature of cardiac lesion by ECHO and assess cardiac functional status according to NYHA
- Assess the mortality risk according to nature of lesion
- Counsel the women against conception, if she is in high risk category
- Counsel for correction of cardiac lesion if correctable, prior to conception for woman with moderate risk/low risk
- Cardiac medication of the patient should be checked and optimized to suit pregnancy
- All potential sources of infection should be looked for and appropriately treated.

Findings in Normal Pregnancy

Symptoms

- Fatigue
- Dyspnea
- Palpitations
- Reduced exercise tolerance
- Orthopnea
- Pedal edema

Physical Examination

- Hyperventilation
- Pedal edema
- Distended neck veins with prominent and v waves
- Increased heart rate and wide pulse pressure
- Upward and leftward deviation of point of maximal impulse
- Flow murmurs (pulmonic and aortic)
- Mammary soufflé (left sternal border, continuous murmur)
- Increased first heart sound and exaggerated splitting of 2nd heart sound
- Pulmonary basilar rales

Electrocardiographic Findings

- Sinus tachycardia
- Leftward axis deviation
- Increased R/S ratio in leads V_1 and V_2
- Repolarization changes

Echocardiographic Findings

- Increased left ventricular diastolic dimension
- Increased left ventricular wall thickness
- Mild increase in contractility
- Moderate increase in size of right atrium, right ventricle, and left atrium
- Functional tricuspid and mitral regurgitation
- Small pericardial effusion

Risk for Maternal Mortality (ACOG 1992)

Group I/Low risk (1–3%)

- ASD
- VSD
- PDA
- Pulmonic and tricuspid disease
- Corrected Fallot's tetralogy
- MS with NYHA class I & II
- MR

Group II/Moderate risk (5–20%)

- MS with NYHA class III/IV

- AS
- Coarctation of aorta with no valvular involvement
- Uncorrected Fallot's tetralogy
- Previous MI
- Marfan's syndrome with normal valve
- MS with atrial fibrillation
- Artificial valve

Group III/ High-risk (20–50%)
- Pulmonary hypertension (Primary/secondary)
- Coarctation of aorta with valve involvement
- Marfan's with aortic involvement

RISK PREDICTORS OF ADVERSE FETAL AND MATERNAL OUTCOME

Predictors for a Maternal Cardiac Event

- Prior cardiac event (heart failure, transient ischemic attack or stroke) or arrhythmia
- Baseline NYHA class >II or cyanosis
- Left heart obstruction (mitral valve area <2 cm^2, aortic valve area <1.5 cm^2, or peak ventricular outflow tract gradient >30 mm Hg by echocardiography)
- Reduced systemic left ventricular function (ejection fraction <40%)

Predictors for Adverse Neonatal Events

- NYHA class >II or cyanosis during the baseline prenatal visit
- Maternal left ventricular obstruction
- Maternal smoking
- Multiple gestation
- Anticoagulation during pregnancy

If no predictive factors at beginning of pregnancy-<5% risk of cardiac complications
1 factor–30% risk
2 or more predictors–70% risk
Frequency of adverse cardiac events:
NYHA Class I, II – 3–69%
NYHA Class III, IV – 85%

Risk of Congenital Heart Defect in Offspring

Congenital heart defect	Neonatal risk
Any defect	5–6
ASD	4–10
VSD	6–10
Tetralogy of Fallot	3–5
Transposition of great arteries	0

Contd...

Contd...

Aortic coarctation	4
Aortic stenosis	4–18
Pulmonary stenosis	3–4
Ebstein's anomaly	4–6

Obstetric Management

Management is a team approach involving the patient's primary care physician, high-risk obstetric team and cardiologist.

Indications for MTP

Absolute:
- Primary pulmonary hypertension
- Eisenmenger's syndrome
- Complex cyanotic congenital heart disease
- Pulmonary veno-occlusive disease
- Corpulmonale
- Single ventricle
- Severe coarctation
- Marfan's with aortic root dilatation
- Severe MS with complications
- Poor residual left ventricular function (EF <40%)

Relative:
- Parous women with NYHA class III or IV lesions
- Class I and II with previous h/o cardiac failure in early months or in between pregnancies

ANC–Every 2 weeks till 28 weeks then weekly till delivery.

During each visit, look for signs and symptoms of cardiac failure and those which aggravate heart failure, treat infections, if any.

Features of failure: Tachycardia, dyspnea, palpitations, basal crepitations, raised JVP, hepatomegaly, pedal edema.

Aggravating factors of failure: Infections (UTI, URTI, dental infections), anemia, obesity, hypertension, arrhythmias, hyperthyroidism, multiple pregnancy, drugs like betamimetics

- Advice regarding rest, dental hygiene
- Asymptomatic bacteruria should be looked for and treated, anemia and hypertension to be treated properly
- Cardiologist to be met before planning for pregnancy and once during pregnancy as baseline, at around 30–32 weeks when chances of failure are more and whenever features of failure appears. 2D echo is indicated in congenital heart disease and valvular heart diseases.

Mode of Delivery

- Spontaneous vaginal delivery preferred.
- No trial of labor.
- Labor to be avoided in decompensated heart disease, wait till patient is stable or deliver by cesarean section.
- Induction of labor done only for obstetric indications. Prostaglandins and high dose oxytocin used for augmentation of labor are not contraindicated. Induction of labor done at 40 weeks of gestation.

Elective cesarean section indicated in–
- Marfan's with aortic involvement
- Severe AS
- Cyanotic heart disease with unfavorable cervix
- Aortic dilatation/ dissection
- Recent myocardial infarction
- Cardiomyopathy
- Primary pulmonary hypertension

Emergency cesarean section indicated for–
- Obstetric indication
- Acute severe decompression in labor despite optimal management

If she is on warfarin and has come in labor, give inj. vit K 1 ml (10 mg) IM and post for cesarean section.

Management in Labor

- Complete history including drug history
- Assess vitals, JVP, edema and confirm NYHA class:1/2 hrly
- Auscultate lungs and cardiovascular system
- Per-abdomen and vaginal examination for diagnosis of labor
- Use pulse oxymeter in all cases to monitor SpO_2 levels
- In critical patients (NYHA class III and IV, pulmonary edema, recent MI, peripartum cardiomyopathy, obstructive cardiomyopathy) monitor with –
  - Continuous ECG monitor
  - CVP line–maintain at 8-10 cm of water
  - Arterial blood gases

First Stage of Labor

- Semirecumbent position with lateral tilt
- Oxygen inhalation at 6–8 liters/minute
- Watch for signs of heart failure

Infective endocarditis prophylaxis: Indicated in women with (AHA 2007)
- Prosthetic heart valves
- Previous infective endocarditis
- Unrepaired cyanotic congenital heart disease (including palliative shunts or conduits)

- Repaired CHD with residual defect at or adjacent to the site of repair
- During first 6 months after repair of congenital heart defects using prosthetic material or device
- Cardiac transplantation recipients who develop cardiac valvulopathy

Prophylactic regimens (AHA 2007)

- Standard prophylaxis
  - Amoxicillin 2 gm per oral 1 hr before vaginal delivery/section
    or
  - Ampicillin 2 gm IV or IM 30 min before vaginal delivery/section
    or
  - Cefazolin or Ceftriaxone 1 gm IV or IM 30 min before vaginal delivery/section
- Penicillin allergy
  - Clindamycin 600 mg per oral 1 hr before vaginal delivery/section
    or
  - Cephalexin 2 gm per oral 1 hr before vaginal delivery/section
    or
  - Azithromycin or clarithromycin 500 mg 1 hr before vaginal delivery/section
- Continue cardiac drugs, e.g.: Digoxin 0.125 mg/day with normal renal functions
- Pain relief:
  - Morphine 3 mg/ IV slowly or 6–8 mg IM (Nalorphine to be available)
  - Epidural analgesia (recommended in most cases if available, but may cause hypotension). It needs strict monitoring of vitals, intake/output.
  - Regional anesthesia is contraindicated in cardiac shunts and where hypotension can be dangerous:
    - Severe AS
    - Severe AR
    - Hypertrophic cardiomyopathy
    - Cyanotic heart disease
    - Pulmonary hypertension

In such individuals where regional anesthesia is contraindicated, general anesthesia must be given.

- Fluid management:
  - Spontaneous labor–Allow oral fluids
  - IV line to be kept ready
  - Induced/Augmented labor–Use fluids cautiously not more than 75 ml/hr (15–18 drops/min) (150 ml /hr fluid-AS)
  - Bolus doses of oxytocin should be avoided as they can cause severe hypotension. Low dose oxytocin infusions are safer.
- ARM-should be avoided unless indicated because of risk of infections
- Fetal monitoring–Continuous FHS monitoring
- Repeated P/V examination avoided. To be done under strict aseptic precautions.
- Diuretics: 20–40 mg IV only if systolic BP is more than 100 mm Hg.

Indications for diuretics–pulmonary edema, LV diastolic dysfunction, anemia

- Obstetric drugs to be avoided:
  - Epidosin (valethamate bromide)

- Drotin (drotaverine)
- Methergine (methylergometrine) as it causes hypertension

Second Stage of Labor

- Propped up position with minimal flexion at hips
- Cut short 2nd stage of labor if indicated (individualize to each patient) by outlet forceps

Why not vacuum – vaccum needs maternal efforts which further aggravates heart failure.

- Cord clamping- delayed clamping is preferred

Third Stage of Labor

- Avoid methylergometrine
- Active management of third stage of labor

Role of active management–prevents extra load on heart so prevents pulmonary edema

Fourth Stage of Labor

- Monitor vitals because of high risk of pulmonary edema for 48 hours.
- Careful hemodynamic monitoring postpartum is typically required for 24–72 hours, but this should be extended to 10–14 days in women with pulmonary hypertension. Multidisciplinary followup should take place 6 weeks after delivery.
- Avoid fluid overload.

Management of Cardiac Failure (In Antepartum/Intrapartum Period)

Signs and Symptoms

- Dyspnea
- Orthopnea
- Paroxysmal nocturnal dyspnea
- Fatigue
- Dizziness
- Palpitations

Physical examination

- Tachycardia
- Tachypnea
- Narrow pulse pressure
- Basal crepitations
- Raised JVP
- Edema, hepatomegaly
- Pulsus alternans
- Third heart sound

Treatment

- Propped up position

- O_2 inhalation
- Fluid restriction
- Morphine 3 mg IV slowly
- Diuretics–IV Frusemide 20–40 mg 8th hrly
- Vasodilators–nitroglycerin (0.4–0.8 mg s/l every 3–5 min)
- Inotropic therapy–If no improvement with the above, temporary hemodynamic support–Dobutamine begun at 2.5–5 μg/kg/min IV every 30 min until desired effect is reached.
- Digoxin 0.125 mg/day orally if patient is already not started on it.
- β-blockers–metoprolol 25 mg orally QID.

Digoxin–Can be given in a dose of 0.06–0.5 mg. Dose must be adjusted in case of renal failure (halve the dose or administer every alternate day).
Indications:
1. Heart failure
2. Arrhythmias
3. AV node re-enterant tachycardia

MANAGEMENT OF SPECIFIC LESIONS

Mitral Stenosis

- Mild stenosis–mitral valve area 1.5–2.5 cm². In these patients pregnancy is usually well-tolerated.
- Moderate stenosis–mitral valve area–1–1.5 cm²
- Critical/severe stenosis–mitral valve surface area <1 cm²

Aim is to reduce the heart rate and left atrial pressure
- Limited physical activity, if symptoms of pulmonary congestion develop further reduction in activity
- Restriction of dietary sodium
- Judicious use of diuretics
- Cardioselective β-bockers preferred
- Digoxin to control the ventricular rate
- If new-onset atrial fibrillation develops, intravenous verapamil 5 to 10 mg is given.
- Thromboprophylaxis throughout pregnancy
- Epidural analgesia for labor is ideal, but with strict attention to avoid fluid overload.
- Vaginal delivery preferable
- Intensive monitoring because the risk of pulmonary edema and atrial fibrillation is more
- Severe MS -pulmonary artery catheterization needed during labor, delivery and immediate postpartum period (12–24 hrs).
- BMV or PMC should be considered in symptomatic severe disease (ideally in second trimester).

If mitral stenosis diagnosed prior to pregnancy patients with critical stenosis or moderate symptomatic stenosis should be offered percutaneous balloon valvuloplasty or valve repair.

Mitral Regurgitation

- Well-tolerated because decreased systemic vascular resistance results in less regurgitation.
- Managed conservatively without any therapy.
- In patients with decompensated heart failure and left ventricular dysfunction – diuretics and digoxin.

Aortic Regurgitation

- AR without left ventricular dysfunction is well tolerated.
- In symptomatic patients, diuretics, digoxin and hydralazine for afterload reduction.

Aortic Stenosis

- Mild stenosis—aortic valve area 1.5–2.5 cm^2. In these patients pregnancy is usually well-tolerated.
- Moderate stenosis—aortic valve area-1–1.5 cm^2.
- Critical/severe stenosis—aortic valve surface area <1 cm^2. It significantly increases the risk of hemodynamic deterioration, heart failure, premature delivery.
    - Asymptomatic woman with aortic stenosis, no treatment except close observation is required
    - Absolute rest
    - If symptoms persist despite bed rest, valve replacement or valvotomy using cardiopulmonary bypass to be considered
    - Intensive hemodynamic monitoring
    - Adequate hydration
    - Narcotic epidural analgesia is ideal
    - Severe AS-pulmonary artery catheterization needed during labor, delivery and immediate postpartum period (12–24 hrs)
    - Minimize blood loss during delivery.

Life expectancy averages only 5 years after exertional chest pain develops, and valve replacement is indicated for symptomatic patients.

Acyanotic Congenital Heart Disease

- Usually won't interfere with pregnancy unless complicated with pulmonary hypertension
- Pregnancy is not advised if associated atrial fibrillation, pulmonary hypertension and large defects
- Surgical correction should be done before pregnancy

- Anticoagulation and strict bed rest is recommended if associated pulmonary hypertension

Cyanotic Congenital Heart Disease

Most common is tetralogy of Fallot. During pregnancy, when peripheral resistance decreases, the shunt increases and cyanosis worsens. Women who have undergone repair, and in whom cyanosis did not reappear, do well in pregnancy.

Women with cyanotic heart disease generally do poorly during pregnancy. With uncorrected Fallot tetralogy, for example, maternal mortality rates approach 10 percent.

It is associated with high rates of premature labor, spontaneous abortion and fetal growth restriction:

- If corrected, TOF pregnancy is well-tolerated
- If uncorrected, strict bed rest and diuretics should be given
- Vaginal delivery is preferred
- Care must be taken to avoid sudden hypotension.
- For labor pain, epidural opiates may suffice
- Controversy exists between general and epidural anesthesia for section.

Risk of fetus developing cardiac defects: 3–17%.

Coarctation of Aorta

Other associated lesions are persistent ductus arteriosus, septal defects and Turner syndrome.

Typical findings include hypertension in the upper extremities but normal or reduced pressures in the lower extremities:

- If corrected before pregnancy, it is well tolerated.
- If uncorrected or even incorrected ones chances of aneurysm, resistant hypertension and rupture are more.
- Poorly controlled hypertension can lead to neonatal growth restriction, placental abruption, premature delivery, and maternal complications like preeclampsia, hypertensive crisis, rupture of intracranial aneurysm.
- BP should be controlled below 130/80 with beta blockers (fetal growth should be monitored because IUGR is more with beta blockers).
- Resection of the coarctation be undertaken during pregnancy to protect against the possibility of a dissecting aneurysm and aortic rupture.
- Cut short second stage to prevent aortic wall stress.
- Cesarean section if aneurysm is present.
- Angioplasty and stenting should not be done during pregnancy because of increased risk of dissection.

Mitral Valve Prolapse

- Mitral valve prolapse is the most common cardiac abnormality in the pregnant population, affecting 12–17% of women of childbearing age.
- Mitral valve prolapse without regurgitation does not affect the cardiovascular response to pregnancy and, thus, seldom gives rise to cardiovascular complications.

Peripartum Cardiomyopathy

- This is a form of dilated cardiomyopathy
- Criteria to diagnose: Heart failure within one month before delivery or 5 months after delivery after other causes of heart failure excluded
- 2D Echo- LVEF <40%, LV end diastolic pressure >2.7 cm/m^2
- Risk factors: multiparity, multiple pregnancy, preeclampsia, eclampsia, postpartum hypertension, cocaine abuse, selenium deficiency.
- 50–60% completely recover within 6 months of delivery
- Mostly symptomatic treatment
- Diuretics, sodium, fluid restriction, β-blockers (to reduce preload)
- Nitrates and digoxin (to reduce afterload)
- Careful hemodynamic monitoring of labor and delivery
- Recurrence is high (50–100%) so avoid further pregnancies
- Angiotensin-converting enzyme inhibitors should be used only in the postpartum period as they are teratogenic and have been associated with renal failure in the fetus.
- Hydralazine is a safe and useful afterload reducing agent in the antepartum period.
- Anticoagulation should be considered in the presence of significantly reduced left ventricular ejection fraction (p35%), intracardiac thrombus or cardiac arrhythmias, such as atrial fibrillation. Before delivery, heparin is the anticoagulant of choice.
- The role of immunosuppressive therapy is unclear but should be restricted to those with biopsy proven myocarditis in the absence of viral particles and those who fail to respond after 2 weeks of standard medical treatment.
- The addition of pentoxifylline, a drug known to inhibit production of tumor necrosis factor-α, to conventional anti-failure treatment, was found to improve outcomes in a small prospective study.
- Cardiac transplantation is a final option for those who continue to deteriorate despite maximal medical therapy.
- Reported mortality from peripartum cardiomyopathy ranges from 15 to 50% often within the first 3 months of diagnosis.
- Death is usually caused by progressive heart failure, arrhythmias or thromboembolic complications.
- Prognosis appears to be related to the extent of recovery of left ventricular size and function within 6 months after delivery. Those who recover usually do so within 6 months of diagnosis and have significantly improved survival. In those with persistent left ventricular dysfunction, the mortality rate in one study was reported to be 85% over 5 years.

Eisenmenger's Syndrome

- Secondary pulmonary hypertension that develops from any cardiac lesion.
- The syndrome develops when pulmonary vascular resistance exceeds systemic resistance, with concomitant right-to-left shunting.
- Maternal deaths often occur during delivery or the first week postpartum. Most deaths are attributable to thromboembolism, hypovolemia or preeclampsia.

- Refractory hypoxemia is often the pre-terminal event.
- Maternal mortality 40% perinatal mortality has, however, decreased from 28% to 8%, reflecting advances in perinatal care.
- For these reasons, women with Eisenmenger's syndrome should be strongly advised against pregnancy or offered therapeutic abortion in the event of pregnancy.
- The most common underlying defects are atrial or ventricular septal defects and persistent ductus arteriosus.
- Anticoagulant therapy from 3rd trimester till 4 weeks postpartum as high risk of thromboembolism.
- For patients who decline termination, hospitalization is advisable from mid-gestation or earlier for bed rest.
- Second stage of labor to be cut short by forceps.
- Antibiotic prophylaxis during delivery.

Primary Pulmonary Hypertension

- It is a hemodynamic observation and not a diagnosis—is defined in nonpregnant individuals as a mean pulmonary pressure 25 mm Hg.
- Causes

  I. Pulmonary arterial hypertension
  - Idiopathic—previously "primary" pulmonary hypertension
  - Familial—e.g., chromosome 2 genes in TGF superfamily
  - Associated with: collagen-vascular disorders, congenital left-to-right cardiac shunts, HIV infection, thyrotoxicosis, sickle hemoglobinopathies, antiphospholipid antibody syndrome, diet, drugs, portal hypertension
  - Persistent pulmonary hypertension of the newborn

  Other

  II. Pulmonary hypertension with left-sided heart disease
  - Left-sided atrial or ventricular disease
  - Left-sided valvular disease

  III. Pulmonary hypertension associated with lung disease
  - Chronic obstructive pulmonary disease
  - Interstitial lung disease

  Other

  IV. Pulmonary hypertension due to chronic thromboembolic disease

  V. Miscellaneous
  - Maternal mortality is appreciable
  - Pregnancy is contraindicated with severe disease, especially those with pulmonary arterial changes—most common class I. With milder degrees of other causes—class II being common—the prognosis is much better.

Management

- Prenatal:
  - Cardiac catheterization is gold standard for determining pulmonary artery pressures

- Termination of pregnancy should be offered to the patient because of maternal risks
- Calcium channel blockers – Cap nifedipine 90–120 mg/day
- Thromboprophylaxis from the time of diagnosis of pregnancy (cardiac activity on USG) to be given as mentioned below.
- From early third trimester—in hospital bed rest, oxygen therapy (upto FiO_2 of 0.4) and frequent monitoring with pulse oximeter.
- Prostacyclin analogues, sildenafil, inhaled nitric oxide, endothelin receptor antagonist but it should be used with caution as animal studies have shown teratogenicity.
- Antepartum fetal surveillance

- Labor and delivery
  - 25% of such babies are growth restricted.
  - Spontaneous labor preferred, cesrean delivery only for obstetric indication.
  - Induction of labor – oxytocin and E-series of prostaglandins preferred at 40 weeks of gestation in well-compensated cases.
  - Continuous SpO_2 monitoring. O_2 by mask 5–6 lt/min
  - Monitor blood pressure
  - Maintain fluid balance
  - Intravenous prostacyclin or inhaled nitric oxide therapy (5–20 ppm) during labor–cause vascular dilatation, inhibit platelet aggregation, lead to improved oxygenation, decreased pulmonary vascular resistance, decreased risk of thromboembolism.
  - Epidural catheter placed early in labor. Intrathecal narcotics decrease hypotensive effect of local anesthetics.
  - Crystalloids to replace volume and maintain preload.
- Postnatal:
  - Thromboprophylaxis and oxygen therapy are continued
  - Close monitoring for 48–72 hrs
  - Nitric oxide is slowly weaned
  - Permanent sterilization offered
  - Progesterone only contraceptives to reduce risks of surgery and anesthetic risks is preferred. Estrogen to be avoided.

Myocardial Infarction in Pregnancy

- Coronary thrombosis without evidence of atherosclerosis 21%
- Coronary dissection 16%
- Aneurysm 4%
- Spasm in 1%
- Troponin I is now the main marker used for diagnosing acute myocardial injury.
- Owing to its cardiac specificity, troponin I levels are not elevated above the upper limits of normal in healthy women 30 minutes, 12 and 24 hours following delivery. The levels are also not affected by prolonged labor or cesarean section.
- Creatinine kinase and the MB isoenzyme, on the other hand, lacks cardiac specificity as they are both present in the uterus. These levels may be elevated

postpartum as a result of uterine contractions and cell breakdown, making them less useful as markers of myocardial damage.
- Echocardiography is useful to demonstrate wall motion abnormalities
- Coronary angiography should be contemplated to ascertain the cause of infarction as this may have implications for management.

Treatment of myocardial infarction during pregnancy is the same as that outside pregnancy, with heparin, beta-blockers and nitrates. Coronary angiography is safe in pregnancy and percutaneous catheter intervention is used as the first-line treatment. Thrombolysis can cause bleeding from the placental site but is still indicated in the management of acute myocardial infarction.

Artificial Valves

- If bioprosthetic valves no need of anticoagulation
- If mechanical values anticoagulation is necessary
- The maternal mortality rate is 3 to 4 percent with mechanical valves, and fetal loss is common.

Factors that determine the risk of prosthetic valve thrombosis:
- Type of valve
- Location
- Presence of atrial fibrillation
- Left atrial size
- Previous episodes of thrombosis
- Adequacy of anticoagulation

Anticoagulation During Pregnancy

Conditions requiring anticoagulation:
- Mechanical prosthetic valves
- Chronic atrial fibrillation
- Acute venous thromboembolism
- Eisenmenger's syndrome
- Antiphospholipid antibody syndrome
- Inherited deficiencies predisposing to thromboembolism (Factor V Leiden mutation)

The three most common agents used during pregnancy are unfractionated heparin, LMWH and warfarin.

There are three potential strategies for anticoagulation during pregnancy (6th ACCP consensus conference).

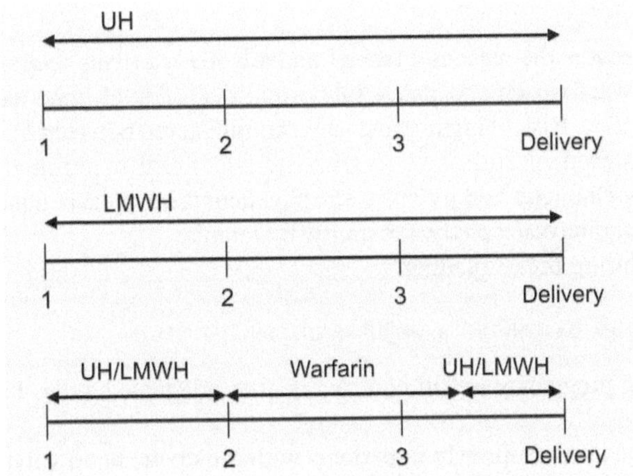

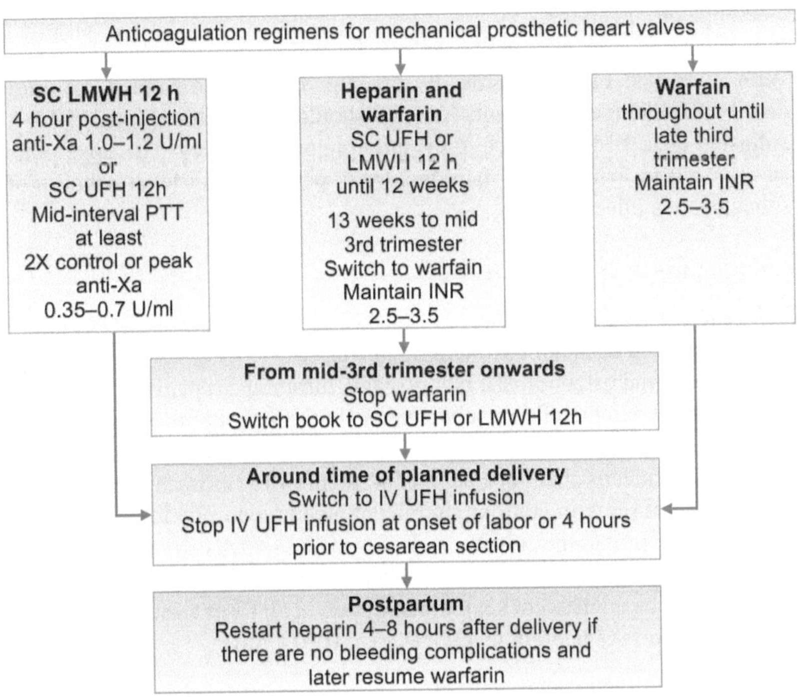

The use of the drugs depends on the preferences of the treating physician after weighing the risks and benefits of each drug.

Warfarin

- It freely crosses the placental barrier and adversely affects fetal development. It causes warfarin embryopathy (abnormalities of fetal bone and cartilage). Risk is 4–10%. Risk being highest when administered between 6th–12th week.
- If administered in 2nd and 3rd trimesters-Conradi syndrome occurs with >5 mg/day characterized by optic atrophy, chondrodysplasia punctata, mental retardation, microencephaly, spasticity, hypotonia.
- It is safe during breast feeding.

Low-Molecular Weight Heparin (LMWH)

- Use during pregnancy is still controversial as adequate studies have not been published.
- It should be used cautiously in patients with prosthetic heart valves.
- Advantage over unfractionated heparin is less incidence of HITT, osteoporosis, bleeding complications.
- It does not cross the placenta hence safe for the fetus.
- With increased blood volume during later half of pregnancy, volume of distribution changes hence anti-Xa level should be monitored (goal = 0.7–1.2)
- Adjusted-dose LMWH twice daily throughout pregnancy. The doses should be adjusted to achieve the manufacturer's peak anti-Xa level 4 hours after subcutaneous injection.

Unfractionated Heparin (UFH)

- It does not cross placenta
- Unlike warfarin does not have teratogenic effect
- Causes maternal osteoporosis, hemorrhage, thrombocytopenia (HITT syn)
- Administered parenterally or subcutaneously throughout pregnancy
- Dose is based on the aPTT levels. It should be 2 to 3 times the control
- Parenteral infusions should be stopped 4 hrs prior to cesarean section
  In the event of preterm labor or significant bleeding during delivery, it may be reversed with protamine sulfate
- Adjusted-dose UFH is administered every 12 hours throughout pregnancy. The doses should be adjusted to keep the midinterval aPTT at least twice of control or attain an anti-Xa heparin level of 0.35 to 0.70 U/mL.

Indications for unfractionated heparin:
- Mechanical prosthetic heart valves
- Cyanotic heart disease
- Artificial shunts
- ASD with pulmonary hypertension

Monitoring of heparin:
- If LMWH antifactor Xa levels may be measured within 4 hrs of starting therapy with a therapeutic goal of 0.6–1 U/ml.
- Because the aPTT levels will be normal, so we can't monitor with these levels
- Frequent monitoring is typically not recommended.

- If UFH, the aPTT should be monitored every 1–2 weeks, target is to keep INR 2–3.
- The initial platelet count followed by day 5, then once in 2–3 days upto 2 weeks or weekly for first 3 weeks.
- Ideally warfarin should be stopped immediately after conception till 12 weeks.
- After 12 weeks switch over to warfarin 2.5–3 mg/day till 36 weeks (if she can't afford heparin throughout pregnancy).
- Switchover to heparin (LMWH 1 mg/kg 12th hourly) after 36 weeks and stop 12–24 hrs prior to cesarean and 6 hrs prior to vaginal delivery.
- 24 hrs after the delivery, restart the heparin along with warfarin and stop heparin when INR is 2–3.
- LMWH or UFH (17,500–20,000 U 12th hrly) until 13 weeks gestation with warfarin substitution until close to delivery when LMWH or UFH is resumed.
- In women judged to be at very high risk of thromboembolism and in whom concerns exist about the efficacy and safety of LMWH or UFH as dosed above—some examples include older-generation prosthesis in the mitral position or history of thromboembolism.

Anticoagulation Dosing

Regimen	Dosing	Monitoring	Therapeutic goal
LMWH throughout pregnancy	Begin with 1 mg/kg enoxaparin q12 hrs	Anti-factor Xa level 4 hrs after dose	Manufacturer's upper therapeutic range
UFH throughout pregnancy	Begin at 17,500–20,000 U q 12 hrs	aPTT or Anti-factor Xa level 4–6 hrs after dose	>2 x control 0.35–0.70U/ml
LMWH or UFH through 13 weeks and after 36 weeks. Warfarin from 14–36 weeks	Heparin q12 hr Warfarin daily (2.5–3 mg/day)	As above for heparin	As above
Aspirin to be added to all above regimens	75–100 mg		

ACC/AHA Guidelines for Selection of Anticoagulation Regimen in Pregnant Patients with Mechanical Prosthetic Valves

Class I (Benefits >>> Risk) Procedure/treatment should be performed or administered	Level of evidence
• All pregnant patients with mechanical prosthetic valves—continuous therapeutic anticoagulation	B
• Patients with mechanical prosthetic valves should be counseled about warfarin, IV/ subcutaneous UFH, subcutaneous LMWH With continuous IV UFH fetal risk is lower but maternal risks of prosthetic valve thrombosis, systemic embolization, infection, osteoporosis and heparin induced thrombocytopenia are relatively higher	C

Contd...

Contd...

• For women with mechanical prosthetic valves who are willing to stop warfarin between 6–12 weeks–continuous IV UFH or subcutaneous LMWH	C
• Anticoagulation in pregnancy should be uninterrupted	C
• In pregnant patients with mechanical valves who receive dose adjusted LMWH, it should be administered twice daily, subcutaneously to maintain anti-Xa level between 0.7–1.2 U/ml 4 hrs after administration	C
• In patients who receive UFH, the aPTT should be twice the control. Those who receive warfarin INR goal should be 3.	C
• In pregnant patients who are receiving warfarin it should be discontinued and continuous IV UFH given 2–3 weeks before planned delivery	C
Class IIa (Benefits >> risk) it is reasonable to perform procedure/ administer treatment	
• In patients with mechanical prosthetic valves, avoid warfarin between 6–12 weeks due to risk of fetal defects	C
• In patients with mechanical valves, resume UFH 4–6 hrs after delivery and begin oral warfarin when there is no bleeding	C
• In patients with mechanical valves, give low dose aspirin (75–100 mg) in 2nd & 3rd trimesters along with warfarin or heparin	C
Class III (Risk ≥ benefis) procedure/treatment should not be performed	
• LMWH should not be administered to patients with mechanical valves unless anti-Xa levels are monitored 4–6 hrs after administration	C
• Dipyridamole should not be used as an alternative to aspirin in patients with mechanical valves due to fetal risks	B

Contraception

- Because of their possible thrombogenic action, estrogen-progestin oral contraceptives are relatively contraindicated in women with prosthetic valves.
- If willing for permanent methods vasectomy is ideal.
  Or
  Tubectomy by minilap method as interval procedure/once hemodynamically stable at least after one week in peurperium under local anesthesia.

Temporary Methods

- Barrier method is ideal
- IUCD under aseptic precautions can be used
- POPs, injectable progesterone like DEPOT injections can be safely used

CHAPTER

40

Diabetes

DEFINITION

Cases with abnormal carbohydrate tolerance with onset or first detected during present pregnancy.
Incidence: 10–15% in Asians.

NICE CRITERIA FOR DIAGNOSIS OF GDM

GDM is diagnosed either by:
- Fasting blood glucose of 7.0 mmol/l (126 mg/dl), or
- A blood glucose of 7.8 mmol/l (140 mg/dl), measured 2 h after a 75 g oral glucose tolerance test (OGTT).

Risk Factors

- Low-risk:
  - Member of ethnic group of low prevalence of GDM
  - No known diabetes in first degree relatives
  - Age <25 yrs
  - Weight normal (BMI <23), before pregnancy
  - No history of abnormal glucose metabolism
  - No history of poor obstetric outcome
- High-risk:
  - Severe obesity, BMI >30, PCOD, Age >35 yrs
  - Strong family history of type 2 diabetes, acanthosis
  - Previous history of GDM, impaired glucose metabolism, or glucosuria, macrosomia
  - Ethnic predisposition (Indians belong to high-risk group)
- Average risk (in between)–women of Hispanic, African, native American, South or east Asia regions.

Screening Protocol

American Diabetes Association (ADA) recommends two-step procedures for screening and diagnosis of diabetes and that too in selective (high risk) population.

Compared with selective screening, universal screening for GDM detects more cases and improves maternal and neonatal prognosis. In the Indian context, screening is essential in all pregnant women as the Indian women have 11-fold increased risk of developing glucose intolerance during pregnancy compared to Caucasian women. The recent data on the prevalence of GDM in our country was 16.55% by WHO criteria of 2 hr PG ≥140 mg/dl. As such Universal screening during pregnancy has become important in our country.

DIPSI Recommended Method

As a pregnant woman walks into the antenatal clinic in the fasting state, she has to be given a 75g oral glucose load and at 2 hrs a venous blood sample is collected for estimating plasma glucose. This one step procedure of challenging women with 75 gm glucose and diagnosing GDM is simple, economical and feasible.

Clarity in Labeling the Different Magnitude of Abnormal Glucose Intolerance on Pregnancy

Increasing maternal carbohydrate intolerance in pregnant women without GDM is associated with a graded increase in adverse maternal and fetal outcomes implying that fetal morbidity starts at a lower maternal glycemic level (<140 mg/dl). The frequency of adverse fetal outcome increases with 2 hr PG >120 mg/dl and taking care of these women had results in a better fetal outcome.

The term 'Impaired Gestational Glucose Tolerance (IGGT)' is used by few authors to indicate pregnant women whose 2 hr PG is > 120 mg/dl. It may be appropriate to use the term 'Decreased Gestational Glucose Tolerance (DGGT)' instead of impaired gestational glucose tolerance. The use of the term 'Decreased' is appropriate as it implies only 'Low' whereas the term 'Impaired' means both high and low. Further, quiet frequently we come across labeling any abnormal value in the OGTT not meeting the diagnostic criteria of GDM as IGT.The use of this term 'IGT' during pregnancy may be confusing, as this terminology is also being used in nonpregnant adult with 2 hr PG >140 mg/dl. This level is also applied to diagnose GDM by WHO criteria. Hence it may be prudent to label 2 hr plasma glucose value >140 mg/dl as GDM and a 2 hr plasma glucose value >120 mg/dl as 'Decreased Gestational Glucose Tolerance' (DGGT). The term IGTshould not be used to denote any abnormal value during pregnancy. The figures suggested below are easy to remember.

With 75 gm OGTT (WHO criteria):

	In Pregnancy	Outside Pregnancy
2 hr ≥200 mg/dl	Diabetes	Diabetes
2 hr ≥140 mg/dl	GDM	IGT
2 hr ≥120 mg/dl	DGGT	—

Gestational Weeks at Which Screening is Recommended

Practically all the pregnant women should undergo screening for glucose intolerance. The usual recommendation for screening is between 24 and 28 weeks of gestation. The recent concept is to screen for glucose intolerance in the first trimester itself as the fetal beta cell recognizes and responds to maternal glycemic level as early as 16th week of gestation. By following the usual recommendation for screening between 24 weeks and 28 weeks of gestation, the chance of detecting unrecognized type 2 diabetes before pregnancy (pre-GDM) is likely to be missed. If the 2-hour PG is > 200 mg/dL in the early weeks of pregnancy, she may be a pre-GDM and A1C of ≥6.5 is confimatory. A pregnant woman found to have normal glucose tolerance (NGT), in the first trimester, should be tested for GDM again around 24th–28th week and finally around 32nd–34th week.

- Low risk-no need of screening
- Average risk—OGCT at 24–28 wks & 32–34 weeks

  if positive → OGTT

  if negative → no need of further screening
- High risk – (Indians will fall under this category) screen at 16 weeks, if negative repeat at 24–28 wks/any time when symptoms and signs of hyperglycemia develop 32–34 wks.

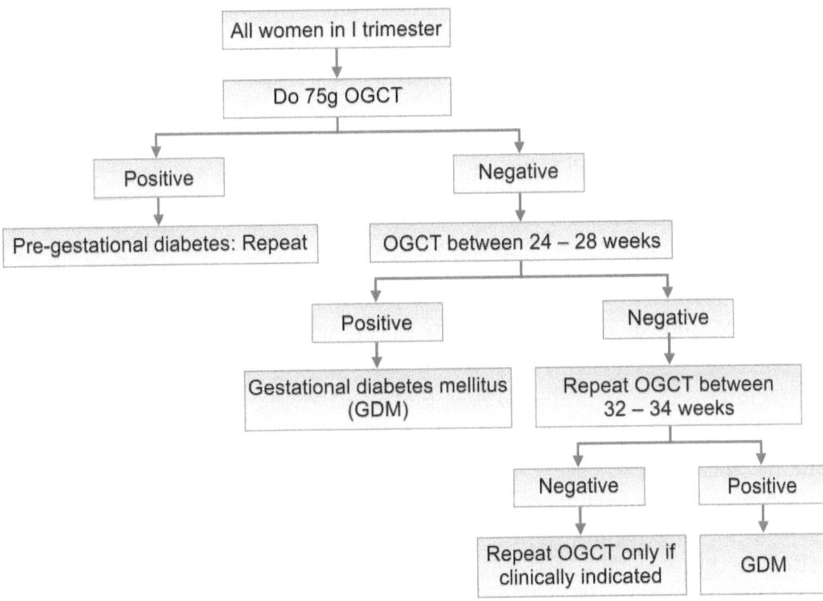

OGCT

- Timing: 24–28 weeks gestation
- Testing state: Irrespective of the fasting state
- Dose of glucose: 75 gm dissolved in glass of water
- Blood to be collected after 2 hrs
- Threshold values: 140 mg/dl

WHO 75 g method

Serum glucose cut-off point	Proportion with positive test	For GDM
>140	14–18%	80%
>130	20–25%	90%

Two-hour plasma glucose	Interpretation
>200 mg/dl	Diabetes mellitus
>140–199 mg/dl	Gestational diabetes mellitus (GDM)
120–139 mg/dl	Gestational glucose intolerance
<120 mg/dl	Normal

OGTT

- Timing: 24–28 weeks if OGCT values >140 mg%
- Testing state: Overnight fast of at least 8 hrs, not more than 14 hrs and at least 3 days of unrestricted diet (150 g carbohydrate/day) and physical activity
- Dose of glucose: 100 gm/75 gm dissolved in a glass of water
- Blood to be tested in the fasting state, 1 hr, 2 hrs, 3 hrs after glucose
- ≥2 values must be abnormal

Time	NDDG 100 g/3 hr	Carpenter & Coustan 100 g/3 hr	ADA/IADPSG 75 g/2 hr	WHO 75 g
Fasting	105	95	92	126
1hr	190	180	180	
2hr	165	155	153	140
3hr	145	140		
GDM	Two/more values to be met	Two/more values to be met	Two/more values to be met	Either of the values to be met

Note: According to DIPSI criteria for developing countries, 75 gm OGCT is considered as 1 step procedure (OGTT) both screening and diagnostic method.

Preconceptual Counseling

Multidisciplinary

- Optimize glycemic control – Aim for HbA1c 6.1% less
- Discuss hypoglycemia
- Review diet & weight loss
    - Diet – carbohydrate – 50 – 60%,
    - Protein – 20%
    - Fats – 25 – 30%
- Discuss complications of pregnancy

Health Risks of Gestational Diabetes

Mother	Fetus	Newborn	Child/Adult
Birth trauma	Hyperinsulinemia	Respiratory distress syndrome	Obesity
Increased cesarean section	Cardiomyopathy	Hypoglycemia	Type 2 diabetes
Preeclampsia/Gestational hypertension	Stillbirth	Hypocalcemia	Metabolic syndrome

Contd...

Contd...

Type 2 diabetes	Large for gestational age/macrosomia	Hypomagnesemia	
Metabolic syndrome	Birth trauma	Hyperviscosity Polycythemia Hyperbilirubinemia Cardiomyopathy	

Pre-conceptional Counseling

- Multidisciplinary
- Optimize glycemic control—Aim for HbA1c 6.1%/less
- Discuss hypoglycemia
- With Type I DM—ketone testing strips for ketonuria/ketonemia – hyperglycemia or unwell
- Review diet, weight loss and exercise
- Discuss how nausea and vomiting can affect glycemic control
- Discuss complications of pregnancy, fetus and need for cesarean section
- Prescribe folic acid 5 mg
- Review renal function and BP
- Retinal assessment, assessment for diabetic nephropathy
- Glycemic targets, glucose monitoring and medications
- Review medications—Statins, ACE inhibitors
- Smoking cessation.

Goals of Treatment

- FBS: 90–99 mg/dl
- 1 hr PPBS: <140 mg/dl
- 2 hr PPBS: <120 mg/dl.

Obstetric Management

- Routine obstetric care
- Record reviewed for glycemic control, urinary ketone bodies
- Insulin dose adjustments
- BP <130/80 mm of Hg
- Dietary adjustments
- Encourage for self-monitoring glucose levels, teach insulin administration
- RFT, urine proteinuria, C/s, thyroid function, ophthalmic examination in 3 trimesters (in pregestational diabetes)
- HbA1c should be checked.

First Trimester

- Accurate dating scan
- HbA1c, routine investigations
- Retinal assessment booking
  - If normal--28 weeks
  - If retinopathy—16 weeks, 6 m postpartum

II, III Trimester

- Obstetric examination
- Targeted USG
  - 18–20 weeks anomaly scan
  - 20–22 weeks—Fetal echo if indicated only (NICE guidelines do not recommend routine ECHO)
- From 28 weeks once in 4–6 weeks to detect IUGR, macrosomia, hydramnios, DFKC, NST, BPP, Doppler velocimetry.

Antepartum Fetal Surveillance

- GDM controlled with diet alone—no need of additional surveillance
- GDM mother on insulin treatment, overt diabetic

Low Risk (Excellent control, no vasculopathy & stillbirth)

- USG @ 4 – 6 wks intervals
- DFKC >28 wks
- NST weekly >32 wks, Twice weekly >34 wks
- BPP if NST Non-reactive
- Doppler if vascular complications suspected/IUGR
- Elective delivery prior to 39 wks

High Risk (poor control – macrosomia, hydramnios, vasculopathy & past h/o stillbirth)

- USG @ 4–6 weeks intervals
- DFKC >28 weeks
- NST > 28 wks twice weekly
- BPP if NST Non-reactive

Frequency of Visits Determined by Degree of Glycemic Control

GDM—Weekly till glycemic control

Self-blood glucose monitoring while fixing dose of insulin–7 values: Preprandial and 2 hrs postprandial after each meal and at 2 am (practically-4 values)

- Once target blood glucose is achieved
  - <28th week—lab monitoring of FBS and PPBS once a month
  - >28th week—lab monitoring once in 2 weeks
  - >32 weeks—lab monitoring once a week till delivery
- Overt
  - Daily till glycemic control
  - Every two weeks till 36 weeks, weekly >36 weeks

Medical Nutritional Therapy

- Diet therapy if FBS <105 mg/dl and PPBS <140 mg/dl
- Insulin if FBS >120 mg/dl
  - ACOG – FBS >95 mg/dl and 2 hr PPBS >120 mg/dl after 2 weeks of medical mutrition therapy—initiating or changing insulin therapy

- Type I DM—test for ketonuria/ketonemia if they become hyperglycemic or unwell.

Goals of Treatment

	mg/dL
Before breakfast	60–90
Before lunch, supper, night snack	60–105
One, two hours after meals	<140, <120
2 am–6 am	>60
HbA1c	<60
Premeal, On average	<100

Recommended calories	BMI	Daily calorie intake
≤80%	<19.8	35–40
80–120%	19.8–26	30
120–150%	26.1–29	25
≥150%	>29	12–18

Daily self-blood glucose monitoring 4 times a day fasting and 1 hr after each meal
3 meals 3 snacks- 20–30 kcal/kg of pre-pregnant wt.
Total calories = 30 kcal/kg/day {Prepregnant wt, nonobese}
BMI >27 kg/m^2 – restrict calorie intake (to 25 kcal/kg/day or less)

- Carbohydrates 40–65%
- Fat—40%
- Proteins—20%

Moderate exercise (of at least 30 minutes daily). Aerobic activities – walking, stationary cycling at least 3 days/wk 20 – 45 min per session of moderate intensity.

Insulin Therapy in GDM

Initiate therapy if FBS >105 mg/dl despite diet therapy.
Insulin requirement per day:

- I trimester (5–12 weeks)–0.7 U/kg/day
- II trimester (12–26 weeks)–0.8 U/kg/day
- III trimester (26–36 weeks)–0.9 U/kg/day
- Term (36–40 weeks)–1 U/kg/day

Total Dose = 60 U.

Ideal insulin is regular insulin given 3 times in a day.
Commonly used 2/3rd intermediate acting insulin and 1/3rd regular insulin.
Of this combination 2/3rd before breakfast and 1/3rd before dinner.

		Regular	Intermediate
Morning dose	40 U	10	30
Evening dose	20 U	5	15

Basal-bolus regime – newer modality of treatment

This regime involves three injections of fast-acting insulin before meals and a single injection of long-acting insulin at bedtime. This gives better control of sugars. Still under study.

Role of OHAs During Pregnancy

- Glibenclamide {Glyburide}—**Cat C**-compared to insulin for treatment gestational diabetes found no significant differences in major outcomes like blood glucose levels, macrosomia, neonatal hypoglycemia, NICU admissions
- Plasma t ½ 4–6 hrs {2nd generation}
- DOA—18–24 hrs
- Starting dose 2.5 mg orally with morning meal
- Increase dose by 2.5 mg/wk increments till 10 mg/day then BD till 20 mg/day.

Metformin—GDM

Metformin with insulin in GDM {MIG Trial} confirmed safety and benefit of metformin after 20 weeks **Cat B.**

Partial placental barrier exists 0.5–2 gm, 2–4 doses/day pharmacological agents for GDM.

- Pharmacological agents.

	Insulin	**Glyburide**	**Metformin**
Mechanism of action	Receptor-mediated glucose uptake; other actions	Stimulates pancreatic beta-cell insulin release	Increases sensitivity to insulin; stimulates insulin induced glucose uptake
Onset of action	Varies	Approximately 1 h	Approximately 1 h
Peak	Varies	4 h	
Dosing	Varies	2.5 mg in AM or every 12 hr, increase weekly by 2.5 mg to a maximum of 10 mg every 12 hr	500 mg in AM or every 12 hr; maximum 1000 mg every 12 hr
Placental transport	Minimal (only antibody bound fraction)	Minimal to none	Yes
FDA pregnancy category	B	C	B
Experience with use in pregnancy	Substantial	Modest	Limited
Failure rate requiring insulin		20%	35%

Timing of Delivery

Small risk of late intrauterine death even with good glycemic control.

- GDM with diet management with excellent gestational dating in a well-controlled patient—wait for spontaneous labor up to 40 weeks

- GDM with insulin treatment—at 38 completed weeks
- Overt diabetic well-controlled with no other complications—at 38 completed weeks
- Uncontrolled diabetes—whenever indicated.

Elective Section Indications:
Sonographically EFW >4.5 kg, IUGR
Advanced DM {vascular disease}, Obstetrics complications

TOLAC is not contraindicated in GDM.

Insulin Management During Labor and Delivery

- Usual dose of intermediate acting insulin given at bedtime
- Morning dose of insulin is withheld
- IV infusion of NS is begun
- Glucose levels checked hourly
- Goal Maternal Blood Glucose {72–126 mg/gl}

Plasma glucose	Insulin/IV Fluids
<70 mg/dl	5% DNS-100 ml/hr
90–120 mg/dl	NS or RL 100 ml/hr
120–140 mg/dl	NS or RL 100 ml/hr plus 4U of regular insulin added with IV fluids
140–180 mg/dl	NS or RL 100 ml/hr plus 6U of regular insulin added with IV fluids
>180 mg/dl	NS or RL 100 ml/hr plus 8U of regular insulin added with IV fluids

Post-delivery

In GDM—insulin requirement mostly nil, but sugars should be monitored 6th hrly for first 24 hrs, once FBS, PPBS after starting on regular diet, then at discharge FBS, PPBS.

Later OGTT after 6 weeks

- *In type-I diabetes*

Insulin requirement reduces immediately after delivery and remains for 48 – 96 hrs, but immediate postop

- Needs of insulin is variable, so GRBS 6th hrly
- According to sliding scale (mostly first 24 hrs)
- After starting on regular diet as before delivery or

1/3rd of III trimester dose, FBS, PPBS after 1 hr of food target FBS is <95 mg/dl, PPBS <120 mg/dl if not increase the insulin dose by 3 units; if less, decrease by 2 units.

Elective LSCS

- Scheduled early morning bedtime NPH insulin given night before
- Nil per oral after midnight
- Morning dose of insulin is withheld, blood glucose monitored every hour before, during surgery

- Blood glucose <70 mg/dl – 5% D started
- Regular insulin IV used for glycemic control
- Epidural analgesia preferred

Indications

Sonographically EFW >4.5 kg, IUGR, advanced DM {vascular disease}, obstetrics complication.

Diabetic Ketoacidosis

- *Symptoms*
  Polyuria, thirst, weight loss, weakness, nausea, vomiting, leg cramp, blurred vision, abdominal pain
- *Signs*
  Dehydration, hypotension, cold extremities, peripheral cyanosis, tachycardia, air hunger {Kussmaul's breathing}
  Acetone smell, hypothermia, confusion, drowsiness coma {10%}

Investigations

- Urine for ketone bodies
- ABG, RFT, S. electrolytes, Blood glucose
- ECG, CBC, CRP, Urine culture
- Done baseline, 1 hr, 2 hrs, 3 hrs, 6 hrs, 12 hrs, 24 hrs
- Hourly BP, PR, RR, Urine output, Capillary blood glucose
- ABG
  - No clinical improvement
  - Plasma HCO_3 <15 mmol/lt

Management

- **Laboratory Assessment**
  Obtain glucose, urine ketone bodies, ABG {acidosis}
- **Insulin**
  - Low dose, IV Infusion
  - Loading dose: 0.2–0.4 U/kg
  - Maintenance: 2.0–10 U/hr
- **Fluids**
  - Isotonic sodium chloride {0.9%}
  - Total replacement in first 12 hrs = 4–6 L
    - 1L—First hour
    - 500–1000 ml/hr for 2–4 hrs
    - 250 ml/hr until 80% replaced.
- **Glucose**
  5% DNS, if RBS <250 mg/dl, 1 lt 8 th hourly
- **Potassium**
  - None in 1st lt IV fluids unless <3 mmol/l

- <3.5 mmol/lt–40 mmol added 1 lt @ 20 mmol/hr
- 5.0 mmol/lt–20 mmol added
- 5 mmol/lt/Anuric–No need

- **Bicarbonate**
  If pH <7.10–Add 1 amp {44 mEq} to 1 lt of 0.45 NS

Congenital Malformations

- 5–10 times more common
- 10–50% perinatal mortality

- **Anomalies**
  Cardiac {VSD, ASD} – 3–5 fold increase in risk
  CNS {2–5 fold increase in risk}, Skeletal, GIT, Renal
  Caudal regression—200-fold increase risk
- **Risk factors:** Poor preconceptual glycemic control, early onset ketoacidosis, vasculopathy, hypoxia
- **Correlation between HbA1c and fetal malformation rate**
  <6.9%–No anomalies
  7–8.5%–5% risk
  >8.5–9.5–20%

Postpartum Follow-up

- Check blood sugars before discharge
- Breastfeeding: helps in weight loss
- Lifestyle modification: exercise, weight reduction
- Oral glucose tolerance test at 6–12 weeks postpartum: classify patients into normal/impaired glucose tolerance and diabetes
- Preconception counseling for next pregnancy

Frequency of Monitoring

- Depends on level of glycemic control
- OGTT after 6 weeks, according to this result like–
- Risk of recurrence 50%

OGTT result	Frequency of monitoring
Normal	Every 3 yrs
IGT	Every 1 yr
Diabetes	Treat

Management of Neonate

- Hypoglycemia <40 mg/dl, Preterm <35 mg/dl, Encourage early breastfeeding
- If symptomatic, give a bolus of 2–4 ml/kg, IV, 10% dextrose
- IV dextrose: 6–8 mg/kg/min infusion
- Check for calcium, if seizure/irritability/RDS.

CHAPTER

41

Epilepsy

DEFINITION

Epilepsy is recurring spontaneous seizures due to sudden excessive and disordered electrical discharge from the neuron of the cerebral cortex.

- 0.5–1% of the general population is affected.

Effect of Anti-Epileptic Drugs on the Fetus

- Increased risk of congenital malformations in fetuses exposed to: phenytoin, carbamazepine, valproic acid, phenobarbital
- Risk of major malformations is 4–6%
- Fetal anticonvulsant syndrome—infants born with congenital anomalies after being exposed to anticonvulsant drugs in utero
- Frequency of anticonvulsant embryopathy with 1 anticonvulsant drug is 20.6% and with 2 drugs is 28%
- The most common congenital anomalies with AEDs are neural tube defects, congenital heart and urinary tract defects, and cleft palate

Mechanism for Teratogenicity

1. Low or deficient epoxide hydroxylase activity which increases levels of teratogenic oxidative metabolites
2. Oxidative damage to DNA from free radical intermediates produced by prostaglandin H synthase bioactivation

Valproate

- Cartegory D drug
- Neural tube defects (spina bifida aperta, open lumbosacral myelocele), meningomyelocele, cardiovascular and urogenital malformations with minor craniofacial, skeletal, genital anomalies
- Facial valproate syndrome–Brachycephaly with high forehead, shallow orbits, small nose, small mouth and low posterior ears. Long overlapping fingers and toes and hyperconvex nails. Cleft palate and congenital heart diseases
- 1–2% affected with monotherapy, and 9–12% with polytherapy
- First trimester maternal exposure increases the risk
- Higer doses were associated with more sever dysmorphia
- Valproate preferably not used as it is associated with higher umbilical than maternal concentrations

- If valprotae is used—high plasma levels (>70 μg/ml) should be avoided
- It should be given in three to four divided doses daily.

Phenytoin

- Category D drug
- Fetal hydantoin syndrome—craniofacial anomaly, upturned nose, long upper lip with thin vermilion border, distal phalanges hypoplasia, fingernail hypoplasia, growth deficiency, developmental delay, cleft lip, cardiac anomalies, urogenital anomalies
- 5–11% are affected

Phenobarbital

- Category D drug
- Cleft lip, cardiac anomaly, urinary tract malformation
- 10–20% are affected

Carbamazepine

- Category D drug
- Fetal hydantoin syndrome–spina bifida
- 1–2% are affected

Newer Anti-epileptics

- Lamotrigine, gabapentin, felbamate, topiramate, tiagabine, levetiracetam, pregabalin
- All belong to category C drugs
- Actual risk of congenital anomalies are not known
- 2.7–3.2% incidence of congenital anomalies after first trimester use of lamotrigine monotherapy
- Lamotrigine is excreted extensively in breast milk. Adverse effects of the high dose not known.

Effect of Epilepsy on Fetus

- Fetal hypoxia due to decreased blood flow during conculsions or post-ictal apnea
- Non-convulsive seizures are less dangerous
- Other risks of seizures—injury to fetus, abruption or miscarriage
- Increase in IUGR (1.9-fold) and low-birth weight (2.79-fold)

Effect of Pregnancy on Seizures

- In 30% of epileptics, seizure frequency increases due to:
  - Enhanced metabolism and increased drug clearance associated with pregnancy can result in decreased serum drug concentration
  - Increased volume of distribution of the AED
  - Increased serum binding proteins
  - Decreased or non-compliance with medication

- Sleep deprivation, hormonal changes of pregnancy (high estrogen), and associated psychological and emotional stress of pregnancy: all lower threshold for seizures
- Nausea and vomiting

Other physiological changes of pregnancy:
- Reduction in FRC with hypercapnea and reduction in cerebral blood flow
- Hyperventilation causing compensation acidosis
- Retention of sodium and water
- Nitrogen sparing effect of pregnancy->changes in aminoacid concentration

- 20% show decrease in seizure frequency due to improved compliance with drug regimen in some patients
- In 50% seizure frequency may remain unchanged
- Risk of seizures during pregnancy is 0.15–10%
- At the time of delivery seizure risk–3.5%

PRE-CONCEPTIONAL COUNSELING

- Epilepsy is not a contraindication for pregnancy.
- Risk of inheritance is four-fold higher in offspring of affected mother (9%) than in father (2%).
- Offsprings typically inherit the seizure type of the parent but at an earlier age.
- Optimize antiepileptic therapy prior to conception. Dosage should be the minimum dose needed to maintain seizure control.
- As there is no concensus on the best anti-epileptic drug, the drug which stops seizures is the one that should be used.
- Discontinue antiepileptic drugs before or during pregnancy if seizures have been well-controlled for 2 years.
- The AED dose should be tapered till stopped completely at least 6 months prior to any planned pregnancy.
- Monotherapy adviced to reduce risk of malformations.
- If family history of neural tube defects, avoid valproate and carbamazepine, unless patient's seizures cannot be controlled by other drugs.
- Delay in conception until epilepsy is well-controlled.
- Folic acid 5 mg/day for 1–3 months prior to conception and throughout pregnancy to reduce neural tube defects.
- Compliance in taking AED must be stressed.

MANAGEMENT DURING PREGNANCY

- If on anti-epileptic drugs, serum and red cell folate levels should be monitored
- Measurement of the free unbound anti-epileptic drug level in maternal serum. But it is not neccesary, because of altered protein binding it is not reliable. Also no evidence that such monitoring improves seizure control so indicated only when recurrence or noncompliance is suspected
- A fall in drug level is common, it doesn't necessitate the incrementation of dose—the change of dosage depends on clinical status with drug levels used to guide such changes

- Real time ultrasound-Anencephaly: 18–20 week, NTD and cleft lip and palate: 18–20 weeks, congenital cardiac defects: 22–24 weeks
- Serum AFP screening by amniocentesis: 14–16 weeks
- Vitamin K: 20 mg per day orally given to mother during last 4 weeks of gestation to decrease the risk of fetal coagulopathy (tablets not available Inj. Vit K 1 ml–2 ampoules–8 mg IM every week in last 4 weeks of pregnancy)

MANAGEMENT OF PREGNANCY IN WOMEN WITH EPILEPSY

Third Stage of Labor and Delivery

- Inform all health care providers that the patient has epilepsy
- Each woman's usual anti-epileptic regimen should be continued during labor. Missed doses, and consequent falls in plasma levels of anti-epileptic drugs are to be avoided
- Women with epilepsy should be offered the same range of methods of pain relief in labor (including epidural analgesia) as is available to other women
- Seizure activity during labor is not an indication for immediate delivery unless fetal bradycardia or status epilepticus develops
- Elective cesarean section in patients refractory to treatment in third trimester or status epilepticus
- *Indications for cesarean section:*
  - Seizures refractory to treatment during third trimester
  - Status epilepticus
  - Repeated seizures during labor
  - Absence or psychomotor seizures which limit maternal awareness and ability to cooperate
  - Obstetric indications
- Manage seizures acutely with intravenous benzodiazepines (2 mg inj. lorazepam repeated at 5 min intervals if required) and then start on inj. phenytoin loading dose as 20 mg/kg as infusion at 50 mg/min
- Avoid prolonged pushing in the second stage. Prophylactic instrumental delivery

Postnatal

- Inj Vit K 1 mg IM to the baby
- Breastfeeding encouraged
- If possible, avoid phenobarbitone, primidone while breastfeeding as it causes neonatal sedation
- Any increase in drugs during pregnancy will need to be decreased slowly to pre-pregnancy doses over 3–4 weeks to avoid toxicity
- During the first postpartum day, 1–2% of women will have tonic-clonic seizures and should be managed as described
- If the mother is breastfeeding, sleep deprivation may be unavoidable. The mother should make up any missed sleep during the infant's daytime naps, whenever possible

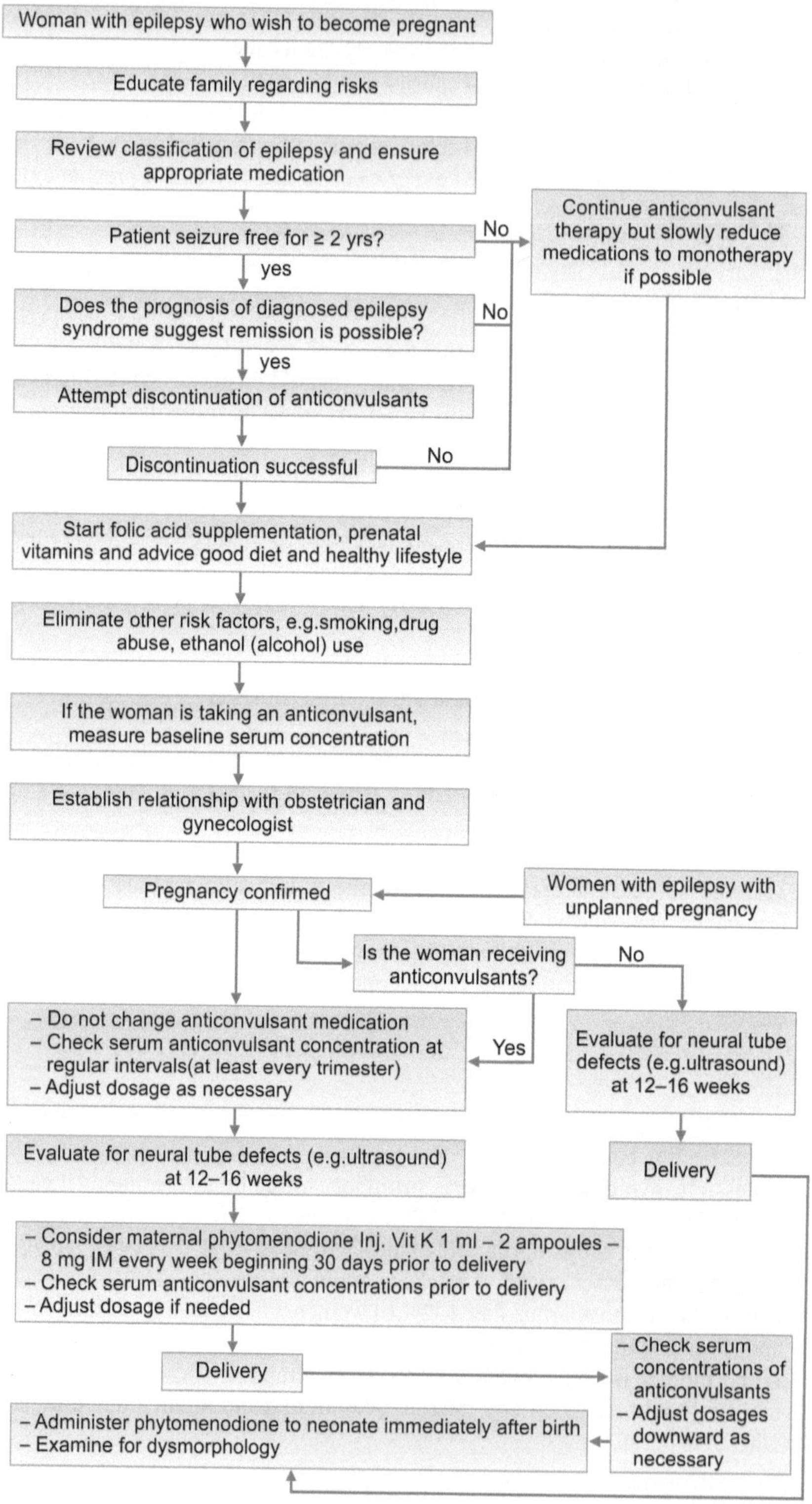
Woman with epilepsy who wish to become pregnant
Educate family regarding risks
Review classification of epilepsy and ensure appropriate medication
Patient seizure free for ≥ 2 yrs?
No
Continue anticonvulsant therapy but slowly reduce medications to monotherapy if possible
yes
Does the prognosis of diagnosed epilepsy syndrome suggest remission is possible?
No
yes
Attempt discontinuation of anticonvulsants
Discontinuation successful
No
Start folic acid supplementation, prenatal vitamins and advice good diet and healthy lifestyle
Eliminate other risk factors, e.g.smoking,drug abuse, ethanol (alcohol) use
If the woman is taking an anticonvulsant, measure baseline serum concentration
Establish relationship with obstetrician and gynecologist
Pregnancy confirmed
Women with epilepsy with unplanned pregnancy
Is the woman receiving anticonvulsants?
No
Yes
– Do not change anticonvulsant medication
– Check serum anticonvulsant concentration at regular intervals(at least every trimester)
– Adjust dosage as necessary
Evaluate for neural tube defects (e.g.ultrasound) at 12–16 weeks
Evaluate for neural tube defects (e.g.ultrasound) at 12–16 weeks
Delivery
– Consider maternal phytomenodione Inj. Vit K 1 ml – 2 ampoules – 8 mg IM every week beginning 30 days prior to delivery
– Check serum anticonvulsant concentrations prior to delivery
– Adjust dosage if needed
Delivery
– Check serum concentrations of anticonvulsants
– Adjust dosages downward as necessary
– Administer phytomenodione to neonate immediately after birth
– Examine for dysmorphology

Contraception

- Barriers and IUDs are recommended
  Many AEDs induce the hepatic cytochrome P-450 system, which is the primary metabolic pathway of the sex steroid hormones. This leads to rapid clearance of steroid hormones and allows ovulation in women taking OCPs or other hormonal forms of birth control
- The newer transdermal patch formulation has a higher failure rate with these AEDs
- IM medroxyprogesterone provides higher dosages of progestin but still may require dosing at 8- to 10-week intervals rather than 12-week intervals
- Antiepileptic drug effects on hormonal contraceptives
  - Lower hormone level–Phenobarbital, Phenytoin, Carbamazepine, Primidone, Topiramate, Oxcarbazepine
  - No significant effect–Ethosuximide, Valproate, Gabapentin, Lamotrigine, Tiagabine, Levetiracetam, Zonisamide

MANAGEMENT OF PATIENTS WITH STATUS EPILEPTICUS

- Establish the ABCs, and check vital signs
- Assess the fetal heart rate
- Rule out eclampsia
- Administer a bolus of lorazepam (0.1 mg/kg, i.e., 5–10 mg) at no faster than 2 mg/min
- Load phenytoin (20 mg/kg, i.e., 1–2 g) at no faster than 50 mg/min, with cardiac monitoring and maintenance on Inj phenytoin 150 mg IV TID
- If this is not successful, load phenobarbital (20 mg/kg, i.e., 1–2 g) at no faster than 100 mg/min
- Hypotension should be avoided in danger of cerebral hypoperfusion
- Check laboratory findings, including electrolytes, AED levels, glucose, and toxicology screen
- If fetal testing results are non-reassuring, move to emergent delivery
- Majority of women will have a safe vaginal delivery without seizure occurrence; provided, the AED is taken before and throughout labor
- Oxygen should be administered to the patient and she should be placed on her left side.

CHAPTER

42

Bronchial Asthma

- Chronic inflammation of airways
- Airway hyper-responsiveness
  - Wheezing, cough, shortness of breath
  - Especially at night or early morning
- Reversible airflow obstruction

EFFECT OF PREGNANCY ON ASTHMA

- 1/3 Improvement
- 1/3 Worsening
- 1/3 Stay same
- Worsen 29–36 weeks
- Last 4 weeks less severe
- Rarely exacerbates in labor

EFFECT OF ASTHMA ON PREGNANCY

- Preeclampsia
- Preterm delivery
- Low-birth weight

LIFE-THREATENING COMPLICATIONS

- Pneumonia
- Cor pulmonale
- Cardiac arrhythmias
- Acute respiratory failure

COUNSELING

Risk of child developing asthma

- 6%–when only 1 parent is asthmatic
- 30%–when both parents are asthmatic

CLASSIFICATION OF ASTHMA SEVERITY

	Intermittent	Persistent		
Component		Mild	Moderate	Severe
Symptoms	<2 days/wk	>2 days/wk, 32 not daily	daily	Throughout day
Nocturnal awakening	<2 times/month	3–4/month	>1/wk, not nightly	Often 7 times /wk
Short-acting β-agonist for symptoms	<2 days/wk	>2 days/wk, but not >1/day	daily	Several times daily
Interference with normal activity	None	Minor limitation	Some limitation	Extremely limited
Lung function	Normal between exacerbations			
FEV1	>80% predicted	>80% predicted	60–80% predicted	<60% predicted
FEV1/FVC	Normal	Normal	Reduced 5%	Reduced >5%

Management of Acute Exacerbations of Asthma During Pregnancy

Rescue Agents

These are those medications used to treat acute bronchospam and provide symptomatic relief but do not treat the underlying inflammation that cause bronchospasm.
(Inhaled β_2 agonist and ipratropium)

Maintenance

Medications that help to control airway hyperactivity and generally treat the underlying inflammation of airway, e.g.: Inhaled steroids, systemic steroids, leukotriene antagonist (disodium cromoglycate)

Home Management

- Decrease in fetal movement early manifestation of asthma exacerbation
- Salbutamol 2–4 puffs every 20 min for up to 1 hr

Hospital Management

- Salbutamol 2.5 mg in 2.5 ml NS with oxygen
- Oxygen saturation >95%
- IV corticosteroids: if no response

Management During Labor and Delivery

- PGE1/2 used for cervical ripening
- Pain management during labor
  - Bronchospasm increases with increased pain
  - Fentanyl, butorphanol indicated
  - Epidural is the preferred method
  - Ketamine, Halogenated anesthetics–GA

- If PPH develops
  - PGF 2 alpha, Methergine contraindicated
  - PGE 2, oxytocin preferred

Acute Asthma Exacerbation

Signs of a severe attack are:
- Tachycardia (>120 bpm)
- Raised respiratory rate
- Peak expiratory flow rate <120 L/min
- Moderate to severe wheeze
- Inability to complete sentences
- SpO_2 >95%

Management

- Inhaled beta 2 adrenergic agonist
- Methylprednisolone 125 mg IV–60 mg q6h/hydrocortisone 80 mg q6h
- Oral prednisolone 60 mg OD reduced over 2 weeks
- Avoid SC epinephrine

Stepwise Therapy of Chronic Asthma During Pregnancy

Severity	Stepwise therapy
Mild intermittent	• No daily treatment necessary
	• Inhaled β-agonists as needed
Mild persistent	• Inhaled β_2 adrenergic agonists as needed
	And
	• Daily treatment with inhaled low dose inhaled corticosteroids
	• Alternatives–Cromolyn, leukotriene antagonists or theophylline
Moderate persistent	• Inhaled β_2 adrenergic agonists
	And
	• Daily treatment with inhaled low-dose inhaled corticosteroids and daily treatment with salmeterol or
	• Daily treatment with inhaled medium dose corticosteroids
	• Alternative–daily low dose (or medium if needed) inhaled steroids and either theophylline or leukotriene antagonists
Severe persistent	• Inhaled β_2 adrenergic agonists as needed
	And
	• Daily treatment with high-dose inhaled corticosteroids
	And
	• Daily treatment with salmeterol if needed
	• Daily treatment with systemic steroids

Postnatal Advice

- Continue asthmatic medication and breastfeeding
- Breastfeeding between 1–6 months reduces prevalence of asthma by 30–50%

CHAPTER

43

Jaundice

LIVER FUNCTION TESTS IN NORMAL PREGNANCY

Aspartate transaminase, alanine transaminase, γ-glutamyl transferase, and total bilirubin each falls during pregnancy, the upper limit of normal being about 25% lower than outside pregnancy. This is mainly as a result of hemodilution. Alkaline phosphatase rises steadily through pregnancy, reaching a peak in the third trimester up to 300% above the nonpregnant range, due to the production of a heat-stable placental isoenzyme: If there is a clinical indication to differentiate the hepatic from the placental form, then the sample can be heat-treated to 60°C for 10 minutes and then reanalyzed, the fall representing the liver isoenzyme.

	Nonpregnant	First trimester	Second trimester	Third trimester
AST u/L	7–40	10–28	11–29	11–30
ALT u/L	0–40	6–32	6–32	6–32
Bili μmol/L	0–17	4–16	3–13	3–14
GGT u/L	11–50	5–37	5–43	5–41
Alk phos u/L	30–130	32–100	43–135	130–418

ALT, alanine aminotransaminase; AST, aspartate aminotransaminase; Bili, bilirubin; GGT, γ-glutamyl transferase; AJK phos, alkaline phosphatase

In the postnatal period, alkaline phosphatase falls steadily, reaching nonpregnant values by day 13 in most women. The transaminases may rise considerably, especially during the first 5 days of the puerperium and can exceed both the pregnant and nonpregnant reference ranges. This is because they are not specific to liver, occurring also in breast, smooth and striated muscle, and red blood cells. The exercise of labor, the trauma of delivery, and breastfeeding may all contribute to this phenomenon.

	Postpartum peak (days)	Mean rise (%)	Range rise (%)
AST	2–5	88	0–500
ALT	5	147	0–1140
GGT	5–10	62	0–450
Alk phos	Predelivery	–	–

ALT, alanine aminotransaminase; AST, aspartate aminotransaminase; GGT, γ-glutamyl transferase; Alk phos, alkaline phosphatase

LIVER FUNCTION TESTS FOLLOWING DELIVERY IN NORMAL PREGNANCY

Disorders of the Liver and Biliary Tract

There are several disorders of the liver which are specific to pregnancy which are important to recognize as they are associated with significant morbidity and mortality for the mother and her fetus and delivery is the only cure. Some pre-existing conditions may only become clinically evident during pregnancy and others such as Hepatitis E have a predilection for pregnant women in whom the prognosis is significantly worse.

Classification

A. The pregnancy-specific causes of jaundice:
1. Acute fatty liver of pregnancy
2. HELLP (hemolysis, elevated liver enzymes, low platelets) syndrome
3. Obstetric cholestasis
4. Hyperemesis gravidarum

B. Non-pregnancy-specific liver disease:
1. Viral hepatitis-Hepatitis A, B, C, or E
   - Cytomegalovirus
   - Epstein-Barr virus
   - Toxoplasmosis
   - Herpes simplex
2. Gallbladder disease (Gallstones and Cholecystitis)
3. Drug reactions (Co-amoxiclav is the commonest cause of cholestatic jaundice)
4. Drug abuse, including alcohol.

Three Pathologic Processes Lead to Jaundice

- Hemolysis
- Congenital hyperbilirubinemia
  - Unconjugated
  - Conjugated
- Cholestasis
  - Intrahepatic
  - Extrahepatic

Serum and Urine Findings in a Jaundiced Patient, Allowing Characterization of the Cause of the Jaundice

	Serum bilirubin		Urine bilirubin			
Cause of jaundice	**Unconjugated**	**Conjugated**	**Bilirubin**	**Urobilinogen**	**Reticulocyte count**	**ALT**
Hemolysis	↑	N	–	↑	↑	N
Gilbert's syndrome	↑↑	N	–	↑	N	N
Crigler-Najjar syndrome	↑↑↑	N	–	↑	N	N

Contd...

Contd...

Dubin-Johnson	N/↑	↑		↑	N	N
Hepatocellular	N/↑	↑		↑/N	N	↑
Hepatocanalicular	N/↑	↑		↑/N	N	↑
Extrahepatic	N/↑	↑		↑/N	N	↑

–, absent; ↑, increased; ↓, decreased; ALT, alanine transaminase; N, normal

Cholestasis of Pregnancy

Obstetric cholestasis is unique to pregnancy.

Prevalence: It is about 0.1% in the USA and ~0.7% in the UK. Women of Indian and Pakistani descent have a two-fold increase in risk.

The cause is multifactorial. Genetic, environmental and hormonal factors and has been associated with:

- Spontaneous or iatrogenic prematurity
- Fetal intracranial bleeding
- Meconium-stained amniotic fluid
- Intrapartum fetal distress
- Intrauterine death.

Maternal morbidity is related to the intense pruritus and consequent sleep deprivation.

- An increased risk of postpartum hemorrhage, secondary to deficiency of vitamin K, has been reported.
- It has an increased incidence of spontaneous and iatrogenic preterm birth and a stillbirth rate comparable to that in the general population; and that the evidence for an increased risk of meconium-stained liquor, cesarean section or postpartum hemorrhage is inconclusive.

Presentation is with severe pruritus affecting the limbs and trunk, particularly, the palms and soles, developing in the second half of pregnancy (usually during the third trimester) with excoriations, but no rash. Insomnia and malaise are common. Complete recovery is usually rapid after delivery, although rarely the condition may worsen postpartum. Abnormal liver function tests may take 4–6 weeks to return to normal in some women.

Clinical signs include dark urine, anorexia, and malabsorption of fat with steatorrhea.

Laboratory investigations involve using pregnancy-specific reference ranges for liver function tests. They show a moderate increase of transaminases (usually less than three-fold) and less commonly of GGT, bilirubin and APS (in excess of the normal pregnancy rise). Total bile acids are elevated and are a sensitive marker for the condition; this may be the only biochemical abnormality. Pruritus may precede the abnormal liver function tests, and serial measurements are advised in women with persistent typical itching.

The **diagnosis** is made by:

- A typical history of pruritus without rash
- Abnormal liver function tests
- Exclusion of other causes of abnormal liver function
- Postnatal resolution of symptoms and liver function tests.

Ultrasound of the liver, viral serology (for hepatitis A, B, and C; Epstein-Barr virus, cytomegalovirus) and liver autoantibodies (anti-smooth muscle antibody for chronic active autoimmune hepatitis; anti-mitochondrial antibodies for primary biliary cirrhosis) should be done to exclude other causes of pruritus and abnormal liver function tests. Pregnancy-specific causes of abnormal liver function tests (e.g. preeclampsia, acute fatty liver of pregnancy) must be excluded.

Monitoring after diagnosis:

- Liver function tests and prothrombin should be measured weekly and bile acids frequently.
- No specific method of monitoring can predict fetal compromise or death.
- The probability of adverse fetal outcome increases by 1–2% for each additional μmol/l of bile acid, and it does not increase until bile acid levels >40 μmol/l.

Commonly a combination of cardiotocography and ultrasound is used, but there is no evidence base: women should be warned of the limitations of existing practice.

Maternal treatment consists of vitamin K and symptom control.

Vitamin K (10 mg po daily) may reduce the risk of maternal and fetal bleeding. It is started at 32 weeks or from diagnosis (if after 32 weeks) because of the increased incidence of preterm labor. Vitamin K, preferably in a water-soluble formulation, is essential for women with a prolonged prothrombin time or receiving cholestyramine therapy.

Topical emollients and antihistamines (e.g. chlorpheniramine 4 mg tds or promethazine 25 mg at night) may help relieve pruritus.

Ursodeoxycholic acid (1000–1500 mg daily in 2–3 doses) is a hydrophilic bile acid that decreases the hydrophobic hepatotoxic bile acids, and may reduce pruritus and abnormal liver function. Ursodeoxycholic acid is not licensed for use in pregnancy, but there are no reports of adverse fetal or maternal effects.

Other: Reduction in symptom severity has also been reported with dexamethasone (12 mg po daily for 7 days), **S-adenosylmethionine** and **cholestyramine**. The latter two are no longer widely used.

Labor: In most centers, in women who do not deliver prematurely, labor is usually induced at 37–38 weeks gestation. This is not supported by evidence, and the theoretical advantages should be considered together with the risks of respiratory morbidity and emergency cesarean section from the earlier delivery/induction of labor. During labor, close monitoring of the mother and fetus should be instigated due to the risks of fetal distress and postpartum hemorrhage. The neonate should receive vitamin K (IV).

Post-delivery: Liver function should be measured post-delivery to ensure resolution. The risk of recurrence in future pregnancies is ~90%, and these women should avoid estrogen-containing oral contraceptives or liver function should be monitored if they are used.

Acute Fatty Liver of Pregnancy (AFLP) and HELLP Syndrome

Preeclampsia, HELLP syndrome and AFLP are related conditions; 20–50% of women with preeclampsia may present with abnormal liver function tests.

HELLP syndrome (Hemolysis Elevated Liver Enzymes and Low Platelets)

Background

HELLP is thought to be a severe form of preeclampsia, affecting 5–20% of these pregnancies, with one-third postpartum. Hepatic damage is thought to occur as a result of increased sinusoidal pressure, hypovolemia and fibrin deposition.

Maternal mortality of ~1% and perinatal mortality of ~10–50% have been reported.

Presentation is with right upper quadrant or epigastric pain (65%), and nausea and vomiting (35%). Hypertension is present in 80% of cases ± proteinuria and metabolic acidosis may be present.

Laboratory investigations show low-grade hemolysis on peripheral blood smear (with associated increased lactate dehydrogenase), low or falling platelets, increased transaminases, and there may be an increase in bilirubin and signs of disseminated intravascular coagulation. A mildly elevated prothrombin time indicates disseminated intravascular coagulation, whereas a gross elevation is seen with hepatic necrosis.

Risks include subcapsular liver hematoma, massive hepatic necrosis, abruption and, more rarely, acute renal failure, pulmonary edema and metabolic acidosis.

Management involves prompt stabilization and delivery. Platelets should be given only for counts $<50 \times 10^9/l$ if there is active bleeding or before an invasive or surgical procedure; fresh frozen plasma should be given for coagulopathy. A transient improvement may be seen with administration of maternal corticosteroids for fetal lung maturity, although attempts to prolong gestation may be fatal. Postpartum deterioration may be seen, and ≤30% of cases may arise postpartum. A rapid and complete recovery is usual. Studies vary on the recurrence rate of HELLP in a future pregnancy, with figures of 2–27% quoted. The risk of preeclampsia is higher, and may be up to 75% if background hypertension is present.

Acute Fatty Liver of Pregnancy (AFLP)

Background: This rare disorder is associated with abnormalities in mitochondrial-oxidation and LCHAD deficiency. There is considerable overlap of the symptoms and signs with preeclampsia and HELLP syndrome.

Incidence: AFLP is rare; the annual incidence in this is 1 case per 7000–16000 population. It usually occurs in the third trimester. It can lead to hepatic failure and encephalopathy and death for the fetus (20–30%) and mother (10–20%) if untreated.

Risk factors include obesity, multiple pregnancy and male fetuses.

Complications–AFLP carries a high maternal and fetal mortality between 2–18% and 7–58% respectively. Maternal complications include disseminated intravascular coagulation, renal failure, pancreatitis and (transient) diabetes insipidus. There is also a risk of progression to hepatic encephalopathy and fulminant liver failure.

Initial manifestations include malaise (100%), anorexia and nausea and vomiting (70%) and abdominal pain (50–80%). Jaundice often follows these non-specific symptoms in 1–2 weeks; this is the phase when the diagnosis is usually made. Transient diabetes insipidus has been described.

The disease may initially appear similar to preeclampsia, but hypertension and proteinuria are usually mild. Transaminases are markedly abnormal, with values higher than those seen in HELLP, and jaundice may be present with increased conjugated bilirubin.

White cell count may be elevated in excess of the normal pregnancy rise (>15 × 10^9/l). Excessive hyperuricemia and hypoglycemia should alert one to the diagnosis of AFLP. Metabolic acidosis may be present. Hepatic failure with disseminated intravascular coagulation and renal failure may ensue in advanced cases.

The diagnosis can be confirmed with liver biopsy, but this is rarely done in those with clotting defects, and a clinical diagnosis is sufficient.

Imaging (ultrasound, MRI, CT) is occasionally employed to exclude organic lesions in liver, liver rupture, infarct or biliary disease.

Swansea criteria for diagnosis of AFLP[a]–six or more of the following features in the absence of another explanation
Vomiting
Polydipsia/polyuria
Abdominal pain
Encephalopathy
Elevated bilirubin (>14 μmol/L)
Hypoglycemia (<4 mmol/L)
Elevated urate (>340 μmol/L)
Leukocytosis (>11 x 10^9l/L)
Ascites or bright liver on ultrasound scan
Microvesicular steatosis on liver biopsy
Elevated transaminases (aspartate aminotransferase or alanine aminotransferase >42 IU/L)
Renal impairment (creatinine >150 μmol/L)
Coagulopathy (prothrombin time >14 s or activated partial thromboplastin time >34 s)

[a]Ch'ng CL, Morgan M, Hainsworth I, Kingham JG. Prospective study of liver dysfunction in pregnancy in Southwest Wales. Gut 2002 Dec;51:876-80.

Management: There is no benefit in conservative management.

Delivery is the only treatment, and a multidisciplinary team (obstetrician, anesthetist, hematologist, pediatrician) should be involved. Resuscitation including correction of coagulopathy and hypoglycemia (hypertonic glucose infusions) should be undertaken before delivery. The fetus is at risk and should be carefully monitored. Hypoglycemia can last for many days or even weeks after recovery begins, and must be watched for until liver function returns to normal. Broad-spectrum antimicrobial therapy (including anti-fungal agents) should be instituted early.

There is almost always early onset of acute renal dysfunction, which is usually reversible, but renal support is often required.

Patients with encephalopathy should be considered for intubation and mechanical ventilation. There is often a worsening of liver function, renal function and coagulopathy for 48 hours after delivery, but improvement should occur after this time. Initially, liver function tests improve, followed by coagulation and renal function, and finally pancreatic function.

Post-delivery most women recover quickly, and management is conservative and supportive. Liver function may take up to 4 weeks to recover and liver transplantation should be considered in those with liver rupture, severe encephalopathy or failure of liver recovery. The recurrence rate for AFLP is around 25% but many women avoid a further pregnancy. The baby should be screened for LCHAD deficiency. Subsequent pregnancies should be monitored with serial liver function tests.

Distinguishing features of acute fatty liver and HELLP[a]

	HELLP	AFLP
Epigastric pain	++	+
Vomiting	±	++
Hypertension	++	+
Proteinuria	++	+
Elevated liver enzymes	+	++
Hypoglycemia	±	++
Hyperuricemia	+	++
DIC	+	++
Thrombocytopenia (without DIC)	++	±
White blood cell count ↑	+	++
Ultrasound/CT	Normal/hepatic hematoma	See text
Multiple pregnancy		+
Primiparous	++	++
Male fetus	50%	70% (M:F = 3:1)

[a]Reproduced by kind permission of Informa Healthcare USA Inc, Nelson Piercy C. Handbook of Obstetric Medicine. Informa Healthcare 2009;231.

Differential Diagnosis of Pruritus and Abnormal Liver Function Tests in Pregnancy

Differential diagnosis	Features to note in the history	Test
Biliary obstruction	Right upper quadrant pain, jaundice, history of gallstones, steatorrhea, dark urine	USS liver, gallbladder and biliary tree
Acute cholecystitis	Severe right upper quadrant pain, nausea, vomiting, systemic malaise, fever	
Viral hepatitis	Systemic malaise	Hepatitis A, B & C, EBV, CMV
Autoimmune liver disease	History of autoimmune disease	Anti-microbial antibodies, anti-smooth muscle antibodies
Congenital (Gilbert's, Dubin Johnson, Rotor)	Family history of jaundice particularly during periods of illness	Isolated hyperbilirubinemia
Pruritus gravidarum	Pruritus with its onset in pregnancy at any gestation, affects 20% of women	Normal LFT, bile acids
Drug reaction	Use of antihypertensives (especially methyldopa but also atenolol and verapamil), antituberculous medication (rifampicin, isoniazid), penicillins (flucloxacillin, ampicillin, amoxicillin, co-amoxiclav), nitrofurantoin, antithyroid medication (propylthiouracil, carbimazole), phenothiazines (e.g. chlorpromazine) and paracetamol in high doses	

Evaluation of Pruritus in Pregnancy

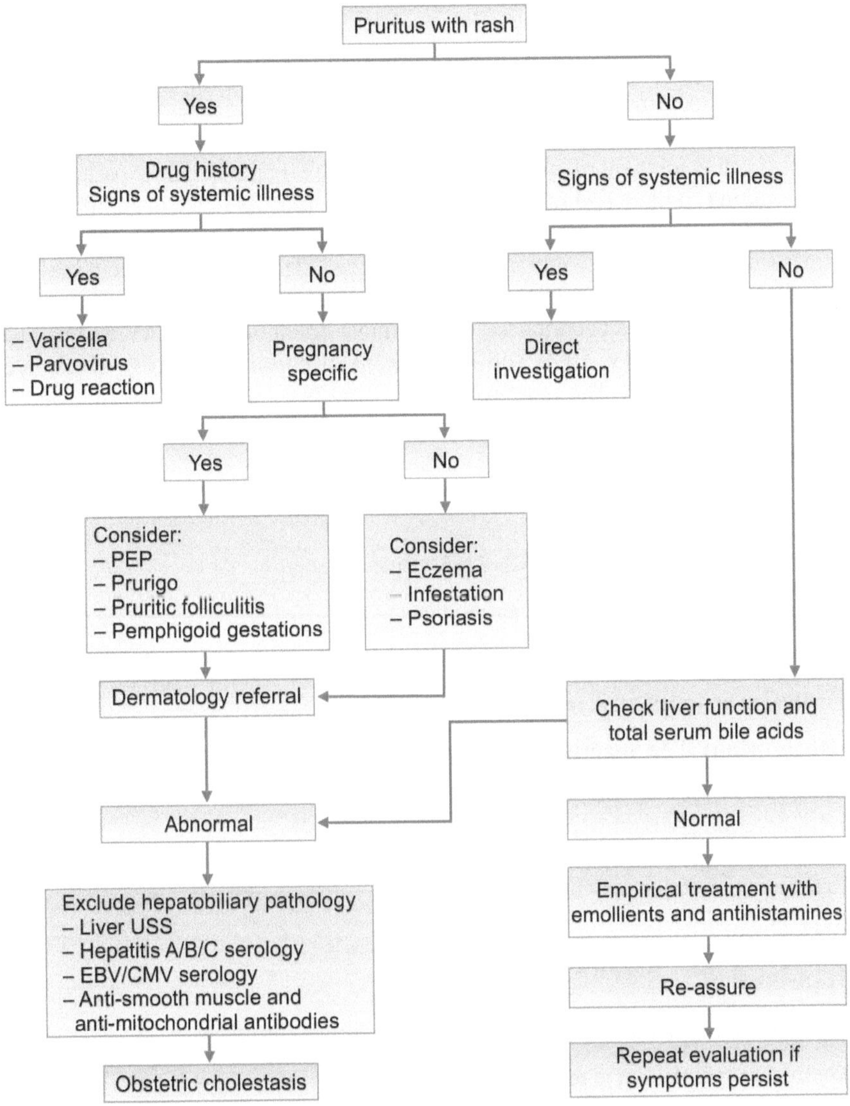

VIRAL INFECTIONS

Hepatitis

Acute viral hepatitis is the commonest cause of jaundice in pregnancy. It is caused by the hepatitis viruses (A, B, C, D, E), cytomegalovirus, Epstein-Barr virus and herpes simplex virus. Many patients are asymptomatic or could complain, even before the development of jaundice, of myalgia, right upper quadrant pain, nausea and vomiting, fatigue and malaise. The course for most patients is unaffected by pregnancy, apart from hepatitis E virus (HEV) and disseminated herpes simplex virus: maternal and fetal mortality are increased. Transaminase levels may be >1000 IU, but APS and GGT are frequently normal. A few patients may develop cholestasis during the acute phase. This is most common with HAV and can be prolonged. Only HBV, HCV and HDV result in chronic hepatitis, which is a histological diagnosis. The course of chronic hepatitis is unaffected by pregnancy. Liver biopsy is often required in the management of chronic liver disease, but should be avoided in pregnancy.

Hepatitis A Virus

Transmission is mainly orofecal. RNA virus.

Diagnosis is by anti-HAV IgM antibodies.

Acute illness is often self-limiting.

Vertical transmission is rare.

Vaccination: The inactivated vaccine against HAV and the postexposure immunoglobulin prophylaxis are safe in pregnancy.

Hepatitis B Virus

Prevalence in pregnancy is 0.1–1%.

DNA virus

Transmission

Mother–Mainly by sexual contact and infected blood products.

Vertical transmission is mainly intrapartum.

Diagnosis: Standard testing is for the surface antigen (HBsAg). Other tests include core antigen (HBc), the e-antigen (HBeAg) and, later in the disease, their antibodies. IgM anti-HBc suggests acute HBV infection. The individual is a carrier of hepatitis B antigen if the antigen is detectable after six months. Persistent e-antigen is associated with high infectivity.

Acute illness is often self-limiting.

Vaccination: Neonates should be given HBV immunoglobulin and vaccine within 24 hours from birth because 95% of vertical transmission occurs intrapartum; this is 85–95% effective at preventing HBV infection and chronic carrier state

(90% risk after neonatal infection). Babies may safely be breastfed if they are immunized.

Hepatitis D Virus

Measures to prevent hepatitis B are effective in preventing hepatitis D because HDV is dependent on coinfection with HBV for replication.

Hepatitis C Virus

Prevalence in pregnancy is 0.2–3%.

RNA Virus

Transmission

Mother: Through infected blood exposure and sexual contact.

The vertical transmission rate is ~5% and increases 3–5-fold if coinfected with HIV and with increasing maternal viral load at the time of birth. It is not influenced by the HCV genotype.

Diagnosis: Testing is by measuring serum anti-HCV antibodies, but acute infection cannot be reliably diagnosed this way because tests may not become positive for up to three months. In chronic disease, detection of antibodies is not sufficient and persisting viral RNA can be detected in the serum by polymerase chain reaction.

Symptoms: 75% of HCV infections are asymptomatic. About 70% of patients develop chronic infection, 20% of whom develop cirrhosis over 10–30 years, and ≤4% hepatocellular carcinoma.

Sequelae: Chronic active HCV is associated with an increased incidence of preterm delivery and intrauterine growth restriction.

Treatment: There is no safe treatment or vaccine for preventing HCV infection during pregnancy.

Contraindication: Pre-natal diagnosis and invasive monitoring in labor (relative contraindication) should be avoided.

Vertical transmission occurs during pregnancy or in the peripartum period. There is no association between gestational age at delivery or chorioamnionitis and the risk of vertical transmission. Data are conflicting regarding duration of ruptured membranes and the risk of vertical transmission but, if this exceeds six hours, the risk may be increased. The planned cesarean section may not prevent or reduce the incidence of vertical transmission.

Breastfeeding is safe; HCV has been detected in milk and colostrum in some studies; breastfeeding with high viral loads should be avoided.

Postnatal follow-up: HCV-IgG antibodies can be detected in baby's blood for ≤18 months. Vertical transmission is diagnosed by a positive serum HCV-RNA on two occasions 3–4 months apart after the infant is at least 2-months-old and/or by the detection of anti-HCV antibodies after the infant is 18-months-old. Early treatment reduces the risk of chronic infection (80 to 50% with treatment) in HCV diagnosed during pregnancy.

Hepatitis E Virus

HEV is transmitted through the orofecal route. During pregnancy, it can cause fulminating hepatitis, mimicking AFLP, with a mortality rate of 16%. It is particularly dangerous if contracted in the third trimester, and can result in hepatic encephalopathy and liver failure. Vertical transmission among HEV-RNA-positive mothers ≤50% and nearly 100% among women with symptomatic infection with significant perinatal mortality and morbidity.

Herpes Simplex Virus Type 2

Herpes simplex virus type 2 is sexually transmitted and can cause fulminant hepatic failure, pneumonitis or encephalitis in pregnancy with a high mortality. Antiviral therapy (acyclovir IV) is recommended.

Epstein-Barr Virus and Cytomegalovirus

Acute hepatitis is common in infections with Epstein-Barr virus, and rare with cytomegalovirus. Jaundice is uncommon.

Epstein-Barr virus is transmitted by close oral contact and may be acquired asymptomatically. If symptoms occur, they are usually a sore-throat and generalized lymphadenopathy. Perinatal transmission does not occur. About 50–60% of women of childbearing age have antibodies to cytomegalovirus, indicating previous infection. Primary infection in the pregnant woman at any gestation may affect the fetus (30–40%), causing congenital abnormalities and growth restriction.

GALLBLADDER DISEASE (GALLSTONES AND CHOLECYSTITIS)

Pregnancy increases the risk of gallstone formation, as estrogen increases the cholesterol content of the liver and progesterone increases bile secretion. This results in increased saturation of the bile with cholesterol and gallstone formation. Cholecystitis should be treated promptly with broad-spectrum intravenous antibiotics and fluids, as it can precipitate pre-term labor. Pancreatitis is another serious complication of gallstones and again management is usually conservative as discussed below. Pancreatitis rarely occurs in pregnancy and is most commonly due to gallstones. Hypertryglyceridemia and hypercalcemia of primary hyperparathyroidism are other causes. The presentation and symptoms are similar to the non-pregnant patient and the diagnosis is usually made when the serum amylase >1000 U/l.

Management is supportive with intravenous fluids and analgesia. Most cases will resolve spontaneously but around 10% will develop severe complications needing ITU support. Careful assessment of renal and liver function, clotting, glucose, full blood count and oxygen saturation will help to distinguish those needing intensive care.

Differential diagnosis of abnormal liver function in pregnancy	
Viral hepatitis (A, B, C, E)	Serology
EBV, CMV, HSV	
Autoimmune hepatitis	ANA, anti-LKM antibodies
Primary biliary cirrhosis	Anti-mitochondrial antibodies, ANF, ANTI-sm
Autoimmune sclerosing cholangitis	Anti-sm, ANCA
Wilson's disease	Serum copper and ceruloplasmin
Hemochromatosis	Ferritin
Gallstones	Ultrasound
Fatty liver	
Cirrhosis	
ANA, antinuclear antibodies; LKM, liver-kidney microsome; ANF, antinuclear factor; sm, smooth muscle	

PREGNANCY FOLLOWING LIVER TRANSPLANTATION

The chance of successful pregnancy in women following transplantation is around 70%, although the risk of complications such as miscarriage, IUGR, pre-term delivery and preeclampsia is increased. Ideally pregnancy should be deferred until at least 1 year following liver transplantation to allow the graft function to stabilize and when lower doses of immunosuppressants can be used. Also there is an increased risk of infection with cytomegalovirus immediately follow transplantation which may result in congenital abnormalities if occurs in early pregnancy. Graft function and survival are not affected by pregnancy though. The immunosuppressant agents Tacrolimus, Prednisolone and Cyclosporine are generally well tolerated in pregnancy and are not associated with fetal malformations. Mycophenolate Mofetil (MMF) is teratogenic in animals and there are reported cases of congenital malformations in babies born to mothers taking this drug and therefore should be avoided. Rates of cesarean section are high amongst this group of women although vaginal delivery is not contraindicated.

CHAPTER

44

Thyroid Disorders

CHANGES IN THYROID PHYSIOLOGY IN PREGNANCY

- Pregnancy has goitrogenic effect because of the increased demand
- TBG increases because of increased synthesis under the influence of of estrogen and reduced clearance, total serum T_3 and T_4 levels increase during pregnancy due to an increase in thyroid binding globulin (TBG) which doubles the non-pregnant levels by 16–20 weeks beginning in the early weeks and increase in plasma volume (Total T_4 increases to 1.5 times its nonpregnant levels, hence nonpregnant values should be multiplied by 1.5 to obtain normal values for pregnancy).
- Free hormone levels remain unchanged
- To maintain a constant T_4 level in the plasma, the production of T_4 increases by 30–50%
- hCG has thyrotropic effect, hence increases free thyroxine levels transiently at 8–10 weeks of gestation. As a result, TSH levels are suppressed and free hormone levels are increased in first trimester. Upper limit of TSH in first trimester is 2.5 mIU/L.
- Iodine requirement increases due to increased synthesis of thyroxine, the transplacental transfer of thyroxine and iodine to fetus and increased iodine excretion during pregnancy due to increased GFR and plasma clearance.
- Mild biochemical hypothyroidism in third trimester may be due to–
  - Physiological dilution
  - Increased breakdown by large placenta [placenta contains the enzyme 3-deiodinase which converts T_4 to reverse T which is an inactive form of the enzyme]
  - Inability to compensate for increased fetal demand
  - Physiological adaptation to conserve energy for parturition.

Hormonal Changes in Pregnancy

	Non-pregnant	1st trimester	2nd trimester	3rd trimester
TSH mu/l	0–4	0–1.6	0.1–1.8	0.7–7.3
FT_4 pmol/l	11–23	11–22	11–19	7–15
FT_3 pmol/l	4–9	4–8	4–7	3–5

HYPOTHYROIDISM

1/600–2000 deliveries

Causes

- Chronic autoimmune thyroid disease (Hashimotos)
- Goitrous (iodine deficiency)
- Atrophic
- Radioiodine-131 ablation
- Thyroidectomy
- Congenital like defect in thyroglobulin synthesis
- Infiltrative disorders like sarcoidosis, amyloidosis, hemochromatosis, etc.

Symptoms: Fatigue, sleepiness, lethargy, mental slowing, depression, cold intolerance (unusual in pregnancy), decreased perspiration, dry skin, sparse thin hair, deeper voice or hoarseness, reduced appetite but weight gain, constipation, arthralgias, muscle ache, stiffness, paresthesias (carpal tunnel syndrome) in 75% cases.

Signs: General slowing (speech, movements), sparse hair, dry skin, deep, voice, horseness, bradycardia, myxedema (nonpitting edema), pale or yellowish skin, hyporeflexia, prolonged relaxation of reflexes. Pulse rate is appropriately slow for pregnancy.

Overt Hypothyroidism

TSH is increased and free T_4 decreased

Implications of hypothyroidism in pregnancy:

- Increased risk of miscarriage
- High-risk of PIH (15–30%)
- Placental abruption and PPH
- Premature delivery (22–44%)
- IUGR
- Fetal distress
- Neurodevelopmental delay
- Anemia
- Myxedematous coma (rare but serious complication with maternal mortality of 20%)

Subclinical Hypothyroidism

- TSH is increased and free T_4 is normal
- Does not affect the pregnancy

Isolated Maternal Hypothyroxinemia

- Free T_4 is low but TSH is normal
- Has no increased adverse pregnancy outcome
- So universal screening for thyroid dysfunction during pregnancy is not recommended unless clinically indicated.

Iodine Deficiency

- Adequate iodine is requisite for fetal neurological development beginning soon after conception and abnormalities are dependent on degree of deficiency
- Mild deficiency causes intellectual impairment
- Moderate deficiency causes various effects on intellectual and psychomotor function
- Severe deficiency causes endemic cretinism
- Recommended supplementation during pregnancy and lactation is 150 μg/day

Treatment

- L-thyroxine
- Initial dose is 50 μg/day if TSH<10 mU/ml
  75 μg/day if TSH<11–20 mU/ml
  100 μg/day if TSH>20 mU/ml
  Reqirement of thyroxine is increased by 25% during pregnancy beginning as early as 5 weeks but routine increase in thyroxine dose in pregnancy is not recommended.
- Patient on thyroxine replacement, TSH and free T_4 is done once in 4 to 6 weeks till we achieve euthyroid state (free T_4 level at the upper end of normal range and TSH at lower end of the normal range), later serum TSH levels once in 3 months.
- After delivery the dosage of thyroxine should be reduced to prepregnancy levels and TSH measured at 6 to 8 weeks postpartum.

Congenital Hypothyroidism

- Universal newborn screening is recommended because the clinical diagnosis of hypothyroidism in neonates is usually missed.
- Screening done within one hour of delivery by cord blood or on 6th day of life using heel prick.
- Early and aggressive thyroxine replacement is critical for infants with congenital hypothyroidism.
- Maternal TSH receptor blocking antibodies can cross the placenta and can cause fetal thyroid dysfunction.
- Antithyroid peroxidase and anti-thyroglobulin antibodies have no effect on fetal thyroid function even though they crossed placenta.
- Prevalence of fetal hypothyroidism in women with Hashimoto thyroiditis is very low.

HYPERTHYROIDISM IN PREGNANCY

Causes of thyrotoxicosis:

1. Autoimmune:
   - Graves disease
   - Subacute thyroiditis
2. Tumors:
   - Thyroid tumors

- Toxic adenoma
- Toxic nodular goiter
- Pituitary thyrotropic adenoma
- Struma ovarii

3. Drugs containing iodine like amiodarone, lithium, etc.
4. Gestational trophoblastic disease

Clinical presentation: Heat intolerance, sweating, tachycardia, dyspnea, nervousness, emotional liability, inability to gain weight

Physical signs: Skin is warm and moist. Cardiovascular signs are pronounced like thrill, tachycardia, diffuse and forceful apex beat and loud S1 and S2 heart sounds. Neurological signs may reveal tremors of hands and proximal muscle weakness and there might be lid lag or globe lag.

Symptoms and signs which help to differentiate between physiological changes and hyperthyroidism are persistent tachycardia >100/min, weight loss inspite of good appetite and eye changes.

Laboratory tests: FT_4, FT_3, serum TSH (pregnancy specific ranges should be considered)

Overt hyperthyroidism: SH decreased, FT_4 increased

Subclinical hyperthyroidism: TSH decreased, FT_4 normal (not associated with adverse pregnancy outcomes, requires only periodic surveillance)

Gestational thyrotoxicosis: Seen in hyperemesis gravidarum–TSH decreased, FT_4 increased because of increased β hCG, it becomes normal by mid-pregnancy so antithyroid drugs are not recommended.

Pre-pregnancy counseling: Dosage of ATD is frequently adjusted

- Goal of keeping free thyroid hormone level in the upper one-third of the normal range
- 30% of the women may be discontinued in the last few weeks of gestation

Anti-Thyroid Drugs

Propylthiouracil (PTU)

Most preferred drug because it partially inhibits conversion of T_4 to T_3 and crosses placenta readily than methimazole (methimazole embryopathy-esophageal/choanal atresia and aplasia cutis) initial dose is 300–450 mg and then reduce to minimum effective dose once euthyroidism is achieved (maintenance dose is 50–300 mg/day).

- Serum FT_4 should be measured 4 weekly
- Dose is adjusted such that FT_4 should be maintained in the upper 1/3rd of the normal range.
- Overdosage may produce fetal goiter and hypothyroidism
- Continue therapy until at least 32 weeks gestation

Side Effects

- Transient leukopenia in 10% (should not stop treatment)
- Agranulocytosis 0.3–0.4% (stop the drug)—it is not dose-related and is acute in onset, so serial leukocyte counts during therapy are not helpful. If fever or

sore-throat develops, stop medication immediately and send for complete blood count
- Hepatotoxicity
- Vasculitis
- Urticaria or rash.

Carbimazole 10–20 mg, BD
Beta blockers: Ameliorate symptoms like palpitations, tachycardia and tremors

Surgery

Subtotal thyroidectomy is indicated in those who don't respond or intolerant to medical treatment or having developed compressive symptoms due to large goiter
Complications: High incidence of hypothyroidism, hypoparathyroidism (1–2%), recurrent laryngeal nerve palsy (1–2%)
- Ablation with radioactive iodine is contraindicated in pregnancy, if taken before conception pregnancy should be avoided for at least 6 months.
- The pregnancy loss associated with general anesthesia and surgery is approximately 8% in first trimester and 6.5% in second trimester.

Thyroid Storm

- Acute life-threatening hyper metabolic state which is rare in pregnancy
- The pregnant women with thyrotoxicosis has minimal cardiac reserve, decompensation is precipitated by preeclampsia, anemia, sepsis

Management

Should be carried out in ICU
- PTU (Propylthiouracil) 1000 mg orally or crushed and given through nasogastric tube, later 200 mg 6th hourly
- After 1 hour of propylthiouracil sodium iodine dose 500–1000 mg IV every 8th hourly should be given to inhibit thyroidal release of T_3, T_4
  Other forms of iodine can be given are:
  - Supersaturated solution of potassium iodide TID or
  - Lugol solution 10 drops orally TID or
  - Lithium carbonate 300 mg 6th hourly (In case of iodine – induced anaphylaxis)
- Most authorities recommend 2 mg dexamethasone IV every 6th hourly 4 doses

Fetal and Neonatal Effects

- Clinical hyperthyroidism occurs in 1% of neonates born to woman with Graves' disease
- Few babies develop goitrous thyrotoxicosis caused by placental transfer of thyroid stimulating immunoglobulin
- Fetal exposure to maternally administered thionamides may cause goitrous hypothyroidism, if it is detected, the fetus can be treated by a reduction in maternal antithyroid medication and injection of intra-amniotic thyroxine if necessary.

Fetal Diagnosis

- To exclude hyperthyroidism secondary to passive antibody transfer and hypothyroidism secondary to antithyroid medications
- Routine fetal thyroid sonographic assessment in women taking thionamide drugs or those with thyroid stimulating antibodies is not recommended
- In fetuses with hydrops, IUGR, goiter or tachycardia then fetal sampling seems appropriate
- After 7–10 days postnatally—hyperthyroidism since the half-life of maternally-derived antithyroid drugs is shorter than that of TSH receptor antibodies.
- Breastfeeding is safe in those receiving propylthiouracil <150 mg/day and carbimazole <15 mg/day

Guidelines for Measurement of Thyroid Stimulating Hormone Receptor Antibodies in Pregnancies

1. An euthyroid pregnant woman without medication but who has previously received antithyroid drugs for Graves disease. The risk for fetal and neonatal hyperthyroidism is negligible. Measurement of TRAbs is not necessary.
2. An euthyroid pregnant women (with or without thyroid hormone substitution therapy) who has previously received radioiodine therapy or undergone thyroid surgery for Graves disease—measure TRAbs in the first trimester
   - If absent or low–no further evaluation is recommended
   - If high—fetus should be followed carefully for the signs of hyperthyroidism, again measure TRAbs in the last trimester to evaluate the risk of neonatal hypothyroidism
3. A pregnant woman who takes antithyroid drugs for Graves disease TRAbs should be measured in the last trimester
   - If absent or low—neonatal hyperthyroidism is ulikely
   - If high—evaluation for neonatal hyperthyroidism is needed (clinical evaluation and thyroid function tests on cord blood and again after 4 to 7 days)

Postpartum thyroiditis: Transient autoimmune thyroiditis found in 5–10% of women during the first year of the child birth

Clinical manifestations: Diagnosed infrequently because it typically develops months after the delivery and have vague and nonspecific symptoms

Clinical phases:

Factor	Thyrotoxicosis	Hypothyroidism
Onset	1–4 months	4–8 months
Incidence	4%	2–5%
Mechanism	Destruction induced hormone release	Thyroid insufficiency
Symptoms	Small painless goiter, fatigue, palpitations	Goiter, fatigue, inability to concentrate
Treatment	β blockers for symptoms	Thyroxine for 6–12 months
Sequelae	1/3rd develop hypothyroidism	1/3rd permanently hypothyroid by 6–7 yrs

Thyroid Nodules

- 2% of pregnant women, usually present with hyperthyroidism.
- 90% of thyroid cancers present as thyroid nodules so it needs evaluation

Diagnosis

USG is the mainstay of investigation
(Radioactive iodine is contraindicated)

Indications for FNAC

- Rapidly enlarging nodules
- Cystic nodules >4 cm
- Solid nodules >2 cm
    - Management of thyroid nodule depends on gestational age
    - Nodule identified at >20 weeks should be biopsied after delivery
    - If biopsy shows low grade, benign, slow growing—surgery is deferred until delivery
    - If biopsy confirms malignancy, surgery is the mainstay, can be safely performed in 2nd trimester.

SECTION 5

INFECTIONS IN PREGNANCY

- HIV Infection
- Hepatitis B Infection
- Malaria
- Urinary Tract Infection
- Tuberculosis
- Syphilis
- Torch Infections
- Bacterial Vaginosis
- Monilial Vaginitis

CHAPTER

45

HIV Infection

HIV/AIDS is a major concern of health care professionals all over the world.

Laboratory diagnosis is the method of defining/establishing HIV status of an individual. HIV infection is spreading rapidly in India. AIDS has shattered the global economy with no successful treatment and vaccine in sight.

INCIDENCE

- The global population of women living with HIV/AIDS grew by 1.2 million between 2004–2006 to a total of 17.7 million, or 48% of total population of adults living with HIV
- The HIV epidemic in India is diverse with the highest burden in 6 states in Maharashtra, Andhra Pradesh, Tamil Nadu, Karnataka, Manipur, Nagaland.
- The prevalence rates for adult females are 0.29% while for males it is 0.43%.
- According to NACO, 27 million pregnancies a year, 0.3% prevalence rate 1,00,000 HIV infected women deliver every year in India.

NATIONAL GUIDELINES ON TESTING ADULTS

- For symptomatic persons: The sample should be reactive with two different kits.
- For asymptomatic persons: The sample should be reactive with three different kits.
- The blood sample collected at one time is tested with the first kit. If it is reactive, it is then retested sequentially with the second and third kits.

SYMPTOMATIC PATIENTS

HIV Strategy II B (blood/plasma/serum)

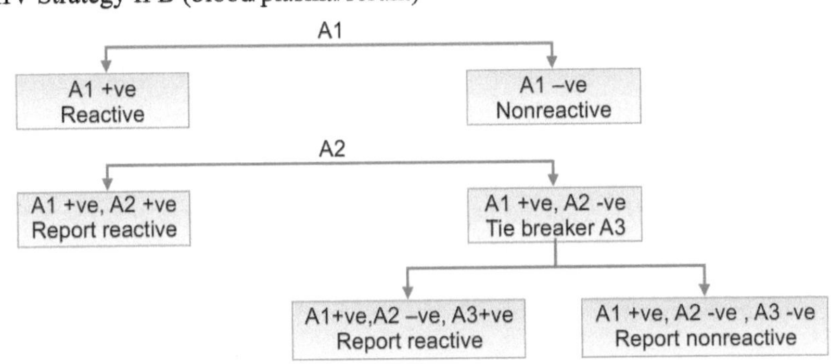

Asymptomatic Patients

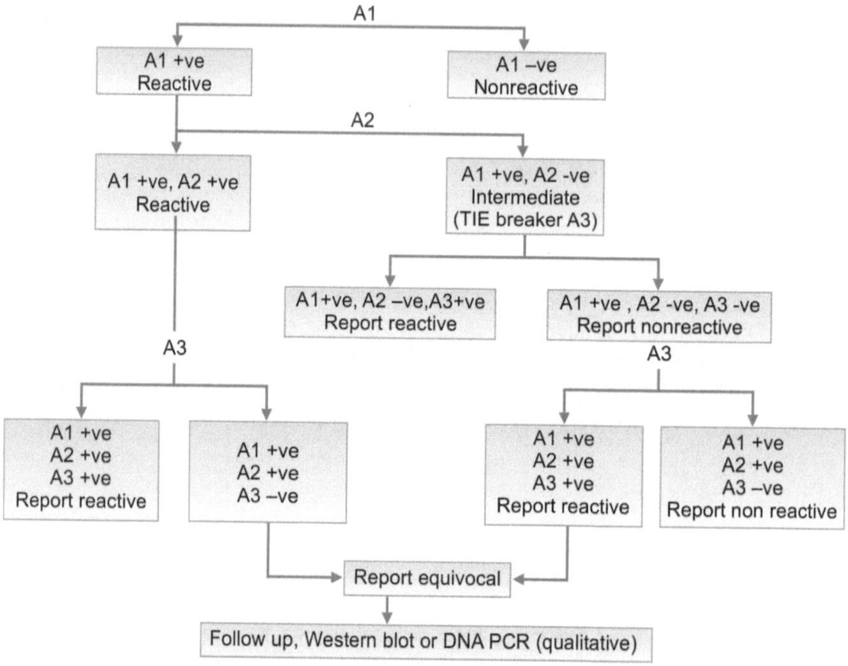

Assessment and Management of HIV Infected Person

- Perform history taking and physical examination
- Evaluate for signs and symptoms of HIV infections or OIs and WHO clinical staging
- Provide appropriate investigations/treatment of OIs
- If pregnant, refer to PPTCT
- Screen for TB
- Screen for STI
- Give patient education on treatment and adherence
- Arrange psychosocial, nutrition and community support
- Start ART
- Arrange follow up and monitoring
- Assess adherence every visit
- Provide positive prevention advice and condoms
- Provide patient information sheet on the ART regimen prescribed

At the beginning of HIV care and prior to starting ART:

- Determine the clinical stage of HIV infection
- Identify history of past illnesses (especially those related to HIV)
- Identify current HIV related illnesses that require treatment
- Determine the need for ART and Opportunistic infections prophylaxis
- Identify coexisting medical conditions and treatments that may influence the choice of therapy

WHO CLINICAL STAGING OF HIV/AIDS FOR ADULTS AND ADOLESCENTS 2010

Clinical Stage 1

- Asymptomatic
- Persistent generalized lymphoadenopathy

Clinical Stage 2

- Unexplained moderate weight loss (<10% of presumed or measured body weight)
- Recurrent respiratory tract infections (sinusitis, tonsillitis, otitis media)
- Herpes zoster
- Angular cheilitis
- Recurrent oral ulceration
- Papular pruritic eruptions
- Seborrheic dermatitis
- Fungal nail infections

Clinical Stage 3

- Unexplained severe weight loss (>10% presumed body weight) (Assessment of body weight in pregnant woman needs to consider expected weight gain of pregnancy)
- Unexplained chronic diarrhea for longer than 1 week
- Unexplained persistent fever (>37.5°C intermittent or constant for longer than 1 month)
- Persistent oral candidiasis
- Oral hairy leukoplakia
- Pulmonary TB
- Severe bacterial infections (pneumonia, empyema, pyomyositis, meningitis)
- Acute necrotizing ulcerative stomatitis, gingivitis or periodontitis
- Unexplained anemia (<8 g /dl), neutropenia ($<0.5 \times 10^9$/litre^3) and or chronic thrombocytopenia ($<50 \times 10^9$/litre^3)

Clinical Stage 4

- HIV wasting syndrome
- Pneumocystis pneumonia (PCP)
- Recurrent severe or radiological bacterial pneumonia
- Extrapulmonary tuberculosis
- HIV encephalopathy
- CNS toxoplasmosis
- Chronic (more than 1 month) or orolabial herpes simplex infection
- Esophageal candidiasis
- Kaposi's sarcoma
- Cytomegaloviral infections (CMV retinitis or infection of organs other than the liver, spleen or lymph nodes)
- Extrapulmonary cryptococcosis
- Disseminated endemic mycoses (e.g., coccidioidomycosis, penicilliosis, histoplasmosis)
- Cryptosporidiosis
- Isosporiasis
- Disseminated non-tuberculous mycobacteria infection

- Tracheal, bronchial or pulmonary candida infection
- Visceral herpes simplex infection
- Acquired HIV-associated rectal fistula
- Cerebral or B cell non-Hodgkin lymphoma
- Progressive multifocal leukoencephalopathy (PML)
- HIV-associated cardiomyopathy or nephropathy

Physical Examination

Physical examination checklist	
Record vital signs, body weight, height and body mass index (BMI), temperature, blood pressure, pulse rate, respiratory rate	
Appearance	• Unexplained moderate or severe weight loss, HIV wasting • Rapid weight loss is suggestive of active OI, especially if associated with fever • Gradual weight loss (not caused by malnutrition or other obvious illness) is suggestive of HIV infection • "Track marks" and soft tissue infections which are common among IDUs
Consider conditions other than HIV skin	• Malaria, tuberculosis, syphilis, gastrointestinal infections, bacterial pneumonia, pelvic inflammatory disease, viral hepatitis • Look for signs of HIV-related and other skin problems. These include diffuse dry skin, typical lesions of PPE, especially on the legs, seborrheic dermatitis on face and scalp • Look for Herpes simplex and Herpes zoster or scarring of previous Herpes zoster (especially multi-dermatome)
Lymph nodes	• Start with posterior cervical nodes • PGL (persistent glandular lymphadenopathy) typically presents as multiple bilateral, soft, non-tender, mobile cervical nodes. Similar nodes may be found in the armpits and groin • Tuberculosis lymph nodes typically present as unilateral, painful, hard, enlarging nodes, with constitutional symptoms such as fever, night sweats and weight loss
Mouth	• Look for signs suggestive of HIV infection including white plaques on tongue, cheeks and roof of mouth (oral candida), white stripped lesions on the side of the tongue (OHL) and cracking at the corners of the mouth (angular cheilitis) • Difficulty in swallowing is commonly caused by esophageal candida
Chest	• The most common problems will be PCP and TB • Signs and symptoms are cough, shortness of breath, hemoptysis, weight loss, fever, congestion or consolidation • Perform a chest X-ray, if symptomatic
Abdomen	• Hepatosplenomegaly, masses and local tenderness • Jaundice may indicate viral hepatitis
Ano-genital	• Herpes simplex and other genital sores/lesions, vaginal or penile discharge • Perform Pap smear, if possible
Neurological examination	• Focus on visual fields and the signs of neuropathy (bilateral peripheral or localized mono-neuropathies) • Assess focal neurological deficit

Note: During each consultation, patient is to be clinically screened for TB (history and physical examination)

Comprehensive Laboratory Evaluation

Rationale of laboratory evaluation in HIV/AIDS	
Essential	**Optional**
Confirm HIV infection: HIV status must be documented. Refer to ICTC if in doubt	**Fasting lipid profile:** May be recommended in patients with established coronary disease risk factors, or if stavudine, efavirenz, protease inhibitor (PI) use is contemplated
Specific investigations: To rule out OIs, depending on the clinical need	**Pregnancy test:** EFV is contraindicated in pregnancy during the first trimester of pregnancy
CD4 counts: All patients should have baseline screening	**Anti-HCV screening:** The prevalence of hepatitis C virus (HCV) is low in HIV-infected patients, except, for example, in the northeastern states of India, where injecting drug use is a risk factor. Such screening is also recommended in HIV-infected hemophiliacs and thalassemics.
CBC: Hb, TLC, DLC, ESR, GBP	**Chest X-ray:** To rule out TB or other pulmonary infection based on symptoms
LFTs: Necessary to find evidence of hepatitis, particularly when NVP use is contemplated	**Plasma viral load (PVL):** A baseline PVL is not necessary. With optimum adherence and a potent regimen, undetectable levels should be achieved at 6 months after ART initiation
Urine routine: To evaluate proteinuria and sugar (may necessitate estimation of blood glucose)	
HBsAg: To rule out concomitant hepatitis B infection as this can influence choice of ARV regimen.The abrupt stopping of anti-HBV drugs such as lamivudine and tenofovir is not recommended in patients with chronic hepatitis B co-infection since it may result in hepatitis B flare-up.This screening is mandatory for IVDUs and those with transfusion-associated HIV infection	
HCV screening: Mandatory for IVDUs and those with transfusion-associated HIV infection **VDRL/TPHA (syphilis screening):** Especially for persons From high-risk behavior groups, those with history of STIs and/or symptoms suggestive of syphilis	
Pap smear: Helps in earlier diagnosis of cervical intraepithelial neoplasia (CIN). Or trichloroacetic acid staining at district facilities where PAP smear is not available	

CD4 Monitoring and Follow-up Schedule

CD4 count	Repeat at
<350 and not on ART	3 months
>350 and not on ART	6 months
On ART (any value)	6 months
>500	Annual screening

Prophylaxis for Opportunistic Infections

Co-trimoxazole (CTX) Prophylaxis in Pregnant Women

Co-trimoxazole Prophylaxis Recommendations, 2006

Commencing primary CPT CD4 not available, CD4 available	CD4 not available	CD4 available
	WHO clinical stage 3 or 4 (This includes all patients with TB)	Any WHO clinical stage and CD4 <200 cells/mm^3 or Any WHO clinical stage, CD4 <350 cells/mm^3 and if patient is symptomatic or WHO stage 3 or 4 irrespective of CD4 count
Commencing secondary CPT	For all patients who have completed successful treatment for PCP until CD4 >200	
Timing the initiation of co-trimoxazole in relation to initiating ART	Start co-trimoxazole prophylaxis first. Start ART about two weeks later if the patient can tolerate co-trimoxazole and has no symptoms of allergy (rash, hepatotoxicity) Meanwhile, make use of the time for adherence and treatment preparation	
Dosage of cotrimoxazole in adults and adolescents	One double-strength tablet or two single-strength tablets once daily. Total daily dose of 960 mg (800 mg SMZ + 160 mg TMP)	
Cotrimoxazole for pregnant women	Women who fulfil the criteria for CPT should continue on it throughout pregnancy. If a woman requires CPT during pregnancy, it should be started regardless of the stage of pregnancy Breastfeeding women should continue CPT where indicated	
Patients allergic to sulpha-based medications	Dapsone 100 mg per day, if available Co-trimoxazole desensitization may be attempted but not in patients with a previous severe reaction to CTX or other sulpha-containing drugs	
Monitoring	No specific laboratory monitoring is required in patients receiving co-trimoxazole	

When to Stop Co-trimoxazole Prophylaxis

When to stop prophylaxis (co-trimoxazole or dapsone) in patients on ART	CD4 count not available	CD4 count available
	Continue prophylaxis indefinitely until CD4 count can be taken	If CD4 count >200 or at least 6 months and If patient is on ART for at least 6 months, is asymptomatic and well

Notes: If CPT is started at CD4 levels between 200–350 cells/mm^3. CD4 counts should have increased, patient is on ART for at least 6 months, is asymptomatic and well; before CPT is stopped.

Recommended Schedule for Starting and Stopping OI Prophylaxis

Opportunistic infection	Primary prophylaxis indicated when CD4 is –	Drug of choice	Discontinue primary prophylaxis when CD4 is –
PCP	<200	TMP-SMX 1 DS od	>200
Toxoplasmosis	<100	TMP-SMX 1 DS od	>200
CMV retinitis	Not indicated	Secondary: oral ganciclovir	Not applicable
Cryptococcus meningitis	Not indicated	Secondary: fluconazole	Not applicable
Oral and esophageal candidiasis	Not indicated	Not applicable	Not applicable

Protocol for Co-trimoxazole Desensitization

Step	Dosage
Day 1	80 mg SMX + 16 mg TMP (2 ml oral suspension)
Day 2	160 mg SMX + 32 mg TMP (4 ml oral suspension)
Day 3	240 mg SMX + 48 mg TMP (6 ml oral suspension)
Day 4	320 mg SMX + 64 mg TMP (8 ml oral suspension)
Day 5	One single-strength SMX-TMP tablet (400 mg SMX + 80 mg TMP)
Day 6	Two single-strength SMX-TMP tablets or one double-strength tablet (800 mg SMZ + 160 mg TMP)
Reference: Guidelines on co-trimoxazole prophylaxis for HIV-related infections among children, adolescents and adults in resource-limited settings: Recommendations for a public health approach. World Health Organization, 2006.	

Note: Co-trimoxazole oral suspension contains 40 mg TMP + 200 mg SMX per 5 ml

ARV DRUGS

Classes of Drugs Available

Nucleoside reverse transcriptase inhibitors (NRTI)	Non-nucleoside reverse transcriptase inhibitors (NNRTI)	Protease inhibitors
Zidovudine (AZT/ZDV)* x*	Nevirapine* (NVP)	Saquinavir* (SQV)
Stavudine (d4T)*	Efavirenz* (EFV)	Ritonavir* (RTV)
Lamivudine (3TC)*	Delavirdine (DLV)	Nelfinavir* (NFV)
Didanosine (ddI)*		Amprenavir* (APV)
Zalcitabine (ddC)*	**Fusion inhibitors (FI)**	Indinavir* (INV)
Abacavir (ABC)*	Enfuvirtide (T-20)	Lopinavir* (LPV)
Emtricitabine (FTC)		Fosamprenavir* (FPV)

Contd...

Contd...

(NtRTI)	**Integrase inhibitors new**	Atazanavir* (ATV)
Tenofavir* (TDF)		Tipranavir (TPV)
	CCR5 entry inhibitor new	

*Available in India

Dosage

AZT (Zidovudine)	300 mg BD
3TC (Lamivudine)	150 mg BD
D4T (Stamivudine)	30 mg BD
NVP (Nevirapine)	200 OD for 14 days followed by BD

Goals of ARV Therapy

- Clinical goals: Prolongation of life and improvement in quality of life
- Virological goals: Greatest possible reduction in viral load for as long as possible
- Immunological goals: Immune reconstitution that is both quantitative and qualitative
- Therapeutic goals: Rational sequencing of drugs in a fashion that achieves clinical, virological and immunological goals while maintaining treatment options, limiting drug toxicity and facilitating adherence
- Reduction of HIV transmission in individuals: Reduction of HIV transmission by suppression of viral load
- The goals of management of HIV in pregnancy are dual:
    - Managing the mother's HIV status
    - Prevention of mother-to-child transmission (PMTCT)

Principles for Selecting the First-line Regimen

1. Choose 3TC (lamivudine) in all regimens
2. Choose one NRTI to combine with 3TC (AZT or d4T)
3. Choose one NNRTI (NVP or EFV)

Prevention of Mother to Child Transmission (PMTCT)

During antenatal period:

- Regular ANC–General measures (good diet, correction of anemia)
- Health education regarding safer sex practices, contraception
- Knowing HIV status after pretest counseling and informed consent
- Choice of MTP or continuation of pregnancy
- Infections to be treated: Malaria, tuberculosis, other RTIs, UTI, recurrent vaginal candidiasis, STIs

Risk of Mother to Child Transmission

Risk of transmission timing	Transmission rate
Pregnancy	5–10%
Labor and delivery	10–15%
Breastfeeding	5–20%
Overall without breastfeeding	15–25%
Overall with breastfeeding for 6 months	20–35%
Overall with breastfeeding for 18 to 24 months	30–45%

Risk of Transmission After Intervention

Intervention	Risk of mother to child transmission-to-child HIV transmission
No ARV, breastfeeding	30–45%
No ARV, No breastfeeding	20–25%
Short course with 1 ARV, breastfeeding	15–25%
Short course with 1 ARV, No breastfeeding	5–15%
Short course with 2 ARVs, No breastfeeding	5%
3 ARVs (ART), no breastfeeding	1%
2 ARVs, breastfeeding	Unknown
3 ARVs (ART), breastfeeding	Unknown

Risk Factors

- In pregnancy–High maternal viral load, viral, bacterial, parasitic infestations (especially malaria), STI, maternal malnutrition (indirectly)
- During labor and delivery–Rupture of membranes >4 hrs, invasive delivery procedures, chorioamnionitis, first infant in multiple gestation
- During feeding: Duration mixed feeding, breast inflammation/abscess/cracked nipples, infant oral disease (DICE).

Situation 1

HIV-infected woman who is receiving ART and becomes pregnant

- Continue current HAART regimen during pregnancy including 1st trimester, labor and after delivery
- Avoid use of EFV or other potentially teratogenic drugs in the 1st trimester and drugs with known adverse potential for mother (combination d4T/ddI)
- HIV antiretroviral drug resistant technique is recommended if the woman has detectable viremia on therapy
- ART for neonate
    - For breastfeeding infants—daily nevirapine from birth until 6 weeks of age
    - For non-breastfeeding—daily AZT or NVP from birth until 6 weeks of age

Situation 2

HIV-infected pregnant woman who is not on antiretroviral but has indications for antiretroviral therapy

- Initiation of ART for her own health is recommended if CD4 count is <350 cells/cumm irrespective of WHO clinical staging and for those with WHO clinical
  staging 3 or 4 irrespective of CD4 count.
- ART should be started irrespective of gestational age irrespective of delivery and thereafter
- 1st line ART–AZT+3TC+NVP/AZT+3TC+EFV
- Alternative regimen–TDF+3TC (or FTC) + NVP/TDF+3TC (or FTC) + EFV
- Avoid use of EFV or other potentially teratogenic drugs in the 1st trimester and drugs with known adverse potential for mother (combination d4T/ddI)
- ART for infants–
  - For breastfeeding infants—daily nevirapine from birth until 6 weeks of age
  - For non-breastfeeding—daily AZT or NVP from birth until 6 weeks of age

Situation 3

HIV-infected pregnant woman who is not on antiretroviral and does not require ART for her own health

- ARV prophylaxis is recommended for prevention of perinatal transmission
- ARV prophylaxis is indicated regardless of viral load
- ARV prophylaxis should be started from 14 weeks of gestation or as soon as possible when women present late in pregnancy and labor and to be continued till 1 week after breastfeeding has ended
- 1st line ARV prophylaxis
  - Daily AZT- Antepartum
  - Sd-NVP at onset of labor
  - AZT+3TC during labor and delivery and 7 days postpartum
- Sd-NVP & AZT+3TC intra- and postpartum can be omitted if mother receives more than 4 weeks of AZT during pregnancy
- Alternative regimens
  - AZT+3TC+LVP/r or
  - AZT+3TC+EFV or
  - AZT+3TC+ABC or
  - TDF+XTC+EFV
- ARV for infants–
  - Breastfeeding—daily NVP from birth until 1 week after breastfeeding has been stopped
  - For non-breastfeeding—daily AZT or NVP from birth until 6 weeks of age

Situation 4

HIV-infected woman who has received no antiretroviral therapy or prophylaxis prior to labor (during labor protocol)

- SdNVP+AZT duing labor

- AZT+3TC for 7 days postpartum (this will reduce the development of NVP resistance)
- Alternative regimen
  - NVP 200 mg at the onset of labor and 1 more dose at least 2 hrs before birth
  - Infant-Sd-NVP 2 mg/kg body weight within 72 hours
- ARV for infants
  - Sd-NVP + AZT for 6 weeks

Situation 5

Infant born to HIV infected woman who has received no antiretroviral therpy or prophylaxis prior to or during labor
- AZT given for 6 weeks to the infant started as soon as possible after birth
- Consultation with the pediatric HIV specialist is recommended
- Evaluate need for initiation of postpartum maternal therapy

Benefits of the New PMTCT Policy Guidelines

- AZT started earlier in pregnancy—significantly reduces rates of intrauterine transmission. Women receive prophylaxis for more of the transmission period
- AZT can now be started at the woman's first visit
- Transmission through breastfeeding will decrease because the baby or mother will receive ARV prophylaxis daily
- Mothers can breastfeed for a longer time because the baby is receiving NVP; hence contributing to "increased HIV free survival" through reduced HIV risk as well as morbidity and mortality from malnutrition

NVP in women with CD4 count of 200–350 cells/mm^3: They face a higher risk of severe hepatotoxicity. This happens most often in the first 6–12 weeks of therapy. It is recommended that such women should undergo the following:
- Close observation over the first 12 weeks of therapy (every 2 weeks)
- Baseline and regular monitoring of liver enzymes (at baseline and at 2, 4, 8 and 12 weeks, followed by symptom-directed evaluation)
- Patient education to encourage them to return if there are problems such as rash, abdominal pain, jaundice and fever
- If the liver enzymes increase to grade 3 or higher (ALT and/or AST >5.1 times the upper normal limit) without an alternative explanation, NVP should be permanently discontinued. If symptoms suggesting hepatic toxicity, including rash, develop in pregnant women, NVP should be discontinued immediately, For those with anemia during pregnancy, the problem should be managed by conservative methods, such as giving ferrous folate, other oral preparations and blood transfusion (if required)
- The preferred NRTIs for use in pregnant women are AZT and 3TC. The combination of ddI and d4T should not be used because of associated increased toxicities in pregnant women. Studies have shown that TDF is associated with decreased fetal growth and bone demineralization
- The preferred NNRTI is NVP, with which there has been extensive clinical experience globally. Its efficacy in reducing mother-to-child transmission has been proven

- SQV/r and Nelfinavir (NLF) are the preferred PIs if the woman needs to take PIs. EFV may be considered after the first trimester. In pregnant women who are on a first-line EFV-based regimen, EFV should be substituted with NVP in the first trimester
- Women with higher CD4 cell counts should be monitored closely
- Women who have previously received single-dose NVP for PPTCT should be considered eligible for the first-line NNRTI-based regimens. Alternatives may be considered for women whose exposure to single-dose NVP has been for less than six months and who require ART for their own health.

Monitoring and Follow-up Schedule for Patients on ART

	Day 0 (baseline) be fore or at start of ART	**At 15 days**	**At 1 month**	**At 2 months**	**At 3 months**	**Every 6 months**	**Consul-tation as needed (symptom directed)**
Clinical and adherence counseling	✓	✓	✓	✓	✓	✓	
Weight	✓	✓	✓	✓	✓	✓	
Hb	✓	✓ (If on AZT)	✓ (If on AZT)		✓	✓	✓
ALT[1]	✓	✓ (If on NVP)	✓ (If on NVP)		✓	✓	✓
Random blood sugar	✓					✓ (if on PI)	✓
CD4	✓					✓	✓
Urine analysis	✓					✓ (if on TDF)	
Lipid profile[2]	✓ (only plan-ning for PI)					✓ (if on PI)	✓
Pregnancy test for woman with reproductive potential	✓ (if planning for EFV)						✓
HBV and HCV screening	✓ (if history of IDU, transfusion related transmis-sion)						

Contd...

Contd...

VDRL/TPHA (syphilis screening)	✓ (if history of high risk behavior, recurrent STIs and/or symptoms suggestive of syphilis)						
Plasma viral load[3]						✓	

1. For patients co-infected with HBV and/or HCV, and on ART; 3–6 monthly monitoring of liver function is recommended.
2. d4T and PIs may cause lipid abnormalities. In patients with significant risk factors for coronary artery disease a fasting lipid may be done at 6 months; otherwise annual screening is sufficient.
3. The national program does not recommend routine viral load monitoring. Viral load measurement is not recommended for decision making for the intiation or regular monitoring of ART in resource limited settings (WHO 2006). It may be considered for the diagnosis of early treatment failure or to assess discordant clinical and CD4 findings in patients in whom failure of ART is suspected.

Side effects and common uses		
Time	**Side effects and toxicities**	**Common causes**
Short-term (the first few weeks)	Gastrointestinal toxicities, including nausea, vomiting and diarrhea	AZT, TDF, PIs
	Rash Most rashes occur within the first 2–3 weeks	NVP, EFV Abacavir PIs (rarely)
	Hepatotoxicity (more common in hepatitis B or C co-infection)	NVP, EFV PIs
	Drowsiness, dizziness, confusion and vivid dreams (normally self-resolving but can take weeks to months)	EFV
Medium term (the first few months)	Anemia and neutropenia Sudden and acute bone marrow suppression can occur within the first weeks of therapy are present as a slow onset of progressive anemia over months	AZT
	Hyper-pigmentaion of skin, nails and mucous membranes	AZT
	Lactic acidosis (more common after the first few months, most commonly associated with d4T)	d4T, ddI, AZT
	Peripheral neuropathy (more common after the first few months)	d4T, ddI
	Pancreatitis (can occur at any time)	ddI
Long-term (after 6–18 months)	Lipodystrophy and lipoatrophy	d4T, ddI, AZT PIs
	Dyslipidemia	d4T, EFV, PIs
	Diabetes	IDV
	Skin hair and nail abnormalities. PIs, especially	IDV

ART Failure

Clinical failure – New or recurrent WHO stage 4 condition, after at least 6 months of ART.

Immunological failure – Fall of CD4 count to pre-therapy baseline (or below)
- 50% fall from the on-treatment peak value (if known)
- Persistent CD4 levels below 100 cells/mm

Virological failure–Plasma viral load >10,000 copies/mL

Indications For Cesarean Section

- Obstetric indications
- Unknown viral load
- RNA >1000 copies/ml at 36 weeks of gestation
- Not taken ARV or antiretroviral therapy during pregnancy
- Rupture of membranes not > 4 hrs

Care During Section

- Should be scheduled at 38 weeks or before rupture of membranes
- Senior obstetrician should perform it
- Immediate cord clamping
- Avoid manual removal of placenta
- Perioperative antibiotic prophylaxis

During Labor

- Minimal PV examinations
- Give prophylactic antibiotics
- HIV per se is not an indication for continuous monitoring
- Avoid prolonged labor, ARM, episiotomy, instrumental deliveries, invasive procedures, unless absolutely indicated
- Safe transfusion practices, with universal precautions conduct delivery (explain universal precaution, PEP), start AZT IV infusion 2 mg/kg in 1 hr loading dose followed by 1 mg/kg in 1 hr as continuous infusion at the onset of labor continue till cord clamping, do early cord clamping under gauze
- Avoid suctioning of baby unless absolutely indicated. Mechanical suction <100 mm of Hg of pressure is preferred rather than mouth operated suction.
- Baby should be dried immediately, NVP drops 2 mg/kg body weight should be given within 72 hrs of delivery, administer vit K, silver nitrate ointment. Good pediatric follow-up is required.

Universal Precautions

a. Wear protective eyewear and mask, if spatter with blood or body fluids is a possibility
b. Also wear gowns and protective leg wear
c. Wear double gloves

d. Handle all linen soiled with blood or fluid as potentially infectious
e. Process all lab specimens as potentially infectious, including blood
f. Handwashing before and after all medical procedures
g. Safe handling and immediate safe disposal of sharps: not recapping needles; using special containers for sharp disposals; using needle cutter/destroyers; using forceps instead of fingers for guiding sutures; using vacutainers where possible
h. Safe decontamination of instruments
i. A health care professional who has a cut or abrasion should cover the wound before providing care
j. Safe disposal of contaminated waste

Postpartum Care

- Continue routine health care including annual Pap smears, monitoring for vaginal infections
- Monitor for signs and symptoms of infection
  - Burning micturition, fever, foul smelling lochia, severe lower abdominal tenderness, redness, pus or drainage from incisions

Feeding

Considering Indian situation (poor hygienic practices, ignorance of mother, lack of enough money for artificial feeds) the chance of baby dying due to GE is higher than the chance of the child dying of HIV.

"AFASS" criteria used to determine whether a mother is able to replacement feed

- Acceptable–Mother perceives no significant cultural or social barriers to replacement feeding
- Feasible–Mother has adequate knowledge, skills, resources, and support to correctly mix formula or milk, and feed the infant up to 12 times in 24 hours
- Affordable–Mother and family can pay the costs of replacement feeding—fuel, clean water, and all ingredients—without compromising the health and nutrition of the family.
- Sustainable–Mother has access to a continuous and uninterrupted supply of all ingredients needed for safe replacement feeding as long as the infant needs it
- Safe replacement feeds are correctly and hygienically stored, prepared, and fed in nutritionally adequate amounts. Infant is fed by clean hands and preferably by cup

Note: Currently options for replacement feeding include commercial infant formula and modified animal milk, however, WHO recommended that animal milk should no longer be used for infants below 6 months.

NEW FEEDING GUIDELINES

- Mothers strongly recommended to exclusively breastfeeding until 6 months of age, and continue breastfeeding while introducing complementary feeds until 12 months of age

- ◆ If mothers cannot provide sufficient animal milk at 12 months, they can continue to breastfeed until able
- Exposed infants receive daily NVP prophylaxis until 1 week after cessation of breastfeeding
- Breastfeeding is the preferred feeding method. However, if mothers still desire to replacement feed, they can, if able to meet the AFASS criteria
- Infants confirmed HIV-positive should breastfeed exclusively for 6 months and continue breastfeeding while adding in complementary feeds until 24 months.

BENEFITS OF GUIDELINES

When mothers breastfeed for 12 months and with ARV prophylaxis:

- Risk of HIV transmission is reduced because ARV prophylaxis is provided throughout the breastfeeding period
- Risk of malnutrition is greatly reduced because babies are receiving breast milk for 12 months—by that age the baby has grown and the malnutrition risk is less
  Dosing schedule for infant NVP prophylaxis

Infant age		NVP daily dose (10 mg/ml formulation)
Birth to 6 weeks	Birth weight 2.0 to 2.5 kg	1 ml once daily
	Birth weight >2.5 kg	1.5 ml once daily
>6 weeks to 6 months		2 ml once daily
>6 months to 9 months		3 ml once daily
>9 months to end of breastfeeding		4 ml once daily

Immunization and Vitamin A Supplementation

HIV-exposed children should be immunized according to the routine national immunization schedule with the following notes:

- BCG should not be given in symptomatic HIV-infected children.
- HiB vaccine should be given to all who are confirmed HIV-infected on the basis of 2 positive DNA PCR tests done at 6 weeks of age.
- Additional vaccines such as pneumococcal, varicella, hepatitis A, influenza virus, etc. may be given as necessary.
- Vitamin A supplementation should be as per the UIP schedule.

Contraception

- Combined oral contraceptives–NVP, ritonavir, nelfinavir, lopinavir/ritonavir and saquinavir/ritonavir result in reduced ethinyl estradiol levels. Estrogens are slightly increased by atazanavir, indinavir and efavirenz (EFV). Thus, women on ART should not use hormonal contraception or should use it with caution and appropriate dose adjustment.
- Medroxyprogesterone acetate (Depo-provera injectable) does not interact with NVP, EFV or NLF. Hence it may be considered for use as a contraceptive.
- Intrauterine contraceptive devices may be used with caution in HIV-infected women with close monitoring because of the risk of intrauterine infection.

- The consistent use of condoms is recommended for all HIV-infected women who are on ART. This is for the prevention of secondary transmission of HIV from/to the partner, as well as the prevention of unplanned pregnancy.
- Sterilization operations are safe and can be performed.

Who and When to Re-test for HIV

Who to Re-test	When to Re-test
Pregnant women who have tested HIV-negative in the 1st or 2nd trimester of pregnancy	Re-test in the 3rd trimester (preferably between 28–36 weeks) *If woman does not return for testing in 3rd trimester, she should be re-tested during labor or just after delivery
Outpatients with a negative HIV test result, but with clinical conditions suggestive of HIV-infection	Re-test 4 weeks after HIV-negative test
Individuals with STIs who have an HIV-negative test result	
TB-infected individuals with an HIV negative test result who have had a new potential HIV exposure	
HIV-negative persons with ongoing risk behaviors (persons with known HIV-positive partner, partner of unknown status, sex workers, and injection drug users)	Re-test at least annually
Persons with a specific incident of known HIV-exposure within the past 3 months, who test negative at the first testing	Re-test 4 weeks after initial HIV- negative test
Persons with specific incidence of possible HIV-exposure within the past 72 hours (should receive post-exposure prophylaxis and baseline HIV test)	Re-test 4 weeks after exposure, and if negative, retest again at 12 weeks post-exposure

Post-exposure Prophylaxis (PEP) in Pregnancy

- Most antiretrovirals are class B or C
- Antiretroviral pregnancy registry has not detected increased teratogenic risk for ARVs in general, nor specifically for AZT and 3TC, in the first trimester
- Avoid efavirenz (anencephaly in monkeys), amprenavir (ossification defects in rabbits), and indinavir in late term (hyperbilirubinemia)

Potentially infectious body fluids	
Exposure to body fluids considered 'at risk'	**Exposure to body fluids considered 'not at risk'**
• Blood • Semen • Vaginal secretions • Cerebrospinal fluid • Synovial, pleural, peritoneal, pericardial fluid • Amniotic fluid • Other body fluids contaminated with visible blood	• Tears • Sweat • Urine and feces • Saliva *Unless these secretions contain visible blood*

HIV Transmission Risk of Different Routes

Exposure route	HIV
Blood transfusion	90–95%
Perinatal	20–40%
Sexual intercourse	0.1 to 10%
Vaginal	0.05–0.1%
Anal	0.065–0.5%
Oral	0.005–0.01%
Injecting drugs use	0.67%
Needle stick exposure	0.3%
Mucous membrane splash to eye, oronasal	0.09%

Disinfectants Effective in Inactivating HIV

Disinfectant	Contact time
Ethanol 70%	3–5 min
Propranolol 70%	3–5 min
Povidine iodine 2%	1–5 min
Formalin 4%	30 min
Glutaraldehyde 2% (Cidex)	30 min 30 min
Hydrogen proxide 6%	30 min
Sodium hypochlorite solution	20 min

Post-exposure Prophylaxis Guidelines for Occupational Exposure (Steps for Managing Occupational Exposure)

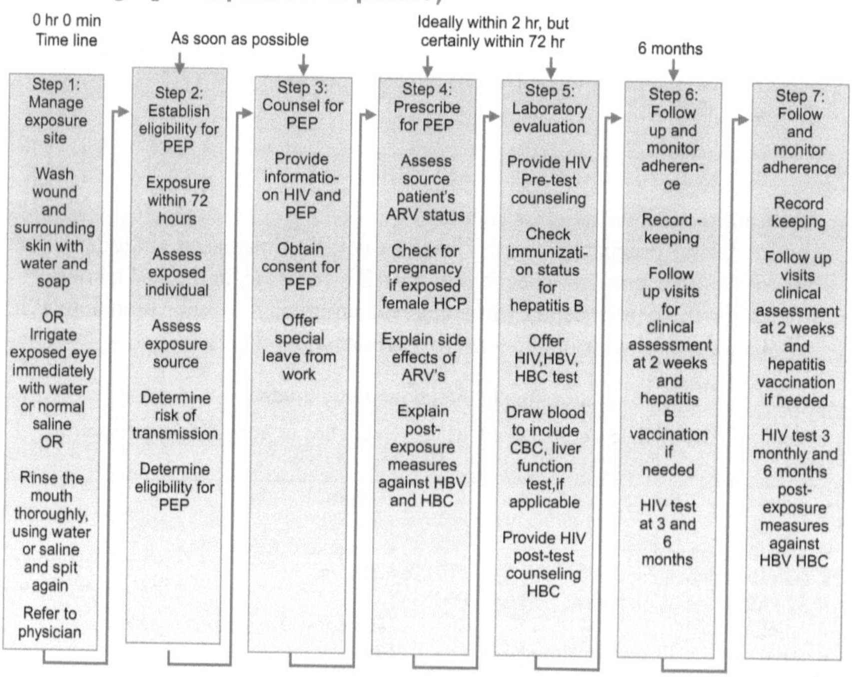

Summary of Do's and Dont's for Management of Exposure Site

Do's	Dont's
Remove gloves, if appropriate	Do not panic
Wash the exposed site thoroughly with running water	Do not put the pricked finger in mouth
Irrigate with water or saline if eyes or mouth have been exposed	Do not squeeze the wound to bleed it
Wash the skin with soap and water	Do not use bleach, chlorine, alcohol, betadine, iodine or other antiseptics/ detergents on the wound

Evaluate Need for Post-exposure Prophylaxis

Exposure	HIV positive and asymptomatic (sc1) low viral load <1500 copies/ml (sc1)	HIV positive and symptomatic (sc2), high viral load, acute seroconversion	HIV status unknown
C0 (intact skin/with non-infectious source material)	No PEP needed	No PEP needed	No PEP needed
C1 (mucous membrane, non intact skin with small volume)	Consider basic regimen	Start basic regimen	Usually no PEP/ Consider basic regimen
C2 (mucous membrane, non intact skin with large volume/several drops, major splash, longer duration) or percutaneous superficial/small volume (e.g. scratch, solid needle)	Start basic regimen	Start expanded regimen	Consider basic regimen
C3 Percutaneous with large volume	Expanded regimen	Expanded regimen	Consider basic regimen

Basic regimen: Zidovudine (AZT)–600 mg in divided doses (300 mg/twice a day or 200 mg/thrice a day for 4 weeks + Lamivudine (3TC)–150 mg twice a day for 4 weeks

2nd choice: Stavudine (d4T)–30 mg twice a day + Lamivudine (3TC)-150 mg twice a day for 4 weeks

Expanded regimen: Basic regimen (+ Indinavir – 800 mg/thrice a day, or any other protease inhibitor for 4 weeks

Duration of PEP

PEP should be started, as early as possible, after an exposure. It has been seen that PEP started after 72 hours of exposure is of no use and hence is not recommended. The optimal course of PEP is not unknown, but 4 weeks of drug therapy appears to provide protection against HIV.

If the HIV test is found to be positive at anytime within 12 weeks, the HCW should be referred to a physician for treatment.

Recommended Follow-up

Timing	In persons taking PEP (standard regimen)	In persons not taking PEP
Weeks 2 and 4	Transaminases—to detect hepatitis Complete blood count—for patients on AZT containing regimens	Clinical monitoring for hepatitis
Week 6	HIV-Ab	HIV-Ab
Month 3	HIV-Ab, anti-HCV, HBsAg transaminases	HIV-Ab, anti-HCV, HBsAg
Month 6	HIV-Ab, anti-HCV, HBsAg transaminases	HIV-Ab, anti-HCV, HBsAg

CHAPTER

46

Hepatitis B Infection

HEPATITIS B

- Double stranded DNA virus
- The virus has 3 antigens – surface antigen (HBsAg); core antigen (HBcAg), and HBeAg, a protein secreted from infected cells
- Incubation period is 4 weeks to 6 months following exposure, depending on viral inoculums
- HBV is transmitted primarily via parenteral routes, sexual transmission, and perinatal exposure.

Clinical Course

- Symptoms are nonspecific.
- Examination may reveal tender hepatosplenomegaly in 10% cases. This may not be made out in the 3rd trimester due to enlarged uterus.
- Acute signs and symptoms resolve in 6 weeks.
- 85 to 90% of patients acutely infected with HBV clear their infection.
- Fewer than 1% of infected patients develop fulminant hepatitis, characterized by massive hepatic necrosis and potentially accompanied by pancreatitis.
- 15% of patients become chronically infected with HBV, and 15 to 30% of these patients will develop liver cirrhosis.
- The incidence of acute HBV infection in pregnancy is 1 to 2 per 1000, and 5 to 15 per 1000 pregnant women have chronic HBV infection.

Effects on Pregnancy

- Increased risk of spontaneous miscarriages and preterm
- Increased incidence of low-birth weight
- Increased risk of intrapartum or postpartum hemorrhage, if PT is deranged as in fulminant hepatic failure

Diagnosis

- Acute HBV infection is diagnosed by detection of HBsAg and IgM to the core antigen (HBc) or by viral load determination.
- Chronic HBV (formerly described as chronic active) is characterized by positive HBsAg and HBeAg, an HBV DNA titer ranging from 10^7 to 10^{11} and positive hepatic nuclear HBcAg
- LFT elevated AST, ALT, serum bilirubin.

Vertical Transmission

- Risk of transmission is 20–30%
- If both antigens positive for HBV (HBsAg and HBeAg) risk is 90% but if HBeAg negative, risk is 25%.
- Acute infection in 1st trimester risk is 10%, 3rd trimester risk is 90%.

Recommendations for Prenatal Screening of Hepatitis

- All pregnant women should be screened routinely for HBsAg at the same time as other routine prenatal testing
- Women at high risk should be screened again before delivery
- Women not tested prenatally should be tested as soon as possible after admission for delivery
- Infants born to HBsAg positive mothers should receive appropriate immunoglobulins along with vaccination beginning within 12 hours of birth
- HBIg 12–40 IU/kg IM soon following exposure and second dose after 1 month.

Serological Markers of Hepatitis B Infection

- HBsAg appears in the blood 4 weeks prior to onset of clinical symptoms and remains detectable for 1–6 weeks. The titers decrease as symptoms diminish.
- HbsAb defines the absence of carrier state. Titers increase slowly during clinical recovery period and continue to increase for 10–12 months after HBsAg is no longer detectable.
- HbcAb begins to appear 3–5 weeks after HbsAg appears in the blood. The titer drops off in the first 1 or 2 years after infection, although it is still detectable for years after the disease.
- HbeAg–It parallels HbsAg.
- HbcAb–It is detectable shortly after the time that HbcAg disappears.

HBsAg	HBsAb	HBcAb	HBeAg	HBeAb	Interpretation
+	–	IgM	+	–	Acute HBV infection, highly infectious
+	–	IgG	+	–	Chronic HBV infection, Highly infectious
+	–	IgG	–	–	Late acute/Chronic HBV infection. Low infectivity
+	+	IgG/IgM	+/–	+/–	1. HBsAg of one subtype and heterotypic anti-HBs (common) 2. Process of sero conversion from HBsAg to anti-HBs (rare)
–	–	IgM	+/–	+/–	1. Acute HBV infection 2. Anti-HBc window
–	–	IgG	–	+/–	1. Low level HBsAg carrier 2. Remote past infection 3. False positive
–	+	IgG	–	+/–	Recovery from HBV infection
–	+	–	–	–	1. Immunization 2. Possible remote infection 3. False positive

PREVENTION

- Hepatitis B vaccine which is given in 3 doses <1 ml for adults, 0.5 ml for neonatal
- Intramuscularly at 0, 1 and 6 months. Now it is part of National Immunization Schedule in India.

Post-exposure Prophylaxis of Susceptible Pregnant Women

- Exposure to persons who have acute hepatitis B when exposure by sexual contact within 14 days, a course of HBV vaccine into deltoid muscle and hepatitis B immunoglobulin 0.06 mL/kg IM into the contralateral arm. Second dose of HB immunoglobulin given 1 month later along with 2nd dose of vaccine.
- Exposure to persons who have chronic infection.
  Active post-exposure prophylaxis with HBV vaccine for all sexual and needle sharing partners.

Antepartum Management of Pregnant Hepatitis B Carriers

- Management is mainly supportive with high calorie diet, bed rest
- Vaccination against HAV
- Avoidance of alcohol and hepatotoxic drugs such as acetaminophen
- Avoid blood donation, sharing of tooth brushes and razors
- The pediatrician and labor room staff should be alerted
- Active and passive immunization of their neonate
- Annual examination by a physician
- Sexual partner of the woman needs to be counseled about the risks of transmission and the need for testing and vaccination

Mode of Delivery

- Cesarean section only for obstetric indications

Prevention of Neonatal Infection

- Passive and active immunizations within 12 hours of birth decrease risk of vertical transmission by 90%.
- Passive immunization-hepatitis B hyperimmunoglobulin 200 IU IM.
- Active immunization-hepatitis B vaccine 0.5 ml 0, 1, 6 months should be given immediately after delivery.
- Antiviral therapy (lamivudine)–to the woman during pregnancy is still experimental.
- Breastfeeding is not contraindicated.

CHAPTER

47

Malaria

Malaria in pregnancy is caused by protozoan *P.vivax, P.ovale, P.falciparum* and *P.malariae*. The first two species are prevalent in India.

DEFINITIONS

Severe and Complicated Malaria

The severe signs of malaria are non-specific and other causes must be excluded before assigning the signs and symptoms to malaria. The parasitemia of severe malaria can be less than 2%. Pregnant women with 2% or more parasitized red blood cells are at higher risk of developing severe malaria and should be treated with the severe malaria protocol.

Uncomplicated Malaria

Uncomplicated malaria is defined as fewer than 2% parasitized red blood cells in a woman with no signs of severity and no complicating features.

Congenital Malaria

Congenital malaria in the very young infant or newborn results from the passage of parasites or infected red blood cells from the mother to the newborn while in utero or during delivery and not by the bite of the female anopheline mosquito.

Resistance

Resistance is defined as the ability of a parasite strain to survive and multiply despite the administration and absorption of a medicine given in doses equal to or higher than those usually recommended but within the tolerance of the subject, with the caveat that the form of the drug active against the parasite must be able to gain access to the parasite or the infected red blood cell for the duration of time necessary for its normal action.

EFFECTS OF PREGNANCY ON MALARIA

- Atypical presentation probably due to the hormonal, immunological and hematological changes of pregnancy.

- Mortality is double, the parasitemia tends to be 10 times higher and as a result, all the complications of falciparum malaria are more common in pregnancy.
- Primigravidae-60–70%
- Highest prevalence in second half of pregnancy
- *Plasmodium falciparum*–More common due to immunosuppression and loss of acquired immunity to malaria
- More atypical

EFFECTS OF MALARIA ON PREGNANCY

- Spontaneous abortion
- Prematurity
- Stillbirth
- Placental insufficiency and IUGR – Placenta is the preferred site of sequestration and development of malarial parasite. Intervillous spaces are filled with parasites and macrophages, interfering with oxygen and nutrient transport to the fetus.
- Fetal distress
- Congenital malaria

The clinical manifestations in pregnancy depend on premunition; that is, the degree of naturally acquired host immunity to malaria. Premunition depends on repeated exposure to infectious anopheline bites.

Clinical Features

- Fever
    - Afebrile to continuous fever, low grade to hyperpyrexia
    - 3 stages: Cold stage, hot stage and sweating stage followed by similar attack in another 24 hrs
    - In 2nd half of pregnancy, there may be more frequent paroxysms due to immunosuppression
- Headache
- Muscle pain
- Nausea
- Vomiting
- Diarrhea
- Cough
- General malaise

Signs

- Jaundice
- Elevated temperature
- Perspiration
- Pallor
- Splenomegaly
- Respiratory distress

Complications

- Cerebral malaria
- Seizures
- Algid fever with persistent vomiting and diarrhea
- Circulatory collapse causing a cold clammy skin
- Black water fever
- Hypoglycemia
- Severe anemia
- Respiratory distress (acidotic breathing, acute respiratory distress syndrome)
- Jaundice
- Acute pulmonary edema
- Jaundice

Diagnosis

- Giemsa staining of peripheral smear–
  - Thick smear–To identify the parasite
  - Thin smear–To identify the species
    Quantitative estimate
    \+ - 1–10 parasites per 100 thick films
    ++ - 11–100 parasites per 100 thick films
    +++ - 1–10 parasites per each thick film field
    ++++ - >10 per each thick film
- Fluorescent microscopy/QBC

A small quantity of blood is spun in the QBC centrifuge. The parasites get concentrated near the tip of RBC column. Pre-coating of the tube with acridine orange induces a fluorescence on the column. But it doesn't quantify or identify species.

In a febrile patient, three negative malaria smears 12–24 hours apart, rule out the diagnosis of malaria

- Rapid malaria test–Rapid detection tests may miss low parasitemia, which is more likely in pregnant women, and rapid detection tests are relatively insensitive in *P. vivax* malaria.
- Immunodiagnosis
  - Parasight F test (HRP-2)
  - Dipstick tests
  - Molecular methods
  - Dot blot assay
  - DNA probes
  - PCR amplification
- Serological test
  - ELISA
  - IHA
  - IFA

Poor Prognostic Parameters

- Severe anemia (Hemoglobin <8.0 g/dl)
- Thrombocytopenia
- Hypoglycemia (<2.2 mmol/l)
- Acidosis (pH <7.3)
- Renal impairment (oliguria <0.4 ml/kg body weight/hour or creatinine >265 μmol/l)
- Hyperlactatemia (correlates with mortality)
- Hyperparasitemia (>2% parasitized red blood cells)
- 'Algid malaria'–Gram-negative septicemia
- Lumbar puncture to exclude meningitis

Management

The 'ABCD' of malaria prevention is a useful formula to remember the components of malaria prevention:

- Awareness of risk
- Bite prevention
- Chemoprophylaxis
- Diagnosis and treatment which must be prompt

Risk

Risk of contracting malaria during a 1 month stay without chemoprophylaxis
Area Risk

- Oceania (Papua New Guinea, Papua, Solomon Islands and Vanuatu) 1:20
- Sub-Saharan Africa 1:50
- Indian subcontinent 1:500
- Southeast Asia 1:500
- South America 1:2500
- Central America and the Caribbean 1:10,000

Bite Prevention

- Repellents—the evidence favors skin repellents containing 50% DEET
- Knock-down mosquito sprays: permethrin and pyrethroids sprays kill resting and flying mosquitoes
- Insecticide treated bed nets: Long-lasting pyrethroid-impregnated bed nets offer significant protection
- Clothing that covers the body and forms a barrier from biting mosquitoes will reduce the risk of malaria
- Room protection: Electrically heated mats will kill mosquitoes in the room

Chemoprophylaxis

- Doxycycline and primaquine are contraindicated as chemoprophylaxis in pregnant women.

Dosing regimen for chemoprophylaxis in pregnancy			
Regimen	**Dose for chemoprophylaxis**	**Usual amount/ tablet (mg)**	**P. falciparum resistance**
Mefloquine	1 tablet weekly	250	Chloroquine resistant
Alovaquone-proguanil[a]	1 tablet daily	250 atovaquone + 100 proguanil	Chloroquine resistant & mefloquine not tolerated or contraindicated or Mefloquine resistant
Proguanilla plus chloroquine	2 tablets daily plus 2 tablets weekly	100 proguanil + 150 (chloroquine; base)	No chloroquine resistance

[a]Folic acid supplements (5 mg daily) need to be taken if proguanil is used in those who are pregnant or seeking to become pregnant

- Doxycyline has been reported to disturb bone growth of the fetus and to cause irreversible teeth coloration when given in the third trimester and congenital cataract has been reported.
- Primaquine can cause hemolysis, particularly, in G6PD deficiency. Fetal red blood cells are more sensitive to hemolysis and the G6PD status of the fetus cannot be determined.
- While chloroquine and proguanil are safe, they are no longer efficacious in areas of chloroquine resistance and provide women with suboptimal prophylaxis if recommended.

Emergency stand by treatment: Within 24 hrs of onset of symptoms:
- Antipyretics should be used for fever.
- Quinine (300 mg tablets, two tablets three times a day for 7 days) and clinda-mycin (150 mg capsules, three capsules three times a day for 5–7 days).
- If a dose is vomited within 30 minutes, the full dose should be repeated and if the dose is vomited after 30–60 minutes, half the dose should be repeated. The treatment should be finished and mefloquine should be commenced 1 week after the last treatment dose.

Treatment

Before treating pregnant woman, consider–
- Place
- Trimester
- Clinical and parasitic situation

The drugs chosen should be effective in the reduction of asexual forms in the blood and placenta.

Admit all with symptoms suggestive of malaria:
- Base-line investigations + antigen test
- Treat dehydration, start antipyretics, check RBS

- TPR/BP charting 4th hrly
- Tepid cold sponging if febrile
- Severe malaria–admit to ICU
- Do not persist with oral therapy if vomiting is persistent.

Antimalarials in Pregnancy

- All trimesters:
  - First line–Chloroquine; Quinine
  - Second line–Artesunate/Artemether/Arteether
- 2nd/3rd trimester: with caution
  - Pyrimethamine + Sulphadoxine; Mefloquine
- Contraindicated:
  - Primaquine; Tetracycline; Doxycycline

NATIONAL DRUG POLICY ON MALARIA

Treatment of Uncomplicated Malaria

Plasmodium falciparum

Uncomplicated:
Oral quinine 600 mg 8 hourly and oral clindamycin 450 mg 8 hourly for 7 days;
If vomiting–Quinine: Loading dose–20 mg/kg infusion over 4 hours
Maintenance dose–10 mg/kg, 3 times a day for 7 days

- Loading dose is not needed if patient has already received quinine or if the treating physician feels it is inappropriate.
- Infusion rate should not exceed 5 mg/kg/hr as it causes hypoglycemia.

Adverse effects–Principally cinchonism, which includes tinnitus, headache, nausea, diarrhea, altered auditory acuity and blurred vision

ACT (Artemisinin-based Combination Therapy) – Not to be given in I trimester

Artesunate 4 mg/kg for 3 days + Sulphadoxine 25 mg/kg + Pyrimethamine 1.25 mg/kg on 1st day

Plasmodium Vivax, Malariae, Ovale

Chloroquine– 600 mg followed by 300 mg 6 hours later.
Day 2–300 mg
Day 3–300 mg

Resistant *P. vivax*–As for uncomplicated malaria *P. falciparum*

- Preventing relapse during pregnancy–Chloroquine oral 300 mg weekly until delivery
- Preventing relapse after delivery–Postpone until 3 months after delivery and G6PD testing
- *P. ovale*–Oral primaquine 15 mg single daily dose for 14 days
- *P. vivax*–Oral primaquine 30 mg single daily dose for 14 days

- G6PD (mild) for *P. vivax* or *P. ovale* Primaquine oral 45–60 mg once a week for 8 weeks

Mixed infection (Vivax + Falciparum)–Full course of ACT

Severe Malaria

Artesunate–2.4 mg/kg IV or IM–0 hours, 12 hrs, 24 hrs. Followed by OD. When the patient is well enough to take oral medication she can be switched to oral artesunate 2 mg/kg (or IM artesunate 2.4 mg/kg) once daily, plus clindamycin.
OR
Artemether–3.2 mg/kg IM on admission and then 1.6 mg/kg for 1 day
OR
Arteether–150 mg IM/day for 3 days
OR
Quinine–Loading dose–20 mg/kg in 5% D infusion over 4 hours

Maintenance dose–10 mg/kg, 3 times a day for 7 days plus clindamycin IV 450 mg every 8 hours (max. dose quinine 1.4 g).

When the patient is well enough to take oral medication she can be switched to oral quinine 600 mg 3 times a day to complete 5–7 days and oral clindamycin 450 mg 3 times a day 7 days.

*Quinine dosing should be reduced to 12-hourly dosing if IV therapy extends more than 48 hours or if the patient has renal or hepatic dysfunction.

Antenatal Management

- If PCV < 20 packed cell transfusion to be given.
- Folic acid daily 10 mg to be given to prevent megaloblastic anemia.
- Prevent mortality from pulmonary edema and acute respiratory distress syndrome by clinical assessment of jugular venous or central venous pressure, aimed at keeping right arterial pressure less than 10 cm H_2O.
- Monitor sugar every 6th hrly when on quinine as hypoglycemia will be exaggerated.
- Monitor electrolytes, renal, liver functions and hematology during treatment.
- After therapy, maintain vigilance/surveillance for IUGR and preterm labor.

Management During Labor

- Falciparum malaria induces uterine contractions, resulting in premature labor. Careful monitoring of maternal and fetal parameters is extremely important.
- Pregnant women with severe malaria are better managed in an intensive care unit.
- Careful fluid management is also very important. Dehydration as well as fluid overload should be avoided, because both could be detrimental to the mother and/or fetus.
- Once the patient is in labor, fetal or maternal distress may indicate the need to shorten the 2nd stage by forceps or vacuum extraction.
- Cesarean section must be considered for obstetric indications.

Postpartum

- Breastfeeding is not a contraindication.
- Vertical transmission to the fetus can occur particularly when there is infection at the time of birth, and the placenta and cord are blood film positive for malaria.
- All neonates whose mothers developed malaria in pregnancy should be screened for malaria with standard microscopy of thick and thin blood films at birth and weekly blood films for 28 days.

Management of Complications

Acute pulmonary edema: Careful fluid management, back rest, oxygen, diuretics ventilation if needed.

Hypoglycemia: 25–50% Dextrose, 50–100 ml IV, followed by 10% dextrose continuous infusion. Blood sugar should be monitored every 4–6 hours for recurrent hypoglycemia.

Anemia: Packed cells should be transfused if hemoglobin is <5 g%.

Renal failure: Renal failure could be pre-renal due to unrecognized dehydration or renal due to severe parasitemia. Treatment involves careful fluid management, diuretics, and dialysis if needed.

CHAPTER

48

Urinary Tract Infection

This is the most common bacterial infection during pregnancy.

PRINCIPAL PRESENTATIONS

- Asymptomatic bacteriuria (3–11%)
- Acute cystitis (1%)
- Pyelonephritis

Asymptomatic Bacteriuria

Persistent actively multiplying bacteria within the urinary tract in women who have no symptoms.

Diagnosis

- Urine culture is gold standard.
- A clean voided specimen containing more than100,000 organisms per milliliter of same species is diagnostic.

Treatment

Single-dose Treatment

- Amoxicillin 3g
- Ampicillin 2g
- Cephalosporin 2g
- Nitrofurantoin 200 mg
- Trimethoprim-sulphamethoxazole 320/1600 mg

Three-day Course

- Amoxicillin 500 mg three times daily
- Ampicillin 250 mg four times daily
- Cephalosporin 250 mg four times daily
- Ciprofloxacin 250 mg twice daily
- Levofloxacin 250 mg daily
- Nitrofurantoin 50 to 100 mg four times daily; 100 mg twice daily
- Trimethoprim-sulfamethoxazole 160/800 mg two times daily

Other

- Nitrofurantoin 100 mg four times daily for 10 days
- Nitrofurantoin 100 mg twice daily for 7 days
- Nitrofurantoin 100 mg at bed time for 10 days

Treatment Failures

- Nitrofurantoin 100 mg four times daily for 21 days
- Suppression for bacterial resistance or recurrence
- Nitrofurantoin 100 mg at bed time for remainder of pregnancy

Suspect underlying anatomical abnormalities or involvement of upper urinary tract if recurrent treatment failures.

CYSTITIS/URETHRITIS

Clinical Features

Dysuria, urgency and frequency with few associated systemic findings.

Diagnosis

Microscopic hematuria is common, occasionally, there is gross hematuria from hemorrhagic cystitis.

Treatment

3-day regimens are 90% effective.

ACUTE PYELONEPHRITIS

- Most commonly develops in 2nd trimester
- In (50% cases) unilateral that to right side is common, 25% bilateral

Clinical Features

Sudden onset with fever with chills, pain in one or both lumbar regions, nausea, vomiting, anorexia, dehydration, tenderness in costovertebral angles.

Management

- Hospitalize patient.
- Obtain urine and blood cultures.
- Evaluate hemogram, serum creatinine, electrolytes.
- Monitor vital signs frequently, including urinary output—consider indwelling catheter.
- Establish urinary output to >50 ml per hour with intravenous crystalloid.
- Administer intravenous antimicrobial therapy. Empirically start either Ampicillin + Gentamicin or Ceftriaxone. Avoid hyperthermia by giving antipyretics (Paracetamol).

- Obtain chest radiograph if there is dyspnea or tachypnea.
- Change to oral antimicrobials when afebrile.
- Discharge when afebrile in 24 hours, consider antimicrobial therapy for 7 to 10 days.
- Repeat urine culture 1 to 2 weeks after antimicrobial therapy completed.
- If no clinical improvement by 48–72 hrs, do sonography to look for urinary tract obstuction. Obstruction should be removed by ureteral stent placement by cystoscopy or percutaneous nephrostomy.

Differential Diagnosis

Chorioamnionitis, appendicitis, placental abruption, infarcted myoma

Effects on Pregnancy

- Anemia
- Preterm
- IUGR
- Low-birth weight babies

CHAPTER

49

Tuberculosis

Causative organism is *Mycobacterium tuberculosis.*

- India is the highest TB burden country accounting for one-fifth of global incidence (20%).
- Annual risk of infection from different parts of India reported to be between 1–2%.
- Prevalence of infection—38–44% of all ages.
- Prevalence of pulmonary TB—20 per 1000 population.
- In pregnancy pulmonary TB is the commonest presentation accounting to 85–90%.

MODE OF SPREAD

- Through the air droplet nuclei measuring 1–5 µm.
- The droplet nuclei will be carried to bronchial tree where ingested by alveolar macrophages.
- It multiplies over 2–12 weeks to become 10^3–10^4 which is sufficient to elicit a cellular response which can be detected by tuberculin skin test (TST).
- **Mother to Child Transmission**

In utero	Hematogenous dissemination (umbilical vein) Aspiration (infected amniotic fluid)
Intrapartum	Aspiration (infected fluid secretions or genital secretions)
Postpartum	Inhalation (respiratory droplets) Ingestion (infected breast milk)

CLINICAL FEATURES

1. Past history of TB or contact with TB patient is often present in about a third of cases.
2. Early cases may often be asymptomatic or complaint of loss of appetite, lassitude, night sweats and evening rise of temperature, cough >3 weeks.
3. With advanced disease, patients complain of cough with expectoration, hemoptysis and weight loss. Abdominal pain is common in ileocecal TB.

Concerns in pregnancy:

- Delay in the diagnosis of TB
- Safety of anti-tubercular drugs
- Need for prophylaxis

PULMONARY TUBERCULOSIS

Symptoms	Pathogenesis
Asymptomatic	Latent infection
Persistent cough–the most common symptom. Initially dry and non-productive but may later become productive. Associated with hemoptysis in some cases when a granuloma erodes into blood vessels	Enlargement of mediastinal nodes which press on the bronchus or inflammation of the airways. It becomes productive, with inflammatory exudates and/or discharging granulomatous lesions
Breathlessness—a late feature	Destruction of substantial lung tissue or significant pleural effusion
Chest pain–relatively uncommon. Dull, ill-localized or pleuritic in nature Localized wheeze	Pleuritic if peripheral granulomatous lesions are present
Signs suggestive of pleural disease, pleural effusion or lung collapse	Collapse of distal lung caused by hilar lymph node or bronchial narrowing secondary to compression by lymph node

EXTRAPULMONARY TUBERCULOSIS

Sites	Clinical features
Central nervous system • Responsible for 5% of non-respiratory TB • Associated with significant morbidity and mortality • TB meningitis responsible for two-thirds of maternal deaths in the last CEMACH report	• Early constitutional symptoms of anorexia and malaise may be associated with headache, vomiting and altered behavior • Focal neurological signs, depending on the site of involvement, i.e. cerebellar signs, extrapyramidal movements, hemiparesis or monoparesis • Decreasing level of consciousness can occur after a few weeks or months
Lymph nodes • The most common site of extrapulmonary disease	• Persistent lymphadenopathy of >4 weeks' duration in people other than white UK=born should be regarded as TB until demonstrated otherwise and investigated appropriately • Gradual painless enlargement of lymph nodes, fluctuant swelling, superficial ulceration and sinus formation with discharge
Bones and joints • Pregnancy can unmask subtle manifestations and hasten progress of the disease	• Lower back pain is often mistaken for a physiological change associated with pregnancy • An isolated lesion of the joint or a mono-arthritis in a woman from an ethnic minority group should raise suspicion of joint TB • Spinal disease is associated with local tenderness, kyphosis, paraspinal abscesses presenting as a loin mass or psoas abscess or signs of spinal cord compression
Gastrointestinal system • The ileocecal area is the most common site • Varied presentations make it difficult to diagnose	• Unexplained lower abdominal, right iliac fossa pain with the systemic features should raise a suspicion of TB • Ileocecal TB can present with acute onset of right iliac fossa pain, simulating acute appendicitis and/or features of acute intestinal obstruction with vomiting, pain and abdominal distension

Contd...

Contd...

	• Some present with constitutional symptoms of fever, malaise, failure to gain weight in pregnancy or weight loss, abdominal pain and abdominal distension or altered bowel habit
Other sites	• Genitourinary, miliary, skin and pericardial TB are very rare in pregnancy. Tuberculosis can also present with cold abscesses in the liver, adrenals and pancreas

THE EFFECTS OF PREGNANCY ON TB

Pregnancy has neither a beneficial nor a detrimental effect on the course of TB, including sputum conversion rate, stabilization of the disease and relapse rate, as long as it is diagnosed and treated appropriately without delay.

THE EFFECTS OF TB ON PREGNANCY

Pulmonary TB, if associated with late diagnosis, increases the obstetric morbidity in the form of preeclampsia or acute respiratory failure and preterm labor.

Extrapulmonary TB has no direct effect on the course of pregnancy, preeclampsia or mode of delivery but is associated with maternal morbidity in the form of recurrent admission rates and disability as well as increased mortality in cases of TB of the central nervous system and other complications.

Perinatal outcome depends on whether TB is pulmonary or extrapulmonary and also whether it is diagnosed late in pregnancy. The perinatal mortality is six times higher. The incidence of prematurity, small for dates and low birth weight is doubled. The rate of adverse effects is higher if maternal TB was diagnosed in the third trimester, disease is in advanced stage or the woman was non-compliant with the treatment.

INVESTIGATIONS FOR DIAGNOSING TB IN PREGNANCY

Investigation	Role	Interpretation
Tuberculin skin testing (Mantoux test) • 0.1 ml (5 tuberculin units) purified protein derivative is regarded as sale in pregnancy • Results are not affected by pregnancy	• Representative of latent infection • False positive: infection with non-TB mycobacteria, previous BCG vaccination, technical errors • False negative: recent or very old TB infection, recent live-virus vaccination, overwhelming TB disease, some viral illnesses	• Reaction is classified by the diameter of induration perpendicular to the long axis of the forearm 0–4 mm: no further action; 5–10 mm: doubtfully positive 10-15 mm: reactive in high risk cases; >15 mm: positive in all cases
Chest X-ray • Radiation exposure of <0.01 mGy (no evidence of any fetal damage at 100 mGy, so can be done safely in pregnancy	• Defines the extent of pulmonary involvement and diagnosis of active disease • Can be used to identify improvement by comparison	• Patch or nodular shadows in the upper zones • Loss of volume and fibrosis with or without cavitation • Primary focus may be present in latent TB

Contd...

Contd...

Other imaging • CT/MRI of spine/ abdomen/brain, etc, to be used with caution after appropriate counseling	• Helps in establishing diagnosis and extent of extrapulmonary TB	• Depends on the site of the lesion
Smear and/or culture sensitivity • Any tissue specimen or tissue fluid, i.e. sputum; gastric, tracheal or bronchial lavage; CSF, etc.	• Gold standard for diagnosis • May be negative in paucibacillary cases, sampling error	• Gram-positive, acid-fast bacilli in the culture
Interferon-gamma release assays; immunological test such as QuantiFERON Gold or T-SPOT.TB	• Currently, there is a lack of evidence for use in pregnancy or long-term safety • Improved specificity over the Mantoux test • Reduced cross-reactivity with the BCG and most non-tuberculous mycobacteria	• QuantiFERON TB Gold In-Tube assay reports a value of ≥35 IU as a positive test • T-SPOT.TB reports a value of ≥6 spots as a positive test • An indeterminate result may be reported in both tests; the laboratory should be contracted for further details

BCG, Bacille Calmette-Guérin; CSF, Cerebrospinal fluid; CT, Computed tomography; MRI, Magnetic resonance imaging

Mantoux Test (TST)

It is considered safe and the detection of latent infection is not affected by pregnancy.

Method–0.1 ml of 5 TU is given intradermally on the forearm. It should be read after 48–72 hrs. Measured as diameter of maximum induration.

Result is classified based on size of the reaction, and patient risk factor.

Interpretation

Positive if ≥5 mm
- Immunocompromised
- Fibrotic lesion on chest X-ray
- Recent contact with infected person

≥10 mm–Pregnancy
- Recent immigrants from endemic areas
- IV drug users

≥15 mm
- Persons with no known risk factors

Sensitivity – 75–95%–Active disease

Specificity – 98–99%

False positive – Prior BCG vaccination

False negative—immunocompromised, malignancy, malnutrition, severe bacterial and viral infections, steroid use, wrong technique

RISK FACTORS FOR TB

- Close contact with infectious cases
- Living in, travel to or receiving visitors from places where TB is still very common, i.e. developing Asian and African countries
- Living in ethnic minority communities originating from places where TB is still very common
- Having an immune system weakened by HIV infection or other medical problems
- Being very young or elderly, as their immune systems are less robust
- Chronic poor health and nutrition because of lifestyle problems such as homelessness, drug abuse or alcoholism, being a migrant worker or their family
- Living in poor or crowded housing conditions, including living in hostels

CONGENITAL TB

Congenital TB is very rare. Typically, infected infants present in the second or third week of life with–

- Hepatosplenomegaly, respiratory distress, fever, low weight gain, irritability and poor feeding.
- Cantwell's diagnostic criteria for congenital TB are:
  Presence of TB lesions in the infant and one of the following:
  - Lesions in the first week of life
  - A primary hepatic complex or caseating granuloma
  - Documented tuberculous infection of the placenta or endometrium
    And/or exclusion of the possibility of postnatal transmission by a thorough investigation of contacts.
- Clinical features in neonate–Usually occurs in 2nd or 3rd week, but may present at birth. Presents with fever, lymphadenopathy, respiratory distress, irritability, abdominal distention, hepatosplenomegaly.

Atypical forms:

- Extrapulmonary TB–20% of the cases.

Lymphadenitis most common–no adverse maternal or fetal outcome.

- Other forms–Intestinal, spinal, endometrial and meningeal TB–associated with increased frequency of maternal disability, FGR and infants with low Apgar.

Management

Indications for treatment are same as for nonpregnant women.

Treatment should not be delayed due to maternal or fetal concerns whatever may be the period of gestation.

1. Rest
2. Nutritious diet
3. Medical management (ATT)

The aims of treatment are to:

- Achieve cure without relapse

- Prevent progression of the disease or occurrence of complications
- Stop transmission to other individuals, healthcare professionals or newborns and prevent emergence of drug resistance.
  - Pregnant women with TB are managed by a multidisciplinary team consisting of a bacteriologist, chest physician, specialist TB nurse and obstetrician.
  - Hospitalization for a brief period may be needed in extremely-ill women and smear positive, highly infectious and multidrug-resistant (MDR)-TB cases. It may also be necessary for those in whom diagnosis is uncertain or to gain cooperation.

Pre-pregnancy and prenatal:

- Positive TST in low risk asymptomatic pregnant patient – Chest X-ray after 12th week of pregnancy.
- If active disease chest X ray should be performed regardless of gestational age.
- If TB positive treat with isoniazid, rifampicin, ethambutol for 9 months.
- Pyrazinamide only if multiresistant strain.
- Streptomycin should be avoided in pregnancy.

Labor and delivery:

- Mask worn by patient more effective than exposed person wearing mask because airborne droplet nuclei are much smaller than parent droplets.
- Droplet nuclei do not settle they remain suspended in air for long time.
- Health care workers should wear respirators capable of filtering particles to 1 μm in diameter with facial leak of 10% or less.
- Health care workers exposed to patients with active disease should have a PPD administered immediately and again in 12 weeks.

Chemotherapy

- Treatment depends on the disease status, i.e. whether it is latent or active TB or whether there is drug resistance.
- It is divided into an **initial intensive phase**, which aims to kill actively growing and semi-dormant bacilli, followed by a **continuation phase**, which eliminates most of the residual bacilli and reduces failures and relapses.
- In the case of active TB, isoniazid, rifampicin and ethambutol are considered to be the first-line antituberculous drugs.
- During pregnancy, a regimen that includes pyrazinamide for the fist 2 months can be considered.
- It is considered that the use of at least two, but usually three or more drugs will prevent the increasing incidence of single-drug-resistant TB and multi-drug-resistant TB.
- In the follow-up, women should be seen regularly to identify improvement and ensure their conversion from being infectious to noninfectious. A worsening chest radiograph on treatment or no improvement of symptoms should prompt exclusion of other differential diagnosis and MDR-TB.
- Follow-up after 3 months is necessary, as relapse can occur within this time.
- Multidrug-resistant cases should be followed for at least 1 year after treatment has been completed.

DOSAGE OF ANTITUBERCULAR DRUGS

Drugs	Daily dose (mg/kg/day)	Twice weekly dose (mg/kg/day)	Maximum daily dose (mg/kg/day)
Isoniazid (H)	10	20	300
Rifampicin (R)	10–20	10–20	600
Ethambutol (E)	15–25	50	2500
Pyrizinamide (Z)	25–35	50	2500

Category	Type of patient	Initial phase	Continuation phase
Cat I	New smear positive PTB New smear negative PTB with extensive parenchymal involvement New cases of severe extrapulmonary PTB	2 (HRZE) 3	4 (HR) 3
Cat II	Sputum smear positive – Relapse – Treatment failure – Treatment after interruption	2 (HRZES) 3/1 (HRZE) 3	5 (HRE) 3
Cat III	New smear negative PTB (othor than in cat I) New less severe forms of extrapulmonary TB	2 (HRZE) 3	4 (HR) 3
Cat IV	MDR-TB cases (and those with rifampicin resistance)	6 drugs–kanamycin, ofloxacin (levofloxacin), ethionamide, pyrazinamide, ethambutol and cycloserine during 6–9 months	4 drugs–ofloxacin (levofloxacin), ethionamide, ethambutol and cycloserine for 18 months. p-aminosalicylic acid (PAS is included in the regimen as a substitute drug if any bactericidal drug (K, Ofl, Z and Eto) or 2 bacteriostatic (E and Cs) drugs are not tolerated

According to RNTCP Guidelines

TB patients are classified into two groups, namely, 'New' or 'Previously Treated', based on the history of previous treatment.

New: 2 HRZE 3/4 HR

Treated: 2 SHRZE/1 HRZE/5 HRE

Drugs	Use	Dosage	Adverse effects	Effects on fetus
Isoniazid	First-line therapy	3–5 mg/kg up to 300 mg/day	Skin rash and fever, rarely hepatitis, peripheral neuropathy in high doses	No increase in malformations or growth restriction Safest in pregnancy Can cross placenta and cause demyelination, so pyridoxine supplementation advised

Contd...

Contd...

Rifampicin	Used in intensive phase	10–20 mg/kg up to 600 mg orally four times daily	Enzyme inducer Hepatitis Cutaneous hypersensitivity Gastrointestinal reactions Thrombo-cytopenic purpura	Theoretical risk of teratogenesis One study: increased risk of central nervous system abnormalities, limb reduction defects and hypoprothrombinemia and hemorrhagic disease of newborn Overall risk of congenital malformations not increased
Ethambutol	Overall relatively safe in pregnancy second to isoniazid	15 mg/kg	Dose-related optic retrobulbar neuritis Arthralgia	It readily crosses the placenta and there have been few reports of animal teratogenicity with its use Theoretical possibility of ocular toxicity
Pyrazinamide	Used with caution in pregnancy	20–30 mg/kg	Anorexia Nausea Photosensitivity Flushing Hepatotoxicity	No significant animal teratogenicity studies or reports of malformations in treated patients are available
Streptomycin	No consistent relationship between gestational age at exposure and ototoxicity–should be avoided throughout the entire gestation period	12–15 mg/kg	Cutaneous hypersensitivity Giddiness Numbness and tinnitus Vertigo Ataxia Deafness	Variable transplacental passage Ototoxicity varying from minor vestibular and/or auditory impairment, to cases of severe, irreversible bilateral loss of hearing and marked vestibular abnormalities
Kanamycin,[a] amikacin, capreomycin, ofloxacin, ciprofloxacin, ethionamide,[a] prothionamide, cycloserine, *para*-amino-salicyclic acid	Safety profile in pregnancy has not been ascertained and should generally be avoided unless necessary for maternal well-being	Second-line drugs useful in multi-drug-resistant cases	Ototoxicity, nephrotoxicity, gastrointestinal reaction	Same potential problems as streptomycin. Inadvertent use does not require termination of pregnancy or invasive diagnostic procedures, but hearing tests should be performed after birth

Latent TB and the Role of Chemoprophylaxis

- The role of treatment in latent TB infection, especially in pregnant women, is controversial.

- Better to delay treatment until after delivery because pregnancy itself does not increase the risk of progression of the disease, and the women in pregnancy and the early postpartum period may be vulnerable to isoniazid hepatotoxicity.

Infection Control in Late Pregnancy and the Puerperium

- Pulmonary TB is potentially infectious, particularly when the index case has sputum that is smear positive for the bacilli on microscopy. These women can be rendered non-infectious by 2 weeks of treatment which include rifampicin and isoniazid.
- If admitted to hospital, the decision about isolation depends on the initial assessment of infectivity, the possibility of multiple-drug resistance and the immune status of the individual.
- Women with suspected or confirmed MDR-TB should be admitted to a negative pressure ventilation room.
- Control of infection in health care settings among patients and health care workers is the responsibility of infection control teams.
- Tuberculosis is a notifiable disease and the clinician in charge of the patient is responsible for notification to the consultant in communicable disease control. If the woman is later found to be negative, they can be denotified.
- If TB is diagnosed postnatally, with the mother being sputum positive for acid-fast bacilli within the 2 weeks following delivery, there is a potential risk of transmission of the disease to the newborn.
- Infants with a mother who has had less than 2 weeks of treatment and who is sputum positive for acid-fast bacilli should be given prophylactic isoniazid (5 mg/kg) and pyridoxine (vitamin B_6) (5–14 mg/kg) and have a tuberculin test at 6–12 weeks. If this is negative then a Bacilli Calmette Guérin (BCG) can be given and the chemoprophylaxis stopped. If the tuberculin test is positive, then extended treatment should be given for a total of 6 months.
- The BCG vaccine is not recommended for the babies of mothers who are HIV-positive until they have been shown to be HIV-negative.
- Contact tracing and screening involves all close family members or other individuals who have had close contact and is done by history, examination, tuberculin testing and chest X-ray. Contacts who are ill should be thoroughly investigated for TB.
- In an adult contact, if the tuberculin test is positive and they are immuno-compromised or they have HIV infection and have not had a BCG, chemoprophylaxis with isoniazid is given.
- In children, a positive tuberculin test is suggestive of infection and treatment is given. A negative tuberculin test is repeated in 6 weeks and if it is still negative then a BCG is given; if it turns positive, it suggests active infection and this needs treatment.
- Breastfeeding is recognized as the healthiest way to feed a baby. Antituberculous drugs cross into the breast milk but the amounts are too small to produce toxicity. Women taking isoniazid should also take pyridoxine supplementation (14–25 mg/day). There are no reports of any adverse effects among infants of nursing mothers receiving anti-TB drugs. If a breastfeeding mother becomes

acutely-ill with TB, breastfeeding may have to be interrupted and breast milk expressed to prevent development of mastitis.

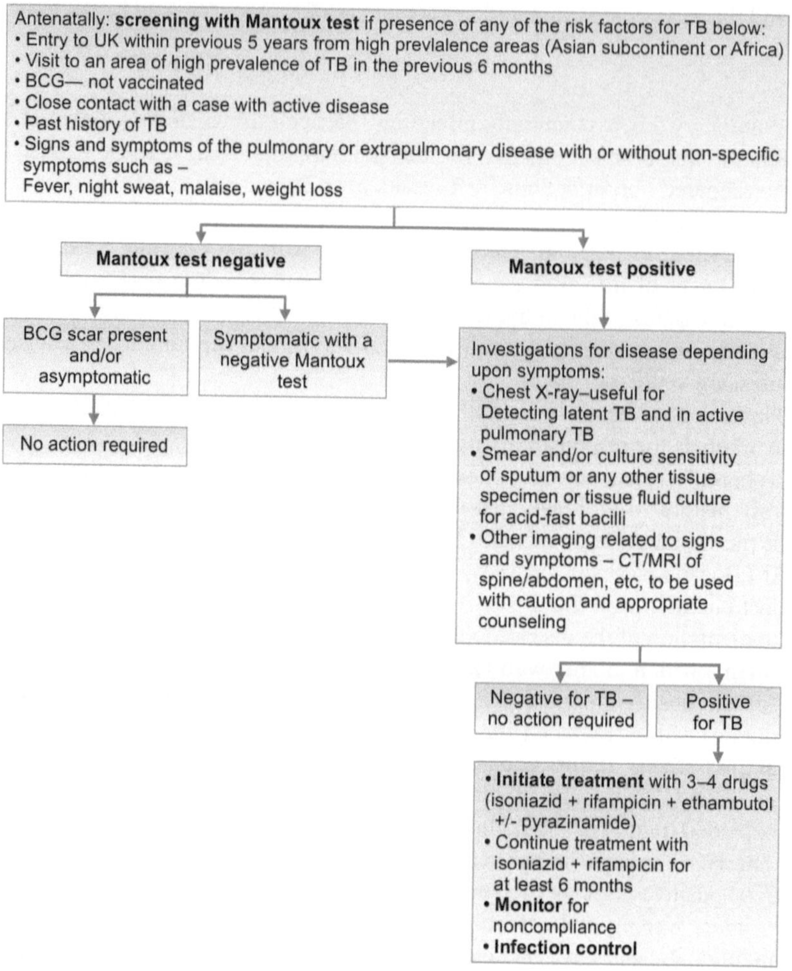

The Role of the BCG Vaccine

- The BCG vaccine contains a live attenuated strain of the bacillus derived from *M. bovis.* No harmful effects on the fetus have been observed from BCG during pregnancy but, as it is a live attenuated vaccine, it should be avoided in pregnancy, particularly in the first trimester, and wherever possible delayed until after delivery.
- Breastfeeding is not a contraindication to the BCG.
- It should be given to all neonates and infants who live in an area with an annual TB incidence of 40 per 100,000 people or with a parent or grandparent from a country where the incidence is 40 per 100,000 population or family history of TB in the previous 5 years.
- It is effective in preventing severe disease in infants and young children.

- The BCG is not recommended for babies of mothers, who are HIV-positive until they have been shown to be HIV-negative, or if a member of the household has suspected or active TB.

Multidrug-resistant TB in Pregnancy

- It is associated with a high mortality rate in the general population.
- There is a lack of evidence-based information in pregnancy.
- Management of these cases should be individualized.
- Multidrug-resistant TB develops if there is non-compliance with the treatment initially. It must be treated with second line antituberculous drugs and for a period of 2 years.

Pregnancy with MDR-TB

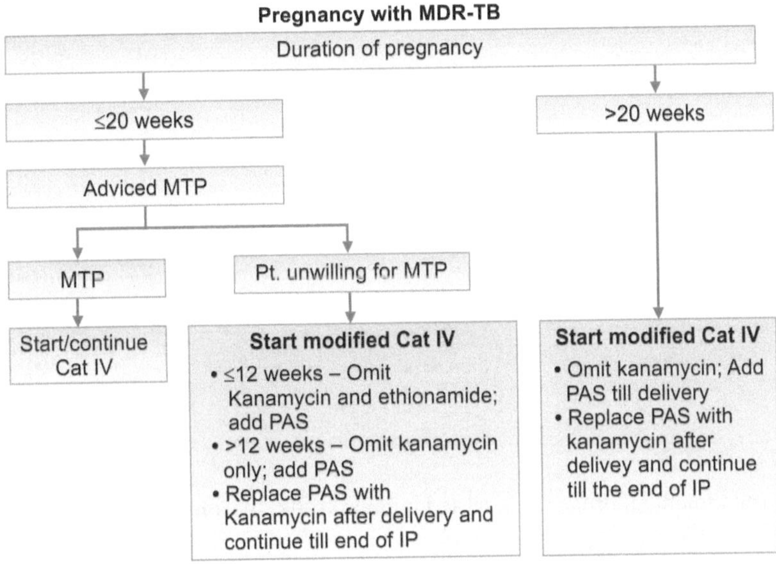

INH PROPHYLAXIS FOR PREGNANT WOMAN

Indication

- Positive tuberculin test with abnormal CXR.
- Recent converters (within 2 years) as the risk of active TB is maximum during the first 2 years.
- Close contacts of a person with active TB.
- Immunocompromised women.

  Dose–5 mg/kg; max 300 mg/day.

Adverse Drug Reactions

Hepatotoxicity (10%). This is increased when associated hepatitis or HIV is present. Hence monthly LFT is advised.

Pyridoxine should be supplemented to avoid the risk of peripheral neuritis.

INH Prophylaxis for Babies

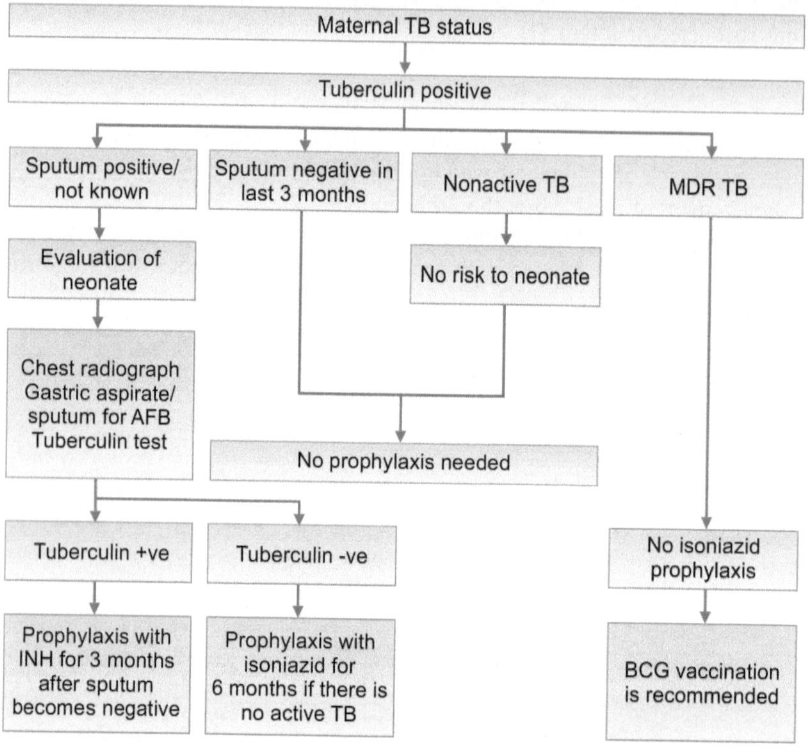

Breastfeeding

- Even though all drugs are excreted in breast milk, the amount is not more than 20% of the dose ingested by mother so breastfeeding is not contraindicated.
- Avoid direct coughing on infant.

Contraception

- OCPs are not advised because of increased metabolism due to simultaneous use of enzyme inducer drug rifampicin.
- Barrier and IUCDs are safe.
- Depot injections can be given.

CHAPTER

50

Syphilis

Causative agent is *Treponema pallidum*, which belongs to spirochete family.

MODE OF TRANSMISSION

- Sexual contact
- Fetus during pregnancy or birth
- Kissing or other of a close contact with an active lesion
- Transfusion of fresh human blood (banked for <24–48 hrs)
- Accidental direct inoculation

A patient cannot spread syphilis by sexual contact four years or more after acquiring the disease.

Within hours or days after *T. pallidum* penetrates the intact mucous membrane or gains access through abraded skin, it enters the lymphatics or blood stream and disseminates through the body.

The median incubation period is 21 days (3–90 days).

The secondary or disseminated stage is 2–12 weeks (6 weeks).

Seventy-five percent vertical transmission rate
Vertical transmission before 16 weeks is rare
Treatment of the mother decreases risk of infection to 1%.

CLINICAL FEATURES

Primary syphilis: Characteristic chancre-painless indurated ulcer with raised edge, firm border and smooth base associated with non-suppurative lymphadenopathy in 50% of cases. The first symptomatology which develops lasts for 4–6 weeks. Chancres heal spontaneously in 3–6 weeks leaving no trace or thin atrophic scar.

Secondary syphilis: Fever, malaise, anorexia, headache, myalgia, arthralgia, diffuse macular rash, plantar and palmar target lesions, patchy alopecia, condyloma lata (flesh colored papules and nodules on perineum and perianal area).

Latent syphilis: Reactive serological tests but resolved clinical manifestations.

Tertiary syphilis: Neurosyphilis, cardiovascular syphilis, gummata (inflammatory fibrous nodules/plaques commonly affect bone and skin).

- Neurosyphilis: Asymptomatic, symptomatic (tabes dorsalis, dementia and meningovascular involvement).
- Cardiovascular syphilis–aortitis (aortic regurgitation, aneurysm and angina).

DIAGNOSIS

Direct Examination

Primary/secondary and early congenital syphilis—dark field examination or immunofluorescence of secretions from chancre for presence of spirochete.

Serologic tests

a. *Non-treponemal tests*
- VDRL
- RPR

b. *Treponemal*
- FTA-abs
- TP-PA
- MHA-TP

- Syphilis reaginic antibodies are IgG and IgM.
- The standard non-treponemal test is VDRL, but most laboratories have adopted RPR.
- RPR test should be non-reactive after successful therapy in primary syphilis and 2 years in secondary syphilis.
- The time taken for VDRL to become non-reactive depends on the duration that the disease has been present before treatment. After secondary stage, it will never become non-reactive even with adequate treatment (Wasserman fastness).
- TPHA once it becomes positive, remains so for life.
- The FTA-ABS is a standard treponemal test but due to difficulty with standardization between laboratories, TPHA is being used now.
- False positive tests seen in acute bacterial or viral infection, vaccination, early HIV infection, other spirochete illness, like relapsing fever, yaws, pinta, leptospirosis or rat bite fever.
- Lyme disease results in FTA–ABS but negative VDRL/RPR.
- Neurosyphilis–CSF examination along with serological tests.

Ultrasound

Ultrasound findings include placentomegaly, IUGR, microcephaly, anemia, hydrops.

Management

Stages of syphilis	Patient without penicillin allergy	Patient with confirmed penicillin allergy
Primary, secondary, or early latent	Penicillin G benzathine (single dose of 2.4 MU IM)	Tetracycline hydrochloride (500 mg PO qid) or doxycycline (100 mg PO bid) for 2 weeks
Late latent (or latent of uncertain duration), cardiovascular or benign tertiary • CSF normal and patient infected with HIV	Lumbar puncture • CSF normal: Pencillin G benzathine (2.4 MU IM weekly for 3 weeks) • CSF abnormal: Treat as neurosyphilis	Lumbar puncture • CSF normal and patient not infected with HIV: Tetracycline hydrochloride (500 mg PO qid) or doxycycline (100 mg PO bid) for 4 weeks. Desensitization and treatment with penicillin. If compliance cannot be ensured, treat as neurosyphilis
Neurosyphilis (asymptomatic or symptomatic)	Aqueous penicillin G (18–24 MU/d IV, given as 3–4 MU 4th hrly or continuous infusion) for 10–14 days	Desensitization and treatment with penicillin

Syphilis during pregnancy-Treatment	
Category	**Treatment**
a. Early syphilis	Benzathine penicillin-G, 2.4 million units IM as single injection—some recommend a second dose one week later
b. More than one year duration	Benzathine penicillin-G 2.4 million units IM weekly for 3 doses
c. Neurosyphilis	Aqueous crystalline penicillin-G 3–4 million units IV every 4 hours for 10–14 days
	OR
	Aqueous procaine penicillin, 2.4 million units IM daily, plus probenecid 500 mg orally 4 times daily, both for 10–14 days

a. Primary, secondary and latent syphilis of less than 1 year duration
b. Latent syphilis of unknown or more than 1 year duration
c. Some recommend benzathine penicillin 2.4 million units IM after completion of neurosyphilis treatment regimens

Women with a history of penicillin allergy should have skin testing to confirm the risk of IgE mediated anaphylaxis, if confirmed, penicillin desensitization followed by benzathine penicillin G treatment.

Prenatal

All women should be screened for syphilis at the first prenatal visit for communities in which prevalance of syphilis is high screening again at 28 weeks and at delivery.

The Jarisch-Herxheimer reaction is a systemic reaction that occurs 1–2 hrs after initial treatment with antibiotics. Consists of abrupt onset of fever, chills, myalgia, headache, tachycardia, hyperventilation, vasodilation with flushing, and mild hypotension. After 24 weeks, they may also present with uterine contractions, and fetal heart rate decelerations. It lasts for 12–24 hrs and may be treated with antipyretics or prednisone.

Labor and Delivery

Any woman who delivers stillborn infant after 20 weeks should be tested for syphilis.

Kasowitz theory–There is progressive improvement in the pregnancy outcome with each consecutive pregnancy.

Abortion → IUD → Stillborn → Preterm → Normal delivery

Postpartum

All patients with early or congenital syphilis should be tested at 3, 6 and 12 months.

- Secondary syphilis for more than 1 year should also be tested at 24 months after treatment.
- Latent syphilis–5 years

Neonatal manifestations–rhinitis (snuffles), diffuse maculopapular, desquamative rash with extensive sloughing on the palms, soles, mouth and anus. Hepatosplenomegaly anemia, thrombocytopenia and jaundice. Neonatal death may be due to liver failure, severe pneumonia, pulmonary hemorrhage. Renal involvement, generalized osteochondritis, perichondritis may be seen.

CHAPTER

51

TORCH Infections

TOXOPLASMOSIS

Caused by *Toxoplasma gondii.*

Transmission

- Ingestion of tissue cysts by handling infected meat or eating undercooked meat/ infective oocysts excreted in feces of infected cat.
- Congenital transmission.
- Rarely through blood or organ transplantation.

Clinical Features

Generally asymptomatic

- Occasionally mild malaise, lethargy and lymphadenopathy (enlarged lymph nodes are discrete, firm, tender/nontender, nonsuppurative).
- Immunocompromised adults may develop hepatitis, chorioretinitis, polymyositis, dermatomyositis, myocarditis.

Effects on Pregnancy

- Primary infection during pregnancy is associated with increased adverse pregnancy outcomes.
- Outcome depends on period of gestation at the time of infection.
- Whereas the risk of congenital transmission—parasites entering fetal circulation by infection of placenta is 0–9% in 1st trimester, 27% in 2nd trimester, 59% in 3rd trimester.
- Severity of congenital infection is greater in early pregnancy.

Four Forms of Congenital Toxoplasmosis

- Symptomatic neonatal disease
- Mild–severe disease in 1st month
- Childhood-adolescent sequelae from previous undiagnosed infection
- Subclinical infections

Prenatal USG: Hydrocephalus, intracranial calcification, ventricular dilatation, hepatic enlargement, ascites, increased placental thickness.
Neonatal manifestations: Hydrocephalus, microcephaly, intracranial calcification, chorioretinitis, blindness, mental retardation, petechiae–thrombocytopenia.

Classical Triad

- Chorioretinitis
- Intracranial calcification
- Hydrocephalus

Diagnosis and Treatment

Indirect detection	Direct detection
IgG and IgM antibodies	PCR
Avidity of IgG antibodies (ELISA, Sabin-Feldman Dye Test)	Cell culture
IFA, Modified Direct Agglutinin Test	

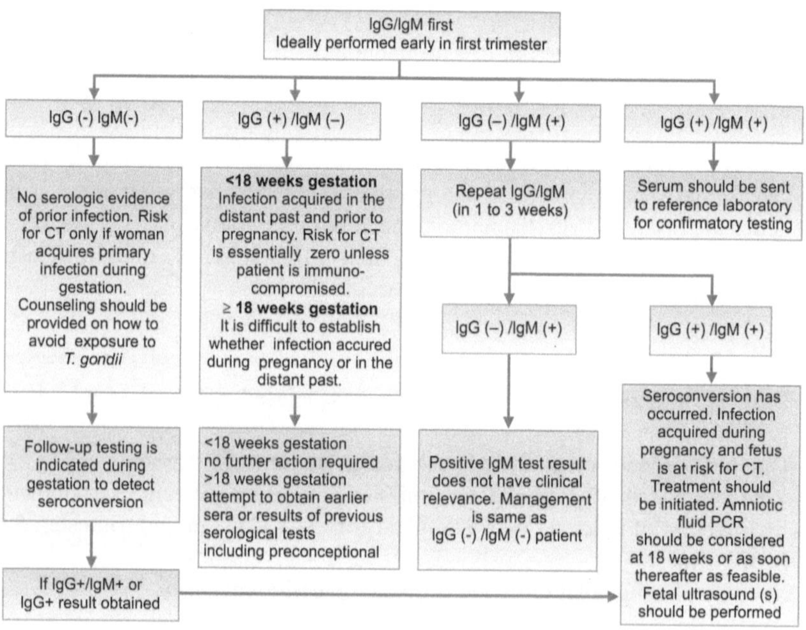

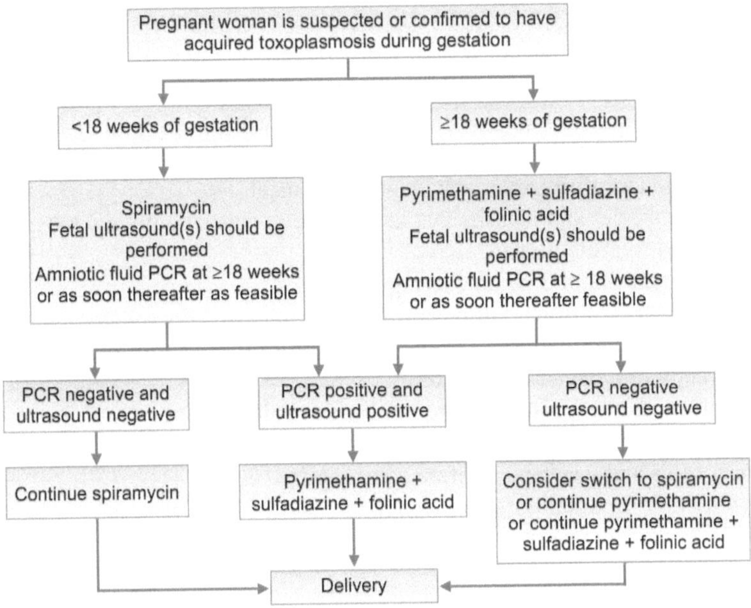

Treatment	Dosage	Comments
Spiramycin	1 g (3 million U) every 8 h (for a total of 3 g or 9 million U per day)	Not teratogenic; does not treat infection in the fetus; indicated for pregnant women suspected of having acquired the infection at <18 weeks of gestation. Spiramycin treatment should be continued until delivery in women with low suspicion of fetal infection or those with documented negative results of amniotic fluid PCR and negative findings on ultrasounds at follow-up. Available in the United States only through the investigational New Drug process at the FDA. Prior consultation with medical consultants[a] is required.
Pyrimethamine, sulfadiazine, and folinic acid	Pyrimethamine: 50 mg every 12 h for 2 days followed by 50 mg daily; sulfadiazine: initial dose of 75 mg/kg, followed by 50 mg/kg every 12 h (maximum, 4 g/day); folinic acid (leucovorin): 10–20 mg daily (during and 1 week after completion of pyrimethamine therapy)	Pyrimethamine is teratogenic; therefore, this combination should not be used before week 18 of gestation (in some centers in Europe, it is used as early as week 14–16). Indicated for women suspected of having acquired infection at 18 weeks of gestation and those with documented fetal infection (positive result of amniotic fluid PCR) or abnormal ultrasound findings suggestive of congenital toxoplasmosis, given when patient is at 18 weeks of gestation.

Prevention Measures

- Cook meat to "well done" or thoroughly to 67°C (153°F). Meat should not be "pink" in the center.
- Note that meat that is smoked, cured in brine, or dried may still be infectious.
- Avoid mucous membrane contact when handling raw meat.
- Wash hands carefully after contact with raw meat.
- Kitchen surfaces and utensils that have come in contact with raw meat should be washed wearing gloves.
- Refrain from skinning or butchering animals.
- Avoid contact with materials potentially contaminated with cat feces, especially when handling cat litter or gardening. Wearing gloves is recommended when these activities cannot be avoided.
- Disinfect emptied cat-litter box with near boiling water for 5 min before refilling.
- Wash fruits and vegetables before consumption.
- Avoid drinking water potentially contaminated with oocysts.

RUBELLA (GERMAN MEASLES)

- It is an infection of school-going age group caused by RNA togavirus, transmitted by nasopharyngeal secretion with incubation period: 12–23 days.
- Once primary infection occurs, it produces life-long immunity.
- 80–85% of women of child-bearing age would have contacted rubella at early age and would have developed IgG antibodies.
- If the mother is negative for rubella antibodies, then she should be immunized during nonpregnant interval.
- Accidental vaccination in early pregnancy is not an indication for termination of pregnancy.
- Usually asymptomatic and goes undetected in majority of the pregnant women.

Effects of Maternal Rubella on Fetus and Newborn

Period of gestation	Risk of infection	Consequence
0–12 weeks	40–50%	100% risk of major congenital abnormalities
13–16 weeks	30–35%	Deafness and retinopathy in 15% spontaneous abortion in 20%
After 16 weeks	10%	Usually normal development with slight risk of deafness and retinopathy

Clinical Manifestations–*In adults*

- Mild febrile illness, generalized maculopapular rash beginning on the face and spreading to trunk and extremities, arthritis and arthralgia, lymphadenopathy, conjunctivitis.

Congenital Rubella Syndrome

Hanshaw classification of clinical features of congenital rubella:

1. Transient features:

- Thrombocytopenic purpura
- Hepatitis
- Hemolytic anemia

2. Developmental features: occur later in life
   - Intellectual impairment
   - Sensory neuronal deafness—most common single defect
   - Diabetes mellitus
3. Permanent features:
   The classical rubella triad (Triad of Gregg):
   - Eye–Congenital cataract, salt and pepper retinopathy, microphthalmia, glaucoma
   - Ear–Bilateral and progressive sensory neural deafness
   - Congenital heart disease–PDA, pulmonary artery stenosis, pulmonary valvular stenosis, rarely ASD, VSD and coarctation of aorta

Extended Rubella Syndrome

One-third of the infants who are asymptomatic at birth, will develop progressive panencephalitis and type-1 diabetes mellitus in 2nd or 3rd decade of life.

Other features–Congenital glaucoma, hepatosplenomegaly and jaundice, radiolucent bone disease.

Lab Diagnosis

1. Serology — mainstay of diagnosis — isolated from urine, nasopharynx and CSF
   - On infecting a person, the virus multiplies in the upper respiratory mucosa and lymph node for 1 week, next week is period of viremia.
   - After 1 week of viremia — facial rashes appear, mother can now transmit virus to the fetus, high risk of congenital damage in fetus if detected in 1st 16 weeks of pregnancy.
   - Rubella specific IgM antibodies appear shortly before the onset of symptoms (during the phase of viremia). Peak levels are noted 1 week later and disappear roughly 1 month after the rash has occurred.
   - Rubella specific IgM differentiates primary infection from reinfection. IgM is present only in primary infection.
   - Should test for both IgG and IgM antibodies.
   - A rising titer in 4 weeks time of IgG antibodies between paired sera is a better indicator of primary infection of rubella during pregnancy than IgM.

   IgG antibodies appear soon after the onset of symptoms, peak levels are achieved in a week and they remain lifetime.

Management of Pregnant Women with Suspected Rubella or a History of Contact with Rubella

Facts to be remembered:

- Incubation period lasts for 2–3 weeks.

- IgM antibodies usually disappear in two months' time.
- Risk to the fetus lies one week before sero-conversion or appearance of rash in the mother. Ex: if mother tests positive for IgM at 16 weeks of pregnancy, viremia in the mother would have occurred anytime between 14 and 15 weeks of gestation and hence puts fetus at very high risk of congenital damage.
- Cord blood for IgM antibodies or PCR on fetal samples indicate fetal infection but do not confirm or rule out fetal damage.
- Gross cardiac anomalies, fetal growth restriction, intracranial calcification, microcephaly and microphthalmia, meconium peritonitis, hepatosplenomegaly can be detected by antenatal USG.

Prevention

- Droplet precaution is for 7 days after the onset of rash
- Vaccination
  - Rubella vaccine should be offered to nonpregnant women of child-bearing age group who do not have the evidence of infection.
  - Should be avoided 1 month before or during pregnancy because vaccine contains attenuated live virus.

Indications of Termination of Pregnancy

- Acute infection–IgM positive or rising titers of IgG demonstrated
- Sonological evidence of congenital anomalies

CYTOMEGALOVIRUS INFECTION

- It is the most common congenital viral infection affecting 1% live births, caused by cytomegalovirus.
- Transmitted by nasopharyngeal secretion, urine, saliva, semen, cervical secretions, blood, intrauterine or intrapartum infection, neonatal infection from breastfeeding.
- The high incidence of CMV infection is because of the fact that the infected mothers can transmit the virus to the fetus, irrespective of the nature of infection whether primary or secondary.

Clinical Manifestations

- Most infections are asymptomatic but 15% infected adults develop mononucleosis like syndrome characterized by–Fever, pharyngitis, lymphadenopathy, polyarthritis
- Immunocompromised women develop–Myocarditis, pneumonitis, hepatitis, retinitis, gastroenteritis, meningoencephalitis

Congenital CMV/Cytomegalic Inclusion Disease

Classical Tetrad

- Mental retardation
- Cerebral calcifications
- Microcephaly
- Chorioretinitis

Other Features

- Growth restriction
- Locomotor retardation
- Sensorineural deficits
- Hepatosplenomegaly
- Jaundice
- Hemolytic anemia
- Thrombocytopenic purpura

2. Infants with asymptomatic congenital infection develop late onset sequelae
    - Sensorineural hearing loss — commonest permanent deficit, typically detected by 2–3 months of age, severe profound hearing loss seen by 3–4 years of age.
    - Neurological deficit
    - Chorioretinitis
    - Psychomotor retardation
    - Learning disabilities
    - Visual impairments—chorioretinitis (19%), optic atrophy (11%)

Strabismus (23%), pigmentary retinopathy (7%), nystagmus (3%) and coloboma (1%) 5–10% of infected babies are symptomatic at birth, and manifest with classical cytomegalic inclusion disease. Out of the symptomatic infants 30% die immediately, 70% survive, of which 90% die within 2 years. 10% survive with developmental errors. 90% remain asymptomatic–in which 10–15% develop late sequelae, sensory neural deafness, chorioretinitis and neurological defects. CMV is not associated with higher incidence of abortions.

Lab Diagnosis

- Primary infection is diagnosed by seroconversion of CMV specific IgG in paired acute and convalescent sera assayed simultaneously and immunoassay for virus specific IgM antibodies.
- There is 4-fold increase in IgG titer in case of primary infection.
- Recurrent infection of CMV does show IgM antibodies.

Abnormal Maternal CMV Screening

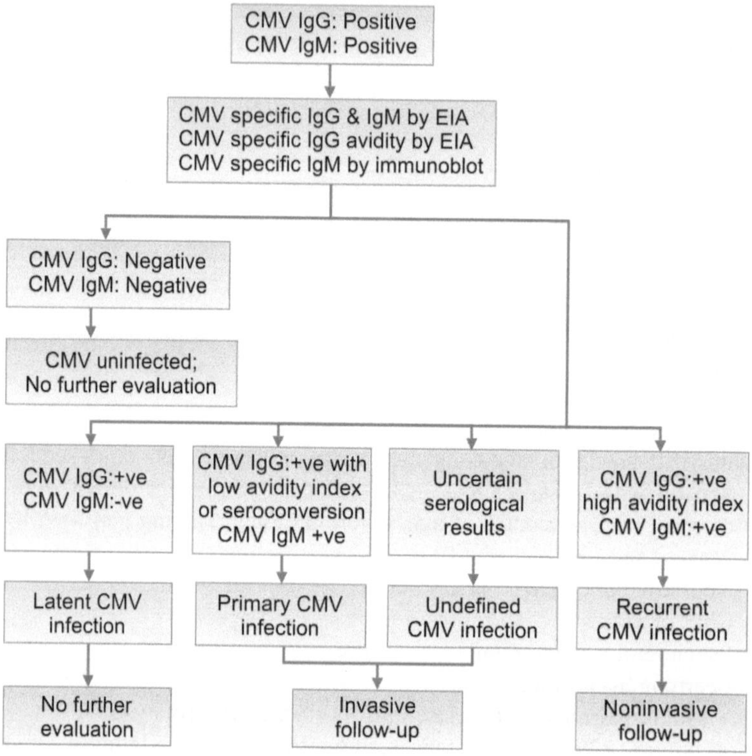

The measurement of specific IgG avidity is valuable in confirming primary CMV infection.

The IgG antibody response matures from low-avidity to high-avidity production over several weeks to months.

Invasive Follow-up

- Amniotic fluid for viral cultures, if facilities available
- Cordocentesis for IgM antibodies, Hb%, platelet count, LFT (particularly for enzymes)

Non-Invasive Follow-up

USG, CT, MRI

- For diagnosing fetal problems such as microcephaly, ventriculomegaly, cerebral calcification and fetal hyperechoic bowel.

Think of CMV Infection in Pregnancy in the Following Situations

- Mother presenting herself with signs of primary infection (rare situation).
- Accidental finding of IgM positive antibodies in pregnant women while she is being investigated for previous stillbirth. Presence of IgM in the index

pregnancy is probably related to this pregnancy only and unrelated to previous stillbirth which could have been due to some other cause.

- USG characters in the fetus might give a clue when one sees an IUGR fetus with hepatosplenomegaly, etc. mentioned above.

Treatment

- There is no accepted treatment modality.
- Use of IV Ganciclovir (analogue of guanosine and a homologue of acyclovir; it is the 1st anti-CMV agent) for 6 weeks to neonates with symptomatic CNS disease prevents hearing deterioration at 6 months and later.
- Foscarnet is another potent drug against CMV but highly toxic causing renal failure, hypocalcemics and seizures and hence not recommended in neonates.

Prophylaxis

- Primary prevention is the only way to prevent CMV infection, i.e. prevention of maternal infection.
- CMV infection typically spreads by droplet infection and also during sexual contact which requires education regarding behavioral pattern, like use of condoms, attention to personal hygiene and avoid contact with children's secretion.
- Passive immunization with CMV specific hyperimmune globulin significantly lowers the risk of congenital CMV infection when given to pregnant women with primary disease.
- There is no CMV vaccine.
- CMV is not a cause of recurrent abortions but in subsequent pregnancy the protective maternal antibodies which are transmitted transplacentally will protect the fetus from infection unless women is contracting repeated infection.

Indications for Termination of Pregnancy

Primary infection in the first half of the pregnancy.

Reinfection and infection in the second half of the pregnancy — only if the fetus is infected or developed anomalies.

HERPES SIMPLEX VIRUS INFECTION

Usually caused by HSV2 and less commonly by type 1.

Clinical Features

1. First Episode Primary Infection: "Classical presentation" characterized by papular eruption with itching or tingling, which then becomes painful and vesicular, tender inguinal lymphadenopathy and systemic symptoms.
2. First Episode Non-Primary Infection: Fewer lesions, few systemic manifestations, less pain with short duration.
3. Reactivation Disease/Recurrent Infection: Lesions are less in number with less duration and may be unilateral.

Diagnosis

Virological tests	Type specific serologic tests
1. Isolation of HSV in cell culture	ELISA-herpes ELISA
2. PCR	Herpe select immunoblot
3. Tzanck preparation	Captita HSV type specific test kit

Antiviral Medications for Herpes Virus Infection

Indication	Pregnancy recommendation
Primary /First episode infection	Acyclovir, 400 mg, orally three times daily for 7–10 days OR Valacyclovir, 1 gm, orally twice daily for 7–10 days
Symptomatic recurrent infection	Acyclovir, 400 mg, orally three times daily for 5 days OR Acyclovir, 800 mg, orally twice daily for 5 days OR Valacyclovir, 500 mg, orally twice daily for 3 days OR Valacyclovir, 1 gm, orally once daily for 5 days
Daily suppression	Acyclovir, 400 mg orally three times daily from 36 weeks until delivery OR Valacyclovir, 500 mg orally twice daily from 36 weeks until delivery

Cesarean Delivery for Women with Genital HSV Lesions

C-section is recommended for all women presenting in labor with Herpes lesions or with prodromal symptoms suggestive of genital herpes, but not indicated for women who develop first episode of genital herpes lesions during first or second trimester.

C-section is justified even if the infected woman has ruptured membranes for more than 4 hours.

Woman who present with first episode of genital herpes lesions within 6 weeks of EDD or onset of preterm labor, elective section is considered at term.

For women like this, who opt for vaginal delivery, invasive procedures like fetal scalp electrode monitoring, fetal blood sampling and instrumental deliveries should be avoided.

Neonatal Herpes

Neonatal infection is caused by contact with infected genital secretions.

Recommended regimen is acyclovir, 20 mg/kg body weight IV every 8 hrs for 21 days for disseminated and CNS disease, or 14 days for disease limited to the skin and mucous membrane.

CHAPTER

52

Bacterial Vaginosis

Bacterial vaginosis is polymicrobial alteration in the vaginal flora causing an increase in vaginal pH, sometimes, associated with a homogeneous discharge, but in the absence of a demonstrable inflammatory response.

ETIOLOGY

Remains unclear. Believed to be due to:

- Smoking, change in sexual partner, black race–risk factors.
- Estrogen—favors disappearance of Lactobacilli and unopposed growth of other organisms.
- Enzymes—mucinase and sialidase breaks down mucosal barrier allowing entry of pathogens.
- Role of phage virus—favors growth of anaerobes decreasing the number of Lactobacilli.

MICROBIOLOGY

- Lactobacilli produce lactic acid, lactacin B, acidolin and hydrogen peroxide deterring the growth of potentially pathogenic bacteria.
- Mobiluncus and bacteroides produce ketoacid, succinate and raise vaginal pH and blunt the chemotactic response of neutrophils and reduce their killing ability.
- Total bacterial count of normal vaginal flora is $<10^6$ organisms/ml, and is up to 10^9 organisms/mL.
- *G. vaginalis*, bacteroides species, *mobiluncus species* and *M. hominis* dominate the flora with reduction in the quality and quantity of the lactobacilli.
- *G. vaginalis* and other anaerobes produce amines and organic acids responsible for fishy odor.

Adverse Sequelae

Obstetric

- Late miscarriage
- PPROM
- Chorioamnionitis
- Spontaneous preterm labor
- Postpartum endometritis

Gynecological

- Pelvic inflammatory disease
- Infertility
- Cervical intraepithelial neoplasia
- Post-hysterectomy vaginal cuff infection

CLINICAL FEATURES

Up to half the women with bacterial vaginosis are asymptomatic.
Symptoms: Non-irritating, malodorous vaginal discharge is characteristic.

Signs: Vagina is usually not erythematous and whitish grey, thin, homogeneous and adherent to the vaginal walls with fishy odor may be noted.

Diagnosis: Three of the four criteria to be met for diagnosis of bacterial vaginosis (Amsel's criteria).

- Homogeneous, grey-white non-inflammatory discharge adherent to the vaginal walls
- pH >4.5
- Positive Whiff's test: (PPV 90% and specificity 70%)
  - One drop of 10% KOH added to the discharge-fishy-amine odor.
- Saline microscopy: Presence of clue cells making up of at least 20% of the cells (Clue cells-shed out vaginal epithelial cells with adherent bacteria).

Nuget's scoring: Gram staining system of vaginal smears to diagnose bacterial vaginosis.
Lactobacillus morphotype–Large Gram-positive rods (scored 0–4)
Gardenella morphotypes–Small Gram-variable rods (scored 0–4)
Mobiluncus morphotypes–Curved variable rods (scored 0–2)

Result: 7–10 consistent with bacterial vaginosis

New Rapid Tests

- Measuring metabolic products–proline aminopeptidase
- DNA probes for *G.vaginalis* genes (Affirm VP III)

TREATMENT

Metronidazole

- Allergy to the drug is rare, more cost-effective and spares lactobacilli.
- Alcohol should be avoided as it causes disulfiram like reaction.
- Vaginal preparation produces systemic levels of drug far below those of the oral preparation and is costlier than oral preparation.
- It is effective against most anaerobes.

Clindamycin

- Most expensive.
- Delays the return of lactobacilli to the vagina compared to metronidazole.

- Side effect is development of pseudomembranous colitis but vaginal cream is associated with lesser side effects.
- It has good activity against *Mobiluncus* species and *G.vaginalis*.

Agent	Dosage
Metronidazole	500 mg orally twice daily for 7 days OR
Metronidazole gel 0.75%	5 g (1 full applicator) intravaginally once daily for 5 days OR
Clindamycin cream 2%	5 g (1 full applicator) intravaginally at bed time for 7 days OR
Clindamycin	300 mg orally twice daily for 7 days

During Pregnancy

- Both the drugs are equally effective and safe during pregnancy.
- When used in first trimester of pregnancy mutagenicity has not been demonstrated although smaller studies have demonstrated facial defects.
- Both the drugs are secreted in the breast milk but but standard treatment doses are not harmful.
- Vaginal preparation of clindamycin may be used as an alternative.
- Pregnant women presenting with symptoms of bacterial vaginosis can benefit from antibiotic treatment and women at high risk of adverse sequelae in pregnancy should be screened and treated.

Recurrent Bacterial Vaginosis

- Recurrent bacterial vaginosis is mostly new episode rather than treatment failure. Repeated antibiotic treatment produces drug resistance and not acceptable to the patients. Use of *Lactobacillus* strains to replace vaginal flora is still being investigated.
- Vaginal capsule containing 10^6 to 10^8 *Lactobacillus crispatus* twice daily for two days may provide short-term benefit but is not evidence based.
- Avoid washing the genital area with soap, shower gel or other alkaline detergents.
- Practice of vaginal douching should be discouraged.
- Treatment of male partner is not necessary.

CHAPTER

53

Monilial Vaginitis

CAUSATIVE AGENTS

Candida albicans–80 to 90%, *Candida tropicalis*, *Candida glabrata*–10%.

Responsible for 85% of vaginal infections in pregnancy.

Saprophytic fungi which can be recovered from vagina in 25–45% of asymptomatic women.

CLINICAL FEATURES

Symptoms: Vulval and vaginal pruritus, soreness, non-malodorous vaginal discharge, superficial dyspareunia, external dysuria.

Signs: Vulval rash and characteristic white "cottage cheese" discharge that adheres to the vaginal wall.

DIAGNOSIS

pH of vaginal discharge is 4.4–4.5.

1. Microscopy—Gram stain—for spores and pseudohyphae
   Saline microscopy—pseudohyphae may be seen.
   10% KOH preparation—to look for pseudohyphae
2. Culture–Sabouraud's glucose agar media is considered. Culture should be done in women in whom candidiasis is suspected but cannot be confirmed by microscopic examination.
3. Latex agglutination test

Classification of Candidal Vaginal Infection		
	Uncomplicated	**Complicated**
Occurrence	90%	10%
Frequency	Sporadic	Recurrent
Severity	Mild to moderate	Severe
Host	Normal	Abnormal (Uncontrolled diabetes)
Organisms	*Candida albicans*	*C.glabaratar, C.tropicalis*

TREATMENT

- Eliminate predisposing factors.
- Topical clotrimazole or miconazole cream.
- Clotrimazole 100 mg intravaginally for 6 days.
- Clotrimazole 200 mg intravaginally for 3 days.
- Clotrimazole 500 mg intravaginally single dose.
- Sertaconazole 500 mg intravaginally single dose.
- Oral therapy (ketoconazole or fluconazole) is contraindicated.

SECTION 6

GYNECOLOGICAL DISORDERS OF PREGNANCY

- Fibroid
- Genital Prolapse
- Carcinoma Cervix
- Ovarian Tumor

CHAPTER

54

Fibroid

Prevalence of fibroids in pregnancy – 0.09–3.9%.

NATURAL HISTORY OF FIBROIDS IN PREGNANCY

49–60% negligible change in volume (defined as <10%).

- 22–32% – growth increases
- 8–27% – size decreases

COMPLICATIONS

- Spontaneous abortion
- RPL
- Threatened abortion
- Preterm labor
- PROM
- Placental abruption
- Preeclampsia
- IUGR
- Malpresentation
- PPH
- Retained placenta
- Postpartum sepsis

MANAGEMENT

During Pregnancy

- Uncomplicated: Usual antenatal care followed by assessment at 38 weeks to formulate the method of delivery.
- Place of cesarean delivery: Cervical or broad ligament fibroid, associated obstetrical complications.
- Myomectomy is contraindicated during cesarean section. Myomectomy is done only if it is pedunculated subserous fibroid or fibroid obscuring the lower uterine segment.

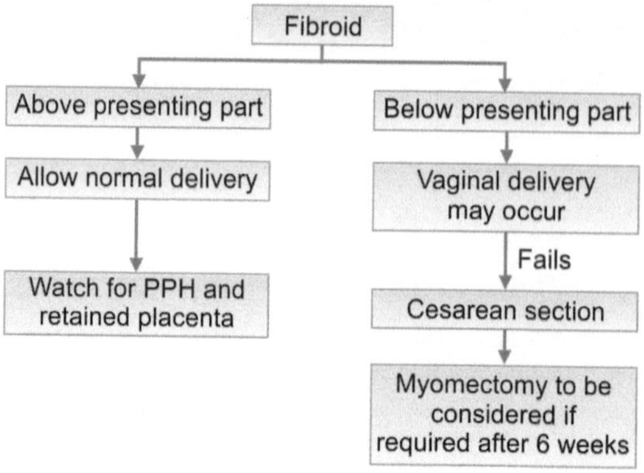
Fibroid
Above presenting part
Below presenting part
Allow normal delivery
Vaginal delivery may occur
Fails
Watch for PPH and retained placenta
Cesarean section
Myomectomy to be considered if required after 6 weeks

CHAPTER

55

Genital Prolapse

INCIDENCE

1 in 250 pregnancies

EFFECTS OF PREGNANCY ON PROLAPSE

- Progression of uterine descent
- Marked hypertrophy and edema of cervix
- Cystocele and rectocele become pronounced
- Constipation, urinary retention
- Aggravation of stress incontinence
- Vaginal discharge may be copious
- Severe backache
- Decubitus ulcer may develop
- Incarceration of the uterus (uterus fails to raise above the pelvis by 16th week of pregnancy).

EFFECTS OF PROLAPSE

During Pregnancy

- Abortion
- Urinary tract infection
- Premature rupture of membranes
- Intrauterine infection

During Labor

- PROM
- Cervical dystocia
- Prolonged labor due to nondilatation of cervix
- Operative interference
- Cervical tears
- PPH

During Puerperium

- Subinvolution
- Uterine sepsis

MANAGEMENT

Antenatal

- Screen for UTI and treat
- The mainstay of the treatment is conservative, i.e. foot end elevation, ring pessary and tampon.
- A new technique called 'Introital tightening' which is safe, simple and effective

Procedure – Local anesthetic agent is infiltrated all around the introitus 2 mm incision is made both at the posterior fourchette and just below the urethra, No.1 vicryl is passed from anterior to posterior submucosally (0.5 cm depth), knot is tied posteriorly tightening the introitus leaving a two-finger space at the vulval introitus which permit adequate drainage of the vulval discharge, easy accessibility to the cervix for examination and coitus. The knot is buried under the vaginal mucosa using chromic catgut 0.

Stitch should be removed at 38 weeks or in the event that the patient goes into preterm labor.

Complications – Hematoma formation and suture may cut through if it is superficial.

Treatment of Edematous and Congested Prolapsed Cervix with Pregnancy

- Foot end elevation at least by 25 cms
- Cover the prolapsed cervix by soaked gauge with glycerine
- Once replaced, patient is allowed to ambulate

Management of Incarcerated Pregnant Uterus

Pregnancy has to be terminated irrespective of period of gestation.

Management of Pregnancy in Women with Previous Conservative Surgeries

Vaginal delivery is not contraindicated.

During Labor

If cervical dilatation fails, then–

At <4 cm in spite of good contraction → Consider emergency LSCS

At 4–7 cm–Hyaluronidase is injected at multiple points on the cervical rim helps in cervical dilatation. If fails, consider emergency LSCS

At >7 cm with good contraction → Duhrssen's incision (2'O and 10'o clock)

↓

Delivery by vacuum/forceps

Postnatal

Consider physiotherapy.

Use pessaries till corrective surgery done after 3 to 6 months.

CHAPTER

56

Carcinoma Cervix

INCIDENCE

1 in 2500 pregnancies

EFFECTS OF PREGNANCY ON CARCINOMA CERVIX

Rapid spread following vaginal delivery and induced abortion.

EFFECTS OF CARCINOMA ON PREGNANCY

- Abortion
- Premature labor
- Secondary cervical dystocia
- Injury to the cervix and lower uterine segment leading to traumatic PPH
- Pyometra
- Uterine sepsis.

DIAGNOSIS

Asymptomatic Cases

- Cytological screening of all pregnant mothers
- Colposcopic directed biopsy for cases showing dyskaryotic smear

Symptomatic Cases

Biopsy from the site of lesion

TREATMENT

Carcinoma in situ
- Vaginal delivery permitted

Invasive carcinoma
- No vaginal delivery

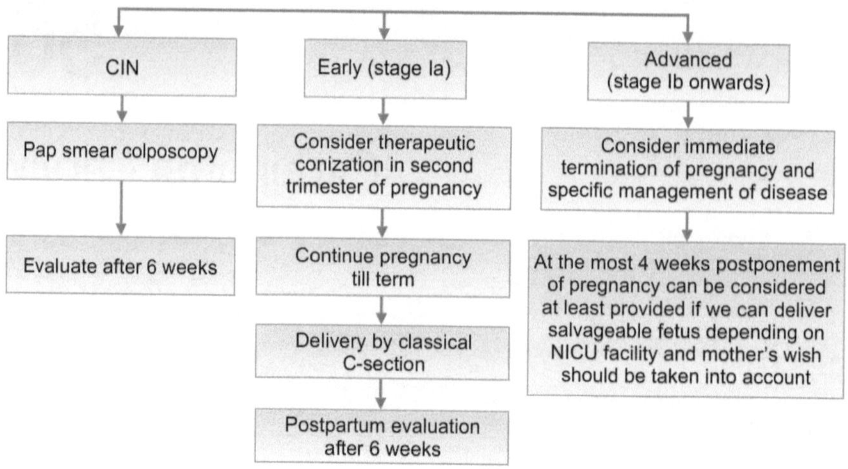
CIN
Pap smear colposcopy
Evaluate after 6 weeks
Early (stage Ia)
Consider therapeutic conization in second trimester of pregnancy
Continue pregnancy till term
Delivery by classical C-section
Postpartum evaluation after 6 weeks
Advanced (stage Ib onwards)
Consider immediate termination of pregnancy and specific management of disease
At the most 4 weeks postponement of pregnancy can be considered at least provided if we can deliver salvageable fetus depending on NICU facility and mother's wish should be taken into account

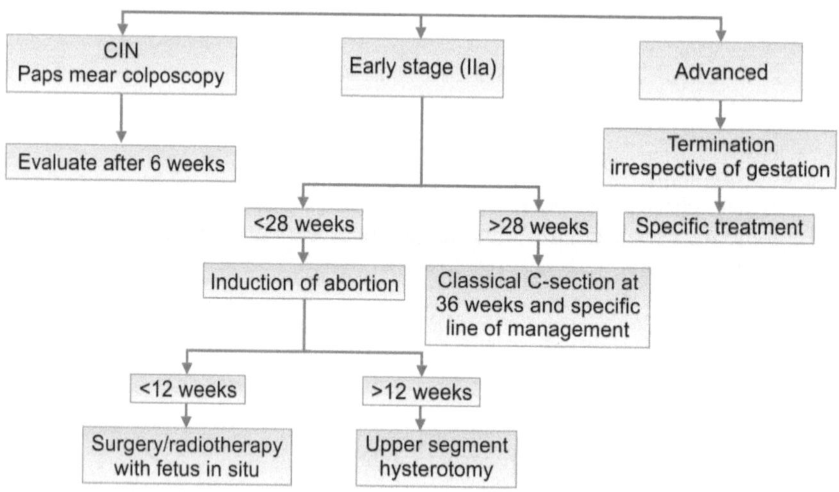
CIN
Paps mear colposcopy
Evaluate after 6 weeks
Early stage (IIa)
<28 weeks
Induction of abortion
<12 weeks
Surgery/radiotherapy with fetus in situ
>12 weeks
Upper segment hysterotomy
>28 weeks
Classical C-section at 36 weeks and specific line of management
Advanced
Termination irrespective of gestation
Specific treatment

CHAPTER

57

Ovarian Tumor

INCIDENCE

1:1000 pregnancy

- Benign tumors are common in pregnancy.
- Benign cyst may undergo torsion causing acute abdomen commonly in puerperium.
- Ovarian malignancy has no effect on pregnancy.
- Pregnancy has no effect on prognosis of ovarian cancer.

DIAGNOSIS

Signs and Symptoms

- Asymptomatic
- Retention of urine
- Mechanical distress due to large cyst
- Acute abdomen
- Cystic mass felt separated from gravid uterus
- Vaginal examination is done to elicit groove in between the the swelling and uterus (Hingorani sign).
- Ultrasonography shows the details of tumors.

Management of benign tumor during pregnancy

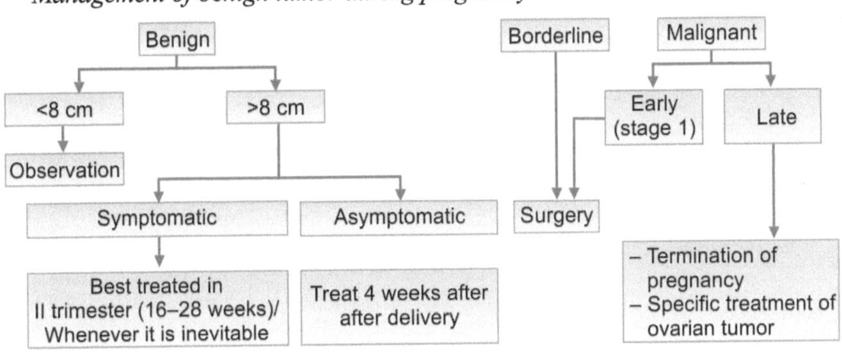

During Labor

- If the tumor is well above the presenting part—watchful expectancy hoping for vaginal delivery is followed.
- If the tumors are impacted in pelvis causing obstruction, cesarean delivery should be done followed by removal of tumor in the same setting.

During Puerperium

On occasion, diagnosis is made following delivery. The tumor should be removed as early in puerperium as possible. Specimen should be sent for histopathological examination.

Bibliography

1. A comprehensive guide to evaluation, management and surgical evaluation.
2. A FOGSI publications – Pregnancy at risk current concepts, 3rd edition.
3. Arias F. Practical guide to high-risk pregnancy and delivery, 3rd edition.
4. Berk and Novak's. Textbook of gynaecology, 14th edition.
5. Desweit Michael.Medical disorders in obstetrics practice, 4th edition.
6. Dutta.Textbook of obstetrics, 7th edition.
7. FOGSI Focus on PPH and Anaemia.
8. Gandhi G, Mehta S, Batra S. Infections in obstetrics and gynaecology.
9. Goel N, Rajaram S. State of the art vaginal surgery, 1st edition 2007.
10. Griffin BP, Topol EJ. Maual of cardiovascular medicine, 3rd edition.
11. Guidelines:
    a. FIGO guidelines, International journal of obstetrics and gynaecology 2007
    b. RCOG 2008
    c. ACOG 2010
    d. NICE 2010
12. Gunasheela.Practical management in obstetrics.
13. Hopkin's Johns. Manual of obstetrics and gynaecology, 4th edition.
14. James DK.High risk pregnancy management options, 3rd edition.
15. Kumar A. Common medical disorders in obstetrics, 1st edition.
16. Kumaran Arul. Normal labour, 2nd edition.
17. MTP Act 2003.
18. Munroker's operative obstetrics, 10th edition.
19. North American clinics medical disorders in pregnancy.
20. Oxorn-Forte Human Labor and birth, 5th edition.
21. Shah MR. Hypertensive disorders in pregnancy, FOGSI publication.
22. Steven G.Gabbe-Obstetrics, 5th edition.
23. Studd John. Progress in obstetrics and gynaecology, volume 15, 16, 17.
24. The California Maternal Quality Care Collaborative (CMQCC).
25. The clinical use of blood in medicine, obstetrics, paediatrics, surgery, anaesthesia, trauma and burns. WHO blood transfusion safety.
26. WHO 2010 FOGSI Focus on APH.
27. Williams obstetrics, 23rd edition.

Index

Page numbers followed by *f* refer to figure, *t* refer to table and *fc* refer to flow chart, respectively.

B

C

D

E

H

I

J

K

L

M

P

U

V

W

Z